EU
O2

THE COMPLETE
INTRODUCTORY
LECTURES ON
PSYCHOANALYSIS

By SIGMUND FREUD

The Complete Introductory Lectures on Psychoanalysis

SIGMUND FREUD

Translated and Edited by

JAMES STRACHEY

NEW YORK

W · W · NORTON & COMPANY · INC ·

ISBN 0 393 01077 5

Library of Congress Catalog Card No. 66-16766

PRINTED IN THE UNITED STATES OF AMERICA

3 4 5 6 7 8 9 0

CONTENTS

TWO
NEW INTRODUCTORY LECTURES
ON PSYCHOANALYSIS 1933

APPENDIXES

NOTE TO

THE COMPLETE INTRODUCTORY LECTURES ON PSYCHOANALYSIS

FREUD published two sets of Introductory Lectures—the first in 1917 and the second more than fifteen years later, in 1933. Between them they cover in outline the whole stretch of his observations and theories. He regarded the two sets as belonging together, which is proved by his having numbered the two series of lectures consecutively. Nevertheless, it is only here, for the first time in any language, that both of them are collected into a single volume.

The text is derived from Volumes XV, XVI and XXIII of the Standard Edition of *The Complete Psychological Works of Sigmund Freud,* in the preparation of which I have enjoyed the advice and assistance of Miss Anna Freud. My thanks are also due to Miss Angela Richards, upon whom many of the details of editorial work have devolved.

James Strachey

One

INTRODUCTORY LECTURES ON
PSYCHOANALYSIS
(1916–17 [1915–17])

EDITOR'S INTRODUCTION

VORLESUNGEN ZUR EINFÜHRUNG IN DIE PSYCHOANALYSE

(*a*) GERMAN EDITIONS:

1916 Part I (separately), *Die Fehlleistungen.* Leipzig and Vienna: Heller.

1916 Part II (separately), *Der Traum.* Same publishers.

1917 Part III (separately), *Allgemeine Neurosenlehre.* Same publishers.

1917 The above, three parts in one volume. Same publishers. Pp. viii + 545.

1918 2nd ed. (With index and inserted list of 40 corrigenda.) Same publishers. Pp. viii + 553.

1920 3rd ed. (Corrected reprint of above.) Leipzig, Vienna and Zurich: Internationaler Psychoanalytischer Verlag. Pp. viii + 553.

1922 4th ed. (Corrected reprint of above.) Same publishers. Pp. viii + 554. (Also Parts II and III separately, under titles *Vorlesungen über den Traum* and *Allgemeine Neurosenlehre.*)

1922 Pocket ed. (No index.) Same publishers. Pp. iv + 495.

1922 Pocket ed. (2nd ed., corrected and with index.) Same publishers. Pp. iv + 502.

1924 *G.S.*, **7**. Pp. 483.

1926 5th ed. (Reprint of *G.S.*) I.P.V. Pp. 483.

1926 Pocket ed. (3rd ed.) Same publishers.

1930 Small 8vo. ed. I.P.V. Pp. 501.

1933 (By licence.) Berlin: Kiepenheuer. Pp. 524.

1940 *G.W.*, **11**, Pp. 495.

(*b*) English Translations:

A General Introduction to Psychoanalysis

1920   New York: Boni & Liveright. Pp. x + 406. (Tr. un-
specified; Foreword G. Stanley Hall.)

Introductory Lectures on Psycho-Analysis

1922   London: Allen & Unwin. Pp. 395. (Tr. Joan Riviere;
without Freud's preface; with preface by Ernest
Jones.)

1929   2nd ed. (revised). Same publishers. Pp. 395.

A General Introduction to Psychoanalysis

1935   New York: Liveright. Pp. 412. (The London ed. under
the title of the old New York one. Tr. Joan Riviere;
with prefaces by Ernest Jones and G. Stanley Hall.
Freud's preface included.)

The present translation is a new one by James Strachey.

This book had a wider circulation than any of Freud's
works, except, perhaps, *The Psychopathology of Everyday Life*.[1] It
is also distinguished by the number of misprints in it. As is
recorded above, 40 were corrected in the second edition; but
there were many more, and a considerable number of slight
variations in the text may be observed in the various editions.
The present translation follows the text of the *Gesammelte Werke*,
which is in fact identical with that of the *Gesammelte Schriften*;
and only the more important deviations from earlier versions
have been recorded.

The actual date of publication of the three parts is not clear.
Part I was certainly out before the end of July, 1916, as is
shown by a reference to it in a letter of Freud's to Lou Andreas-
Salomé of July 27, 1916 (cf. Freud, 1960). In the same letter he

---

[1] The *Lectures* were certainly the most translated of any. In Freud's lifetime (apart from English) they appeared in Dutch (1917), French (1922),
Italian (1922), Russian (1922–3), Spanish (1923), Japanese (1928),
Norwegian (1929), Hebrew (1930), Hungarian (1932), Serbo-Croatian
(1933), Chinese (1933), Polish (1935) and Czech (1936). They had probably also appeared by then in Portuguese, Swedish, and later in Arabic.

also speaks of Part II as being on the point of appearing. Part III seems to have been published in May, 1917.

The academic year of the University of Vienna fell into two parts: a winter term (or semester) running from October to March, and a summer one from April to July. The lectures printed here were delivered by Freud in two successive winter terms during the first World War: 1915–16 and 1916–17.[1] The fullest account of the circumstances leading to their publication will be found in the second volume of Ernest Jones's biography (1955, 245 ff.).

Although, as Freud himself remarked in his preface to the *New Introductory Lectures*, his membership of the University of Vienna had only been 'a peripheral one', he had nevertheless, from the time of his appointment as Privatdozent (University Lecturer) in 1885 and as Professor Extraordinarius (Assistant Professor) in 1902, given many courses of University lectures. These remained unrecorded, though some accounts of them may be found—for instance, by Hanns Sachs (1945, 39 ff.) and Theodor Reik (1942, 19 ff.), as well as by Ernest Jones (1953, 375 ff.). Freud decided that the series beginning in the autumn of 1915 should be the last, and it was at Otto Rank's suggestion that he agreed upon their publication. In his preface to the *New Introductory Lectures* which has just been quoted Freud tells us that the first half of the present, earlier, series 'were improvised, and written out immediately afterwards' and that 'drafts of the second half were made during the intervening summer vacation, at Salzburg, and delivered word for word in the following winter'. He adds that at that time he 'still possessed a phonographic memory', for, however carefully his lectures might have been prepared, his actual delivery of them was invariably extempore[2] and usually without notes. There is general agreement upon his technique of lecturing: that he was never rhetorical and that his tone was always one of quiet and

---

[1] The opening lecture of the series was delivered, according to Ernest Jones, on October 23, 1915, but according to a contemporary notice (*Int. Z. Psychoan.*, **3**, 376) on October 16. It is agreed that they were given on Saturdays.

[2] A single exception to this rule is recorded in the case of his Budapest Congress paper (1919*a*); cf. Jones (1953, 375 *n.*).

even intimate conversation. But it must not be supposed from this that there was anything slovenly or disordered about his lectures. They almost always had a definite form—a head, body and tail—and might often give the hearer the impression of possessing an aesthetic unity.

It has been said (Reik, 1942, 19) that he disliked lecturing, but it is difficult to reconcile this, not only with the number of lectures he delivered in the course of his life, but with the remarkably high proportion of his actually published work which is in the form of lectures. There is, however, a possible explanation of this inconsistency. Examination shows that among his publications it is predominantly the *expository* works that appear as lectures: for instance, the early lecture on 'The Aetiology of Hysteria' (1896*c*), the somewhat later one 'On Psychotherapy' (1905*a*), as well, of course, as the *Five Lectures* delivered in America (1910*a*) and the present series. But beyond this, when, many years afterwards, he undertook an exposition of the later developments of his views, he, for no obvious reason, once more threw them into lecture form and published his *New Introductory Lectures* (1933*a*), though there was never any possibility of their being delivered as such. Thus lectures as a method of putting forward his opinions evidently appealed to Freud, but only subject to a particular condition: he must be in a lively contact with his real or supposed audience. Readers of the present volume will discover how constantly Freud retains this contact—how regularly he puts objections into his audience's mouth and how frequently there are imaginary arguments between him and his hearers. He in fact carried over this method of stating his case to some of his works which are not lectures at all: the whole of *The Question of Lay Analysis* (1926*e*) and the greater part of *The Future of an Illusion* (1927*c*) take the form of dialogues between the author and a critical listener. Contrary, perhaps, to some mistaken notions, Freud was entirely opposed to laying down his views in an authoritarian and dogmatic fashion: 'I shall not tell it you', he says to his audience at one point below (p. 431), 'but shall insist on your discovering it for yourselves.' Objections were not to be shouted down but brought into the open and examined. And this, after all, was no more than an extension of an essential feature of the technique of psycho-analysis itself.

The *Introductory Lectures* may justly be regarded as a stock-taking of Freud's views and the position of psycho-analysis at the time of the first World War. The secessions of Adler and Jung were already past history, the concept of narcissism was some years old, the epoch-making case history of the 'Wolf Man' had been written (with the exception of two passages) a year before the lectures began, though it was not published till later. So, too, the great series of 'metapsychological' papers on fundamental theory had been finished a few months earlier, though only three had been published. (Two more of them appeared soon after the lectures, but the remaining seven disappeared without leaving a trace.) These latter activities, and no doubt the production of the lectures as well, had been facilitated by the slackening in Freud's clinical work imposed by war conditions. A watershed had apparently been reached and the time seemed to have come for a halt. But in fact fresh creative ideas were in preparation which were to see the light in *Beyond the Pleasure Principle* (1920*g*), *Group Psychology* (1921*c*) and *The Ego and the Id* (1923*b*). Indeed, the line must not be drawn too sharply. Already, for instance, hints may be detected of the notion of the 'compulsion to repeat' (p. 274), and the beginnings of the analysis of the ego are quite apparent (pp. 422 and 428), while the difficulties over the multiple senses of the term 'unconscious' (see p. 227*n.* 1) are paving the way towards the new structural account of the mind.

In his preface to these lectures Freud speaks a little depreciatively of the lack of novelty in their contents. But no one, however well-read in psycho-analytic literature, need feel afraid of being bored by them or could fail to find plenty in them that is not to be found elsewhere. The discussions on anxiety (Lecture XXV) and on primal phantasies (Lecture XXIV), which Freud himself singles out in his preface as fresh material, are not the only ones he might have mentioned. The review of symbolism in Lecture X is probably his most complete. Nowhere does he give such a clear summary of the formation of dreams as in the last pages of Lecture XIV. There are no more understanding commentaries on the perversions than those in Lectures XX and XXI. Finally, there is no rival to the analysis of the process of psycho-analytic therapy given in the last lecture of all. And even where the subjects would seem to be well-worn, such as the mechanism of parapraxes and of dreams, they are approached from unexpected directions and throw fresh illumination on what might have seemed depressingly familiar ground. The *Introductory Lectures* have thoroughly deserved their popularity.[1]

[1] From their very nature these lectures touch upon a large variety of subjects, into some of which Freud (as he himself remarks in the last paragraph of the final lecture) has been unable to enter very deeply. Many readers, and especially students who find in this work their first approach to psycho-analysis, are likely to come upon some point about which they would wish to learn more. An attempt has accordingly been made in the footnotes of this edition to give particularly generous references to others of Freud's writings in which the topic in the text is dealt with at greater length.

PREFACE [1]
[1917]

WHAT I am here offering the public as an 'Introduction to Psycho-Analysis' [2] is not designed to compete in any way with such general accounts of this field of knowledge as are already in existence, e.g. those of Hitschmann (1913), Pfister (1913), Kaplan (1914), Régis and Hesnard (1914) and Meijer (1915). This volume is a faithful reproduction of the lectures which I delivered [at the University] during the two Winter Terms 1915/16 and 1916/17 before an audience of doctors and laymen of both sexes.

Any peculiarities of this book which may strike its readers are accounted for by the conditions in which it originated. It was not possible in my presentation to preserve the unruffled calm of a scientific treatise. On the contrary, the lecturer had to make it his business to prevent his audience's attention from lapsing during a session lasting for almost two hours. The necessities of the moment often made it impossible to avoid repetitions in treating some particular subject—it might emerge once, for instance, in connection with dream-interpretation and then again later on in connection with the problems of the neuroses. As a result, too, of the way in which the material was arranged, some important topics (the unconscious, for instance) could not be exhaustively treated at a single point, but had to be taken up repeatedly and then dropped again until a fresh opportunity arose for adding some further information about it.

Those who are familiar with psycho-analytic literature will find little in this 'Introduction' that could not have been known to them already from other much more detailed publications. Nevertheless, the need for rounding-off and summarizing the subject-matter has compelled the author at certain points (the

[1] [This Preface was omitted from the 1922 English translation and its re-issues.]

[2] [A literal translation of the German title of the book would be 'Lectures to Serve as an Introduction to Psycho-Analysis'.]

aetiology of anxiety and hysterical phantasies) to bring forward material that he has hitherto held back.

FREUD

VIENNA, *Spring* 1917

PREFACE TO THE
HEBREW TRANSLATION[1]
[1930]

THESE lectures were delivered in 1916 and 1917; they gave a
fairly accurate account of the position of the young science at
that period and they contained more than their title indicated.
They provided not only an introduction to psycho-analysis but
covered the greater part of its subject-matter. This is naturally
no longer true. Advances have in the meantime taken place in
its theory and important additions have been made to it, such
as the division of the personality into an ego, a super-ego and
an id, a radical alteration in the theory of the instincts, and
discoveries concerning the origin of conscience and the sense of
guilt. These lectures have thus become to a large extent incomplete; it is in fact only now that they have become truly
'introductory'. But in another sense, even to-day they have not
been superseded or become obsolete. What they contain is still
believed and taught, apart from a few modifications, in psycho-
analytic training schools.

Readers of Hebrew and especially young people eager for
knowledge are presented in this volume with psycho-analysis
clothed in the ancient language which has been awakened to a
new life by the will of the Jewish people. The author can well
picture the problem which this has set its translator. Nor need
he suppress his doubt whether Moses and the Prophets would
have found these Hebrew lectures intelligible. But he begs
their descendants (among whom he himself is numbered), for
whom this book is designed, not to react too quickly to their
first impulses of criticism and dislike by rejecting it. Psycho-
analysis brings forward so much that is new, and among it so
much that contradicts traditional opinions and wounds deeply-
rooted feelings, that it is bound at first to provoke denial. A

---

[1] [This preface was first published in German in *G.S.*, **12** (1934),
383–4, and reprinted in *G.W.*, **16** (1950), 274–5. It is here translated
into English for the first time by James Strachey. The Hebrew translation was published by the Verlag Stybel in Jerusalem in 1930.]

reader who suspends his judgement and allows psycho-analysis as a whole to make its impression on him will perhaps become open to a conviction that even this undesired novelty is worth knowing and is indispensable for anyone who wishes to understand the mind and human life.

VIENNA, *December* 1930

PART I
PARAPRAXES
(1916[1915])

LECTURE I

INTRODUCTION

LADIES AND GENTLEMEN,—I cannot tell how much knowledge about psycho-analysis each one of you has already acquired from what you have read or from hearsay. But the wording of my prospectus—'Elementary Introduction to Psycho-Analysis' —obliges me to treat you as though you knew nothing and stood in need of some preliminary information.

I can, however, assume this much—that you know that psycho-analysis is a procedure for the medical treatment of neurotic patients. And here I can at once give you an instance of how in this field a number of things take place in a different way—often, indeed, in an opposite way—from what they do elsewhere in medical practice. When elsewhere we introduce a patient to a medical technique which is new to him, we usually minimize its inconveniences and give him confident assurances of the success of the treatment. I think we are justified in this, since by doing so we are increasing the probability of success. But when we take a neurotic patient into psycho-analytic treatment, we act differently. We point out the difficulties of the method to him, its long duration, the efforts and sacrifices it calls for; and as regards its success, we tell him we cannot promise it with certainty, that it depends on his own conduct, his understanding, his adaptability and his perseverance. We have good reasons, of course, for such apparently wrong-headed behaviour, as you will perhaps come to appreciate later on.

Do not be annoyed, then, if I begin by treating you in the same way as these neurotic patients. I seriously advise you not to join my audience a second time. To support this advice, I will explain to you how incomplete any instruction in psycho-analysis must necessarily be and what difficulties stand in the way of your forming a judgement of your own upon it. I will show you how the whole trend of your previous education and all your habits of thought are inevitably bound to make you into opponents of psycho-analysis, and how much you would

have to overcome in yourselves in order to get the better of this
instinctive opposition. I cannot, of course, foretell how much
understanding of psycho-analysis you will obtain from the
information I give you, but I can promise you this: that by
listening to it you will not have learnt how to set about a
psycho-analytic investigation or how to carry a treatment
through. If, however, there should actually turn out to be one
of you who did not feel satisfied by a fleeting acquaintance with
psycho-analysis but was inclined to enter into a permanent relationship to it, I should not merely dissuade him from doing so
but actively warn him against it. As things stand at present, such
a choice of profession would ruin any chance he might have of
success at a University, and, if he started in life as a practising
physician, he would find himself in a society which did not
understand his efforts, which regarded him with distrust and
hostility, and unleashed upon him all the evil spirits lurking
within it. And the phenomena accompanying the war that is
now raging in Europe will perhaps give you some notion of
what legions of these evil spirits there may be.

Nevertheless, there are quite a number of people for whom,
in spite of these inconveniences, something that promises to
bring them a fresh piece of knowledge still has its attraction. If
a few of you should be of this sort and in spite of my warnings
appear here again for my next lecture, you will be welcome.
All of you, however, have a right to learn the nature of the
difficulties of psycho-analysis to which I have alluded.

I will begin with those connected with instruction, with
training in psycho-analysis. In medical training you are accustomed to *see* things. You see an anatomical preparation, the
precipitate of a chemical reaction, the shortening of a muscle as
a result of the stimulation of its nerves. Later on, patients are
demonstrated before your senses—the symptoms of their illness,
the products of the pathological process and even in many cases
the agent of the disease in isolation. In the surgical departments
you are witnesses of the active measures taken to bring help to
patients, and you may yourselves attempt to put them into
effect. Even in psychiatry the demonstration of patients with
their altered facial expressions, their mode of speech and their
behaviour, affords you plenty of observations which leave a

deep impression on you. Thus a medical teacher plays in the main the part of a leader and interpreter who accompanies you through a museum, while you gain a direct contact with the objects exhibited and feel yourselves convinced of the existence of the new facts through your own perception.

In psycho-analysis, alas, everything is different. Nothing takes place in a psycho-analytic treatment but an interchange of words between the patient and the analyst. The patient talks, tells of his past experiences and present impressions, complains, confesses to his wishes and his emotional impulses. The doctor listens, tries to direct the patient's processes of thought, exhorts, forces his attention in certain directions, gives him explanations and observes the reactions of understanding or rejection which he in this way provokes in him. The uninstructed relatives of our patients, who are only impressed by visible and tangible things—preferably by actions of the sort that are to be witnessed at the cinema—never fail to express their doubts whether 'anything can be done about the illness by mere talking'. That, of course, is both a short-sighted and an inconsistent line of thought. These are the same people who are so certain that patients are 'simply imagining' their symptoms. Words were originally magic and to this day words have retained much of their ancient magical power. By words one person can make another blissfully happy or drive him to despair, by words the teacher conveys his knowledge to his pupils, by words the orator carries his audience with him and determines their judgements and decisions. Words provoke affects and are in general the means of mutual influence among men. Thus we shall not depreciate the use of words in psychotherapy and we shall be pleased if we can listen to the words that pass between the analyst and his patient.[1]

But we cannot do that either. The talk of which psychoanalytic treatment consists brooks no listener; it cannot be demonstrated. A neurasthenic or hysterical patient can of course, like any other, be introduced to students in a psychiatric lecture. He will give an account of his complaints and symptoms, but of nothing else. The information required by analysis will be given by him only on condition of his having a special

[1] [Cf. a parallel passage near the beginning of *The Question of Lay Analysis* (1926e), (Norton, 1950).]

emotional attachment to the doctor; he would become silent as soon as he observed a single witness to whom he felt indifferent. For this information concerns what is most intimate in his mental life, everything that, as a socially independent person, he must conceal from other people, and, beyond that, everything that, as a homogeneous personality, he will not admit to himself.

Thus you cannot be present as an audience at a psycho-analytic treatment. You can only be told about it; and, in the strictest sense of the word, it is only by hearsay that you will get to know psycho-analysis. As a result of receiving your instruction at second hand, as it were, you find yourselves under quite unusual conditions for forming a judgement. That will obviously depend for the most part on how much credence you can give to your informant.

Let us assume for a moment that you were attending a lecture not on psychiatry but on history, and that the lecturer was telling you of the life and military deeds of Alexander the Great. What grounds would you have for believing in the truth of what he reported? At a first glance the position would seem to be even more unfavourable than in the case of psycho-analysis, for the Professor of History no more took part in Alexander's campaigns than you did. The psycho-analyst does at least report things in which he himself played a part. But in due course we come to the things that confirm what the historian has told you. He could refer you to the reports given by ancient writers, who were either themselves contemporary with the events under question or, at any rate, were comparatively close to them—he could refer you, that is to say, to the works of Diodorus, Plutarch, Arrian, and so on. He could put reproductions before you of coins and statues of the king which have survived and he could hand round to you a photograph of the Pompeian mosaic of the battle of Issus. Strictly speaking, however, all these documents only prove that earlier generations already believed in Alexander's existence and in the reality of his deeds, and your criticism might start afresh at that point. You would then discover that not all that has been reported about Alexander deserves credence or can be confirmed in its details; but nevertheless I cannot think that you would leave the lecture-room in doubts of the reality of Alexander the Great. Your decision would be determined essentially by two considerations: first, that the lecturer had no conceivable motive for assuring you of the reality of something he himself did not think real, and secondly, that all the available history books describe the events in approximately similar terms. If you went on to examine the older sources, you would take the same factors into account— the possible motives of the informants and the conformity of the witnesses to one another. The outcome of your examination would undoubtedly be reassuring in the case of Alexander, but would probably be different where figures such as Moses or Nimrod were concerned. Later opportunities will bring to light clearly enough what doubts you may feel about the credibility of your psycho-analytic informant.

But you will have a right to ask another question. If there is no objective verification of psycho-analysis, and no possibility of demonstrating it, how can one learn psycho-analysis at all, and convince oneself of the truth of its assertions? It is true that psycho-analysis cannot easily be learnt and there are not many people who have learnt it properly. But of course there is a practicable method none the less. One learns psycho-analysis on oneself, by studying one's own personality. This is not quite the same thing as what is called self-observation, but it can, if necessary, be subsumed under it. There are a whole number of very common and generally familiar mental phenomena which, after a little instruction in technique, can be made the subject of analysis upon oneself. In that way one acquires the desired sense of conviction of the reality of the processes described by analysis and of the correctness of its views. Nevertheless, there are definite limits to progress by this method. One advances much further if one is analysed oneself by a practised analyst and experiences the effects of analysis on one's own self, making use of the opportunity of picking up the subtler technique of the process from one's analyst. This excellent method is, of course, applicable only to a single person and never to a whole lecture-room of students together.

Psycho-analysis is not to be blamed for a second difficulty in your relation to it; I must make you yourselves responsible for it, Ladies and Gentlemen, at least in so far as you have been students of medicine. Your earlier education has given a particular direction to your thinking, which leads far away from psycho-analysis. You have been trained to find an anatomical basis for the functions of the organism and their disorders, to explain them chemically and physically and to view them biologically. But no portion of your interest has been directed to psychical life, in which, after all, the achievement of this marvellously complex organism reaches its peak. For that reason psychological modes of thought have remained foreign to you. You have grown accustomed to regarding them with suspicion, to denying them the attribute of being scientific, and to handing them over to laymen, poets, natural philosophers[1] and mystics. This limitation is without doubt detrimental to your medical activity, since, as is the rule in all human relationships, your patients will begin by presenting you with their mental *façade*, and I fear that you will be obliged as a punishment to leave a part of the therapeutic influence you[2] are seeking to the lay practitioners, nature curers and mystics whom you so much despise.

I am not unaware of the excuse that we have to accept for this defect in your education. No philosophical auxiliary science exists which could be made of service for your medical purposes. Neither speculative philosophy, nor descriptive psychology, nor what is called experimental psychology (which is closely allied to the physiology of the sense-organs), as they are taught in the Universities, are in a position to tell you anything serviceable of the relation between body and mind or to provide you with the key to an understanding of possible disturbances of the mental functions. It is true that psychiatry, as a part of medicine, sets about describing the mental disorders it observes and collecting them into clinical entities; but at favourable moments the psychiatrists themselves have doubts of whether their purely descriptive hypotheses deserve the name of a science. Nothing is known of the origin, the mechanism or the mutual relations of the symptoms of which these clinical entities are composed; there are either *no* observable changes in the anatomical organ

---

[1] [In the sense of followers of Schelling's pantheistic 'philosophy of nature', which prevailed in Germany during the earlier part of the nineteenth century.]

[2] ['*Sie* (you)' in the earlier German editions; '*sie* (they)' in *G.S.* and *G.W.*]

of the mind to correspond to them, or changes which throw no light upon them. These mental disorders are only accessible to therapeutic influence when they can be recognized as subsidiary effects of what is otherwise an organic illness.

This is the gap which psycho-analysis seeks to fill. It tries to give psychiatry its missing psychological foundation. It hopes to discover the common ground on the basis of which the convergence of physical and mental disorder will become intelligible. With this aim in view, psycho-analysis must keep itself free from any hypothesis that is alien to it, whether of an anatomical, chemical or physiological kind, and must operate entirely with purely psychological auxiliary ideas; and for that very reason, I fear, it will seem strange to you to begin with.

I shall not hold you, your education or your attitude of mind responsible for the next difficulty. Two of the hypotheses of psycho-analysis are an insult to the entire world and have earned its dislike. One of them offends against an intellectual prejudice, the other against an aesthetic and moral one. We must not be too contemptuous of these prejudices; they are powerful things, precipitates of human developments that were useful and indeed essential. They are kept in existence by emotional forces and the struggle against them is hard.

The first of these unpopular assertions made by psycho-analysis declares that mental processes are in themselves unconscious and that of all mental life it is only certain individual acts and portions that are conscious.[1] You know that on the contrary we are in the habit of identifying what is psychical with what is conscious. We look upon consciousness as nothing more nor less than the *defining* characteristic of the psychical, and psychology as the study of the contents of consciousness. Indeed it seems to us so much a matter of course to equate them in this way that any contradiction of the idea strikes us as obvious non-

---

[1] ['*Unbewusst*' and '*bewusst*'. It should be realized from the first that in German these words have a passive grammatical form and, generally speaking, a passive sense. In English 'conscious' and 'unconscious' *may* be used passively but as often as not are used *actively*: 'I am conscious of a pain in my toe' or 'he was unconscious of his hatred'. The German usage would rather speak of the *pain* as conscious and the *hatred* unconscious, and this is the usage adopted regularly by Freud.]

sense. Yet psycho-analysis cannot avoid raising this contradiction; it cannot accept the identity of the conscious and the mental.[1] It defines what is mental as processes such as feeling, thinking and willing, and it is obliged to maintain that there is unconscious thinking and unapprehended willing. In saying this it has from the start frivolously forfeited the sympathy of every friend of sober scientific thought, and laid itself open to the suspicion of being a fantastic esoteric doctrine eager to make mysteries and fish in troubled waters. But you, Ladies and Gentlemen, naturally cannot understand as yet what right I have to describe as a prejudice a statement of so abstract a nature as 'what is mental is conscious'. Nor can you guess what development can have led to a denial of the unconscious—should such a thing exist—and what advantage there may have been in that denial. The question whether we are to make the psychical coincide with the conscious or make it extend further sounds like an empty dispute about words; yet I can assure you that the hypothesis of there being unconscious mental processes paves the way to a decisive new orientation in the world and in science.

You cannot have any notion, either, of what an intimate connection there is between this first piece of audacity on the part of psycho-analysis and the second one, which I must now tell you of. This second thesis, which psycho-analysis puts forward as one of its findings, is an assertion that instinctual impulses which can only be described as sexual, both in the narrower and wider sense of the word, play an extremely large and never hitherto appreciated part in the causation of nervous and mental diseases. It asserts further that these same sexual impulses also make contributions that must not be underestimated to the highest cultural, artistic and social creations of the human spirit.[2]

In my experience antipathy to this outcome of psychoanalytic research is the most important source of resistance which it has met with. Would you like to hear how we explain that fact? We believe that civilization has been created under the pressure of the exigencies of life at the cost of satisfaction of

---

[1] [The first section of Freud's paper on 'The Unconscious' (1915e), discusses this question at great length.]

[2] [The sexual instincts form the topic of Lecture XX.]

the instincts; and we believe that civilization is to a large extent being constantly created anew, since each individual who makes a fresh entry into human society repeats this sacrifice of instinctual satisfaction for the benefit of the whole community. Among the instinctual forces which are put to this use the sexual impulses play an important part; in this process they are sublimated—that is to say, they are diverted from their sexual aims and directed to others that are socially higher and no longer sexual. But this arrangement is unstable; the sexual instincts are imperfectly tamed, and, in the case of every individual who is supposed to join in the work of civilization, there is a risk that his sexual instincts may refuse to be put to that use. Society believes that no greater threat to its civilization could arise than if the sexual instincts were to be liberated and returned to their original aims.[1] For this reason society does not wish to be reminded of this precarious portion of its foundations. It has no interest in the recognition of the strength of the sexual instincts or in the demonstration of the importance of sexual life to the individual. On the contrary, with an educational aim in view, it has set about diverting attention from that whole field of ideas. That is why it will not tolerate this outcome of psycho-analytic research and far prefers to stamp it as something aesthetically repulsive and morally reprehensible, or as something dangerous. But objections of this sort are ineffective against what claims to be an objective outcome of a piece of scientific work; if the contradiction is to come into the open it must be restated in intellectual terms. Now it is inherent in human nature to have an inclination to consider a thing untrue if one does not like it, and after that it is easy to find arguments against it. Thus society makes what is disagreeable into what is untrue. It disputes the truths of psycho-analysis with logical and factual arguments; but these arise from emotional sources and it maintains these objections as prejudices, against every attempt to counter them.

We, however, Ladies and Gentlemen, can claim that in asserting this controversial thesis we have had no tendentious aim in view. We have merely wished to give expression to a

[1] [The antagonism between civilization and the instinctual forces received its fullest treatment by Freud in *Civilization and its Discontents* (1930a), (Norton, 1962).]

matter of fact which we believe we have established by our painstaking labours. We claim, too, the right to reject without qualification any interference by practical considerations in scientific work, even before we have enquired whether the fear which seeks to impose these considerations on us is justified or not.

Such, then, are a few of the difficulties that stand in the way of your interest in psycho-analysis. They are perhaps more than enough for a start. But if you are able to overcome the impression they make on you, we will proceed.

LECTURE II

PARAPRAXES

LADIES AND GENTLEMEN,—We will not start with postulates but with an investigation. Let us choose as its subject certain phenomena which are very common and very familiar but which have been very little examined, and which, since they can be observed in any healthy person, have nothing to do with illnesses. They are what are known as 'parapraxes',[1] to which everyone is liable. It may happen, for instance, that a person who intends to say something may use another word instead (a *slip of the tongue* [*Versprechen*]), or he may do the same thing in writing, and may or may not notice what he has done. Or a person may read something, whether in print or manuscript, different from what is actually before his eyes (a *misreading* [*Verlesen*]), or he may hear wrongly something that has been said to him (a *mishearing* [*Verhören*])—on the assumption, of course, that there is no organic disturbance of his powers of hearing. Another group of these phenomena has as its basis *forgetting* [*Vergessen*]—not, however, a permanent forgetting but only a temporary one. Thus a person may be unable to get hold of a *name* which he nevertheless knows and which he recognizes at once, or he may forget to carry out an *intention*, though he remembers it later and has thus only forgotten it at that particular moment. In a third group the temporary character is absent—for instance in the case of *mislaying* [*Verlegen*], when a person has put something somewhere and cannot find it again,

[1] ['*Fehlleistungen*', literally 'faulty acts' or 'faulty functions'. The general concept did not exist before Freud, and an English term was invented for its translation. The whole of *The Psychopathology of Everyday Life* (1901*b*), (Norton, 1965), is devoted to a discussion of them. Freud often used them in his didactic writings (as he does here) as the most suitable material for an introduction to his theories. They were, indeed, among the earliest subjects of his own psychological investigations. Some account of the history of his interest in them will be found in the Editor's Introduction to the sixth volume of the *Standard Edition*. Since there will be a large number of references to that work in the present lectures, the abbreviation '*P.E.L.*' will be used here in order to economize space. The page references in all such cases will be to the *Standard Ed.* and the Norton edition.]

or in the precisely analogous case of *losing* [*Verlieren*]. Here we have a forgetting which we treat differently from other kinds of forgetting, one at which we are surprised or annoyed instead of finding it understandable. In addition to all this there are particular sorts of *errors* [*Irrtümer*], in which the temporary character is present once more; for in their instance we believe for a time that something is the case which both before and afterwards we know is not so. And there are a number of other similar phenomena known by various names.

All these are occurrences whose internal affinity with one another is expressed in the fact that [in German] they begin with the syllable '*ver*'.[1] They are almost all of an unimportant kind, most of them are very transitory, and they are without much significance in human life. Only rarely does one of them, such as losing an object, attain some degree of practical importance. For that reason, too, they attract little attention, give rise to no more than feeble emotions, and so on.

It is to these phenomena, then, that I now propose to draw your attention. But you will protest with some annoyance: 'There are so many vast problems in the wide[2] universe, as well as within the narrower confines of our minds, so many marvels in the field of mental disorders, which require and deserve to have light thrown upon them, that it does really seem gratuitous to waste labour and interest on such trivialities. If you could make us understand why a person with sound eyes and ears can see and hear in broad daylight things that are not there, why another person suddenly thinks he is being persecuted by the people of whom he has hitherto been most fond, or puts forward the cleverest arguments in support of delusional beliefs which any child could see were nonsensical, then we should have some opinion of psycho-analysis. But if it can do no more than ask us to consider why a speaker at a banquet uses one word instead of another or why a housewife has mislaid her keys, and similar futilities, then we shall know how to put our time and interest to better uses.'

I should reply: Patience, Ladies and Gentlemen! I think your criticism has gone astray. It is true that psycho-analysis cannot

[1] [The English syllable 'mis' has a similar sense.]
[2] [In the editions from 1922 onwards this word is omitted.]

boast that it has never concerned itself with trivialities. On the contrary, the material for its observations is usually provided by the inconsiderable events which have been put aside by the other sciences as being too unimportant—the dregs, one might say, of the world of phenomena. But are you not making a confusion in your criticism between the vastness of the problems and the conspicuousness of what points to them? Are there not very important things which can only reveal themselves, under certain conditions and at certain times, by quite feeble indications? I should find no difficulty in giving you several examples of such situations. If you are a young man, for instance, will it not be from small pointers that you will conclude that you have won a girl's favour? Would you wait for an express declaration of love or a passionate embrace? Or would not a glance, scarcely noticed by other people, be enough? a slight movement, the lengthening by a second of the pressure of a hand? And if you were a detective engaged in tracing a murder, would you expect to find that the murderer had left his photograph behind at the place of the crime, with his address attached? or would you not necessarily have to be satisfied with comparatively slight and obscure traces of the person you were in search of? So do not let us under-estimate small indications; by their help we may succeed in getting on the track of something bigger. Furthermore, I think like you that the great problems of the universe and of science have the first claim on our interest. But it is as a rule of very little use to form an express intention of devoting oneself to research into this or that great problem. One is then often at a loss to know the first step to take. It is more promising in scientific work to attack whatever is immediately before one and offers an opportunity for research. If one does so really thoroughly and without prejudice or preconception, and if one has luck, then, since everything is related to everything, including small things to great, one may gain access even from such unpretentious work to a study of the great problems. That is what I should say in order to retain your interest, when we deal with such apparent trivialities as the parapraxes of healthy people.

Let us now call in someone who knows nothing of psycho-analysis, and ask him how he explains such occurrences. His first reply will certainly be: 'Oh! that's not worth explaining: they're just small chance events.' What does the fellow mean by this? Is he maintaining that there are occurrences, however small, which drop out of the universal concatenation of events —occurrences which might just as well not happen as happen? If anyone makes a breach of this kind in the determinism of natural events at a single point, it means that he has thrown overboard the whole *Weltanschauung* of science. Even the *Weltanschauung* of religion, we may remind him, behaves much more consistently, since it gives an explicit assurance that no sparrow falls from the roof without God's special will. I think our friend will hesitate to draw the logical conclusion from his first reply; he will change his mind and say that after all when he comes to study these things he can find explanations of them. What is in question are small failures of functioning, imperfections in mental activity, whose determinants can be assigned. A man who can usually speak correctly may make a slip of the tongue (1) if he is slightly indisposed and tired, (2) if he is excited and (3) if he is too much occupied with other things. It is easy to confirm these statements. Slips of the tongue do really occur with particular frequency when one is tired, has a headache or is threatened with migraine. In the same circumstances proper names are easily forgotten. Some people are accustomed to recognize the approach of an attack of migraine when proper names escape them in this way.[1] When we are excited, too, we often make mistakes over words—and over *things* as well, and a 'bungled action' follows. Intentions are forgotten and a quantity of other undesigned actions become noticeable if we are absent-minded—that is, properly speaking, if we are concentrated on something else. A familiar example of this absent-mindedness is the Professor in *Fliegende Blätter*[2] who leaves his umbrella behind and takes the wrong hat because he is thinking about the problems he is going to deal with in his next book. All of us can recall from our own experience instances of how we can forget intentions we have formed and promises we have made because in the meantime we have had some absorbing experience.

This sounds quite reasonable and seems safe from contradic-

---

[1] [This was a personal experience of Freud's. *P.E.L.*, 21.]
[2] [The comic weekly.]

tion, though it may not be very interesting, perhaps, and not what we expected. Let us look at these explanations of parapraxes more closely. The alleged preconditions for the occurrence of these phenomena are not all of the same kind. Being ill and disturbances of the circulation provide a physiological reason for the impairment of normal functioning; excitement, fatigue and distraction are factors of another sort, which might be described as psycho-physiological. These last admit of easy translation into theory. Both fatigue and distraction, and perhaps also general excitement, bring about a division of attention which may result in insufficient attention being directed to the function in question. If so, the function can be disturbed with especial ease, or carried out inaccurately. Slight illness or changes in the blood-supply to the central nervous organ can have the same effect, by influencing the determining factor, the division of attention, in a similar manner. In all these cases, therefore, it would be a question of the effects of a disturbance of attention, whether from organic or psychical causes.

This does not appear to promise much for our psycho-analytic interest. We might feel tempted to drop the subject. If, however, we examine the observations more closely, what we find does not tally entirely with this attention theory of parapraxes, or at least does not follow from it naturally. We discover that parapraxes of this kind and forgetting of this kind occur in people who are *not* fatigued or absent-minded or excited, but who are in all respects in their normal state—unless we choose to ascribe *ex post facto* to the people concerned, purely on account of their parapraxis, an excitement which, however, they themselves do not admit to. Nor can it be simply the case that a function is ensured by an increase in the attention directed upon it and endangered if that attention is reduced. There are a large number of procedures that one carries out purely automatically, with very little attention, but nevertheless performs with complete security. A walker, who scarcely knows where he is going, keeps to the right path for all that, and stops at his destination without having *gone astray* [*vergangen*]. Or at all events this is so as a rule. An expert pianist strikes the right keys without thinking. He may, of course, make an occasional mistake; but if automatic playing increased the danger of bungling, that danger would be at its greatest for a virtuoso, whose playing, as a result of prolonged practice, has become *entirely* automatic. We know, on the contrary, that many procedures are carried out with quite particular certainty if they are not the object of a specially high degree of attention,[1] and that the mishap of a parapraxis is liable to occur precisely if special importance is attached to correct functioning and there has therefore certainly been no distraction of the necessary attention. It could be argued that this is the result of 'excitement', but it is difficult to see why the excitement should not on the contrary *increase* the attention directed to what is so earnestly intended. If by a slip of the tongue someone says the opposite of what he intends in an important speech or oral communication, it can scarcely be explained by the psycho-physiological or attention theory.

There are, moreover, a number of small subsidiary phenomena in the case of parapraxes, which we do not understand and on which the explanations so far given shed no light. For instance, if we have temporarily forgotten a name, we are annoyed about it, do all we can to remember it and cannot leave the business alone. Why in such cases do we so extremely seldom succeed in directing our attention, as we are after all anxious to do, to the word which (as we say) is 'on the tip of our tongue' and which we recognize at once when we are told it? Or again: there are cases in which the parapraxes multiply, form chains, and replace one another. On a first occasion one has missed an appointment. On the next occasion, when one has firmly decided not to forget *this* time, it turns out that one has made a note of the wrong hour. Or one tries to arrive at a forgotten word by roundabout ways and thereupon a second name escapes one which might have helped one to find the first. If one searches for this second name, a third disappears, and so on. As is well known, the same thing can happen with misprints, which are to be regarded as the parapraxes of the compositor. An obstinate misprint of this kind, so it is said, once slipped into a social-democrat newspaper. Its report of some ceremonial included the words: 'Among those present was to be noticed His Highness the *Kornprinz*.' Next day an attempt was

---

[1] [Freud has often suggested elsewhere that functions may be performed more accurately in the absence of conscious attention. See *P.E.L.*, 132.]

made at a correction. The paper apologized and said: 'We should of course have said "the *Knorprinz*".' [1] People speak in such cases of a 'demon of misprints' or a 'type-setting fiend'— terms which at least go beyond any psycho-physiological theory of misprints. [2]

Perhaps you are familiar, too, with the fact that it is possible to *provoke* slips of the tongue, to produce them, as it were, by suggestion. An anecdote illustrates this. A stage neophyte had been cast for the important part in [Schiller's] *Die Jungfrau von Orleans* of the messenger who announces to the King that 'der Connétable schickt sein Schwert zurück [the Constable sends back his sword]'. A leading actor amused himself during the rehearsal by repeatedly inducing the nervous young man to say, instead of the words of the text: 'der Komfortabel schickt sein Pferd zurück [the cab-driver sends back his horse].' [3] He achieved his aim: the wretched beginner actually made his début at the performance with the corrupt version, in spite of having been warned against it, or perhaps *because* he had been warned.

No light is thrown on these small features of parapraxes by the theory of withdrawal of attention. The theory need not on that account be wrong, however; it may merely lack something, some addition, before it is entirely satisfying. But some of the parapraxes, too, can themselves be looked at from another point of view.

Let us take *slips of the tongue* as the most suitable sort of parapraxis for our purpose—though we might equally well have chosen slips of the pen or misreading.[4] We must bear in mind

---

[1] [What was intended was the '*Kronprinz* (Crown Prince)'. '*Korn*' means 'corn' and '*Knorr*' 'protuberance'.]

[2] [Cf. *P.E.L.*, 130–1.]

[3] [There seems to be some confusion here. Actually (in Act I, Scene 2 of the play) it is the King himself who announces the Constable's defection.]

[4] [It is most unfortunate from the point of view of the translator that Freud chose slips of the tongue as his most frequent examples of parapraxes in all three of these lectures, since they are from their very nature peculiarly resistant to translation. We have, however, followed our invariable practice in the *Standard Edition* and kept Freud's instances, with footnote and square bracket explanations, rather than replace them by extraneous English ones. Plenty of the latter will be found elsewhere, especially in papers by A. A. Brill (1912) and Ernest Jones (1911).]

that so far we have only asked when—under what conditions—people make slips of the tongue, and it is only to that question that we have had an answer. But we might direct our interest elsewhere and enquire why it is that the slip occurred in this particular way and no other; and we might take into account what it is that emerges in the slip itself. You will observe that, so long as this question is unanswered and no light thrown on the product of the slip, the phenomenon remains a chance event from the psychological point of view, even though it may have been given a physiological explanation. If I make a slip of the tongue, I might obviously do so in an infinite number of ways, the right word might be replaced by any of a thousand others, it might be distorted in countless different directions. Is there something, then, that compels me in the particular case to make the slip in one special way, or does it remain a matter of chance, of arbitrary choice, and is the question perhaps one to which no sensible answer at all can be given?

Two writers, Meringer and Mayer (a philologist and a psychiatrist), in fact made an attempt in 1895 to attack the problem of parapraxes from this angle. They collected examples and began by treating them in a purely descriptive way. This, of course, provides no explanation as yet, though it might pave the way to one. They distinguish the various kinds of distortions imposed by the slip on the intended speech as 'transpositions', 'pre-sonances [anticipations]', 'post-sonances [perseverations]', 'fusions (contaminations)' and 'replacements (substitutions)'. I will give you some examples of these main groups proposed by the authors. An instance of transposition would be to say '*the Milo of Venus*' instead of 'the Venus of Milo' (a transposition of the order of the words); an instance of a pre-sonance [anticipation] would be: 'es war mir *auf der Schwest* . . . auf der Brust so schwer';[1] and a post-sonance [perseveration] would be exemplified by the well-known toast that went wrong: 'Ich fordere Sie *auf, auf* das Wohl unseres Chefs *auf*zustossen' [instead of *an*zustossen].[2] These three forms of slip of the tongue are not

[1] [The phrase intended was : 'it lay on my breast so heavily.' The meaningless '*Schwest*' was a distortion of '*Brust* (breast)' owing to an anticipation of the '*schw*' of '*schwer* (heavily)'. This and the preceding example are also in *P.E.L.*, 53–4.]

[2] ['I call on you to *hiccough to*' (instead of 'drink to') 'the health of

exactly common. You will come on much more numerous examples in which the slip results from contraction or fusion. Thus, for instance, a gentleman addressed a lady in the street in the following words: 'If you will permit me, madam, I should like to *begleit-digen* you.' The composite word,[1] in addition to the '*begleiten* [to accompany]', evidently has concealed in it '*beleidigen* [to insult]'. (Incidentally, the young man was not likely to have much success with the lady.) As an example of a substitution Meringer and Mayer give the case of someone saying: 'Ich gebe die Präparate in den *Brief*kasten' instead of '*Brüt*kasten'.[2]

The attempted explanation which these authors base on their collection of instances is quite peculiarly inadequate. They believe that the sounds and syllables of a word have a particular 'valency' and that the innervation of an element of high valency may have a disturbing influence on one that is less valent. Here they are clearly basing themselves on the far from common cases of pre-sonance and post-sonance; these preferences of some sounds over others (if they in fact exist) can have no bearing at all on other effects of slips of the tongue. After all, the commonest slips of the tongue are when, instead of saying one word, we say another very much like it; and this similarity is for many people a sufficient explanation of such slips. For instance, a Professor declared in his inaugural lecture: 'I am not '*geneigt* [inclined]' (instead of '*geeignet* [qualified]') to appreciate the services of my highly esteemed predecessor.' Or another Professor remarked: 'In the case of the female genitals, in spite of many *Versuchungen* [temptations]—I beg your pardon, *Versuche* [experiments]. . . .'[3]

The most usual, and at the same time the most striking kind of slips of the tongue, however, are those in which one says the precise opposite of what one intended to say. Here, of course, we are very remote from relations between sounds and the effects of similarity; and instead we can appeal to the fact that

our Chief.' This, too, occurs in *P.E.L.*, 54, where, however, the translation is slightly different.]

[1] [A meaningless one.]

[2] ['I put the preparation into the letter-box' instead of 'incubator', literally, 'hatching-box'. These last two examples occur in *P.E.L.*, 68 and 54.]

[3] [*P.E.L.*, 69 and 78-9.]

contraries have a strong conceptual kinship with each other and stand in a particularly close psychological association with each other.[1] There are historical examples of such occurrences. A President of the Lower House of our Parliament once opened the sitting with the words: 'Gentlemen, I take notice that a full quorum of members is present and herewith declare the sitting *closed*.' [2]

Any other familiar association can act in the same insidious fashion as a contrary one, and can emerge in quite unsuitable circumstances. Thus, on the occasion of a celebration in honour of the marriage of a child of Hermann von Helmholtz to a child of Werner von Siemens, the well-known inventor and industrialist, it is said that the duty of proposing the young couple's health fell to the famous physiologist Du Bois-Reymond. No doubt he made a brilliant speech, but he ended with the words: 'So, long life to the new firm of Siemens and Halske!' That was, of course, the name of the *old* firm. The juxtaposition of the two names must have been as familiar to a Berliner as Fortnum and Mason would be to a Londoner.[3]

We must therefore include among the causes of parapraxes not only relations between sounds and verbal similarity, but the influence of word-associations as well. But that is not all. In a number of cases it seems impossible to explain a slip of the tongue unless we take into account something that had been said, or even merely thought, in an earlier sentence. Once again, then, we have here a case of perseveration, like those insisted upon by Meringer, but of more distant origin.—I must confess that I feel on the whole as though after all this we were further than ever from understanding slips of the tongue.

Nevertheless I hope I am not mistaken in saying that during this last enquiry we have all of us formed a fresh impression of

---

[1] [Cf. below, p. 178 ff.]

[2] [*P.E.L.*, 59. The example was also used by Freud in one of his very last writings, the unfinished 'Some Elementary Lessons in Psycho-Analysis' (1940*b* [1938]).]

[3] [In the original: 'as Riedel and Beutel would be to a Viennese'. This last was a well-known outfitter's shop in Vienna. Siemens and Halske were, of course, the great electrical engineers.]

these instances of slips of the tongue, and that it may be worth while to consider that impression further. We examined the conditions under which in general slips of the tongue occur, and afterwards the influences which determine the kind of distortion which the slip produces. But we have so far paid no attention whatever to the *product* of the slip considered by itself, without reference to its origin. If we decide to do so, we are bound in the end to find the courage to say that in a few examples what results from the slip of the tongue has a sense of its own. What do we mean by 'has a sense'? That the product of the slip of the tongue may perhaps itself have a right to be regarded as a completely valid psychical act, pursuing an aim of its own, as a statement with a content and significance. So far we have always spoken of 'parapraxes [faulty acts]', but it seems now as though sometimes the faulty act was itself quite a *normal* act, which merely took the place of the other act which was the one expected or intended.

The fact of the parapraxis having a sense of its own seems in certain cases evident and unmistakable. When the President of the Lower House with his first words *closed* the sitting instead of opening it, we feel inclined, in view of our knowledge of the circumstances in which the slip of the tongue occurred, to recognize that the parapraxis had a sense. The President expected nothing good of the sitting and would have been glad if he could have brought it to an immediate end. We have no difficulty in pointing to the sense of this slip of the tongue, or, in other words, in interpreting it. Or, let us suppose that one lady says to another in tones of apparent admiration: 'That smart new hat—I suppose you *aufgepatzt* [a non-existent word instead of *aufgeputzt* (trimmed)] it yourself?' Then no amount of scientific propriety will succeed in preventing our seeing behind this slip of the tongue the words: 'This hat is a *Patzerei* [botched-up affair].' Or, once more, we are told that a lady who was well-known for her energy remarked on one occasion: 'My husband asked his doctor what diet he ought to follow; but the doctor told him he had no need to diet: he could eat and drink what I want.' Here again the slip of the tongue has an unmistakable other side to it: it was giving expression to a consistently planned programme.[1]

[1] [These two last examples appear in *P.E.L.*, 87 and 70.]

If it turned out, Ladies and Gentlemen, that not only *a few*
instances of slips of the tongue and of parapraxes in general
have a sense, but a considerable number of them, the *sense* of
parapraxes, of which we have so far heard nothing, would inevitably become their most interesting feature and would push
every other consideration into the background. We should then
be able to leave all physiological or psycho-physiological factors
on one side and devote ourselves to purely psychological investigations into the sense—that is, the meaning or purpose—of
parapraxes. We shall therefore make it our business to test this
expectation on a considerable number of observations.

But before carrying out this intention I should like to invite
you to follow me along another track. It has repeatedly happened that a creative writer has made use of a slip of the tongue
or some other parapraxis as an instrument for producing an
imaginative effect. This fact alone must prove to us that he regards the parapraxis—the slip of the tongue, for instance—as
having a sense, since he has produced it deliberately. For what
has happened is not that the author has made an accidental slip
of the pen and has then allowed it to be used by one of his
characters as a slip of the tongue; he intends to bring something
to our notice by means of the slip of the tongue and we can
enquire what that something is—whether perhaps he wants to
suggest that the character in question is absent-minded and
fatigued or is going to have an attack of migraine. If the author
uses the slip as though it had a sense, we have no wish, of
course, to exaggerate the importance of this. After all, a slip
might in fact be without a sense, a chance psychical event, or
it might have a sense in only quite rare cases, but the author
would still retain his right to intellectualize it by *furnishing* it
with a sense so as to employ it for his own purposes. Nor would
it be surprising if we had more to learn about slips of the tongue
from creative writers than from philologists and psychiatrists.
An example of this kind is to be found in [Schiller's] *Wallenstein* (*Piccolomini*, Act I, Scene 5). In the preceding scene Max
Piccolomini has ardently espoused the Duke's [Wallenstein's]
cause, and has been passionately describing the blessings of
peace, of which he has become aware in the course of a journey
while escorting Wallenstein's daughter to the camp. As he

leaves the stage, his father [Octavio] and Questenberg, the emissary from the Court, are plunged in consternation. Scene 5 continues:

QUESTENBERG   Alas, alas! and stands it so?
                     What, friend! and do we let him go away
                     In this delusion—let him go away?
                     Not call him back immediately, not open
                     His eyes upon the spot?
OCTAVIO (*recovering himself out of a deep study*) He now has open'd mine,
                     And I see more than pleases me.
QUEST.   What is it?
OCT.   Curse on this journey!
QUEST.   But why so? What is it?
OCT.   Come, come along friend! I must follow up
                     The ominous track immediately. Mine eyes
                     Are open'd now, and I must use them. Come!
                         (*Draws Q. on with him.*)
QUEST.   What now? *Where* go you then?
OCT.   To her . . .
QUEST.   To—
OCT. (*correcting himself*) To the Duke. Come let us go.
                           [Coleridge's translation.]

Octavio had meant to say 'to him', to the Duke. But he makes a slip of the tongue, and, by saying 'to her' he betrays to *us* at least that he has clearly recognized the influence that has made the young warrior into an enthusiast for peace.[1]

A still more impressive example has been discovered by Otto Rank [1910*a*] in Shakespeare. It is from *The Merchant of Venice*, in the famous scene in which the fortunate lover chooses between the three caskets, and perhaps I cannot do better than read you Rank's short account of it:

'A slip of the tongue occurs in Shakespeare's *Merchant of Venice* (Act III, Scene 2), which is from the dramatic point of view extremely subtly motivated and which is put to brilliant technical use. Like the slip in *Wallenstein* to which Freud has drawn attention, it shows that dramatists have a clear understanding of the mechanism and meaning of this kind of parapraxis and assume that the same is true of their audience. Portia, who by her father's will has been bound to the choice of a husband by lot, has so far escaped all her unwelcome suitors by a fortunate chance. Having at last found in Bassanio

[1] [This example and the following one also occur in *P.E.L.*, 96–8.]

the suitor who is to her liking, she has cause to fear that he too will choose the wrong casket. She would very much like to tell him that even so he could rest assured of her love; but she is prevented by her vow. In this internal conflict the poet makes her say to the suitor she favours:

> I pray you tarry; pause a day or two
> Before you hazard: for, in choosing wrong,
> I lose your company; therefore forbear a while:
> There's something tells me (*but it is not love*)
> I would not lose you . . . .
>   . . . I could teach you
> How to choose right, but then I am forsworn;
> So will I never be; so may you miss me;
> But if you do you'll make me wish a sin,
> That I have been forsworn. Beshrew your eyes,
> They have o'erlooked me, and divided me;
> *One half of me is yours, the other half yours,—*
> *Mine own, I would say*; but if mine, then yours,
> And so all yours.

The thing of which she wanted to give him only a very subtle hint, because she should have concealed it from him altogether, namely, that even before he made his choice she was *wholly* his and loved him—it is precisely this that the poet, with a wonderful psychological sensitivity, causes to break through openly in her slip of the tongue; and by this artistic device he succeeds in relieving both the lover's unbearable uncertainty and the suspense of the sympathetic audience over the outcome of his choice.'

Observe, too, how skilfully Portia in the end reconciles the two statements contained in her slip of the tongue, how she solves the contradiction between them and yet finally shows that it was the slip that was in the right:

> 'But if mine, then yours,
> And so all yours.'

It has occasionally happened that a thinker whose field lies outside medicine has, by something he says, revealed the sense of a parapraxis and anticipated our efforts at explaining them. You all know of the witty satirist Lichtenberg (1742–99), of whom Goethe said: 'Where he makes a jest a problem lies concealed.' Sometimes the jest brings the *solution* of the problem to light as well. In Lichtenberg's *Witzige und Satirische Einfälle*

[Witty and Satirical Thoughts, 1853] we find this: 'He had read so much Homer that he always read "*Agamemnon*" instead of "*angenọmmen* [supposed]".' Here we have the whole theory of misreading.[1]

We must see next time whether we can go along with these writers in their view of parapraxes.

[1] [Lichtenberg was a favourite author of Freud's and many of his epigrams are discussed in *Jokes and their Relation to the Unconscious* (1905c), (Norton, 1960). The Agamemnon remark is further considered below, p. 70. It is quoted in the book on jokes (p. 93) as well as in *P.E.L.*, 112, where Goethe's comment also appears (*P.E.L.*, 218).]

LECTURE III

PARAPRAXES (*continued*)

LADIES AND GENTLEMEN,—We arrived last time at the idea of considering parapraxes not in relation to the intended function which they disturbed but on their own account; and we formed an impression that in particular cases they seemed to be betraying a sense of their own. We then reflected that if confirmation could be obtained on a wider scale that parapraxes have a sense, their sense would soon become more interesting than the investigation of the circumstances in which they come about.

Let us once more reach an agreement upon what is to be understood by the 'sense' of a psychical process. We mean nothing other by it than the intention it serves and its position in a psychical continuity. In most of our researches we can replace 'sense' by 'intention' or 'purpose'.[1] Was it, then, merely a deceptive illusion or a poetic exaltation of parapraxes when we thought we recognized an intention in them?

We will continue to take slips of the tongue as our examples. If we now look through a considerable number of observations of that kind, we shall find whole categories of cases in which the intention, the sense, of the slip is plainly visible. Above all there are those in which what was intended is replaced by its contrary. The President of the Lower House [p. 34] said in his opening speech: 'I declare the sitting closed.' That is quite unambiguous. The sense and intention of his slip was that he wanted to close the sitting. 'Er sagt es ja selbst'[2] we are tempted to quote: we need only take him at his word. Do not interrupt

---

[1] [It has been thought best to translate the German word '*Tendenz*' by 'purpose' throughout these lectures. The meanings of the two words do not, however, coincide, and in a few passages some such rendering as 'trend' would be preferable. '*Tendenz*' is almost never equivalent to 'tendency', though the adjective '*tendenziös*' has become naturalized in the English form of 'tendentious', as applied, for instance, to a play 'with a purpose'.]

[2] ['He says so himself.' This is a line from the standard German translation of a phrase in *Figaro* which occurs repeatedly in the sextet in Act III.]

40

me at this point by objecting that that is impossible, that we know that he did not want to close the sitting but to open it, and that he himself, whom we have just recognized as the supreme court of appeal, could confirm the fact that he wanted to open it. You are forgetting that we have come to an agreement that we will begin by regarding parapraxes on their own account; their relation to the intention which they have disturbed is not to be discussed till later. Otherwise you will be guilty of a logical error by simply evading the problem that is under discussion—by what is called in English 'begging the question'.

In other cases, where the slip does not express the precise contrary, an opposite sense can nevertheless be brought out by it. 'I am not *geneigt* [inclined] to appreciate the services of my predecessor' [p. 33]. *Geneigt* is not the contrary of *geeignet* [qualified], but it expresses openly something which contrasts sharply with the situation in which the speech was to be made.

In yet other cases the slip of the tongue merely adds a second sense to the one intended. The sentence then sounds like a contraction, abbreviation or condensation of several sentences. Thus, when the energetic lady said: 'He can eat and drink what I want' [p. 35], it was just as though she had said: 'He can eat and drink what he wants; but what has *he* to do with wanting? *I* will want instead of him.' A slip of the tongue often gives the impression of being an abbreviation of this sort. For instance, a Professor of Anatomy at the end of a lecture on the nasal cavities asked whether his audience had understood what he said and, after general assent, went on: 'I can hardly believe that, since even in a city with millions of inhabitants, those who understand the nasal cavities can be counted *on one finger*. . . . I beg your pardon, on the fingers of one hand.' The abbreviated phrase has a sense too—namely, that there is only one person who understands them.[1]

In contrast to these groups of cases, in which the parapraxis itself brings its sense to light, there are others in which the parapraxis produces nothing that has any sense of its own, and which therefore sharply contradict our expectations. If someone twists a proper name about by a slip of the tongue or puts an abnormal series of sounds together, these very common events

[1] [Repeated from *P.E.L.*, 78.]

alone seem to give a negative reply to our question whether all parapraxes have some sort of sense. Closer examination of such instances, however, shows that these distortions are easily understood and that there is by no means so great a distinction between these more obscure cases and the earlier straight-forward ones.

A man who was asked about the health of his horse replied: 'Well, it *draut* [a meaningless word] . . . it *dauert* [will last] another month perhaps.' When he was asked what he had really meant to say, he explained that he had thought it was a '*traurige* [sad]' story. The combination of '*dauert*' and '*traurig*' had produced '*draut*'.[1]

Another man, speaking of some occurrences he disapproved of, went on: 'But then facts came to *Vorschwein* [a non-existent word, instead of *Vorschein* (light)]. . . .' In reply to enquiries he confirmed the fact that he had thought these occurrences '*Schweinereien*' ['disgusting', literally 'piggish']. '*Vorschein*' and '*Schweinereien*' combined to produce the strange word '*Vor-schwein*'.[2]

You will recall the case of the young man who asked the unknown lady if he might '*begleitdigen*' her [p. 33]. We ventured to divide up this verbal form into '*begleiten* [accompany]' and '*beleidigen* [insult]', and we felt certain enough of this interpretation not to need any confirmation of it. You will see from these examples that even these obscurer cases of slips of the tongue can be explained by a convergence, a mutual '*interference*', between two different intended speeches; the differences between these cases of slips arise merely from the fact that on some occasions one intention takes the place of the other completely (becomes a substitute for it), as in slips of the tongue that express the contrary, whereas on other occasions the one intention has to be satisfied with distorting or modifying the other, so that composite structures are produced, which make sense, to a greater or lesser degree, on their own account.

We seem now to have grasped the secret of a large number of slips of the tongue. If we bear this discovery in mind, we shall be able to understand other groups as well which have puzzled us hitherto. In cases of distortion of names, for instance, we

[1] Meringer and Mayer. [*P.E.L.*, 58.]
[2] Meringer and Mayer. [*P.E.L.*, 57.]

cannot suppose that it is always a matter of competition between two similar but different names. It is not difficult, however, to guess the second intention. The distortion of a name occurs often enough apart from slips of the tongue; it seeks to give the name an offensive sound or to make it sound like something inferior, and it is a familiar practice (or malpractice) designed as an insult, which civilized people soon learn to abandon, but which they are *reluctant* to abandon. It is still often permitted as a 'joke', though a pretty poor one. As a blatant and ugly example of this way of distorting names, I may mention that in these days [of the first World War] the name of the President of the French Republic, Poincaré, has been changed into '*Schweinskarré*'.[1] It is therefore plausible to suppose that the same insulting intention is present in these slips of the tongue and is trying to find expression in the distortion of a name. Similar explanations suggest themselves along the same lines for certain instances of slips of the tongue with comic or absurd results. 'I call on you to hiccough [*aufzustossen*] to the health of our Chief [p. 32].' Here a ceremonial atmosphere is unexpectedly disturbed by the intrusion of a word which calls up an unsavoury idea, and, on the model of certain insulting and offensive phrases, we can scarcely avoid a suspicion that a purpose was trying to find expression which was in violent contradiction to the ostensibly respectful words. What the slip seems to have been saying was something like: 'Don't you believe it! I don't mean this seriously! I don't care a rap for the fellow!' Just the same thing applies to slips of the tongue which turn innocent words into indecent or obscene ones: thus, '*Apopos*' for '*à propos*' or '*Eischeissweibchen*' for '*Eiweissscheibchen*'.[2]

Many people, as we know, derive some pleasure from a habit like this of deliberately distorting innocent words into obscene ones; such distortions are regarded as funny, and when we hear one we must in fact first enquire from the speaker whether he

[1] [The Viennese term for a pork chop.]

[2] Both from Meringer and Meyer. [They are also in *P.E.L.*, 82. In the first of these untranslatable examples '*Apopos*' is a non-existent word; but '*Popo*' is a nursery word for 'bottom'. In the second example the nonsense word means literally 'egg-shit-female', while the intended word means 'small slices of white of egg.']

uttered it intentionally as a joke or whether it happened as a slip of the tongue.

Well, it looks now as though we have solved the problem of parapraxes, and with very little trouble! They are not chance events but serious mental acts; they have a sense; they arise from the concurrent action—or perhaps rather, the mutually opposing action—of two different intentions. But now I see too that you are preparing to overwhelm me with a mass of questions and doubts which will have to be answered and dealt with before we can enjoy this first outcome of our work. I certainly have no desire to force hasty decisions upon you. Let us take them all in due order, one after the other, and give them cool consideration.

What is it you want to ask me? Do I think that this explanation applies to *all* parapraxes or only to a certain number? Can this same point of view be extended to the many other kinds of parapraxis, to misreading, slips of the pen, forgetting, bungled actions, mislaying, and so on? In view of the psychical nature of parapraxes, what significance remains for the factors of fatigue, excitement, absent-mindedness and interference with the attention? Further, it is clear that of the two competing purposes in a parapraxis one is always manifest, but the other not always. What do we do, then, in order to discover the latter? And, if we think we have discovered it, how do we prove that it is not merely a probable one but the only correct one? Is there anything else you want to ask? If not, I will go on myself. You will recall that we do not set much store by parapraxes themselves, and that all we want is to learn from studying them something that may be turned to account for psycho-analysis. I therefore put this question to you. What are these intentions or purposes which are able to disturb others in this way? And what are the relations between the disturbing purposes and the disturbed ones? Thus, no sooner is the problem solved than our work begins afresh.

First, then, is this the explanation of *all* cases of slips of the tongue? I am very much inclined to think so, and my reason is that every time one investigates an instance of a slip of the tongue an explanation of this kind is forthcoming. But it is also true that there is no way of proving that a slip of the tongue cannot occur without this mechanism. It may be so; but theoretically it is a matter of indifference to us, since the conclusions we want to draw for our introduction to psycho-analysis remain, even though—which is certainly not the case—our view holds good of only a minority of cases of slips of the tongue. The next question—whether we may extend our view to other sorts of parapraxis—I will answer in advance with a 'yes'. You will be able to convince yourselves of this when we come to examining instances of slips of the pen, bungled actions, and so on. But for technical reasons I suggest that we should postpone this task till we have treated slips of the tongue themselves still more thoroughly.

A more detailed reply is called for by the question of what significance remains for the factors put forward by the authorities—disturbances of the circulation, fatigue, excitement, absent-mindedness and the theory of disturbed attention—if we accept the psychical mechanism of slips of the tongue which we have described. Observe that we are not denying these factors. It is in general not such a common thing for psycho-analysis to *deny* something asserted by other people; as a rule it merely adds something new—though no doubt it occasionally happens that this thing that has hitherto been overlooked and is now brought up as a fresh addition is in fact the essence of the matter. The influence on the production of slips of the tongue by physiological dispositions brought about by slight illness, disturbances of the circulation or states of exhaustion, must be recognized at once; daily and personal experience will convince you of it. But how little they explain! Above all, they are not necessary preconditions of parapraxes. Slips of the tongue are just as possible in perfect health and in a normal state. These somatic factors only serve therefore, to facilitate and favour the peculiar mental mechanism of slips of the tongue. I once used an analogy to describe this relation,[1] and I will repeat it here since I can think of none better to take its place. Suppose that one dark night I went to a lonely spot and was there attacked by a rough who took away my watch and purse. Since I did not see the robber's face clearly, I laid my complaint at the nearest police station with the words: 'Loneliness and darkness have just robbed me of my valuables.' The police officer might then say to me: 'In

[1] [*P.E.L.*, 21.]

what you say you seem to be unjustifiably adopting an extreme mechanistic view. It would be better to represent the facts in this way: "Under the shield of darkness and favoured by loneliness, an unknown thief robbed you of your valuables." In your case the essential task seems to me to be that we should find the thief. Perhaps we shall then be able to recover the booty.'

Such psycho-physiological factors as excitement, absentmindedness and disturbances of attention will clearly help us very little towards an explanation. They are only empty phrases, screens behind which we must not let ourselves be prevented from having a look. The question is rather what it is that has been brought about here by the excitement, the particular distracting of attention. And again, we must recognize the importance of the influence of sounds, the similarity of words and the familiar associations aroused by words. These facilitate slips of the tongue by pointing to the paths they can take. But if I have a path open to me, does that fact automatically decide that I shall take it? I need a motive in addition before I resolve in favour of it and furthermore a force to propel me along the path. So these relations of sounds and words are also, like the somatic dispositions, only things that *favour* slips of the tongue and cannot provide the true explanation of them. Only consider: in an immense majority of cases my speech is not disturbed by the circumstance that the words I am using recall others with a similar sound, that they are intimately linked with their contraries or that familiar associations branch off from them. Perhaps we might still find a way out by following the philosopher Wundt, when he says that slips of the tongue arise if, as a result of physical exhaustion, the inclination to associate gains the upper hand over what the speaker otherwise intends to say. That would be most convincing if it were not contradicted by experience, which shows that in one set of cases the *somatic* factors favouring slips of the tongue are absent and in another set of cases the *associative* factors favouring them are equally absent.

I am particularly interested, however, in your next question: how does one discover the two mutually interfering purposes? You do not realize, probably, what a momentous question this is. One of the two, the purpose that is disturbed, is of course unmistakable: the person who makes the slip of the tongue knows it and admits to it. It is only the other, the disturbing purpose, that can give rise to doubt and hesitation. Now, we have already seen, and no doubt you have not forgotten, that in a number of cases this other purpose is equally evident. It is indicated by the *outcome* of the slip, if only we have the courage to grant that outcome a validity of its own. Take the President of the Lower House, whose slip of the tongue said the contrary of what he intended. It is clear that he wanted to open the sitting, but it is equally clear that he also wanted to close it. That is so obvious that it leaves us nothing to interpret. But in the other cases, in which the disturbing purpose only *distorts* the original one without itself achieving complete expression, how do we arrive at the disturbing purpose from the distortion?

In a first group of cases this is done quite simply and securely —in the same way, in fact, as with the *disturbed* purpose. We get the speaker to give us the information directly. After his slip of the tongue he at once produces the wording which he originally intended: 'It *draut* . . . no, it *dauert* [will last] another month perhaps.' [p. 42]. Well, in just the same way we get him to tell us the *disturbing* purpose. 'Why', we ask him, 'did you say "*draut*"?' He replies: 'I wanted to say "It's a *traurige* [sad] story".' Similarly, in the other case, where the slip of the tongue was '*Vorschwein*' [p. 42], the speaker confirms the fact that he had wanted at first to say 'It's a *Schweinerei* [disgusting]', but had controlled himself and gone off into another remark. Here then the distorting purpose is as securely established as the distorted one. My choice of these examples has not been un-intentional, for their origin and solution come neither from me nor from any of my followers. And yet in both these cases active measures of a kind were necessary in order to bring about the solution. The speaker had to be asked why he had made the slip and what he could say about it. Otherwise he might perhaps have passed over his slip without wanting to explain it. But when he was asked he gave the explanation with the first thing that occurred to him.[1] And now please observe that this small

[1] [The phrase 'thing that occurred to him' here stands for the German word '*Einfall*', for which there is no satisfactory English equivalent. The word appears constantly in the course of these lectures—two or three times in the present passage, repeatedly in Lecture VI, and at many

active step and its successful outcome are already a psycho-analysis and are a model for every psycho-analytic investigation which we shall embark upon later.

Am I too mistrustful, however, if I suspect that at the very moment at which psycho-analysis makes its appearance before you resistance to it simultaneously raises its head? Do you not feel inclined to object that the information given by the person of whom the question was asked—the person who made the slip of the tongue—is not completely conclusive? He was naturally anxious, you think, to fulfil the request to explain the slip, so he said the first thing that came into his head which seemed capable of providing such an explanation. But that is no proof that the slip did in fact take place in that way. It *may* have been so, but it may just as well have happened otherwise. And something else might have occurred to him which would have fitted in as well or perhaps even better.

It is strange how little respect you have at bottom for a psychical fact! Imagine that someone had undertaken the chemical analysis of a certain substance and had arrived at a particular weight for one component of it—so and so many milligrammes. Certain inferences could be drawn from this weight. Now do you suppose that it would ever occur to a chemist to criticize those inferences on the ground that the isolated substance might equally have had some other weight? Everyone will bow before the fact that this was the weight and

points elsewhere—so that some comment on it will be useful. It is customarily translated 'association'—an objectionable term, since it is ambiguous and question-begging. If a person is thinking of something and we say that he has an '*Einfall*', all that this implies is that something else has occurred to his mind. But if we say that he has an 'association', it seems to imply that the something else that has occurred to him is in some way connected with what he was thinking of before. Much of the discussion in these pages turns on whether the second thought is in fact connected (or is necessarily connected) with the original one—whether the '*Einfall*' is an 'association'. So that to translate '*Einfall*' by 'association' is bound to prejudge the issue. Nevertheless it is not always easy to avoid this, more especially as Freud himself sometimes uses the German '*Assoziation*' as a synonym for '*Einfall*', especially in the term '*freie Assoziation*', which must inevitably be translated 'free association'. Every endeavour will be made in the present discussion to avoid ambiguity, even at the cost of some unwieldy phraseology; later on, the need to avoid the word 'association' will become less pressing.]

none other and will confidently draw his further inferences from it. But when you are faced with the psychical fact that a particular thing occurred to the mind of the person questioned, you will not allow the fact's validity: something else might have occurred to him! You nourish the illusion of there being such a thing as psychical freedom, and you will not give it up. I am sorry to say I disagree with you categorically over this.

You will break off at that, but only to take up your resistance again at another point. You proceed: 'It is the special technique of psycho-analysis, as we understand, to get people under analysis themselves to produce the solution of their problems. [Cf. p. 101 below.] Now let us take another example—the one in which a speaker proposing the toast of honour on a ceremonial occasion called on his audience to hiccough [*aufzustossen*] to the health of the Chief [p. 32]. You say [p. 43] that the disturbing intention in this case was an insulting one: that was what was opposing the speaker's expression of respect. But this is pure interpretation on your part, based upon observations apart from the slip of the tongue. If in this instance you were to question the person responsible for the slip, he would not confirm your idea that he intended an insult; on the contrary, he would energetically repudiate it. Why, in view of this clear denial, do you not abandon your unprovable interpretation?'

Yes. You have lighted on a powerful argument this time. I can imagine the unknown proposer of the toast. He is probably a subordinate to the Chief of the Department who is being honoured—perhaps he himself is already an Assistant Lecturer, a young man with excellent prospects in life. I try to force him to admit that he may nevertheless have had a feeling that there was something in him opposing his toast in honour of the Chief. But this lands me in a nice mess. He gets impatient and suddenly breaks out: 'Just you stop trying to cross-question me or I shall turn nasty. You're going to ruin my whole career with your suspicions. I simply said "*aufstossen* [hiccough to]" instead of "*anstossen* [drink to]" because I'd said "*auf*" twice before in the same sentence. That's what Meringer calls a perseveration and there's nothing more to be interpreted about it. D'you understand? *Basta!*'—H'm! That was a surprising reaction, a truly energetic denial. I see there's nothing more to be done with the young man. But I also reflect that he shows a strong personal interest in insisting on his parapraxis not having a sense. You may also feel that there was something wrong in his being quite so rude about a purely theoretical enquiry. But, you will think, when all is said and done he must know what he wanted to say and what he didn't.

But must he? Perhaps that may still be the question.

Now, however, you think you have me at your mercy. 'So that's your technique', I hear you say. 'When a person who has made a slip of the tongue says something about it that suits you, you pronounce him to be the final decisive authority on the subject. "He says so himself! [p. 40]". But when what he says doesn't suit your book, then all at once you say he's of no importance—there's no need to believe him.'[1]

That is quite true. But I can put a similar case to you in which the same monstrous event occurs. When someone charged with an offence confesses his deed to the judge, the judge believes his confession; but if he denies it, the judge does not believe him. If it were otherwise, there would be no administration of justice, and in spite of occasional errors we must allow that the system works.

'Are you a judge, then? And is a person who has made a slip of the tongue brought up before you on a charge? So making a slip of the tongue is an offence, is it?'[2]

Perhaps we need not reject the comparison. But I would ask you to observe what profound differences of opinion we have reached after a little investigation of what seemed such innocent problems concerning the parapraxes—differences which at the moment we see no possible way of smoothing over. I propose a provisional compromise on the basis of the analogy with the judge and the defendant. I suggest that you shall grant me that there can be no doubt of a parapraxis having a sense if the subject himself admits it. *I* will admit in return that we cannot arrive at a direct proof of the suspected sense if the subject refuses us information, and equally, of course, if he is not at hand to give us the information. Then, as in the case of the

[1] [A long discussion of this difficulty will be found in one of Freud's last papers, on 'Constructions in Analysis' (1937*d*).]

[2] [The German words are on the same pattern: '*Versprechen*' and '*Vergehen*'.]

administration of justice, we are obliged to turn to circumstantial evidence, which may make a decision more probable in some instances and less so in others. In the law courts it may be necessary for practical purposes to find a defendant guilty on circumstantial evidence. We are under no such necessity; but neither are we obliged to disregard the circumstantial evidence. It would be a mistake to suppose that a science consists entirely of strictly proved theses, and it would be unjust to require this. Only a disposition with a passion for authority will raise such a demand, someone with a craving to replace his religious catechism by another, though it is a scientific one. Science has only a few apodeictic propositions in its catechism: the rest are assertions promoted by it to some particular degree of probability. It is actually a sign of a scientific mode of thought to find satisfaction in these approximations to certainty and to be able to pursue constructive work further in spite of the absence of final confirmation.

But if the subject does not himself give us the explanation of the sense of a parapraxis, where are we to find the starting-points for our interpretation—the circumstantial evidence? In various directions. In the first place from analogies with phenomena apart from parapraxes: when, for instance, we assert that distorting a name when it occurs as a slip of the tongue has the same insulting sense as a deliberate twisting of a name. Further, from the psychical situation in which the parapraxis occurs, the character of the person who makes the parapraxis, and the impressions which he has received before the parapraxis and to which the parapraxis is perhaps a reaction. What happens as a rule is that the interpretation is carried out according to general principles: to begin with there is only a suspicion, a suggestion for an interpretation, and we then find a confirmation by examining the psychical situation. Sometimes we have to wait for subsequent events as well (which have, as it were, announced themselves by the parapraxis) before our suspicion is confirmed.

I cannot easily give you illustrations of this if I limit myself to the field of slips of the tongue, though even there some good instances are to be found. The young man who wanted to '*begleitdigen*' a lady [p. 33] was certainly a timid character. The lady whose husband could eat and drink what *she* wanted [p. 35] is known to me as one of those energetic women who wear the breeches in their home. Or let us take the following example: At the General Meeting of the 'Concordia'[1] a young member made a speech of violent opposition, in the course of which he addressed the committee as '*Vorschussmitglieder* [lending members]', a word which seems to be made up of '*Vorstand* [directors]' and '*Ausschuss* [committee]'. We shall suspect that some disturbing purpose was at work in him, acting against his violent opposition, based on something connected with a loan. And in fact we learnt from our informant that the speaker was constantly in financial difficulties and just at that time had applied for a loan. The disturbing intention could therefore be replaced by the thought: 'Moderate your opposition; these are the same people who will have to sanction your loan.'

But I can give you a large selection of circumstantial evidence of this kind if I pass over to the wide field of the other parapraxes.

If anyone forgets a proper name which is familiar to him normally or if, in spite of all his efforts, he finds it difficult to keep it in mind, it is plausible to suppose that he has something against the person who bears the name so that he prefers not to think of him. Consider, for instance, what we learn in the following cases about the psychical situation in which the parapraxis occurred.

'A Herr Y. fell in love with a lady, but he met with no success, and shortly afterwards she married a Herr X. Thereafter, Herr Y., in spite of having known Herr X. for a long time and even having business dealings with him, forgot his name over and over again, so that several times he had to enquire what it was from other people when he wanted to correspond with Herr X.' Herr Y. evidently wanted to know nothing of his more fortunate rival: 'never thought of shall he be.'[2]

Or: A lady enquired from her doctor for news of a common acquaintance, but called her by her maiden name. She had

[1] [The Society of Journalists in Vienna. This anecdote will be found in *P.E.L.*, 88; it was originally supplied by Max Graf.]

[2] From Jung [1907, 52. This appears in *P.E.L.*, 25–6. The quotation at the end, 'Nicht gedacht soll seiner werden', forms the first line and a repeated refrain in a poem of Heine's from the *Nachlese*, 'Aus der Matratzengruft', No. IV.]

forgotten her friend's married name. She admitted afterwards that she had been very unhappy about the marriage and disliked her friend's husband.[1]

We shall have a good deal to say about forgetting names in other connections [p. 74 f. below]; for the moment we are principally interested in the psychical situation in which the forgetting occurs.

The forgetting of intentions can in general be traced to an opposing current of thought, which is unwilling to carry out the intention. But this view is not only held by us psycho-analysts; it is the general opinion, accepted by everyone in their daily lives and only denied when it comes to theory. A patron who gives his *protégé* the excuse of having forgotten his request fails to justify himself. The *protégé* immediately thinks: 'It means nothing to him; it's true he promised, but he doesn't really want to do it.'[2] For that reason forgetting is banned in certain circumstances of ordinary life; the distinction between the popular and the psycho-analytic view of these parapraxes seems to have disappeared. Imagine the lady of the house receiving her guest with the words: 'What? have you come to-day? I'd quite forgotten I invited you for to-day.' Or imagine a young man confessing to his *fiancée* that he had forgotten to keep their last *rendez-vous*. He will certainly not confess it; he will prefer to invent on the spur of the moment the most improbable obstacles which prevented his appearing at the time and afterwards made it impossible for him to let her know. We all know too that in military affairs the excuse of having forgotten something is of no help and is no protection against punishment, and we must all feel that that is justified. Here all at once everyone is united in thinking that a particular parapraxis has a sense and in knowing what that sense is. Why are they not consistent enough to extend this knowledge to the other parapraxes and to admit them fully? There is of course an answer to this question too.

Since laymen have so little doubt about the sense of this forgetting of intentions, you will be the less surprised to find writers employing this sort of parapraxis in the same sense. Any of you who have seen or read Bernard Shaw's *Caesar and*

---

[1] From Brill [1912, 191; also *P.E.L.*, 224].

[2] [This situation is considered further below, p. 72 f.]

Cleopatra will remember that in the last scene Caesar, as he is leaving Egypt, is haunted by the idea that there is something else he had intended to do but has forgotten. In the end it turns out what this was: he had forgotten to say good-bye to Cleopatra. The dramatist is seeking by this little contrivance to ascribe to the great Caesar a superiority which he did not in fact possess and which he never desired. For historical sources will tell you that Caesar made Cleopatra follow him to Rome, that she was living there with her little Caesarion when Caesar was murdered, and that she thereupon fled from the city.[1]

Cases of forgetting an intention are in general so clear that they are not of much use for our purpose of obtaining circumstantial evidence of the sense of a parapraxis from the psychical situation. Let us therefore turn to a particularly ambiguous and obscure kind of parapraxis—to losing and mislaying. You will no doubt find it incredible that we ourselves can play an intentional part in what is so often the painful accident of losing something. But there are plenty of observations like the following one. A young man lost a pencil of his of which he had been very fond. The day before, he had received a letter from his brother-in-law which ended with these words: 'I have neither the inclination nor the time at present to encourage you in your frivolity and laziness.' The pencil had actually been given to him by this brother-in-law. Without this coincidence we could not, of course, have asserted that a part was played in the loss by an intention to get rid of the thing.[2] Similar cases are very common. We lose an object if we have quarrelled with the person who gave it to us and do not want to be reminded of him; or if we no longer like the object itself and want to have an excuse for getting another and better one instead. The same intention directed against an object can also play a part, of course, in cases of dropping, breaking or destroying things. Can we regard it as a matter of chance when a schoolchild immediately before his birthday loses, ruins or smashes some of his personal belongings, such as his satchel or his watch?

Nor will anyone who has sufficiently often experienced the torment of not being able to find something that he himself has

---

[1] [This quotation from Shaw appears also in *P.E.L.*, 154*n*.]
[2] From Dattner. [*P.E.L.*, 207.]

put away feel inclined to believe that there is a purpose in mislaying things. Yet instances are far from rare in which the circumstances attendant on the mislaying point to an intention to get rid of the object temporarily or permanently.

Here is the best example, perhaps, of such an occasion. A youngish man told me the following story: 'Some years ago there were misunderstandings between me and my wife. I found her too cold, and although I willingly recognized her excellent qualities we lived together without any tender feelings. One day, returning from a walk, she gave me a book which she had bought because she thought it would interest me. I thanked her for this mark of "attention", promised to read the book and put it on one side. After that I could never find it again. Months passed by, in which I occasionally remembered the lost book and made vain attempts to find it. About six months later my dear mother, who was not living with us, fell ill. My wife left home to nurse her mother-in-law. The patient's condition became serious and gave my wife an opportunity of showing the best side of herself. One evening I returned home full of enthusiasm and gratitude for what my wife had accomplished. I walked up to my desk, and without any definite intention but with a kind of somnambulistic certainty opened one of the drawers. On the very top I found the long-lost book I had mislaid.'[1] With the extinction of the motive the mislaying of the object ceased as well.

Ladies and Gentlemen, I could multiply this collection of examples indefinitely; but I will not do so here. You will in any case find a profusion of case material for the study of parapraxes in my *Psychopathology of Everyday Life* (first published in 1901).[2] All these examples lead to the same result: they make it probable that parapraxes have a sense, and they show you how that sense is discovered or confirmed by the attendant circumstances. I will be briefer to-day, because we have adopted the limited aim of using the study of these phenomena as a help towards a preparation for psycho-analysis. There are only two

[1] [This appears in *P.E.L.*, 49.]
[2] See also similar collections by Maeder [1906–7] (in French), Brill [1912] (in English), Jones [1911] (in English) and J. Stärcke [1916] (in Dutch), etc.

groups of observations into which I need enter more fully here: accumulated and combined parapraxes and the confirmation of our interpretations by subsequent events.

Accumulated and combined parapraxes are without doubt the finest flower of their kind. If we had only been concerned to prove that parapraxes have a sense we should have confined ourselves to them from the first, for in their case the sense is unmistakable even to the dull-witted and forces itself on the most critical judgement. An accumulation of these phenomena betrays an obstinacy that is scarcely ever a characteristic of chance events but fits in well with something intentional. Finally, the mutual interchangeability between different species of parapraxes demonstrates what it is in parapraxes that is important and characteristic: not their form or the method which they employ but the purpose which they serve and which can be achieved in the most various ways. For this reason I will give you an instance of repeated forgetting. Ernest Jones [1911, 483] tells us that once, for reasons unknown to him, he left a letter lying on his desk for several days. At last he decided to send it off, but he had it returned to him by the Dead Letter Office[1] since he had forgotten to address it. After he had addressed it he took it to the post, but this time it had no stamp. And then at last he was obliged to admit his reluctance to sending the letter off at all.

In another case a bungled action is combined with an instance of mislaying. A lady travelled to Rome with her brother-in-law, who was a famous artist. The visitor was received with great honour by the German community in Rome, and among other presents he was given an antique gold medal. The lady was vexed that her brother-in-law did not appreciate the lovely object sufficiently. When she returned home (her place in Rome having been taken by her sister) she discovered while unpacking that she had brought the medal with her—how, she did not know. She at once sent a letter with the news to her brother-in-law, and announced that she would send the article she had walked off with back to Rome next day. But next day the medal had been so cleverly mislaid that it could not be found and sent off; and it was at this point, that the meaning

[1] [In English in the original. This example and the next two appear *P.E.L.*, 230–1.]

of her 'absent-mindedness' dawned on the lady: she wanted to keep the object for herself.[1]

I have already given you an example of a combination of a forgetting with an error, the case of someone forgetting an appointment and on a second occasion, having firmly decided not to forget *this* time, turning up at the wrong hour [p. 30]. An exactly similar case was reported to me from his own experience by a friend with literary as well as scientific interests. 'Some years ago', he told me, 'I allowed myself to be elected to the committee of a certain literary society, as I thought that the organization might one day be able to help me to have my play produced; and I took a regular part, though without being much interested, in the meetings which were held every Friday. Then, a few months ago, I was given the promise of a production at the theatre at F.; and since then I have regularly *forgotten* the meetings of the society. When I read your book on the subject I felt ashamed of my forgetfulness. I reproached myself with the thought that it was shabby behaviour on my part to stay away now that I no longer needed these people, and resolved on no account to forget the next Friday. I kept on reminding myself of this resolution until I carried it into effect and stood at the door of the room where the meetings were held. To my astonishment it was locked; the meeting was over. I had in fact made a mistake over the day; it was now Saturday!'

It would be agreeable to add further, similar examples. But I must proceed, and give you a glimpse of the cases in which our interpretation has to wait for the future for confirmation. The governing condition of these cases, it will be realized, is that the present psychical situation is unknown to us or inaccessible to our enquiries. Our interpretation is consequently no more than a suspicion to which we ourselves do not attach too much importance. Later, however, something happens which shows us how well-justified our interpretation had been. I was once the guest of a young married couple and heard the young woman laughingly describe her latest experience. The day after her return from the honeymoon she had called for her unmarried sister to go shopping with her as she used to do, while her husband went to his business. Suddenly she noticed

[1] Reported by R. Reitler.

a gentleman on the other side of the street, and nudging her sister had cried: 'Look, there goes Herr L.' She had forgotten that this gentleman had been her husband for some weeks. I shuddered as I heard the story, but I did not dare to draw the inference. The little incident only occurred to my mind some years later when the marriage had come to a most unhappy end.[1]

Maeder tells of a lady who, on the eve of her wedding had forgotten to try on her wedding-dress and, to her dressmaker's despair, only remembered it late in the evening. He connects this forgetfulness with the fact that she was soon divorced from her husband. I know a lady now divorced from her husband, who in managing her money affairs frequently signed documents in her maiden name, many years before she in fact resumed it.—I know of other women who have lost their wedding-rings during the honeymoon, and I know too that the history of their marriages has given a sense to the accident.— And now here is one more glaring example, but with a happier ending. The story is told of a famous German chemist that his marriage did not take place, because he forgot the hour of his wedding and went to the laboratory instead of to the church. He was wise enough to be satisfied with a single attempt and died at a great age unmarried.

The idea may possibly have occurred to you that in these examples parapraxes have taken the place of the omens or auguries of the ancients. And indeed some omens were nothing else than parapraxes, as, for instance, when someone stumbled or fell down. Others of them, it is true, had the character of objective happenings and not of subjective acts. But you would hardly believe how difficult it sometimes is to decide whether a particular event belongs to the one group or to the other. An act so often understands how to disguise itself as a passive experience.

All those of us who can look back on a comparatively long experience of life will probably admit that we should have spared ourselves many disappointments and painful surprises if we had found the courage and determination to interpret small parapraxes experienced in our human contacts as auguries and to make use of them as indications of intentions that were still

[1] [This example and the two next will be found *P.E.L.*, 203–4.]

concealed. As a rule we dare not do so; it would make us feel as though, after a détour through science, we were becoming superstitious again. Nor do all auguries come true, and you will understand from our theories that they do not all need to come true.

PARAPRAXES (*concluded*)

LADIES AND GENTLEMEN,—We may take it as the outcome of
our efforts so far and the basis of our further investigations that
parapraxes have a sense. Let me insist once again that I am
not asserting—and for our purposes there is no need to do so—
that every single parapraxis that occurs has a sense, even
though I regard that as probably the case. It is enough for us
if we can point to such a sense relatively often in the different
forms of parapraxis. Moreover, in this respect these different
forms behave differently. Cases of slips of the tongue and of the
pen, etc., may occur on a purely physiological basis. I cannot
believe that this is so in the types depending on *forgetting* (forgetting names or intentions, mislaying, etc.). It is very probable
that there are cases of *losing* which can be regarded as unintended. It is in general true that only a certain proportion
of the *errors* that occur in ordinary life can be looked at from
our point of view. You should bear these limitations in mind
when henceforward we start from the assumption that parapraxes are psychical acts and arise from mutual interference
between two intentions.

This is the first product of psycho-analysis. Psychology has
hitherto known nothing of the occurrence of such mutual interferences or of the possibility that they might result in such
phenomena. We have made a quite considerable extension to
the world of psychical phenomena and have won for psychology phenomena which were not reckoned earlier as belonging
to it.

Let us pause a moment longer over the assertion that parapraxes are 'psychical acts'. Does this imply more than what we
have said already—that they have a sense? I think not. I think,
rather, that the former assertion [that they are psychical acts]
is more indefinite and more easily misunderstood. Anything
that is observable in mental life may occasionally be described
as a mental phenomenon. The question will then be whether the
particular mental phenomenon has arisen immediately from

somatic, organic and material influences—in which case its investigation will not be part of psychology—or whether it is derived in the first instance from other mental processes, somewhere behind which the series of organic influences begins. It is this latter situation that we have in view when we describe a phenomenon as a mental process, and for that reason it is more expedient to clothe our assertion in the form: 'the phenomenon has a sense.' By 'sense' we understand 'meaning', 'intention,' 'purpose' and 'position in a continuous psychical context'. [Cf. p. 40.]

There are a number of other phenomena which are closely akin to parapraxes but to which that name is no longer appropriate. We call them chance and symptomatic actions. Like the others, they have the character of being without a motive, insignificant and unimportant; but they have in addition, more clearly, that of being unnecessary. They are distinguished from parapraxes by their lack of another intention with which they are in collision and which is disturbed by them. On the other hand, they merge insensibly into the gestures and movements which we regard as expressions of the emotions. These chance actions include all sorts of manipulations with our clothing, or parts of our body or objects within our reach, performed as though in play and apparently with no purpose, or, again, the omission of these manipulations; or, further, tunes that we hum to ourselves. I suggest that all these phenomena have a sense and can be interpreted in the same way as parapraxes, that they are small indications of more important mental processes and are fully valid psychical acts. But I do not propose to linger over this fresh extension of the field of mental phenomena; I shall return to the parapraxes, in connection with which problems important for psycho-analysis can be worked out with far greater clarity.[1]

The most interesting questions which we have raised about parapraxes and not yet answered are perhaps these. We have said that parapraxes are the product of mutual interference between two different intentions, of which one may be called the disturbed intention and the other the disturbing one. The

[1] [Symptomatic and chance actions form the subject of Chapter IX of *P.E.L.*]

disturbed intentions give no occasion for further questions, but concerning the latter we should like to know, first, what sort of intentions emerge as a disturbance to others, and secondly what is the relation of the disturbing intentions to the disturbed ones?

If you will allow me, I will once more take slips of the tongue as representatives of the whole class and I will reply to the second question before the first.

In a slip of the tongue the disturbing intention may be related in its content to the disturbed one, in which case it will contradict it or correct it or supplement it. Or—the more obscure and more interesting case—the content of the disturbing intention may have nothing to do with that of the disturbed one.

We shall have no difficulty in finding evidence of the former relation in instances we already know and in similar ones. In almost every case in which a slip of the tongue reverses the sense, the disturbing intention expresses the contrary to the disturbed one and the parapraxis represents a conflict between two incompatible inclinations. 'I declare the sitting opened, but I should prefer it to be already closed' is the sense of the President's slip of the tongue [p. 34]. A political periodical which had been accused of corruption defended itself in an article the climax of which should have been: 'Our readers will bear witness to the fact that we have always acted in the most *unself-seeking* manner for the good of the community.' But the editor entrusted with the preparation of the article wrote 'in the most *self-seeking* manner'. That is to say, he was thinking: 'This is what I am obliged to write; but I have different ideas.' A [German] member of parliament who was insisting that the truth should be told to the Emperor '*rückhaltlos* [unreservedly]' evidently heard an inner voice that was shocked at his boldness and, by a slip of the tongue, changed the word into '*rückgratlos* [spinelessly]'.[1]

In the instances already familiar to you which give an impression of being contractions or abbreviations, what we have before us are corrections, additions or continuations, by means of which a second purpose makes itself felt alongside of the

[1] This was in the German Reichstag in November 1908. [A fuller account of this appears *P.E.L.*, 95–6. The preceding slip will be found *P.E.L.*, 120–1.]

first. 'Facts came to *Vorschein* [light]—better to say it straight out—they were *Schweinereien* [disgusting]; well then, facts came to *Vorschwein* [p. 42].' 'Those who understand this can be counted *on the fingers of one hand*—no, there's really only *one* person who understands it, so: can be counted *on one finger* [p. 41].' Or: 'My husband can eat and drink what he wants. But, as you know, *I* don't put up with his wanting anything at all, so: he can eat and drink what *I* want [p. 35].' In all these cases, then, the slip of the tongue arises from the content of the disturbed intention itself or is connected with it.

The other sort of relation between the two mutually interfering intentions seems puzzling. If the disturbing intention has nothing to do with the disturbed one, where can it have come from and why is it that it makes itself noticeable as a disturbance at this particular point? The observation which can alone give us the answer to this shows that the disturbance arises from a train of thought which has occupied the person concerned a short time before and, whether it has already been expressed in speech or not, produces this subsequent effect. It must in fact, therefore, be described as a perseveration, though not necessarily as the perseveration of spoken words. In this case too an associative link between the disturbing and the disturbed intentions is present; but it does not lie in their content but is artificially constructed, often along extremely forced associative paths.

Here is a simple example of this, derived from my own observation. I once met two Viennese ladies in the lovely Dolomites, who were dressed in walking clothes. I accompanied them part of the way, and we discussed the pleasures and also the trials of spending a holiday in that way. One of the ladies admitted that spending the day like that entailed a good deal of discomfort. 'It is certainly not at all pleasant', she said, 'if one has been tramping all day in the sun and has perspired right through one's blouse and chemise.' In this sentence she had to overcome a slight hesitation at one point. Then she continued: 'But then when one gets "nach *Hose*" and can change. . . .' This slip of the tongue was not analysed but I expect you can understand it easily. The lady's intention had obviously been to give a more complete list of her clothes: blouse, chemise and *Hose* [drawers]. Reasons of propriety led her to omit any mention of the '*Hose*'. But in the next sentence, with its quite independent content, the unspoken word emerged as a distortion of the similar-sounding 'nach *Hause* [home]'.[1]

We can now turn, however, to the main question, which we have long postponed, of what sort of intentions these are, which find expression in this unusual fashion as disturbers of other intentions. Well, they are obviously of very different sorts, among which we must look for the common factor. If we examine a number of examples with this in view, they will soon fall into three groups. The first group contains those cases in which the disturbing purpose is known to the speaker and more-over had been noticed by him before he made the slip of the tongue. Thus, in the '*Vorschwein*' slip [p. 42] the speaker admitted not only that he had formed the judgement '*Schwein-ereien*' about the events in question, but also that he had had the intention, from which he afterwards drew back, of express-ing his judgement in words. A second group is made up of other cases in which the disturbing purpose is equally recognized as his by the speaker, but in which he was unaware that it was active in him just before he made the slip. Thus, he accepts our interpretation of his slip, but nevertheless remains to some extent surprised at it. Instances of this kind of attitude can perhaps be found in other sorts of parapraxes more easily than in slips of the tongue. In a third group the interpretation of the disturbing intention is vigorously rejected by the speaker; he not only denies that it was active in him before he made the slip, but seeks to maintain that it is entirely foreign to him. You will recall the example of the 'hiccough' [p. 49] and the positively rude denial which I brought on myself from the speaker by uncovering his disturbing intention. As you know, we have not yet come to any agreement in our views on these cases. *I* should pay no attention to the denial put forward by the proposer of the toast and should persist in my interpretation unruffled, while *you*, I suppose, are still affected by his protest and raise the question of whether we ought not to give up interpreting parapraxes of this kind and regard them as purely physiological acts in the pre-analytic sense. I can well imagine what it is that deters you. My interpretation carries with it the hypothesis that

[1] [Freud later included this anecdote in the 1917 edition of *P.E.L.*, 64–5.]

intentions can find expression in a speaker of which he himself knows nothing but which I am able to infer from circumstantial evidence. You are brought up short in the face of such a novel and momentous hypothesis. I can understand that, and I see your point so far as that goes. But one thing is certain. If you want to apply consistently the view of parapraxes which has been confirmed by so many examples, you will have to make up your mind to accept the strange hypothesis I have mentioned. If you cannot do that, you will have once more to abandon the understanding of parapraxes which you have only just achieved.

Let us consider for a moment what it is that unites the three groups, what it is that the three mechanisms of slips of the tongue have in common. It is fortunately unmistakable. In the first two groups the disturbing purpose is recognized by the speaker; furthermore, in the first group that purpose announces itself immediately before the slip. But in both cases *it is forced back. The speaker decides not to put it into words, and after that the slip of the tongue occurs: after that, that is to say, the purpose which has been forced back is put into words against the speaker's will, either by altering the expression of the intention which he has permitted, or by mingling with it, or by actually taking its place.* This, then, is the mechanism of a slip of the tongue.

On my view, I can bring what happens in the *third* group into complete harmony with the mechanism I have described. I have only to assume that what distinguishes these three groups from one another is the differing extent to which the intention is forced back. In the first group the intention is there and makes itself noticed before the speaker's remark; only then is it rejected; and it takes its revenge in the slip of the tongue. In the second group the rejection goes further: the intention has already ceased to be noticeable before the remark is made. Strangely enough, this does not in the least prevent it from playing its part in causing the slip. But this behaviour makes it easier for us to explain what happens in the third group. I shall venture to assume that a purpose can also find expression in a parapraxis when it has been forced back and not noticed for a considerable time, for a very long time perhaps, and can for that reason be denied straight out by the speaker. But even if you leave the problem of the third group on one side, you are bound to conclude from the observations we have made in the other cases that *the suppression of the speaker's intention to say something is the indispensable condition for the occurrence of a slip of the tongue.*

We may now claim to have made further advances in our understanding of parapraxes. We know not only that they are mental acts, in which we can detect sense and intention, not only that they come about through mutual interference between two different intentions, but beyond this we know that one of these intentions must have been in some way forced back from being put into effect before it can manifest itself as a disturbance of the other intention. It must itself have been disturbed before it can become a disturber. This does not mean, of course, that we have yet achieved a complete explanation of the phenomena which we call parapraxes. We see further questions immediately cropping up, and we suspect in general that the further our understanding goes the more occasions there will be for raising fresh questions. We may ask, for instance, why things should not be much simpler. If the intention is to force back a particular purpose instead of carrying it into effect, the forcing back should be successful, so that the purpose does not manifest itself at all; or on the other hand the forcing back might fail, so that the purpose that was to have been forced back would manifest itself completely. But parapraxes are the outcome of a compromise: they constitute a half-success and a half-failure for each of the two intentions; the intention which is being challenged is neither completely suppressed nor, apart from special cases, carried through quite unscathed. We may conclude that special conditions must prevail in order that an interference or compromise of this kind shall come about, but we can form no conception of what they can be. Nor do I think that we could discover these unknown factors by going deeper into the study of parapraxes. It will be necessary, rather, to examine first yet other obscure regions of mental life: it is only from analogies which we shall meet with there that we shall find the courage to set up the hypotheses necessary for throwing a more penetrating light upon parapraxes. And one thing more. Working from small indications, as we are constantly in the habit of doing in the present field, brings its own dangers. There is a mental disease, 'combinatory paranoia', in which the exploitation of small indications like these is carried to unlimited lengths; and I will not of course claim that conclusions built on such foundations are invariably correct. We can only be guarded against these risks by the broad basis of our observations, the repetition of similar impressions from the most varied spheres of mental life.

At this point, therefore, we will leave the analysis of parapraxes. But there is one point more to which I would draw your attention. I would ask you to bear in mind as a model the manner in which we have treated these phenomena. From this example you can learn the aims of our psychology. We seek not merely to describe and to classify phenomena, but to understand them as signs of an interplay of forces in the mind, as a manifestation of purposeful intentions working concurrently or in mutual opposition. We are concerned with a *dynamic view* of mental phenomena. On our view the phenomena that are perceived must yield in importance to trends which are only hypothetical.

We shall therefore not enter more deeply into parapraxes, but we may still undertake a cursory survey of the extent of this field, in the course of which we shall come once more upon things we already know but shall also discover some novelties. In this survey I shall keep to the division into three groups which I proposed to begin with:[1] slips of the tongue together with their cognate forms (slips of the pen, misreading and mishearing); forgetting, subdivided according to the objects forgotten (proper names, foreign words, intentions or impressions); and bungled actions, mislaying and losing. Errors, in so far as they concern us, fall under the headings partly of forgetting and partly of bungled actions.

We have already treated *slips of the tongue* in great detail, but there are a few more points to be added. Slips of the tongue are accompanied by certain minor emotional phenomena which are not quite without interest. No one likes making slips of the

[1] [At the beginning of Lecture II (p. 25). These 'three groups' are not to be confused with the 'three groups' discussed on pp. 64–5, which relate to the quite other matter of the attitude towards slips of the tongue adopted by those who make them.]

tongue, and we often fail to hear our own slips, though never other people's. Slips of the tongue are also in a certain sense contagious; it is not at all easy to talk about slips of the tongue without making slips of the tongue oneself. The most trivial forms of such slips, precisely those which have no special light to throw on hidden mental processes, have reasons which are nevertheless not hard to penetrate. For instance, if someone has pronounced a long vowel short on account of a disturbance affecting the word for some reason or other, he will soon afterwards pronounce a subsequent short vowel long, thus making a fresh slip of the tongue to compensate for the earlier one. In the same way, if he pronounces a diphthong incorrectly and carelessly (for instance pronouncing an 'eu' or 'oi' as 'ei')he will try to make up for it by changing a subsequent 'ei' into an 'eu' or 'oi'. The decisive factor here seems to be consideration of the impression made on the audience, who are not to suppose that it is a matter of indifference to the speaker how he treats his mother-tongue. The second, compensating distortion actually has the purpose of directing the hearer's attention to the first one and of assuring him that the speaker has noticed it too. The commonest, simplest and most trivial slips of the tongue are contractions and anticipations [cf. p. 32] which occur in insignificant parts of speech. For instance, in a longish sentence one may make a slip of the tongue which anticipates the last word of what one intends to say. This gives an impression of impatience to be finished with the sentence, and is evidence in general of a certain antipathy against communicating the sentence or against the whole of one's remarks. We thus arrive at marginal cases in which the distinctions between the psycho-analytic view of slips of the tongue and the ordinary physiological one melt into one another. It is to be assumed that a purpose of disturbing the intention of the speech is present in these cases but that it can only announce its presence and not what it itself has in view. The disturbance it produces then proceeds in accordance with certain phonetic influences or associative attractions and can be regarded as a distraction of the attention from the intention of the speech. But neither this disturbance of the attention nor the inclinations to associate which have become operative touch on the essence of the process. This remains, in spite of everything, the indication of the existence of an intention which is disturbing to the intention of the speech, though the *nature* of this disturbing intention cannot be guessed from its consequences, as is possible in all the better defined cases of slips of the tongue.

Slips of the pen, to which I now pass, are so closely akin to slips of the tongue that we have nothing new to expect from them. Perhaps we may glean one little further point. The extremely common small slips of the pen, contractions and anticipations of later words (especially of final words) point, once again, to a general dislike of writing and impatience to be done with it. More marked products of miswriting enable one to recognize the nature and aim of the disturbing purpose. If one finds a slip of the pen in a letter, one knows in general that there was something the matter with its author, but one cannot always discover what was going on in him. A slip of the pen is just as often overlooked by the person responsible as is a slip of the tongue. The following is a noteworthy observation. There are, as we know, people who are in the habit of reading through every letter they write before sending it off. Others do not do this as a rule; but if, as an exception, they do so they always come across some conspicuous slip of the pen, which they can then correct. How is this to be explained? It looks as though these people knew that they had made a mistake in writing the letter. Are we really to believe this?

An interesting problem attaches to the *practical* importance of slips of the pen. You may perhaps remember the case of a murderer, H., who found the means of obtaining cultures of highly dangerous pathogenic organisms from scientific institutes by representing himself as a bacteriologist. He then used these cultures for the purpose of getting rid of his near connections by this most modern of methods. Now on one occasion this man complained to the Directors of one of these institutes that the cultures that had been sent to him were ineffective; but he made a slip of the pen, and instead of writing 'in my experiments on mice or guinea-pigs' he wrote quite clearly 'in my experiments on men'.[1] The doctors at the institute were struck by the slip, but, so far as I know, drew no conclusions from it. Well, what do you think? Should not the doctors, on the contrary, have taken the slip of the pen as a confession and started

[1] ['*Menschen*' instead of '*Mäusen oder Meerschweinchen*'.]

an investigation which would have put an early stop to the murderer's activities? Was not ignorance of our view of parapraxes responsible in this case for an omission of practical significance? Well, I think a slip of the pen like this would certainly have seemed to me most suspicious; but something of great importance stands in the way of using it as a confession. The matter is not as simple as all that. The slip was certainly a piece of circumstantial evidence; but it was not enough in itself to start an investigation. It is true that the slip of the pen said that he was concerned with thoughts of infecting men, but it did not make it possible to decide whether these thoughts were to be taken as a clear intention to injure or as a phantasy of no practical importance. It is even possible that a man who had made a slip like this would have every subjective justification for denying the phantasy and would repudiate it as something entirely foreign to him. You will understand these possibilities still better when later on we come to consider the distinction between psychical and material reality.[1] But this is another instance of a parapraxis acquiring importance from subsequent events. [Cf. p. 57 f. above.]

With *misreading* we come to a psychical situation which differs sensibly from that in slips of the tongue or pen. Here one of the two mutually competing purposes is replaced by a sensory stimulation and is perhaps on that account less resistant. What one is going to read is not a derivative of one's own mental life like something one proposes to write. In a great majority of cases, therefore, a misreading consists in a complete substitution. One replaces the word that is to be read by another, without there necessarily being any connection of content between the text and the product of the misreading, which depends as a rule on verbal similarity. The best member of this group is Lichtenberg's '*Agamemnon*' for '*angenommen*' [p. 39 above]. If we want to discover the disturbing purpose which produced the misreading we must leave the text that has been misread entirely aside and we may begin the analytic investigation with the two questions: what is the first association to the product of the misreading? and in what situation did the misreading occur? Occasionally a knowledge of the latter is alone enough to explain the misreading. For instance, a man under the

---

[1] [See the discussion in Lecture XXIII, p. 368 below.]

pressure of an imperious need was wandering about in a strange town when he saw the word '*Closet-House*' on a large notice-board on the first storey of a building. He had just enough time to feel surprised at the notice-board being placed so high up before discovering that, strictly speaking, what he should have read was '*Corset-House*'.[1] In other cases a misreading precisely of the kind which is quite independent of the content of the text may call for a detailed analysis which cannot be carried through without practice in the technique of psycho-analysis and without reliance on it. As a rule, however, it is not so hard to find the explanation of a misreading: the word substituted immediately betrays, as in the Agamemnon example, the circle of ideas from which the disturbance has arisen. In this time of war, for instance, it is a very usual thing for the names of towns and generals and the military terms that are constantly buzzing around us to be read wherever a similar word meets our eyes. Whatever interests and concerns us puts itself in the place of what is strange and still uninteresting. After-images of [earlier] thoughts trouble new perceptions.

With misreading, too, there is no lack of cases of another sort, in which the text of what is read itself arouses the disturbing purpose, which thereupon, as a rule, turns it into its opposite. What we ought to read is something unwished-for, and analysis will convince us that an intense wish to reject what we have read must be held responsible for its alteration.

In the more frequent cases of misreading which we mentioned first, we miss two factors to which we have assigned an important role in the mechanism of parapraxes: a conflict between two purposes and a forcing-back of one of them which takes its revenge by producing a parapraxis. Not that anything contrary to this occurs in misreading. But the prominence of the thought that leads to the misreading is far more noticeable than the forcing-back which it may have experienced previously.

It is these two factors which we meet with most markedly in the different situations in which parapraxes of forgetting occur. *The forgetting of intentions* is quite unambiguous; as we have already seen [p. 53], its interpretation is not disputed even by laymen. The purpose which disturbs the intention is in every

[1] [Later included in the 1917 edition of *P.E.L.*, 113–14.]

instance a counter-intention, an unwillingness; and all that remains for us to learn about it is why it has not expressed itself in some other and less disguised manner. But the presence of this counter-will[1] is unquestionable. Sometimes, too, we succeed in guessing something of the motives which compel this counter-will to conceal itself; acting surreptitiously by means of the parapraxis it always achieves its aim, whereas it would be sure of repudiation if it emerged as an open contradiction. If some important change in the psychical situation takes place between the forming of the intention and its carrying-out, as a result of which there is no longer any question of the intention being carried out, then the forgetting of the intention drops out of the category of parapraxes. It no longer seems strange to have forgotten it, and we realize that it would have been unnecessary to remember it: thereafter it becomes permanently or temporarily extinct. The forgetting of an intention can only be called a parapraxis if we cannot believe that the intention has been interrupted in this latter way.

The instances of forgetting an intention are in general so uniform and so perspicuous that for that very reason they are of no interest for our investigation. Nevertheless there are two points at which we can learn something new from a study of these parapraxes. Forgetting—that is, failure to carry out— an intention points, as we have said, to a counter-will that is hostile to it. This is no doubt true; but our enquiries show that the counter-will can be of two kinds—direct or indirect. What I mean by the latter will best appear from one or two examples. If a patron forgets to put in a word with a third person on behalf of his *protégé*, this may happen because he is not really very much interested in the *protégé* and therefore has no great desire to speak on his behalf. In any case, that is how the *protégé* will understand the patron's forgetting [cf. p. 53]. But things may be more complicated. The counter-will in the patron against carrying out the intention may come from another direction and may be aimed at quite a different point. It may have nothing to do with the *protégé* but may perhaps be directed

[1] [The concept of a 'counter-will' played a prominent part in some of Freud's very first papers on psychopathology, e.g., in 'A Case of Successful Treatment by Hypnotism' (1892–3). It reappears at several points in *P.E.L.*]

against the third person to whom the recommendation was to have been made. So you see from this once more [cf. p. 70] the doubts that stand in the way of a practical application of our interpretations. In spite of the correct interpretation of the forgetting, the *protégé* is in danger of being too distrustful and of doing his patron a grave injustice. Or, supposing someone forgets an appointment which he has promised someone else to keep, the most frequent reason for it will be, no doubt, a direct disinclination to meeting this person. But in such a case analysis might show that the disturbing purpose did not relate to him but was directed against the place at which the meeting was planned to happen and was avoided on account of a distressing memory attaching to it. Or, again, if someone forgets to post a letter, the counter-purpose may be based on the contents of the letter; but it is by no means out of the question that the letter may be harmless in itself and may only be subject to the counter-purpose because something about it recalls another letter which had been written on some earlier occasion and which offered the counter-will a direct point of attack. It can be said, therefore, that here the counter-will was transferred from the earlier letter, which justified it, to the present one, which it had in fact no grounds for concern about. You see, then, that we must practise restraint and foresight in applying our interpretations, justified as they are: things that are psychologically equivalent may in practice have a great variety of meanings.

Phenomena such as these last may seem to you most unusual, and you will perhaps be inclined to suppose that an 'indirect' counter-will already indicates that the process is a pathological one. But I can assure you that it occurs as well within the limits of what is normal and healthy. Moreover you should not misunderstand me. I am far from admitting that our analytic interpretations are untrustworthy. The ambiguities in the forgetting of intentions which I have been mentioning exist only so long as we have not made an analysis of the case and are only making our interpretations on the basis of our general assumptions. If we carry out an analysis upon the person in question, we invariably learn with sufficient certainty whether the counter-will is a direct one or what other origin it may have.

The second point I have in mind [cf. p. 72] is this. If in a large majority of instances we find confirmation of the fact that the forgetting of an intention goes back to a counter-will, we grow bold enough to extend the solution to another set of instances in which the person under analysis does not confirm but denies the counter-will we have inferred. Take as examples of this such extremely common events as forgetting to return books one has been lent or to pay bills or debts. We shall venture to insist to the person concerned that an intention exists in him to keep the books and not to pay the debts, while he will deny this intention but will not be able to produce any other explanation of his behaviour. Thereupon we shall go on to say that he has this intention but knows nothing about it, but that it is enough for us that it reveals its presence by producing the forgetting in him. He may repeat to us that he has in fact forgotten. You will now recognize the situation as one in which we found ourselves once before [p. 64]. If we want to pursue our interpretations of parapraxes, which have so frequently proved justified, to a consistent conclusion, we are forced to the inescapable hypothesis that there are purposes in people which can become operative without their knowing about them. But this brings us into opposition to all the views that dominate both ordinary life and psychology.

The forgetting of proper names and foreign names, as well as of foreign words, can similarly be traced back to a counter-intention, which is aimed either directly or indirectly against the name concerned. I have already given you several instances of direct dislike [p. 52]. But indirect causation is particularly frequent in these cases and can usually only be established by careful analyses. For instance, during the present war, which has obliged us to give up so many of our former enjoyments, our power of remembering proper names has suffered greatly as the result of the strangest associations. A short time ago I found that I was unable to reproduce the name of the innocent Moravian town of *Bisenz*; and analysis showed that what was responsible for this was not any direct hostility to it but its resemblance in sound to the name of the Palazzo *Bisenzi* in Orvieto which I had repeatedly enjoyed visiting in the past.[1] Here for the first time, in this reason for objecting to remembering a name, we come across a principle which will later on reveal its enormous importance for the causation of neurotic

[1] [This example was added in 1917 to *P.E.L.*, 34.]

symptoms: the memory's disinclination to remembering any-thing which is connected with feelings of unpleasure and the reproduction of which would renew the unpleasure. This in-tention to avoid unpleasure arising from a recollection or from other psychical acts, this psychical flight from unpleasure, may be recognized as the ultimate operative motive not only for the forgetting of names but for many other parapraxes, such as omissions, errors, and so on.

The forgetting of names, however, seems particularly facili-tated psycho-physiologically, and for that reason cases occur in which interference by the unpleasure motive cannot be confirmed. If someone has a tendency to forget names, analytic investigation will show that names escape him not only because he does not like them themselves or because they remind him of something disagreeable, but also because in his case the same name belongs to another circle of associations with which he is more intimately related. The name is, as it were, anchored there and is kept from contact with the other associations which have been momentarily activated. If you recall the tricks of mnemotechnics,[1] you will realize with some surprise that the same chains of association which are deliberately laid down in order to *prevent* names from being forgotten can also *lead* to our forgetting them. The most striking example of this is afforded by the proper names of persons, which naturally possess quite different psychical importance for different people. Let us, for instance, take a first name such as Theodore. To one of you it will have no special meaning, to another it will be the name of his father or brother or of a friend, or his own name. Analytic experience will then show you that the first of these people is in no danger of forgetting that a particular stranger bears this name, whereas the others will be constantly inclined to withhold from strangers a name which seems to them reserved for intimate connections. If you now bear in mind that this associa-tive inhibition may coincide with the operation of the unpleasure principle[2] and, besides that, with an indirect

---

[1] [Artificial methods of improving the memory—e.g. 'Pelman-ism'.]

[2] [Since the time of *The Interpretation of Dreams* (1900a) where the principle is so named, Freud had almost invariably spoken of the 'pleasure principle'. It is discussed under this latter name in Lecture XXII, p. 356 f. below.]

mechanism, you will be in a position to form an adequate idea of the complications in the causation of the temporary forgetting of a name. An appropriate analysis will however unravel every one of these tangles for you.

The forgetting of impressions and experiences demonstrates much more clearly and exclusively than the forgetting of names the operation of the purpose of keeping disagreeable things out of memory. The whole field of this kind of forgetting does not, of course, fall within the class of parapraxes, but only such cases as, measured by the standard of our usual experience, seem to us striking and unjustified: for instance, when the forgetting affects impressions that are too fresh or important, or when the missing memory tears a gap in what is otherwise a well-remembered chain of events. Why and in what way we are able to forget in general, and among other things experiences which have certainly left the deepest impression upon us, such as the events of our earliest childhood years,—that is quite another problem, in which fending off unpleasurable impulses plays a certain part but is far from being the whole explanation.[1] It is an undoubted fact that disagreeable impressions are easily forgotten. Various psychologists have noticed it and the great Darwin was so much impressed by it that he made it 'a golden rule' to note down with especial care any observations which seemed unfavourable to his theory, since he had convinced himself that precisely they would not remain in his memory.[2]

A person who hears for the first time of this principle of the fending off of unpleasurable memories by forgetting rarely fails to object that on the contrary it has been his experience that distressing things are particularly hard to forget but keep on returning to torment him against his will—memories, for instance, of insults and humiliations. This is also a true fact, but the objection is not to the point. It is important to begin in good time to reckon with the fact that mental life is the arena and battle-ground for mutually opposing purposes or, to put

[1] [Infantile amnesia is discussed in Lecture XIII, p. 199 f. below. For a discussion of forgetting in general, see a long footnote added to *P.E.L.*, 274, in 1907.]

[2] [The whole passage from Darwin's autobiography (1958, 123) is quoted *P.E.L.*, 148.]

it non-dynamically, that it consists of contradictions and pairs of contraries. Proof of the existence of a particular purpose is no argument against the existence of an opposite one; there is room for both. It is only a question of the attitude of these contraries to each other, and of what effects are produced by the one and by the other.

Losing and mislaying are of particular interest to us owing to the many meanings they may have—owing, that is, to the multiplicity of the purposes which can be served by these parapraxes. All cases have in common the fact that there was a wish to lose something; they differ in the basis and aim of that wish. We lose a thing when it is worn out, when we intend to replace it by a better one, when we no longer like it, when it originates from someone with whom we are no longer on good terms or when we acquired it in circumstances we no longer want to recall. [Cf. p. 54.] Dropping, damaging or breaking the object can serve the same purpose. In the sphere of social life experience is said to have shown that unwanted and illegitimate children are far more frail than those legitimately conceived. The crude technique of baby-farmers[1] is not necessary for bringing about this result; a certain amount of neglect in looking after the children should be quite sufficient. The preserving of *things* may be subject to the same influences as that of children.

Things may, however, be condemned to be lost without their value having suffered any diminution—when, that is, there is an intention to sacrifice something to Fate in order to ward off some other dreaded loss. Analysis tells us that it is still quite a common thing among us to exorcize Fate in this way; and thus our losing is often a voluntary sacrifice. In the same way, losing may also serve the purpose of defiance or self-punishment. In short, the more remote reasons for the intention to get rid of a thing by losing it are beyond number.

Bungled actions, like other errors, are often used to fulfil wishes which one ought to deny oneself. Here the intention disguises itself as a lucky accident. For instance, as happened to one of my friends, a man may be due, obviously against his will,

---

[1] [In the original literally: 'what are known as angel-makers'.]

to go by train to visit someone near the town where he lives, and then, at a junction where he has to change, may by mistake get into a train that takes him back to where he came from. Or someone on a journey may be anxious to make a stop at an intermediate station but may be forbidden from doing so by other obligations, and he may then overlook or miss some connection so that he is after all obliged to break his journey in the way he wished. Or what happened to one of my patients: I had forbidden him to telephone to the girl he was in love with, and then, when he meant to telephone to me, he asked for the wrong number 'by mistake' or 'while he was thinking of something else' and suddenly found himself connected to the girl's number.[1] A good example of an outright blunder, and one of practical importance, is provided by an observation made by an engineer in his account of what preceded a case of material damage:

'Some time ago I worked with several students in the laboratory of the technical college on a series of complicated experiments in elasticity, a piece of work which we had undertaken voluntarily but which was beginning to take up more time than we had expected. One day as I returned to the laboratory with my friend F., he remarked how annoying it was to him to lose so much time on that particular day as he had so much else to do at home. I could not help agreeing with him and added half jokingly, referring to an incident the week before: "Let us hope that the machine will go wrong again so that we can stop work and go home early."

'In arranging the work it happened that F. was given the regulation of the valve of the press; that is to say, he was, by cautiously opening the valve, to let the fluid under pressure flow slowly out of the accumulator into the cylinder of the hydraulic press. The man conducting the experiment stood by the manometer and when the right pressure was reached called out a loud "Stop!" At the word of command F. seized the valve and turned it with all his might—to the left! (All valves without exception are closed by being turned to the right.) This caused the full pressure of the accumulator to come suddenly on to the press, a strain for which the connecting-pipes are not designed, so that one of them immediately burst—quite

[1] [These last three examples are described much more fully *P.E.L.*, 222 and 226-8.]

a harmless accident to the machine, but enough to oblige us to suspend work for the day and go home.

'It is characteristic, by the way, that when we were discussing the affair some time later my friend F. had no recollection whatever of my remark, which I recalled with certainty.'[1]

This may lead you to suspect that it is not always just an innocent chance that turns the hands of your domestic servants into dangerous enemies of your household belongings. And you may also raise the question whether it is always a matter of chance when people injure themselves and risk their own safety. These are notions whose value you may care to test, if occasion arises, by analysing observations of your own.

This, Ladies and Gentlemen, is far from being all that might be said about parapraxes. Much remains that might be examined and discussed. But I am satisfied if our discussion of the subject so far has to some extent shaken your previous views and has made you a little prepared to accept new ones. I am content, for the rest, to leave you faced with an unclarified situation. We cannot establish all our doctrines from a study of parapraxes and we are not obliged to draw our evidence from that material alone. The great value of parapraxes for our purposes lies in their being very common phenomena which, moreover, can easily be observed in oneself, and which can occur without the slightest implication of illness. There is only one of your unanswered questions which I should like to put into words before I end. If, as we have found from many instances, people come so close to an understanding of para- praxes and so often behave as though they grasped their sense, how is it possible that they none the less set down these same phenomena as being in general chance events without sense or meaning, and that they can oppose the psycho-analytic elucida- tion of them with so much vigour?

You are right. This is a remarkable fact and it calls for an explanation. But I will not give you one. Instead, I will introduce you by degrees to fields of knowledge from which the explanation will force itself upon you without any con- tribution of mine.

[1] [Reproduced from *P.E.L.*, 174.]

PART II
DREAMS
(1916 [1915–16])

DIFFICULTIES AND FIRST APPROACHES

LADIES AND GENTLEMEN,—It was discovered one day that the pathological symptoms of certain neurotic patients have a sense.[1] On this discovery the psycho-analytic method of treatment was founded. It happened in the course of this treatment that patients, instead of bringing forward their symptoms, brought forward dreams. A suspicion thus arose that the dreams too had a sense.[2]

We will not, however, follow this historical path, but will proceed in the opposite direction. We will demonstrate the sense of dreams by way of preparing for the study of the neuroses. This reversal is justified, since the study of dreams is not only the best preparation for the study of the neuroses, but dreams are themselves a neurotic symptom, which, moreover, offers us the priceless advantage of occurring in all healthy people.[3] Indeed, supposing all human beings were healthy, so long as they dreamt we could arrive from their dreams at almost all the discoveries which the investigation of the neuroses has led to.

Dreams, then, have become a subject of psycho-analytic

[1] By Josef Breuer in the years 1880–2. Cf. the lectures delivered by me in America in 1909 (*Five Lectures on Psycho-Analysis* [1910a]) and 'On the History of the Psycho-Analytic Movement' (1914d), (Norton, 1966).]

[2] [Freud's major work on the subject of dreams was, of course, *The Interpretation of Dreams* (1900a). There is, however, scarcely one of his writings in which the topic did not emerge, but a list of the principal discussions of it is given in an Appendix to that work. A considerable number of references to it will be found in editorial footnotes to the present set of lectures; and, to save space, the abbreviation '*I. of D.*' will be used, with application in every case to Volumes IV and V of the *Standard Edition*. It may be noted that the pagination of the text of the latest separate editions of the work (London: Allen and Unwin, 1955, and New York: Basic Books, 1955) is identical with that of the *Standard Edition* volumes.]

[3] [Freud discussed this further towards the end of the last lecture of the series (p. 456 f., below).]

research: once again ordinary phenomena, with little value set
on them, and apparently of no practical use—like parapraxes,
with which indeed they have in common the fact of occurring
in healthy people. But apart from this the conditions for our
work are a good deal less favourable here. Parapraxes had
merely been neglected by science, little attention had been paid
to them; but at least there was no harm in concerning oneself
with them. 'No doubt', people would say, 'there are more
important things. But something may possibly come of it.' But
to concern oneself with dreams is not merely unpractical and
uncalled-for, it is positively disgraceful. It brings with it the
odium of being unscientific and rouses the suspicion of a personal inclination to mysticism. Imagine a medical man going
in for dreams when there are so many more serious things even
in neuropathology and psychiatry—tumours as big as apples
compressing the organ of the mind, haemorrhages, chronic
inflammation, in all of which the changes in the tissues can be
demonstrated under the microscope! No, dreams are much too
trivial, and unworthy to be an object of research.

And there is something else which from its very nature frus-
trates the requirements of exact research. In investigating
dreams one is not even certain about the object of one's research. A delusion, for instance, meets one squarely and with
definite outlines. 'I am the Emperor of China', says the patient
straight out. But dreams? As a rule no account at all can be
given of them. If anyone gives an account of a dream, has he
any guarantee that his account has been correct, or that he may
not, on the contrary, have altered his account in the course of
giving it and have been obliged to invent some addition to it
to make up for the indistinctness of his recollection? Most
dreams cannot be remembered at all and are forgotten except
for small fragments. And is the interpretation of material of
this kind to serve as the basis of a scientific psychology or as a
method for treating patients?

An excess of criticism may make us suspicious. These objections to dreams as an object of research are obviously carried
too far. We have already dealt with the question of unimpor-
tance in connection with parapraxes [p. 26 f.]. We have told
ourselves that big things can show themselves by small indications. As regards their indistinctness—that is one of the charac-

teristics of dreams, like any other: we cannot lay down for things what their characteristics are to be. And incidentally there are clear and distinct dreams as well. There are, moreover, other objects of psychiatric research which suffer from the same characteristic of indistinctness—in many instances, for example, obsessions, and these have been dealt with, after all, by respected and esteemed psychiatrists.[1] I recall the last such case that I came across in my medical practice. This was a woman patient who introduced herself with these words: 'I have a sort of feeling as though I had injured or had wanted to injure some living creature—a child?—no, more like a dog—as though I may have thrown it off a bridge, or something else.' We can help to overcome the defect of the uncertainty in remembering dreams if we decide that whatever the dreamer tells us must count as his dream, without regard to what he may have forgotten or have altered in recalling it. And finally it cannot even be maintained so sweepingly that dreams are unimportant things. We know from our own experience that the mood in which one wakes up from a dream may last for the whole day; doctors have observed cases in which a mental disease has started with a dream and in which a delusion originating in the dream has persisted; historical figures are reported to have embarked on momentous enterprises in response to dreams. We may therefore ask what may be the true source of the contempt in which dreams are held in scientific circles.

It is, I believe, a reaction against the overvaluation of dreams in earlier days. The reconstruction of the past is, as we know, no easy matter, but we may assume with certainty, if I may put it as a joke, that our ancestors three thousand or more years ago already had dreams like ours. So far as we know, all the peoples of antiquity attached great significance to dreams and thought they could be used for practical purposes. They deduced signs for the future from them and searched in them for auguries. For the Greeks and other oriental nations, there may have been times when a campaign without dream-interpreters seemed as

---

[1] [The tendency of obsessional neurotics to uncertainty and vagueness had been discussed by Freud in Section B of Part II of his 'Notes upon a Case of Obsessional Neurosis' (1909d). See also the account of that form of illness in Lecture XVII, p. 258 ff. below.]

impossible as one without air-reconnaissance seems to-day.
When Alexander the Great started on his conquests, his train
included the most famous dream-interpreters. The city of
Tyre, which at that time still stood on an island, offered the
king such a stiff resistance that he considered the possibility of
raising the siege. Then one night he had a dream of a satyr who
seemed to be dancing in triumph, and when he reported it to
his dream-interpreters they informed him that it foretold his
conquest of the city. He ordered an assault and captured Tyre.[1]
Among the Etruscans and Romans other methods of foretelling
the future were in use; but throughout the whole of the Hel-
lenistic-Roman period the interpretation of dreams was practised and highly esteemed. Of the literature dealing with the
subject the principal work at least has survived: the book by
Artemidorus of Daldis, who probably lived during the reign of
the Emperor Hadrian.[2] How it came about after this that the
art of interpreting dreams declined and that dreams fell into
discredit I cannot tell you. The spread of enlightenment cannot
have had much to do with it, for many things more absurd than
the dream-interpretation of antiquity were faithfully preserved
in the obscurity of the Middle Ages. The fact remains that
interest in dreams gradually sank to the level of superstition and
could survive only among the uneducated classes. The final
abuse of dream-interpretation was reached in our days with
attempts to discover from dreams the numbers fated to be
drawn in the game of lotto.[3] On the other hand the exact
science of to-day has repeatedly concerned itself with dreams
but always with the sole aim of applying its physiological
theories to them. Medical men, of course, looked on dreams as
non-psychical acts, as the expression in mental life of somatic
stimuli. Binz (1878,[35]) pronounced that dreams are 'somatic
processes, which are in every case useless and in many cases
positively pathological, to which the soul of the universe and
immortality are as sublimely superior as the blue sky above
some weed-grown, low-lying stretch of sand.' Maury [1878,
50] compares dreams to the disordered twitchings of St. Vitus's

---

[1] [The explanation of this dream is given in Lecture XV, p. 236
below.]

[2] [Some account of this work appears in Chapter II of *I. of D.*]

[3] [Something very similar to what is now known as 'Bingo'.]

dance as contrasted with the co-ordinated movements of a healthy man. According to an old analogy, the contents of a dream are like the sounds produced when 'the ten fingers of a man who knows nothing of music wander over the keys of a piano' [Strümpell, 1877, 84].

Interpreting means finding a hidden sense in something; there can of course be no question of doing that if we adopt this last estimate of the function of dreams. Look at the description of dreams given by Wundt [1874], Jodl [1896], and other more recent philosophers. They content themselves with enumerating the respects in which dream-life differs from waking thought, always in a sense depreciatory to dreams—emphasizing the fact that associations are broken apart, that the critical faculty ceases to work, that all knowledge is eliminated, as well as other signs of diminished functioning. The only valuable contribution to the knowledge of dreams for which we have to thank exact science relates to the effect produced on the content of dreams by the impact of somatic stimuli during sleep. A recently deceased Norwegian author, J. Mourly Vold, published two stout volumes of experimental researches into dreams (German translation, 1910 and 1912), which are devoted almost exclusively to the consequences of alterations in the posture of the limbs. They have been recommended to us as models of exact research into dreams. Can you imagine what exact science would say if it learnt that we want to make an attempt to discover the *sense* of dreams? Perhaps it has already said it. But we will not let ourselves be frightened off. If it was possible for parapraxes to have a sense, dreams can have one too; and in a great many cases parapraxes *have* a sense, which has escaped exact science. So let us embrace the prejudice of the ancients and of the people and let us follow in the footsteps of the dream-interpreters of antiquity.

We must begin by finding our bearings in the task before us and taking a general survey of the field of dreams. What, then, is a dream? It is hard to answer in a single sentence. But we will not attempt a definition when it is enough to point to something familiar to everyone.[1] We should, however, bring the essential feature of dreams into prominence. Where is that

---

[1] [Cf., however, some remarks on this in Lecture XIV, p. 223 below.]

to be found, though? There are such immense differences within
the frame that comprises our subject—differences in every
direction. The essential feature will presumably be something
that we can point to as common to all dreams.

The first thing common to all dreams would seem to be, of
course, that we are asleep during them. Dreaming is evidently
mental life during sleep—something which has certain resemblances to waking mental life but which, on the other hand, is
distinguished from it by large differences. This was, long ago,
Aristotle's definition.[1] It may be that there are still closer
connections between dreams and sleep. We can be woken by a
dream; we very often have a dream when we wake up spontaneously or if we are forcibly aroused from sleep. Thus dreams
seem to be an intermediate state between sleeping and waking.
So our attention is turned to sleep. Well, then, what is sleep?

That is a physiological or biological problem about which
much is still in dispute. On that we can come to no conclusion;
but we ought, I think, to try to describe the psychological
characteristics of sleep. Sleep is a state in which I want to know
nothing of the external world, in which I have taken my interest
away from it. I put myself to sleep by withdrawing from the
external world and keeping its stimuli away from me. I also go
to sleep when I am fatigued by it. So when I go to sleep I say
to the external world: 'Leave me in peace: I want to go to
sleep.' On the contrary, children say: 'I'm not going to sleep
yet; I'm not tired, and I want to have some more experiences.' The biological purpose of sleep seems therefore to be
rehabilitation, and its psychological characteristic suspense of
interest in the world. Our relation to the world, into which
we have come so unwillingly, seems to involve our not being
able to tolerate it uninterruptedly. Thus from time to time we
withdraw into the premundane state, into existence in the
womb. At any rate, we arrange conditions for ourselves very
like what they were then: warm, dark and free from stimuli.
Some of us roll ourselves up into a tight package and, so as to
sleep, take up a posture much as it was in the womb. The world,
it seems, does not possess even those of us who are adults completely, but only up to two thirds; one third of us is still quite
unborn. Every time we wake in the morning it is like a new

[1] [Cf. Chapter I of *I. of D.*]

birth. Indeed, in speaking of our state after sleep, we say that we feel as though we were newly born. (In saying this, incidentally, we are making what is probably a very false assumption about the general sensations of a new-born child, who seems likely, on the contrary, to be feeling very uncomfortable.) We speak, too, of being born as 'first seeing the light of day'.[1]

If this is what sleep is, dreams cannot possibly form part of its programme, but seem on the contrary to be an unwelcome addition to it. In our opinion too, a dreamless sleep is the best, the only proper one. There ought to be no mental activity in sleep; if it begins to stir, we have not succeeded in establishing the foetal state of rest: we have not been able entirely to avoid residues of mental activity. Dreaming would consist in these residues. But if so, it would really seem that there is no need for dreams to have any sense. It was different with parapraxes; they, after all, were activities during waking life. But if I am asleep and have stopped mental activity completely and have merely failed to suppress some residues of it, then there is no need whatever for these residues to have any sense. I cannot even make use of any such sense, since the rest of my mental life is asleep. So it really can only be a matter of reactions, in the nature of 'twitchings', of mental phenomena such as result directly from a somatic stimulus. Dreams would accordingly be residues of waking mental activity which were disturbing sleep, and we might well decide to drop the subject at once, as not being suited to psycho-analysis.

Even if dreams are superfluous, however, they do exist, and we can try to account for their existence. Why does mental life fail to go to sleep? Probably because there is something that will not allow the mind any peace. Stimuli impinge upon it and it must react to them. A dream, then, is the manner in which the mind reacts to stimuli that impinge upon it in the state of sleep. And here we see a way of access to an understanding of dreams. We can take various dreams and try to discover what the stimulus was which was seeking to disturb sleep and to which the reaction was a dream. Our examination of the first thing common to all dreams seems to have taken us so far.

Is there anything else common to them? Yes, something
[1] [In German, literally, 'seeing the light of the world'.]

unmistakable but much harder to grasp and to describe. Mental processes in sleep have a quite different character from those of waking life. We experience every sort of thing in dreams and believe in it, whereas nevertheless we experience nothing, except, perhaps, the single disturbing stimulus. We experience it predominantly in visual images; feelings may be present too, and thoughts interwoven in it as well; the other senses may also experience something, but nonetheless it is predominantly a question of images. Part of the difficulty of giving an account of dreams is due to our having to translate these images into words. 'I could draw it', a dreamer often says to us, 'but I don't know how to say it.' This is not, however, a *reduced* mental activity, like that of a feeble-minded person as compared to that of a genius: it is *qualitatively* different, though it is hard to say where the difference lies. G. T. Fechner once voiced a suspicion that the scene of action of dreams (in the mind) is different from that of waking ideational life.[1] Though we do not understand this and do not know what we are to make of it, it does in fact reproduce the impression of strangeness which most dreams make on us. The comparison between dream-activity and the effects of an unmusical hand on the piano [p. 87] does not help us here. The piano will after all respond with the same sounds, though not with tunes, to any chance pressure on its keys. Let us carefully bear this second thing common to all dreams in mind, even though we may not have understood it.

Are there any other things common to them? I cannot discover any; I can see nothing anywhere but differences, and differences in all kinds of ways: in their apparent duration, as well as in their clarity, in the amount of affect accompanying them, in the possibility of retaining them, and so on. This variety is not in fact what we might expect to find in a mere defensive reaction to a stimulus, something mechanically imposed, an empty thing, like the twitchings of St. Vitus's dance. As regards the dimensions of dreams, some are very short and comprise only a single image or a few, a single thought, or even a single word; others are uncommonly rich in their

[1] [The psycho-physiologist Fechner (1801–87) had a great influence on Freud's theories (see Chapter V of his *Autobiographical Study* (1925d), (Norton, 1963). The present remark is discussed in the section on Regression in Chapter VII of *I. of D.*]

content, present whole novels and seem to last a long time. There are dreams which are as clear as [waking] experience, so clear that quite a time after waking we do not realize that they were dreams; and there are others which are indescribably dim, shadowy and blurred. Indeed in one and the same dream excessively definite portions may alternate with others of scarcely discernible vagueness. Dreams may be entirely sensible or at least coherent, witty even, or fantastically beautiful; others, again, are confused, feeble-minded as it were, absurd, often positively crazy. There are dreams that leave us quite cold and others in which affects of all kinds are manifest—pain to the point of tears, anxiety to the point of waking us up, astonishment, delight, and so on. Dreams are usually quickly forgotten after waking, or they may last through the day, remembered more and more dimly and incompletely till evening; others, again—for instance, childhood dreams—are so well preserved that after thirty years they remain in the memory like some fresh experience. Dreams may appear, like individuals, on a single occasion only and never again, or they may recur in the same person unchanged or with small divergences. In short, this fragment of mental activity during the night has an immense repertory at its disposal; it is capable, in fact, of all that the mind creates in daytime—yet it is never the same thing.

We might try to account for these many variations in dreams by supposing that they correspond to different intermediate stages between sleeping and waking, different degrees of incomplete sleep. Yes, but if this were so, the value, content and clarity of a dream's product—and the awareness, too, of its being a dream—would have to increase in dreams in which the mind was coming near to waking; and it would not be possible for a clear and rational fragment of dream to be immediately followed by one that was senseless and obscure and for this in turn to be followed by another good piece. The mind could certainly not alter the depth of its sleep so quickly as that. So this explanation is of no help: there can be no short cut out of the difficulty.

We will for the moment leave on one side the 'sense' of dreams, and try to make our way to a better understanding of them from what we have found is common to them. We inferred

from the relation of dreams to the state of sleep that dreams are
the reaction to a stimulus which disturbs sleep. We have learnt
that this too is the single point on which exact experimental
psychology is able to come to our assistance: it brings us evidence that stimuli which impinge during sleep make their
appearance in dreams. Many investigations of this kind have
been made, most recently those by Mourly Vold which I have
already mentioned [p. 87]; and each of us, no doubt, has been
in a position to confirm this finding from personal observation.
I will select a few of the earlier experiments. Maury [1878] had
some experiments performed on himself. He was given some
eau-de-cologne to smell in his sleep. He dreamt he was in
Cairo, in Johann Maria Farina's shop, and some further absurd
adventures followed. Or, he was pinched lightly on the neck;
he dreamt of a mustard plaster being applied to him and of a
doctor who had treated him as a child. Or again, a drop of
water was dropped on his forehead; he was in Italy, was sweating violently and was drinking white Orvieto wine.[1]

The striking thing about these experimentally produced
dreams will perhaps be even more plainly visible in another
series of stimulus-dreams. They are three dreams reported by
an intelligent observer, Hildebrandt [1875], all of them reactions to the ringing of an alarm-clock:

'I dreamt, then, that one spring morning I was going for a
walk and was strolling through the green fields till I came to a
neighbouring village, where I saw the villagers in their best
clothes, with hymn-books under their arms, flocking to the
church. Of course! It was Sunday, and early morning service
would soon be beginning. I decided I would attend it; but
first, as I was rather hot from walking, I went into the church-
yard which surrounded the church, to cool down. While I was
reading some of the tombstones, I heard the bell-ringer climbing up the church tower and at the top of it I now saw the little
village bell which would presently give the signal for the beginning of devotions. For quite a while it hung there motionless,
then it began to swing, and suddenly its peal began to ring out
clear and piercing—so clear and piercing that it put an end to
my sleep. But what was ringing was the alarm-clock.

[1] [For these and several other of Maury's experiments see the
section on the Stimuli and Sources of Dreams in Chapter I of
I. of D.]

'Here is another instance. It was a bright winter's day and the streets were covered with deep snow. I had agreed to join a party for a sleigh-ride; but I had to wait a long time before news came that the sleigh was at the door. Now followed the preparations for getting in—the fur rug spread out, the foot-muff put ready—and at last I was sitting in my seat. But even then the moment of departure was delayed till a pull at the reins gave the waiting horses the signal. Then off they started, and, with a violent shake, the sleigh bells broke into their familiar jingle—with such violence, in fact, that in a moment the cobweb of my dream was torn through. And once again it was only the shrill sound of the alarm-clock.

'And now yet a third example. I saw a kitchenmaid, carrying several dozen plates piled on one another, walking along the passage to the dining-room. The column of china in her arms seemed to me in danger of losing its balance. "Take care," I exclaimed, "or you'll drop the whole load." The inevitable rejoinder duly followed: she was quite accustomed to that kind of job, and so on. And meanwhile my anxious looks followed the advancing figure. Then—just as I expected—she stumbled at the threshold and the fragile crockery slipped and rattled and clattered in a hundred pieces on the floor. But the noise continued without ceasing, and soon it seemed no longer to be a clattering; it was turning into a ringing—and the ringing, as my waking self now became aware, was only the alarm-clock doing its duty.'[1]

These are very nice dreams, entirely sensible and by no means as incoherent as dreams are usually apt to be. I am not objecting to them on that account. What they have in common is that in each case the situation ends in a noise, which, when the dreamer wakes up, is recognized as being made by the alarm-clock. So we see here how a dream is produced; but we learn something more than this. The dream does not recognize the alarm-clock—nor does it appear in the dream—but it replaces the noise of the alarm-clock by another; it interprets the stimulus which is bringing sleep to an end, but it interprets it differently each time. Why does it do that? There is no answer to this; it seems a matter of caprice. Understanding the dream would mean being able to say why this particular noise and

[1] [Also quoted in the last mentioned section.of *I. of D.*]

none other was chosen for the interpretation of the stimulus from the alarm-clock. We may make an analogous objection to Maury's experiments: we can see quite clearly that the impinging stimulus appears in the dream; but why it should take this particular form we are not told, and it does not seem by any means to follow from the nature of the stimulus that disturbed sleep. In Maury's experiments, too, a quantity of other dream-material usually appears in addition to the direct effect of the stimulus—for instance, the 'absurd adventures' in the eau-de-cologne dream—, which cannot be accounted for.

And now consider that *arousal* dreams offer the best chance of establishing the influence of external sleep-disturbing stimuli. In most other cases it will become more difficult. We do not wake out of every dream, and if we remember a dream of the past night in the morning, how are we to discover a disturbing stimulus which may perhaps have made its impact on us during the night? I once succeeded in identifying a sound-stimulus of that kind retrospectively, but only, of course, owing to special circumstances. I woke up one morning in a mountain resort in the Tyrol, knowing I had had a dream that the Pope was dead. I could not explain the dream to myself; but later on my wife asked me if I had heard the fearful noise made by the pealing of bells towards morning which had broken out from all the churches and chapels. No, I had heard nothing, my sleep is more resistant than hers; but thanks to her information I understood my dream.[1] How often may stimuli of this kind instigate dreams in a sleeper without his getting news of them afterwards? Perhaps very often, but perhaps not. If the stimulus can no longer be pointed to, we cannot be convinced of its existence. And in any case we have changed our view of the importance of external stimuli that disturb sleep since we learnt that they can explain only a small portion of the dream and not the whole dream-reaction.

There is no need to give up this theory entirely on that account. Moreover it is capable of extension. It is obviously a matter of indifference what it is that disturbs sleep or instigates the mind to dream. If it cannot invariably be a sensory stimulus coming from outside, there may instead be what is called a somatic stimulus, arising from the internal organs. This is a

[1] [Told at greater length in the discussion of The Somatic Sources of Dreams in Chapter V of *I. of D.*]

very plausible notion and agrees with the most popular view of the origin of dreams: 'dreams come from indigestion', people often say. Here too unluckily we must often suspect that there are cases when a somatic stimulus which has impinged on a sleeper during the night is no longer manifest after waking and can therefore not be proved to have occurred. But we shall not overlook the number of clear experiences which support the origin of dreams from somatic stimuli. In general, there can be no doubt that the condition of the internal organs can influence dreams. The relation of the content of some dreams to an over-full bladder or to a state of excitation of the genital organs is too plain to be mistaken. These clear cases lead to others in which the content of the dreams give rise to a justifiable suspicion that there has been an impact from somatic stimuli because there is something in the content which can be regarded as a working-over, a representation or an interpretation of such stimuli. Scherner (1861), who made researches into dreams, argued particularly strongly in favour of this derivation of dreams and brought forward some good examples of it. For instance, in one dream he saw 'two rows of pretty boys with fair hair and delicate complexions facing one another in pugnacious array, making an onset and attacking one another, and then drawing back and taking up their old position again, and then starting the whole business once more.' His interpretation of these two rows of boys as teeth is plausible in itself and seems fully confirmed when we learn that after this scene the dreamer 'pulled a long tooth out of his jaw.'[1] Similarly, the interpretation of 'long, narrow, winding passages' as derived from an intestinal stimulus seems valid, and confirms the assertion by Scherner that dreams seek above all to represent the organ that sends out the stimulus by objects resembling it.

Thus we must be prepared to admit that internal stimuli can play the same part in dreams as external ones. Any estimate of their importance is unfortunately open to the same objections. In a large number of cases an interpretation pointing to a somatic stimulus is uncertain or unprovable. Not all dreams, but only a certain number of them give rise to a suspicion that internal organic stimuli had a share in their origin. And lastly, internal somatic stimuli are as little able as external sensory

[1] [I. of D.]

stimuli to explain more of a dream than what corresponds in it
to a direct reaction to the stimulus. Where the rest of the dream
comes from remains obscure.

Let us notice, however, one peculiarity of dream-life which
comes to light in this study of the effects of stimuli. Dreams do
not simply reproduce the stimulus; they work it over, they
make allusions to it, they include it in some context, they
replace it by something else. This is a side of the dream-work[1]
which is bound to interest us since it may perhaps bring us
nearer to the essence of dreams. When a person constructs
something as a result of a stimulus, the stimulus need not on
that account exhaust the whole of the work. Shakespeare's
Macbeth, for instance, was a *pièce d'occasion* composed to celebrate
the accession of the king who first united the crowns of the
three kingdoms. But does this immediate historical occasion
cover the content of the tragedy? Does it explain its greatnesses
and its enigmas? It may be that the external and internal
stimuli, too, impinging on the sleeper, are only the *instigators*
of the dream and will accordingly betray nothing to us of its
essence.

The second thing that is common to dreams, their psychical
peculiarity [p. 89 f.], is on the one hand hard to grasp and on the
other offers us no starting-point for further enquiry. We experience things in dreams as a rule in visual forms. Can the stimuli
throw any light on this? Is what we experience in fact the
stimulus? But, if so, why is the experience visual, while it is only
in the rarest cases that optical stimulation has instigated the
dream? Or if we dream spoken words, can it be shown that
during sleep a conversation, or some noise resembling one,
made its way into our ears? I venture to dismiss that possibility
decisively.

If we can get no further with what is common to dreams, let
us see whether their differences can help us. Dreams are, of
course, often senseless, confused and absurd; but there are also
sensible, matter-of-fact, and reasonable ones. Let us enquire
whether the latter, the sensible ones, can throw any light on
the senseless ones. Here is the latest reasonable dream that I

---

[1] [The process which transforms the latent thoughts behind the dream
into its manifest form. This is the subject of Lecture XI below.]

have had reported to me. It was dreamt by a young man: 'I went for a walk along the Kärntnerstrasse[1] and met Herr X. there and joined him for a time. Then I went into a restaurant. Two ladies and a gentleman came and sat at my table. I was annoyed at this to begin with and wouldn't look at them. Then I did look and found that they were quite nice.' The dreamer commented on this that on the evening before the dream he had in fact walked along the Kärntnerstrasse, which is the way he usually goes, and had met Herr X. there. The other part of the dream was not a direct recollection, and only had some similarity to an experience a considerable time earlier. Or here is another matter-of-fact dream, this time a lady's: 'Her husband asked her: "Don't you think we ought to have the piano tuned?" And she replied: "It's not worth while; the hammers need reconditioning in any case." '[2] This dream repeated, without much alteration, a conversation which had taken place between her and her husband the day before the dream. What do we learn from these two reasonable dreams? Nothing except that they contain repetitions from daily life or things connected with it. That would already be something, if it could be said of dreams generally. But there is no question of that; it applies only to a minority, and in most dreams there is no sign of a connection with the day before,[3] and no light is thrown by this on the senseless and absurd dreams. It only shows that we have come upon a new task. We not only want to know what a dream says, but, if it speaks clearly, as it does in these examples of ours, we also want to know why and for what purpose this familiar material, only recently experienced, has been repeated in the dream.

I think that, like me, you must be tired of pursuing enquiries like those we have so far been making. All one's interest in a problem is evidently insufficient unless one knows as well of a path of approach that will lead to its solution. We have not yet found such a path. Experimental psychology has brought us nothing but some very valuable information on the significance of stimuli as instigators to dreaming. We have nothing to expect

[1] [The principal shopping street in Vienna.]
[2] [See Chapter V of *I. of D.*]
[3] [A qualification of this statement is to follow shortly (p. 106).]

from philosophy except that it will once again haughtily point
out to us the intellectual inferiority of the object of our study.
Nor have we any wish to borrow anything from the occult
sciences. History and popular opinion tell us that dreams have
a sense and a meaning: that they look into the future—which
is hard to accept and certainly incapable of proof. So our first
effort leaves us completely at a loss.

Unexpectedly, a hint reaches us from a direction in which we
have not so far looked. Linguistic usage, which is no chance
thing, but the precipitate of old discoveries, though, to be sure,
it must not be employed incautiously—our language, then, is
acquainted with things that bear the strange name of 'day-
dreams'. Day-dreams are phantasies (products of the imagination); they are very general phenomena, observable, once more,
in healthy as well as in sick people, and are easily accessible to
study in our own mind. The most remarkable thing about
these imaginative structures is that they have been given the
name of 'day-dreams', for there is no trace in them of the two
things that are common to dreams [p. 88 ff.]. Their relation to
sleep is already contradicted by their name; and, as regards the
second thing common to dreams, we do not experience or
hallucinate anything in them but imagine something, we know
that we are having a phantasy, we do not see but think. These
day-dreams appear in the prepubertal period, often in the
later part of childhood even; they persist until maturity is
reached and are then either given up or maintained till the
end of life. The content of these phantasies is dominated by a
very transparent motive. They are scenes and events in which
the subject's egoistic needs of ambition and power or his erotic
wishes find satisfaction. In young men the ambitious phantasies are the most prominent, in women, whose ambition is
directed to success in love, the erotic ones. But in men, too,
erotic needs are often enough present in the background: all
their heroic deeds and successes seem only to aim at courting
the admiration and favour of women. In other respects these
day-dreams are of many different kinds and pass through
changing vicissitudes. They are either, each one of them,
dropped after a short time and replaced by a fresh one, or they
are retained, spun out into long stories and adapted to the
changes in the circumstances of the subject's life. They go along

with the times, so to speak, and receive a 'date stamp' which bears witness to the influence of the new situation. They are the raw material of poetic production, for the creative writer uses his day-dreams, with certain remodellings, disguises and omissions, to construct the situations which he introduces into his short stories, his novels or his plays. The hero of the day-dreams is always the subject himself, either directly or by an obvious identification with someone else.[1]

It may be that day-dreams bear their name on account of having the same relation to reality—in order to indicate that their content is to be looked on as no less unreal than that of dreams. But perhaps they share this name because of some psychical characteristic of dreams which is still unknown to us, one which we are in search of. It is also possible that we are being quite wrong in trying to make use of this similarity of name as something significant. Only later will it be possible to clear this up.

[1] [Freud's chief discussion of phantasies and of their relation to artistic creation will be found in two of his earlier papers: 'Creative Writers and Day-Dreaming' (1908*e*) and 'Hysterical Phantasies and their Relation to Bisexuality' (1908*a*). He returns to the subject below, in the later part of Lecture XXIII.]

LECTURE VI

THE PREMISSES AND TECHNIQUE
OF INTERPRETATION

LADIES AND GENTLEMEN,—What we need, then, is a new path, a method which will enable us to make a start in the investigation of dreams. I will put a suggestion to you which presents itself. Let us take it as a premiss from this point onwards that *dreams are not somatic but psychical phenomena.* You know what that means, but what justifies our making the assumption? Nothing: but there is nothing either to prevent our making it. Here is the position: if dreams are somatic phenomena they are no concern of ours, they can only interest us on the assumption that they are mental phenomena. We will therefore work on the assumption that they really are, to see what comes of it. The outcome of our work will decide whether we are to hold to this assumption and whether we may then go on to treat it in turn as a proved finding. But what is it actually that we want to arrive at? What is our work aiming at? We want something that is sought for in all scientific work—to understand the phenomena, to establish a correlation between them and, in the latter end, if it is possible, to enlarge our power over them.

We proceed with our work, accordingly, on the supposition that dreams are psychical phenomena. In that case they are products and utterances of the dreamer's, but utterances which tell us nothing, which we do not understand. Well, what do you do if I make an unintelligible utterance to you? You question me, is that not so? Why should we not do the same thing to the dreamer—*question him as to what his dream means?*

As you will remember, we found ourselves in this situation once before. It was while we were investigating certain parapraxes—a case of a slip of the tongue. Someone had said [p. 42]: 'Then facts came to *Vorschwein*' and we thereupon asked him—no, it was luckily not we but some other people who had no connection at all with psycho-analysis—these other people, then, asked him what he meant by this unintelligible remark. And he replied at once that he had intended to say

100

'these facts were *Schweinereien* [disgusting]', but had forced this intention back in favour of the milder version 'then facts came to *Vorschein* [light]'. I pointed out to you at the time [p. 48] that this piece of information was the model for every psycho-analytic investigation, and you will understand now that psycho-analysis follows the technique of getting the people under examination so far as possible themselves to produce the solution of their riddles [p. 49]. Thus, too, it is the dreamer himself who should tell us what his dream means.

But, as we know, things are not so simple with dreams. With parapraxes it worked all right in a number of cases; but then others came along in which the person who was questioned would say nothing, and even indignantly rejected the answer we proposed to him. With dreams cases of the first sort are entirely lacking; the dreamer always says he knows nothing. He cannot reject our interpretation as we have none to offer him. Are we to give up our attempt then? Since he knows nothing and we know nothing and a third person could know even less, there seems to be no prospect of finding out. If you feel inclined, then, give up the attempt! But if you feel otherwise, you can accompany me further. For I can assure you that it is quite possible, and highly probable indeed, that the dreamer *does* know what his dream means: *only he does not know that he knows it and for that reason thinks he does not know it.*

You will point out to me that I am once more introducing an assumption, the second already in this short argument, and that in doing so I am enormously reducing my procedure's claim to credibility: 'Subject to the premiss that dreams are psychical phenomena, and subject to the further premiss that there are mental things in a man which he knows without knowing that he knows them . . .' and so on. If so, one has only to consider the internal improbability of each of these two premisses, and one can quietly divert one's interest from any conclusions that may be based on them.

I have not brought you here, Ladies and Gentlemen, to delude you or to conceal things from you. In my prospectus, it is true, I announced a course of 'Elementary Lectures to Serve as

an Introduction to Psycho-Analysis',[1] but what I had in mind
was nothing in the nature of a presentation *in usum Delphini*,[2]
which would give you a smooth account with all the difficulties
carefully concealed, with the gaps filled in and the doubts
glossed over, so that you might believe with an easy mind that
you had learnt something new. No, for the very reason of your
being beginners, I wanted to show you our science as it is, with
its unevennesses and roughnesses, its demands and hesitations.
For I know that it is the same in all sciences and cannot possibly
be otherwise, especially in their beginnings. I know also that
ordinarily instruction is at pains to start out by concealing such
difficulties and incompletenesses from the learner. But that will
not do for psycho-analysis. So I have in fact laid down two premisses, one within the other; and if anyone finds the whole
thing too laborious and too insecure, or if anyone is accustomed
to higher certainties and more elegant deductions, he need go
no further with us. I think, however, that he should leave
psychological problems entirely alone, for it is to be feared that
in this quarter he will find impassable the precise and secure
paths which he is prepared to follow. And, for a science which
has something to offer, there is no necessity to sue for a hearing
and for followers. Its findings are bound to canvass on its behalf
and it can wait until these have compelled attention to it.

But for those who would like to persist in the subject, I can
point out that my two assumptions are not on a par. The first,
that dreams are psychical phenomena, is the premiss which we
seek to prove by the outcome of our work; the second one has
already been proved in another field, and I am merely ven-
turing to bring it over from there to our own problems.

Where, then, in what field, can it be that proof has been
found that there is knowledge of which the person concerned
nevertheless knows nothing, as we are proposing to assume of
dreamers? After all, this would be a strange, surprising fact and
one which would alter our view of mental life and which would
have no need to hide itself: a fact, incidentally, which cancels
itself in its very naming and which nevertheless claims to be

[1] [The 'elementary' was dropped from the title of the lectures in their
published form. See footnote 2, p. 9.]

[2] ['For the use of the Dauphin'—an edition of the Classics prepared for
his son by order of Louis XIV: 'bowdlerized'.]

something real—a contradiction in terms. Well, it does not hide itself. It is not its fault if people know nothing about it or do not pay enough attention to it. Any more than we are to blame because judgement is passed on all these psychological problems by people who have kept at a distance from all the observations and experiences which are decisive on the matter.

The proof was found in the field of hypnotic phenomena. When, in 1889, I took part in the extraordinarily impressive demonstrations by Liébeault and Bernheim at Nancy,[1] I witnessed the following experiment among others. If a man was put into a state of somnambulism, was made to experience all kinds of things in a hallucinatory manner, and was then woken up, he appeared at first to know nothing of what had happened during his hypnotic sleep. Bernheim then asked him straight out to report what had happened to him under hypnosis. The man maintained that he could remember nothing. But Bernheim held out against this, brought urgent pressure to bear on him, insisted that he knew it and must remember it. And, lo and behold! the man grew uncertain, began to reflect, and recalled in a shadowy way one of the experiences that had been suggested to him, and then another piece, and the memory became clearer and clearer and more and more complete, and finally came to light without a break. Since, however, he knew afterwards what had happened and had learnt nothing about it from anyone else in the interval, we are justified in concluding that he had known it earlier as well. It was merely inaccessible to him; he did not know that he knew it and thought he did not know it. That is to say, the position was exactly the same as what we suspected in our dreamer.

I hope you will be surprised that this fact has been established and will ask me: 'Why did you omit to bring this proof forward earlier, in connection with the parapraxes, when we came to the point of attributing to a man who had made a slip of the tongue an intention to say things of which he knew nothing and which he denied? If a person thinks he knows nothing of experiences the memory of which he nevertheless has within him, it is no longer so improbable that he knows nothing of other mental processes within him. This argument would certainly have impressed us, and helped us to understand parapraxes.' Of course

[1] [Freud returns to this on p. 277.]

I could have brought it forward then, but I reserved it for another place, where it was more needed. The parapraxes explained themselves in part, and in part left us with a suggestion that, in order to preserve the continuity of the phenomena concerned, it would be wise to assume the existence of mental processes of which the subject knows nothing. In the case of dreams we are compelled to bring in explanations from elsewhere and moreover I expect that in their case you will find it easier to accept my carrying over of the explanations from hypnosis. The state in which a parapraxis occurs is bound to strike you as being the normal one; it has no similarity with the hypnotic state. On the other hand there is an obvious kinship between the hypnotic state and the state of sleep, which is a necessary condition of dreaming. Hypnosis, indeed, is described as an artificial sleep. We tell the person we are hypnotizing to sleep, and the suggestions we make are comparable to the dreams of natural sleep. The psychical situations in the two cases are really analogous. In natural sleep we withdraw our interest from the whole external world; and in hypnotic sleep we also withdraw it from the whole world, but with the single exception of the person who has hypnotized us and with whom we remain in rapport. Incidentally, the sleep of a nursing mother, who remains in rapport with her child and can be woken only by him, is a normal counterpart of hypnotic sleep. So it scarcely seems a very bold venture to transpose a situation from hypnosis to natural sleep. The assumption that in a dreamer too a knowledge about his dreams is present, though it is inaccessible to him so that he himself does not believe it, is not something entirely out of the blue. It should be noticed, moreover, that a third line of approach to the study of dreams is opened at this point: from the stimuli which disturb sleep, from day-dreams, and now in addition from the suggested dreams of the hypnotic state.

We may now go back to our task with increased confidence perhaps. It is very probable, then, that the dreamer knows about his dream; the only question is how to make it possible for him to discover his knowledge and communicate it to us. We do not require him to tell us straight away the sense of his dream, but he will be able to find its origin, the circle of thoughts and interests from which it sprang. You will recall that in the case of the parapraxis the man was asked how he had arrived at the wrong word '*Vorschwein*' and the first thing that occurred to him[1] gave us the explanation. Our technique with dreams, then, is a very simple one, copied from this example. We shall once more ask the dreamer how he arrived at the dream, and once more his first remark is to be looked on as an explanation. Thus we disregard the distinction between his thinking or not thinking that he knows something, and we treat both cases as one and the same.

This technique is certainly very simple, but I fear it will rouse your liveliest opposition. You will say: 'A fresh assumption! the third! And the most unlikely of all! If I ask the dreamer what occurs to him in connection with the dream, is precisely the first thing that occurs to him going to bring the explanation we are hoping for? But nothing at all may occur to him, or heaven knows what may occur to him. I cannot see what an expectation of that kind is based on. That is really showing too much trust in Providence at a point where rather more exercise of the critical faculty would be appropriate. Besides, a dream is not a single wrong word; it consists of a number of elements. So which association are we to take up?'

You are correct on all your minor points. A dream differs from a slip of the tongue, among other things, in the multiplicity of its elements. Our technique must take this into account. I therefore suggest to you that we should divide the dream into its elements and start a separate enquiry into each element; if we do this, the analogy with a slip of the tongue is re-established. You are also right in thinking that when the dreamer is questioned about the separate elements of the dream he may reply that nothing occurs to him. There are some instances in which we let this reply pass, and you will later hear which these are [cf. p. 149]; strangely enough, they are instances in which definite ideas may occur to us ourselves. But in general if the dreamer asserts that nothing occurs to him we contradict him; we bring urgent pressure to bear on him, we insist that something must occur to him—and we turn out to be right. He will produce an idea—some idea, it is a matter of indifference to us which. He will give us certain pieces of information,

[1] [See footnote, p. 47 f.]

which may be described as 'historical', with particular ease. He may say: 'That's something that happened yesterday' (as was the case in our two 'matter-of-fact' dreams [p. 97]), or: 'That reminds me of something that happened a short time ago'—and we shall discover in this way that dreams are connected with impressions of the last day or two much more often than we thought to begin with [loc. cit.]. And finally he will also recall, starting from the dream, events from further back and even perhaps from the far distant past.

But on your main point you are wrong. If you think it is arbitrary to assume that the first thing that occurs to the dreamer is bound to bring what we are looking for or to lead us to it, if you think that what occurs to him might be anything in the world and might have no connection with what we are looking for, and that it is only exhibiting my trust in Providence if I expect something different—then you are making a great mistake. Once before [p. 49] I ventured to tell you that you nourish a deeply rooted faith in undetermined psychical events and in free will, but that this is quite unscientific and must yield to the demand of a determinism whose rule extends over mental life. I beg you to respect it as a fact that *that* is what occurred to the man when he was questioned and nothing else. But I am not opposing one faith with another. It can be proved that the idea produced by the man was not arbitrary nor indeterminable nor unconnected with what we were looking for. Indeed, not long ago I learnt—without, I may say, attaching too much importance to the fact—that experimental psychology too had brought up evidence to that effect.[1]

In view of the importance of the matter, I will ask for your special attention. If I ask someone to tell me what occurs to him in response to a particular element of a dream, I am asking him to surrender himself to free association *while keeping an idea in mind as a starting-point*. This calls for a special attitude of the attention which is quite different from reflection and which excludes reflection. Some people achieve this attitude with ease; others show an incredibly high degree of clumsiness when they attempt it. There is, however, a higher degree of freedom of

[1] [A footnote dealing with this was added by Freud in 1919 to his discussion of Recent and Indifferent Material in Dreams in *I. of D.*]

association: that is to say, I may drop the insistence on keeping an initial idea in mind and only lay down the sort or kind of association I want—I may, for instance, require the experimenter to allow a proper name or a number to occur to him freely. What then occurs to him would presumably be even more arbitrary and more indeterminable than with our own technique. It can be shown, however, that it is always strictly determined by important internal attitudes of mind which are not known to us at the moment at which they operate—which are as little known to us as the disturbing purposes of parapraxes and the provoking ones of chance actions [p. 61].

I and many others after me have repeatedly made such experiments with names and numbers thought of at random, and a few of these have been published.[1] Here the procedure is to produce a series of associations to the name which has emerged; these latter associations are accordingly no longer completely free but have a link, like the associations to the elements of dreams. One continues doing this until one finds the impulse exhausted. But by then light will have been thrown both on the motive and the meaning of the random choice of the name. These experiments always lead to the same result; reports on them often cover a wealth of material and call for extensive expositions. The associations to *numbers* chosen at random are perhaps the most convincing; they run off so quickly and proceed with such incredible certainty to a hidden goal that the effect is really staggering. I will give you only one example of an analysis like this of a name, since dealing with it calls for a conveniently small amount of material.

In the course of treating a young man I had occasion to discuss this topic, and mentioned the thesis that, in spite of an apparently arbitrary choice, it is impossible to think of a name at random which does not turn out to be closely determined by the immediate circumstances, the characteristics of the subject of the experiment and his situation at the moment. Since he was sceptical, I suggested that he should make an experiment of the kind himself on the spot. I knew that he carried on particularly numerous relationships of every kind with married women and

[1] [Several examples are given in Section A of Chapter XII of *The Psychopathology of Everyday Life* (1901*b*), (Norton, 1965), where the whole topic is discussed at length.]

girls, so I thought he would have a specially large choice open
to him if it were to be a woman's name that he was asked to
choose. He agreed to this. To my astonishment, or rather, perhaps, to his, no avalanche of women's names broke over me; he
remained silent for a moment and then admitted that only a
single name had come into his head and none other besides:
'Albine'.—How curious! But what does that name mean to you?
How many 'Albines' do you know?—Strange to say, he knew no
one called 'Albine' and nothing further occurred to him in
response to the name. So it might be thought that the analysis
had failed. But not at all: it was already complete, and no
further associations were needed. The man had an unusually
fair complexion and in conversation during the treatment I had
often jokingly called him an albino. We were engaged at the
time in determining the feminine part of his constitution. So
it was he himself who was this 'Albine', the woman who was the
most interesting to him at the moment.

In the same way tunes that come into one's head without
warning turn out to be determined by and to belong to a train
of thought which has a right to occupy one's mind though
without one's being aware of its activity. It is easy to show then
that the relation to the tune is based on its text or its origin.
But I must be careful not to extend this assertion to really
musical people, of whom, as it happens, I have had no experience. It may be that for such people the musical content of
the tune is what decides its emergence. The earlier case is certainly the commoner one. I know of a young man, for instance,
who was positively persecuted for a time by the tune (incidentally a charming one) of Paris's song in [Offenbach's] *La belle
Hélène*, till his analysis drew his attention to a contemporary
competition in his interest between an 'Ida' and a 'Helen'.[1]

If then things that occur to one quite freely are determined
in this way and form parts of a connected whole, we shall no
doubt be justified in concluding that things that occur to one
with a single link—namely their link with the idea which serves
as their starting-point—cannot be any less determined. Investigation shows, in fact, that, apart from the link we have given

[1] [Paris, who eloped with Helen, was at one time a shepherd on
Mount Ida, where he delivered his judgement between three competing
goddesses.]

them with the initial idea, they are found to be dependent as well on groups of strongly emotional thoughts and interests, 'complexes', whose participation is not known at the moment —that is to say, is unconscious.

The occurrence of ideas with links of this kind has been the subject of very instructive experimental researches, which have played a notable part in the history of psycho-analysis. The school of Wundt had introduced what are known as association-experiments, in which a *stimulus word* is called out to the subject and he has the task of replying to it as quickly as possible with any *reaction* that occurs to him. It is then possible to study the interval that passes between the stimulus and the reaction, the nature of the answer given as a reaction, possible errors when the same experiment is repeated later, and so on. The Zurich school, led by Bleuler and Jung, found the explanation of the reactions that followed in the association-experiment by getting the subjects to throw light on their reactions by means of subsequent associations, if those reactions had shown striking features. It then turned out that these striking reactions were determined in the most definite fashion by the subject's complexes. In this manner Bleuler and Jung built the first bridge from experimental psychology to psycho-analysis.

Having learnt thus much, you will be able to say: 'We acknowledge now that thoughts that occur to one freely are determined and not arbitrary as we supposed. We admit that this is also true of thoughts occurring in response to the elements of dreams. But that is not what we are concerned with. You assert that what occurs to the dreamer in response to the dream-element will be determined by the psychical background (unknown to us) of that particular element. This does not seem to us to be proved. We quite expect that what occurs to the dreamer in response to the dream-element will turn out to be determined by one of the dreamer's complexes, but what good does that do us? This does not lead us to an understanding of dreams but, like the association-experiment, to a knowledge of these so-called complexes. But what have they got to do with dreams?'

You are right, but you are overlooking one factor. Moreover it is precisely the factor on account of which I did not choose

the association-experiment as the starting-point of this exposition. In that experiment the single determinant of the reaction—that is, the stimulus-word—is arbitrarily chosen by us.
The reaction is in that case an intermediary between the
stimulus-word and the complex which has been aroused in the
subject. In dreams the stimulus-word is replaced by something
that is itself derived from the dreamer's mental life, from sources
unknown to him, and may therefore very easily itself be a 'derivative of a complex'. It is therefore not precisely fantastic to
suppose that the further associations linked to the dream-elements will be determined by the same complex as that of the
element itself and will lead to its discovery.

Let me show you from another instance that the facts are as
we expect. The forgetting of proper names is actually an excellent model of what happens in dream-analysis; the difference is
only that events that are shared between two people in dream-
analysis are combined in a single person in the parapraxis. If I
forget a name temporarily, I nevertheless feel in myself a certainty that I know it—a certainty which in the case of the
dreamer we only arrived at by the round-about path of the
Bernheim experiment [p. 103]. The name which I have forgotten but which I know is, however, not accessible to me. Experience soon teaches me that thinking about it, with however
much effort, is of no help. But in place of the forgotten name I
can always call up one or several substitute names. It is only
after a substitute name of this kind has occurred to me spontaneously that the conformity of this situation with that of
dream-interpretation becomes obvious. Like this substitute
name, the dream-element is not the right thing, but only takes
the place of something else—of the genuine thing which I do
not know and which I am to discover by means of the dream-
analysis. The difference is once more only that in the case of
forgetting the name, I recognize the substitute unhesitatingly as
something ungenuine, whereas we had to acquire this view
laboriously in the case of the dream-element. Now in the case
of forgetting a name there is also a method by which we can
start from the substitute and arrive at the unconscious genuine
thing, the forgotten name. If I direct my attention to the substitute names and allow further ideas in response to them to
occur to me, I arrive by shorter or longer détours at the for-

gotten name, and I find when this happens that both the spontaneous substitute name and the ones that I have called up are connected with the forgotten one and were determined by it.

I will describe an analysis of this kind to you. I noticed one day that I could not recall the name of the small country on the Riviera, of which Monte Carlo is the chief town. It was very tiresome, but so it was. I summoned up all that I knew about that country. I thought of Prince Albert of the House of Lusignan, of his marriages, of his devotion to deep-sea researches, and everything else I could bring together, but it was of no avail. So I gave up reflection and allowed substitute names to occur to me instead of the lost one. They came rapidly: Monte Carlo itself, then Piedmont, Albania, Montevideo, Colico. Of this series I was struck first by Albania, which was at once replaced by Montenegro, no doubt because of the contrast between white and black.[1] I then saw that four of these substitute names contained the same syllable 'mon', then suddenly I had the forgotten word and exclaimed aloud: 'Monaco!' So the substitute names had in fact arisen from the forgotten one: the first four came from its first syllable while the last reproduced its syllabic structure and its whole last syllable. Moreover I was able to discover quite easily what it was that had temporarily deprived me of the name. Monaco is also the Italian name for Munich; and it was that town which exerted the inhibitory influence.[2]

No doubt this example is a good one, but it is too simple. In other cases it would have been necessary to call up a longer string of ideas in response to the first substitute name. I have had experiences of that sort too. On one occasion a stranger had invited me to drink some Italian wine with him, but when we were in the inn it turned out that he had forgotten the name of the wine which he intended to order because of his very agreeable recollections of it. From a quantity of substitute ideas of different kinds which came into his head in place of the forgotten name, I was able to infer that thoughts about someone called Hedwig had made him forget the name. And he not only confirmed the fact that he had first tasted this wine when he

[1] ['*Albus*' the Latin for 'white', and '*negro*' the Italian for 'black'.]

[2] [This episode is decribed more briefly in *The Psychopathology of Everyday Life*, p. 55.]

was with someone of that name, but with the help of this discovery he recalled the name of the wine. He was happily married at the present time and this Hedwig belonged to earlier
days which he had no wish to remember.

But if it is possible in the case of forgetting a name, it must
also be possible in interpreting dreams to proceed from the substitute along the chain of associations attached to it and so to
obtain access to the genuine thing which is being held back.
From the example of the forgotten name we may conclude that
the associations to the dream-element will be determined both
by the dream-element and also by the unconscious genuine
thing behind it. In this way, then, we seem to have produced
some justification of our technique.

LECTURE VII

THE MANIFEST CONTENT OF DREAMS AND THE LATENT DREAM-THOUGHTS

LADIES AND GENTLEMEN,—As you see, our study of parapraxes has not been unprofitable. Thanks to our labours over them we have, subject to the premisses I have explained to you,[1] achieved two things: a conception of the nature of dream-elements and a technique for interpreting dreams. The conception of dream-elements tells us that they are ungenuine things [p. 110], substitutes for something else that is unknown to the dreamer (like the purpose of a parapraxis), substitutes for something the knowledge of which is present in the dreamer but which is inaccessible to him. We are in hopes that it will be possible to carry over the same conception to whole dreams, which are made up of such elements. Our technique lies in employing free association to these elements in order to bring about the emergence of other substitutive structures, which will enable us to arrive at what is concealed from view.

I now propose that we should introduce a change into our nomenclature which will give us more freedom of movement. Instead of speaking of 'concealed', 'inaccessible', or 'ungenuine',[2] let us adopt the correct description and say 'inaccessible to the dreamer's consciousness' or '*unconscious*'.[3] I mean nothing else by this than what may be suggested to you when you think of a word that has escaped you or the disturbing purpose in a parapraxis—that is to say, I mean nothing else than '*unconscious at the moment*'. In contrast to this, we can of course speak of the dream-elements themselves, and the substitutive ideas that have been newly arrived at from them by association, as '*conscious*'. This nomenclature so far involves no

[1] [See pp. 100 and 101.]

[2] ['*Uneigentlich*' in all the German editions. The sense would seem to require '*eigentlich* (genuine)'.]

[3] [Cf. Lecture I, p. 21; the discussion is continued below in Lecture XIII, p. 212.]

theoretical construction. No objection can be made to using the word 'unconscious' as an apt and easily understandable description.

If we carry over our conception of the separate elements to the whole dream, it follows that the dream as a whole is a distorted substitute for something else, something unconscious, and that the task of interpreting a dream is to discover this unconscious material. From this, however, there at once follow three important rules, which we must obey during the work of interpreting dreams.

(1) We must not concern ourselves with what the dream *appears* to tell us, whether it is intelligible or absurd, clear or confused, since it cannot possibly be the unconscious material we are in search of. (An obvious limitation to this rule will force itself on our notice later [p. 126].) (2) We must restrict our work to calling up the substitutive ideas for each element, we must not reflect about them, or consider whether they contain anything relevant, and we must not trouble ourselves with how far they diverge from the dream-element. (3) We must wait till the concealed unconscious material we are in search of emerges of its own accord, exactly as the forgotten word 'Monaco' did in the experiment I have described [p. 111].

Now, too, we can understand to what extent it is a matter of indifference how much or how little the dream is remembered and, above all, how accurately or how uncertainly. For the remembered dream is not the genuine material but a distorted substitute for it, which should assist us, by calling up other substitutive images, to come nearer to the genuine material, to make what is unconscious in the dream conscious. If our memory has been inaccurate, therefore, it has merely made a further distortion of this substitute—a distortion, moreover, which cannot have been without a reason.

The work of interpreting can be performed on one's own dreams just as on other people's. In fact one learns more from one's own: the process carries more conviction. If, then, we make the attempt, we notice that something is opposing our work. It is true that ideas occur to us, but we do not allow all of them to count; testing and selecting influences make themselves felt. In the case of one idea we may say to ourselves: 'No, this is not relevant, it does not belong here'; in the case of

another: 'this is too senseless' and of a third: 'this is totally unimportant'. And we can further observe how with objections of
this sort we may smother ideas and finally expel them altogether, even before they have become quite clear. Thus on the
one hand we keep too close to the idea which was our starting-
point, the dream-element itself; and on the other hand we interfere with the outcome of the free associations by making a
selection. If we are not by ourselves while interpreting the
dream, if we get someone else to interpret it, we become very
clearly aware of yet another motive which we employ in
making this illicit selection, for sometimes we say to ourselves: 'No, this idea is too disagreeable; I will not or cannot
report it.'

These objections are obviously a threat to the success of our
work. We must guard against them, and in our own case we do
so by firmly resolving not to give way to them. If we are
analysing someone else's dream, we do so by laying it down as
an inviolable rule that he must not hold back any idea from us,
even if it gives rise to one of the four objections—of being too
unimportant or too senseless or of being irrelevant or too distressing to be reported.[1] The dreamer promises to obey the rule,
and we may be annoyed afterwards to find how badly he keeps
his promise when the occasion arises. We may explain this to
ourselves to begin with by supposing that, in spite of our
authoritative assurance, he has not yet realized the justification
for free association, and we may perhaps have the notion of first
convincing him theoretically by giving him books to read or by
sending him to lectures which may convert him into a supporter
of our views on free association. But we shall be held back from
blunders like this when we consider that in the case of ourselves, as to the strength of whose convictions we can, after all,
hardly be in doubt, the same objections arise to certain ideas
and are only set aside subsequently—by a court of appeal, as
it were.

Instead of being annoyed by the dreamer's disobedience, we
may take advantage of these experiences by learning something
new from them—something which is all the more important the

[1] [Freud returns to this 'fundamental technical rule of analysis' in
Lecture XIX, p. 287 below, where an Editor's footnote gives further
references.]

less we are expecting it. We perceive that the work of interpreting dreams is carried out in the face of a *resistance*, which
opposes it and of which the critical objections are manifestations.[1] This resistance is independent of the dreamer's theoretical conviction. We learn still more, indeed. We discover that a
critical objection of this kind never turns out to be justified. On
the contrary, the ideas which people try to suppress in this way
turn out *invariably* to be the most important ones and those
which are decisive in our search for the unconscious material.
It amounts, in fact, to a special distinguishing mark, if an idea
is accompanied by an objection like this.

This resistance is something entirely new: a phenomenon
which we have come upon in connection with our premises
[p. 101 f.], but one which was not included among them. The
appearance of this new factor in our reckoning comes to us as a
not altogether pleasant surprise. We suspect at once that it is
not going to make our work any easier. It might mislead us into
abandoning our whole concern with dreams: something so unimportant as a dream and, on top of that, all these difficulties
instead of a simple straightforward technique! But, on the other
hand, the difficulties might act precisely as a stimulus and make
us suspect that the work will be worth the trouble. We regularly
come up against resistance when we try to make our way forward from the substitute which is the dream-element to the unconscious material hidden behind it. So we may conclude that
there must be something of importance concealed behind the
substitute. Otherwise, what is the point of the difficulties that
are trying to keep the concealment going? If a child refuses to
open his clenched fist to show what he has in it, we may feel
sure that it is something wrong—something he ought not to
have.

The moment we introduce the dynamic idea of a resistance
into the facts of the case, we must simultaneously reflect that
this factor is something variable in quantity. There may be
greater and smaller resistances, and we are prepared to find
these differences showing themselves during our work as well.
We may perhaps be able to link with this another experience
we also meet with during the work of interpreting dreams:
sometimes it requires only a single response, or no more than a

[1] [The subject of 'resistance' is fully dealt with in Lecture XIX.]

few, to lead us from a dream-element to the unconscious material behind it, while on other occasions long chains of associations and the overcoming of many critical objections are required for bringing this about. We shall conclude that these differences relate to the changing magnitude of the resistance, and we shall probably turn out to be right.[1] If the resistance is small, the substitute cannot be far distant from the unconscious material; but a greater resistance means that the unconscious material will be greatly distorted and that the path will be a long one from the substitute back to the unconscious material.

And now perhaps it is time to take a dream and try our technique upon it and see whether our expectations are confirmed. Yes, but what dream are we to choose for the purpose? You cannot imagine how hard I find it to decide; nor can I yet make the nature of my difficulties plain to you. There must obviously be dreams which have on the whole been subjected to only a little distortion, and the best plan would be to begin with them. But what dreams have been least distorted? The ones that are intelligible and not confused, two examples of which I have already put before you [p. 97]? That would be leading us quite astray. Investigation shows that such dreams have been subjected to an extraordinarily high degree of distortion. If, however, I were to disregard particular requirements and were to select a dream at haphazard, you would probably be greatly disappointed. We might have to notice or record such a profusion of ideas in response to the separate dream-elements that we should be unable to make head or tail of the work. If we write down a dream and then make a note of all the ideas that emerge in response to it, these may prove to be many times longer than the text of the dream. The best plan would therefore seem to be to choose out a number of short dreams for analysis, each of which will at least tell us something or confirm some point. So we will make up our minds to take that course, unless experience may perhaps show us where we can really find dreams that have been only slightly distorted.[2]

[1] [Freud discussed the effects on dream-interpretation of a high or low pressure of resistance in Section II of his 'Remarks on the Theory and Practice of Dream-Interpretation' (1923c).]

[2] [See the following lecture.]

I can however think of something else that will make things easier for us—something, moreover, which lies along our path. Instead of starting on the interpretation of *whole* dreams, we will restrict ourselves to a few dream-elements, and we will trace out in a number of examples how these can be explained by applying our technique to them.

(*a*) A lady reported that she very often dreamt when she was a child that *God wore a paper cocked-hat on his head.* What can you make of that without the dreamer's help? It sounds completely nonsensical. But it ceases to be nonsense when we hear from the lady that she used to have a hat of that sort put on her head at meals when she was a child, because she could never resist taking furtive glances at her brothers' and sisters' plates to see whether they had been given larger helpings than she had. So the hat was intended to act like a pair of blinkers. This, incidentally, was a piece of historical information [p. 105 f.] and was given without any difficulty. The interpretation of this element and at the same time of the whole short dream was easily made with the help of a further idea that occurred to the dreamer: 'As I had heard that God was omniscient and saw everything', she said, 'the dream can only mean that I knew everything and saw everything, even though they tried to prevent me.' [1] Perhaps this example is too simple.

(*b*) A sceptical woman patient had a longish dream in the course of which some people told her about my book on jokes [1905*c*] and praised it highly. Something came in then about *a 'channel', perhaps it was another book that mentioned a channel, or something else about a channel . . . she didn't know . . . it was all so indistinct.*

No doubt you will be inclined to expect that the element 'channel', since it was so indistinct, would be inaccessible to interpretation. You are right in suspecting a difficulty; but the difficulty did not arise from the indistinctness: both the difficulty and the indistinctness arose from another cause. Nothing occurred to the dreamer in connection with 'channel', and *I* could of course throw no light on it. A little later—it was the next day, in point of fact—she told me that she had thought of

[1] [This dream is reported in Section F of Chapter VI of *I. of D.*]

something that *might* have something to do with it. It was a joke, too,—a joke she had heard. On the steamer between Dover and Calais a well-known author fell into conversation with an Englishman. The latter had occasion to quote the phrase: 'Du sublime au ridicule il n'y a qu'un pas. [It is only a step from the sublime to the ridiculous.]' 'Yes,' replied the author, '*le Pas de Calais*'—meaning that he thought France sublime and England ridiculous. But the *Pas de Calais* is a channel —the English Channel. You will ask whether I think this had anything to do with the dream. Certainly I think so; and it provides the solution of the puzzling element of the dream. Can you doubt that this joke was already present before the dream occurred, as the unconscious thought behind the element 'channel'? Can you suppose that it was introduced as a subsequent invention? The association betrayed the scepticism which lay concealed behind the patient's ostensible admiration; and her resistance against revealing this was no doubt the common cause both of her delay in producing the association and of the indistinctness of the dream-element concerned. Consider the relation of the dream-element to its unconscious background: it was, as it were, a fragment of the background, an allusion to it, but it was made quite incomprehensible by being isolated.[1]

(*c*) As part of a longish dream a patient dreamt that *several members of his family were sitting round a table of a peculiar shape*, etc. It occurred to him in connection with the table that he had seen a piece of furniture of the kind when he was on a visit to a particular family. His thoughts then went on to say that there was a peculiar relationship between the father and son in this family; and he soon added that the same thing was true of the relationship between himself and his own father. So the table had been taken into the dream in order to point out this parallel.

This dreamer had been long familiar with the requirement of dream-interpretation. Another person might perhaps have taken objection to such a trivial detail as the shape of a table being made the subject of investigation. But in fact we regard nothing in a dream as accidental or indifferent, and we expect

[1] [The whole of this example (*b*) was inserted by Freud into *I. of D.* as a footnote in 1919. See Section A of Chapter VII.]

to obtain information precisely from the explanation of such trivial and pointless details. You may perhaps also feel surprised that the thought that 'the same thing was true of us and of them' should have been expressed by, in particular, the choice of a table [*Tisch*]. But this too becomes clear when you learn that the name of the family in question was *Tischler* [literally, 'carpenter']. By making his relations sit at this *Tisch*, he was saying that they too were *Tischlers*. Incidentally, you will notice how inevitably one is led into being indiscreet when one reports these dream-interpretations. And you will guess that this is one of the difficulties I have hinted at over the choice of examples. I could easily have taken another example in place of this one, but I should probably merely have avoided *this* indiscretion at the price of committing another.

The moment seems to me to have arrived for introducing two terms, which we could have made use of long ago. We will describe what the dream actually tells us as the *manifest dream-content*, and the concealed material, which we hope to reach by pursuing the ideas that occur to the dreamer, as the *latent dream-thoughts*. Thus we are here considering the relations between the manifest content of the dream and the latent dream-thoughts as shown in these examples. These relations may be of very many different kinds. In examples (*a*) and (*b*) the manifest element is also a constituent of the latent thoughts, though only a small fragment of them. A small piece of the large and complicated psychical structure of unconscious dream-thoughts has made its way into the manifest dream as well—a fragment of them, or, in other cases, an allusion to them, a caption, as it were, or an abbreviation in telegraphic style. It is the business of the work of interpretation to complete these fragments or this allusion into a whole—which was achieved particularly nicely in the case of example (*b*). Thus one form of the distortion which constitutes the dream-work is replacement by a fragment or an allusion. In example (*c*) another kind of relation is to be observed in addition; and we shall find this expressed in a purer and clearer form in the examples which follow.

(*d*) The dreamer *was pulling a lady* (a particular one, of his acquaintance) *out from behind a bed*. He himself found the meaning of this dream-element from the first idea that occurred to him. It meant that he was giving this lady preference.[1]

(e) Another man dreamt that *his brother was in a box* [*Kasten*]. In his first response '*Kasten*' was replaced by '*Schrank* [cupboard]', and the second gave the interpretation: his brother was restricting himself ['*schränkt sich ein*'].[2]

(f) The dreamer *climbed to the top of a mountain, which commanded an unusually extensive view*. This sounds quite rational and you might suppose that there is nothing to interpret in it and that all we have to do is to enquire what memory gave rise to the dream and the reason for its being stirred up. But you would be wrong. It turned out that this dream stood in need of interpreting just as much as any other, more confused one. For none of his own mountain climbs occurred to the dreamer, but he thought of the fact that an acquaintance of his was the editor of a 'Survey', dealing with our relations with the most remote parts of the earth. Thus the latent dream-thought was an identification of the dreamer with the 'surveyor'.

Here we have a new type of relation between the manifest and latent dream-elements. The former is not so much a distortion of the latter as a representation of it, a plastic, concrete, portrayal of it, taking its start from the wording. But precisely on that account it is once more a distortion, for we have long since forgotten from what concrete image the word originated and consequently fail to recognize it when it is replaced by the image. When you consider that the manifest dream is made up predominantly of visual images and more rarely of thoughts and words, you can imagine what importance attaches to this kind of relation in the construction of dreams. You will see, too, that in this way it becomes possible in regard to a large number of abstract thoughts to create pictures to act as substitutes for them in the manifest dream while at the same time serving the purpose of concealment. This is the technique of the familiar

___

[1] [This example, like the next, depends on a purely verbal point: the resemblance between the German words for 'pulling out' (*hervorziehen*) and 'preferring' (*vorziehen*). See Section F of Chapter VI of *I. of D.*]

[2] [This and the next example are also from Section F of Chapter VI of *I. of D.*]

picture-puzzles. Why it is that these representations have an appearance of being jokes is a special problem into which we need not enter here.[1]

There is a fourth kind of relation between the manifest and latent elements, which I must continue to hold back from you until we come upon its key-word in considering technique.[2] Even so I shall not have given you a full list; but it will serve our purpose.

Do you feel bold enough now to venture upon the interpretation of a *whole* dream? Let us make the experiment, to see whether we are well enough equipped for the task. I shall of course not select one of the most obscure ones; nevertheless, it will be one that gives a well-marked picture of the attributes of a dream.[3]

Very well then. A lady who, though she was still young, had been married for many years had the following dream: *She was at the theatre with her husband. One side of the stalls was completely empty. Her husband told her that Elise L. and her fiancé had wanted to go too, but had only been able to get bad seats—three for 1 florin 50 kreuzers[4]—and of course they could not take those. She thought it would not really have done any harm if they had.*

The first thing the dreamer reported to us was that the precipitating cause of the dream was touched on in its manifest content. Her husband had in fact told her that Elise L., who was approximately her contemporary, had just become engaged. The dream was a reaction to this information. We know already [p. 106] that it is easy in the case of many dreams to point to a precipitating cause like this from the previous day, and that the dreamer is often able to trace this for us without any difficulty. The dreamer in the present case put similar in-

---

[1] [See the discussion of the point in Chapter VI of Freud's book on jokes (1905c), (Norton, 1960), p. 173; cf. also p. 235 f. below.]

[2] [See below, p. 151.]

[3] [The dream which follows had been analysed, but very much less elaborately, in *I. of D.*, Chap. VI (F). It is also discussed in Chapters VII and VIII of the short work *On Dreams* (1901a), (Norton, 1952). Freud returns to it in these lectures at several points: pp. 139–40, 178, 219–21 and 224–5 below.]

[4] [This had at the time been worth approximately 2s. 6d. or 62½ cents.]

formation at our disposal for other elements of the manifest dream as well.—Where did the detail come from about one side of the stalls being empty? It was an allusion to a real event of the previous week. She had planned to go to a particular play and had therefore bought her tickets *early*—so early that she had had to pay a booking fee. When they got to the theatre it turned out that her anxiety was quite uncalled-for, since *one side of the stalls was almost empty*. It would have been early enough if she had bought the tickets on the actual day of the performance. Her husband had kept on teasing her for having been in too much of a hurry.—What was the origin of the 1 florin 50 kreuzers? It arose in quite another connection, which had nothing to do with the former one but also alluded to some information from the previous day. Her sister-in-law had been given a present of 150 florins by her husband and had been in a great hurry—the silly goose—to rush off to the jewellers' and exchange the money for a piece of jewellery.—Where did the 'three' come from? She could think of nothing in connection with that, unless we counted the idea that her newly-engaged friend, Elise L., was only three months her junior, though she herself had been a married woman for nearly ten years.—And the absurd notion of taking three tickets for only two people? She had nothing to say to that, and refused to report any further ideas or information.

But all the same, she had given us so much material in these few associations that it was possible to guess the latent dream-thoughts from them. We cannot help being struck by the fact that periods of time occur at several points in the information she gave us about the dream, and these provide a common factor between the different parts of the material. She took the theatre tickets *too early*, bought them *over-hurriedly* so that she had to pay more than was necessary; so too her sister-in-law had been *in a hurry* to take her money to the jewellers and buy some jewellery with it, as though otherwise she would *miss it*. If, in addition to the 'too early' and 'in a hurry' which we have stressed, we take into account the precipitating cause of the dream—the news that her friend, though only three months *her junior*, had nevertheless got an excellent husband—and the criticism of her sister-in-law expressed in the idea that it was *absurd* of her to be in such a hurry, then we find ourselves presented almost spontaneously with the following construction of the latent dream-thoughts, for which the manifest dream is a severely distorted substitute:

'Really it was *absurd* of me to be in such a hurry to get married! I can see from Elise's example that *I* could have got a husband later too.' (Being in too great a hurry was represented by her own behaviour in buying the tickets and by her sister-in-law's in buying the jewellery. Going to the play appeared as a substitute for getting married.) This would seem to be the main thought. We may perhaps proceed further, though with less certainty, since the analysis ought not to have been without the dreamer's comments at these points: 'And I could have got one a hundred times better with the money!' (150 florins is a hundred times more than 1 florin 50.) If we were to put her dowry in place of the money, it would mean that her husband was bought with her dowry: the jewellery, and the bad tickets as well, would be substitutes for her husband. It would be still more satisfactory if the actual element 'three tickets' had something to do with a husband. [Cf. below, p. 220.] But we have not got so far as that in our understanding of the dream. We have only discovered that the dream expresses the *low value* assigned by her to her own husband and her regret at having *married so early*.

We shall, I fancy, be more surprised and confused than satisfied by the outcome of this first dream-interpretation. We have been given too much in one dose—more than we are yet able to cope with. We can already see that we shall not exhaust the lessons of this interpretation of a dream. Let us hasten to single out what we can recognize as established new discoveries.

In the first place, it is a remarkable thing that the main emphasis in the latent thoughts lies on the element of being in too great a hurry; nothing of the sort is to be found in the manifest dream. Without the analysis, we should have had no suspicion that that factor plays any part. It seems, therefore, to be possible for what is in fact the main thing, the centre of the unconscious thoughts, to be absent in the manifest dream. This means that the impression made by the whole dream must be fundamentally altered. In the second place, there is an absurd combination in the dream: three for 1 florin 50. We detected in the dream-thoughts the assertion that 'it was absurd (to marry so early)'. Can it be doubted that this thought, 'it was absurd', is represented by the inclusion of an absurd element in the manifest dream? And in the third place, a glance of comparison shows us that the relation between the manifest and latent elements is no simple one; it is far from being the case that one manifest element always takes the place of one latent one. It is rather that there is a group-relation between the two layers, within which one manifest element can replace several latent ones or one latent element can be replaced by several manifest ones. [Cf. below, p. 173.]

As regards the meaning of the dream and the dreamer's attitude to it, we might point out much that is similarly surprising. She agreed to the interpretation indeed, but she was astonished at it. She was not aware that she assigned such a low value to her husband; nor did she know *why* she should set such a low value on him. So there is still much that is unintelligible about it. It really seems to me that we are not yet equipped for interpreting a dream and that we need first to be given some further instruction and preparation.

LECTURE VIII

CHILDREN'S DREAMS

LADIES AND GENTLEMEN,—I am under the impression that we have advanced too quickly. Let us go back a little. Before we made our last attempt at overcoming the difficulty of distortion in dreams by the help of our technique, we were saying [p. 117] that our best plan would be to get round the difficulty by keeping to dreams in which there was no distortion or only a very little—if such dreams exist. This will once more mean a divergence from the historical development of our discoveries [cf. p. 83]; for actually it was only after the technique of interpretation had been consistently applied and distorted dreams had been completely analysed that the existence of dreams that are free from distortion came to our notice.

The dreams we are in search of occur in children.[1] They are short, clear, coherent, easy to understand and unambiguous; but they are nevertheless undoubtedly dreams. You must not suppose, however, that all children's dreams are of this kind. Dream-distortion sets in very early in childhood, and dreams dreamt by children of between five and eight have been reported which bear all the characteristics of later ones. But if you limit yourselves to ages between the beginning of observable mental activity and the fourth or fifth year, you will come upon a number of dreams which possess the characteristics that can be described as 'infantile' and you will find a few of the same kind in later years of childhood. Indeed, under certain conditions even adults have dreams which are quite similar to the typically infantile ones.

From these children's dreams we can draw conclusions with great ease and certainty on the essential nature of dreams in general, and we can hope that those conclusions will prove decisive and universally valid.

(1) No analysis, no application of any technique is necessary

[1] [There is no separate chapter on children's dreams in *I. of D.*, but they are dealt with in Chapter III, where the examples in the present lecture will be found again.]

126

in order to understand these dreams. There is no need to question a child who tells us his dream. One has, however, to add a piece of information to it from the events of the child's life. There is invariably some experience of the previous day which explains the dream to us. The dream is the reaction of the child's mental life in his sleep to this experience of the previous day.

We will take a few examples on which to base our further conclusions.

(*a*) A boy of 22 months was told to hand over a basket of cherries to someone as a birthday present. He was obviously very unwilling to do it, although he was promised that he should have a few of them for himself. Next morning he reported having dreamt: '*Hermann eaten all the chewwies!*'

(*b*) A girl of 3¼ years was taken across the lake for the first time. At the landing-stage she did not want to leave the boat and wept bitterly. The crossing had been too short for her. Next morning she announced: '*Last night I went on the lake.*' We may safely add that this crossing had lasted longer.

(*c*) A boy of 5¼ years was taken on an excursion up the Echerntal near Hallstatt.[1] He had been told that Hallstatt was at the foot of the Dachstein. He had shown great interest in this mountain. There was a fine view of it from where he was staying at Aussee, and the Simony Hut on it could be made out through a telescope. The child had often tried to see it through the telescope—with what success was not known. The excursion began in an atmosphere of cheerful expectation. Whenever a fresh mountain came into view the boy asked: 'Is that the Dachstein?' and he became more and more depressed the more often he was told it was not. Finally he fell completely silent and refused to go with the rest of the party up the short ascent to the waterfall, and it was thought that he must be overtired. But next morning he said with a radiant face: 'Last night I dreamt *we were at the Simony Hut.*' So that had been what he expected to do on the excursion. He gave no further details except something he had heard before: 'You have to climb up steps for six hours.'

These three dreams will give us all the information we require.

(2) As we can see, these children's dreams are not senseless. They are intelligible, completely valid mental acts. You will

[1] [In the Salzkammergut district of Upper Austria.]

recall what I told you of the medical view of dreams and of the analogy with unmusical fingers wandering over the keys of a piano [p. 87]. You cannot fail to observe how sharply these children's dreams contradict this view. It would really be too strange if *children* could perform complete mental functions in their sleep while *adults* were content under the same conditions with reactions which were no more than 'twitchings'. Moreover, we have every reason to think that children's sleep is sounder and deeper.

(3) These dreams are without any dream-distortion, and therefore call for no interpretative activity. Here the manifest and the latent dream coincide. *Thus dream-distortion is not part of the essential nature of dreams.* I expect this will be a weight off your minds. But when we examine these dreams more closely, we shall recognize a small piece of dream-distortion even in them, a certain distinction between the manifest content of the dream and the latent dream-thoughts.

(4) A child's dream is a reaction to an experience of the previous day, which has left behind it a regret, a longing, a wish that has not been dealt with. *The dream produces a direct, undisguised fulfilment of that wish.* Let us recall now our discussions on the part played by somatic stimuli from outside and from within as disturbers of sleep and instigators of dreams [p. 91 ff.]. In that connection we came to know some quite undoubted facts, but by their means we were only able to explain a small number of dreams. In these children's dreams, however, there is nothing that points to the operation of somatic stimuli of that kind; we could not be mistaken in this, for the dreams are completely intelligible and easy to grasp. But this does not mean that we need abandon the stimulus aetiology of dreams. We can only ask how it has happened that from the first we have forgotten that besides somatic stimuli there are *mental* stimuli that disturb sleep. We know, after all, that it is excitations of this kind that are chiefly responsible for disturbing the sleep of an adult by preventing him from establishing the mood required for falling asleep—the withdrawing of interest from the world. He does not want to interrupt his life but would rather continue his work on the things he is concerned with, and for that reason he does not fall asleep. In the case of children, therefore, the stimulus that disturbs sleep is a mental one—the wish that has

not been dealt with—and it is to this that they react with the dream.

(5) This gives us the most direct approach to understanding the function of dreams. In so far as a dream is a reaction to a psychical stimulus, it must be equivalent to dealing with the stimulus in such a way that it is got rid of and that sleep can continue. We do not yet know how this dealing with the stimulus by the dream is made possible dynamically, but we see already that *dreams are not disturbers of sleep*, as they are abusively called, but *guardians of sleep which get rid of disturbances of sleep*. We think we should have slept more soundly if there had been no dream, but we are wrong; in fact, without the help of the dream we should not have slept at all. It is due to it that we have slept as soundly as we have. It could not avoid disturbing us a little, just as the night-watchman often cannot help making a little noise while he chases away the disturbers of the peace who seek to waken us with their noise.

(6) What instigates a dream is a wish, and the fulfilment of that wish is the content of the dream—this is one of the chief characteristics of dreams. The other, equally constant one, is that a dream does not simply give expression to a thought, but represents the wish fulfilled as a hallucinatory experience.[1] '*I should like to go on the lake*' is the wish that instigates the dream. The content of the dream itself is: '*I am going on the lake.*' Thus even in these simple children's dreams a difference remains between the latent and the manifest dream, there is a distortion of the latent dream-thought: *the transformation of a thought into an experience.* In the process of interpreting a dream this alteration must first be undone. If this turns out to be the most universal characteristic of dreams, the fragment of dream which I reported to you earlier [p. 121] 'I saw my brother in a box [*Kasten*]' is not to be translated 'my brother is restricting himself [*schränkt sich ein*]' but 'I should like my brother to restrict him-self: *my brother must restrict himself.*' Of the two general characteristics of dreams which I have here brought forward, the second clearly has more prospect of being accepted without

[1] [It will be noted that the two 'chief characteristics' or 'general characteristics of dreams' considered in what follows are not the same as the two 'things common to all dreams' discussed in Lecture V, p. 88 ff. above.]

contradiction than the first. It is only by means of far-reaching investigations that we shall be able to establish the fact that what instigates dreams must always be a wish and cannot be a worry or an intention or a reproach; but this will not affect the other characteristic—that the dream does not simply reproduce this stimulus, but removes it, gets rid of it, deals with it, by means of a kind of experience.

(7) On the basis of these characteristics of dreams, we can return once more to a comparison between a dream and a parapraxis. In the latter we distinguished between a disturbing purpose and a disturbed one [p. 61 ff.], and the parapraxis was a compromise between them. A dream can be fitted into the same pattern. The disturbed purpose can only be that of sleeping. We may replace the disturbing one by the psychical stimulus, or let us say by the wish which presses to be dealt with, since we have not learnt so far of any other psychical stimulus that disturbs sleep. Here the dream, too, is the result of a compromise. One sleeps, but one nevertheless experiences the removing of a wish; óne satisfies a wish, but at the same time one continues to sleep. Both purposes are partly achieved and partly abandoned.

(8) You will recall that at one point [p. 98] we hoped to approach an understanding of the problems of dreams from the fact that certain imaginative structures which are very transparent to us are known as 'day-dreams'. Now these day-dreams are in fact wish-fulfilments, fulfilments of ambitions and erotic wishes which are well known to us; but they are *thought*, even though vividly imagined, and never experienced as hallucinations. Of the two chief characteristics of dreams, then, the less well assured is preserved here, while the other, since it depends on the state of sleep and cannot be realized in waking life, is entirely absent. Linguistic usage, therefore, has a suspicion of the fact that wish-fulfilment is a chief characteristic of dreams. Incidentally, if our experience in dreams is only a modified kind of imagining made possible by the conditions of the state of sleep—that is, a 'nocturnal day-dreaming'—we can already understand how the process of constructing a dream can dispose of the nocturnal stimulus and bring satisfaction, since daydreaming too is an activity bound up with satisfaction and is only practised, indeed, on that account.

But other usages of language express the same sense. There are familiar proverbs such as 'Pigs dream of acorns and geese dream of maize' or 'What do hens dream of?—Of millet.'[1] So proverbs go even lower than we do—below children to animals —and assert that the content of dreams is the satisfaction of a need. Numbers of figures of speech seem to point in the same direction: 'lovely as a dream', 'I shouldn't have dreamt of such a thing', 'I haven't imagined it in my wildest dreams'. In this, linguistic usage is evidently taking sides. For there are anxiety-dreams as well, and dreams with a distressing or indifferent content; but linguistic usage has been unmoved by them. It is true that it knows of 'bad dreams', but a dream pure and simple is only the sweet fulfilment of a wish. Nor is there any proverb which might tell us that pigs or geese dream of being slaughtered.

It is inconceivable, of course, that the wish-fulfilling characteristic of dreams should not have been noticed by writers on the subject. On the contrary, it has often been noticed; but it has not occurred to any of them to recognize this characteristic as a universal one and to make it into a corner-stone for the explanation of dreams. We can well imagine what it is that has held them back from it and we shall go into the matter later on.

But consider what a large amount of light has been thrown on things by our examination of children's dreams, and with scarcely any effort: the functions of dreams as the guardians of sleep; their origin from two concurrent purposes, one of which, the desire for sleep, remains constant, while the other strives to satisfy a psychical stimulus; proof that dreams are psychical acts with a sense; their two chief characteristics—wish-fulfilment and hallucinatory experience. And in discovering all this we were almost able to forget that we were engaged on psycho-analysis. Apart from its connection with parapraxes, our work has carried no specific mark. Any psychologist, knowing nothing of the postulates of psycho-analysis, might have been able to give this explanation of children's dreams. Why have they not done so?

If dreams of the infantile kind were the only ones, the problem would be solved and our task finished, and that without

[1] [A Hungarian and a Jewish proverb respectively. Cf., the end of Chapter III of *I. of D.*]

our questioning the dreamer or bringing in the unconscious or resorting to free association. This is evidently where a continuation of our task lies ahead. We have already found repeatedly that characteristics which were claimed as being of general validity have turned out to apply only to a particular sort and number of dreams. The question for us is therefore whether the general characteristics we inferred from children's dreams have a firmer footing, whether they also hold good of dreams which are not transparently clear and whose manifest content gives no sign of being connected with a wish left over from the previous day. It is our view that these other dreams have undergone a far-reaching distortion and for that reason cannot be judged at a first glance. We suspect too that to explain this distortion we shall need the psycho-analytic technique which we have been able to do without in the understanding we have just gained of children's dreams.

In any case, there is yet another class of dreams which are undistorted and, like children's dreams, can easily be recognized as wish-fulfilments. These are the dreams which all through life are called up by imperative bodily needs—hunger, thirst, sexual need—that is, they are wish-fufilments as reactions to internal somatic stimuli. Thus I have a note of a dream dreamt by a little girl of nineteen months, which consisted of a *menu*, to which her own name was attached: '*Anna F., stwawbewwies, wild stwawbewwies, omblet, pudden!*' This was a reaction to a day without food, owing to a digestive upset, which had actually been traced back to the fruit which appeared twice in the dream. The little girl's grandmother—their combined ages came to seventy years—was simultaneously obliged to go without food for a whole day on account of a disturbance due to a floating kidney. She dreamt the same night that she had been 'asked out' and had been served with the most appetizing delicacies.

Observations on prisoners who have been compelled to starve, and on people who have been subjected to privations on travels and explorations, teach us that under these conditions the satisfaction of their needs is regularly dreamt of. Thus Otto Nordenskjöld (1904, **1**, 336 f.) writes as follows of the members of his expedition while they were wintering in the Antarctic: 'The direction taken by our innermost thoughts was very clearly shown by our dreams, which were never more vivid or numerous than at this time. Even those of us who otherwise dreamt but rarely had long stories to tell in the morning when we exchanged our latest experiences in this world of the imagination. They were all concerned with the outside world which was now so remote from us, though they were often adapted to our actual circumstances. . . . Eating and drinking, however, were the pivot round which our dreams most often revolved. One of us, who had a special gift for attending large luncheon parties during the night, was proud if he was able to report in the morning that he had "got through a three-course dinner". Another of us dreamt of tobacco, of whole mountains of tobacco; while a third dreamt of a ship in full sail coming in across open water. Yet another dream is worth repeating. The postman brought round the mail and gave a long explanation of why we had had to wait so long for it: he had delivered it at the wrong address and had only succeeded in recovering it with great difficulty. We dreamt, of course, of still more impossible things. But there was a most striking lack of imaginativeness shown by almost all the dreams I dreamt myself or heard described. It would certainly be of great psychological interest if all these dreams could be recorded. And it will easily be understood how much we longed for sleep, since it could offer each one of us everything that he most eagerly desired.' So too, according to Du Prel [1885, 231], 'Mungo Park, when he was almost dying of thirst on one of his African journeys, dreamt unceasingly of the well-watered valleys and meadows of his home. Similarly, Baron Trenck, suffering torments of hunger while he was a prisoner in the fortress at Magdeburg, dreamt of being surrounded by sumptuous meals; and George Back, who took part in Franklin's first expedition, when he was almost dying of starvation as a result of his fearful privations, dreamt constantly and regularly of copious meals.' [1]

Anyone who has eaten some highly-spiced dish at dinner and develops a thirst during the night is very likely to dream that he is drinking. [2] It is of course impossible to get rid of a fairly strong need for food or drink by means of a dream. One

[1] [These two quotations appear in a footnote in Chapter III of *I. of D.*]

[2] [A detailed analysis of a dream of this kind is given at the beginning of Chapter III of *I. of D.*]

wakes up from a dream of this sort still feeling thirsty, and has to have a drink of real water. The effect produced by the dream is in this instance trivial from the practical point of view; but it is none the less clear that it was produced with the aim of protecting one's sleep against a stimulus that was urging one to wake up and take action. When the need is of less intensity dreams of satisfaction often help one to get over it.

In the same way, dreams create satisfactions under the influence of sexual stimuli, but these show peculiarities which deserve mention. Since it is characteristic of the sexual instinct to be a degree less dependent on its object than hunger and thirst, the satisfaction in dreams of emission can be a real one; and in consequence of certain difficulties (which I shall have to mention later) in its relation to its object, it happens with special frequency that the real satisfaction is nevertheless attached to a dream content which is obscure or distorted. This characteristic of dreams of emission (as Otto Rank [1912a] has pointed out) makes them particularly favourable subjects for the study of dream-distortion.[1] Furthermore, all adult dreams arising from bodily needs usually contain, in addition to the satisfaction, other material which is derived from purely psychical sources of stimulation and requires interpretation before it can be understood.

Moreover I do not mean to assert that the wish-fulfilment dreams of adults which are constructed on infantile lines only appear as reactions to the imperative needs that I have mentioned. We are acquainted as well with short, clear dreams of this sort which, under the influence of some dominant situation, arise out of what are unquestionably psychical sources of stimulation. There are, for instance, dreams of impatience: if someone has made preparations for a journey, for a theatrical performance that is important to him, for going to a lecture or paying a visit, he may dream of a premature fulfilment of his expectation; he may, during the night before the event, see himself arrived at his destination, present at the theatre, in conversation with the person he is going to visit. Or there are what are justly known as dreams of convenience, in which a person who would like to sleep longer dreams that he is already up and is washing, or is already at school, whereas he is really

---

[1] [This is discussed more fully in Section E of Chapter VI in *I. of D.*]

still sleeping and would rather get up in a dream than in reality.[1] The wish to sleep, which we have recognized as regularly playing a part in the construction of dreams, comes into the open in these dreams and reveals itself in them as the essential dream-constructor. There is good reason for ranking the need to sleep alongside of the other great bodily needs.

Here is a reproduction of a picture by Schwind in the Schack Gallery in Munich [see Frontispiece], which shows how correctly the artist grasped the way in which dreams arise from the dominant situation. Its title is 'The Prisoner's Dream', a dream whose content is bound to be his escape. It is a happy point that he is to escape through the window, for it is the stimulus of the light pouring in by the window that is putting an end to the prisoner's sleep. The gnomes who are clambering up on one another no doubt represent the successive positions which he himself would have had to take as he climbed up to the level of the window; and, if I am not mistaken and am not attributing too much deliberation to the artist, the topmost of the gnomes, who is sawing through the bars—that is, who is doing what the prisoner would like to do—has the same features as himself.

In all dreams other than children's dreams and those of an infantile type our path is, as I have said, obstructed by dream-distortion. We cannot tell, to begin with, whether these other dreams too are wish-fulfilments as we suspect, we cannot guess from their manifest content to what psychical stimulus they owe their origin, and we cannot prove that they too are endeavouring to get rid of that stimulus or in some way deal with it. They must be interpreted—that is, translated—,their distortion must be undone, and their manifest content replaced by their latent one, before we can form a judgement as to whether what we have found in infantile dreams can claim to be valid for all dreams.

[1] [A dream of this type is reported at the beginning of Chapter III in *I. of D.*]

LECTURE IX

THE CENSORSHIP OF DREAMS

LADIES AND GENTLEMEN,—The study of the dreams of children has taught us the origin, the essential nature and the function of dreams. *Dreams are things which get rid of (psychical) stimuli disturbing to sleep, by the method of hallucinatory satisfaction.* We have, however, only been able to explain one group of the dreams of adults—those which we have described as dreams of an infantile type. What the facts are about the others we cannot yet say, but we do not understand them. We have arrived at a provisional finding, however, whose importance we must not under-estimate. Whenever a dream has been completely intelligible to us, it has turned out to be the hallucinated fulfilment of a wish. This coincidence cannot be a chance one nor a matter of indifference.

We have assumed of dreams of another sort [p. 113 f.], on the basis of various considerations and on the analogy of our views on parapraxes, that they are a distorted substitute for an unknown content, and that the first thing is to trace them back to it. Our immediate task, then, is an enquiry which will lead to an understanding of this *distortion in dreams.*

Dream-distortion is what makes a dream seem strange and unintelligible to us. We want to know a number of things about it: firstly, where it comes from—its dynamics—, secondly, what it does and, lastly, how it does it. We can also say that dream-distortion is carried out by the dream-work; and we want to describe the dream-work and trace it back to the forces operating in it.[1]

And now listen to this dream. It was recorded by a lady belonging to our group,[2] and, as she tells us, was derived from a highly-esteemed and cultivated elderly lady. No analysis was made of the dream; our informant remarks that for a psychoanalyst it needs no interpreting. Nor did the dreamer herself interpret it, but she judged it and condemned it as though she

[1] [The dream-work is discussed in Lecture XI.]
[2] Frau Dr. von Hug-Hellmuth [1915].

understood how to interpret it; for she said of it: 'And disgusting, stupid stuff like this was dreamt by a woman of fifty, who has no other thoughts day and night but worry about her child!' [1]

Here, then, is the dream—which deals with 'love services' in war-time.[2] *'She went to Garrison Hospital No. 1 and informed the sentry at the gate that she must speak to the Chief Medical Officer (mentioning a name that was unknown to her) as she wanted to volunteer for service at the hospital. She pronounced the word "service" in such a way that the N.C.O. at once understood that she meant "love service". Since she was an elderly lady, after some hesitation he allowed her to pass. Instead of finding the Chief Medical Officer, however, she reached a large and gloomy apartment in which a number of officers and army doctors were standing and sitting round a long table. She approached a staff surgeon with her request, and he understood her meaning after she had said only a few words. The actual wording of her speech in the dream was: "I and many other women and girls in Vienna are ready to . . ." at this point in the dream her words turned into a mumble ". . . for the troops—officers and other ranks without distinction." She could tell from the expressions on the officers' faces, partly embarrassed and partly sly, that everyone had understood her meaning correctly. The lady went on: "I'm aware that our decision must sound surprising, but we mean it in bitter earnest. No one asks a soldier in the field whether he wishes to die or not." There followed an awkward silence of some minutes. The staff surgeon then put his arm round her waist and said: "Suppose, madam, it actually came to . . . (mumble)." She drew away from him, thinking to herself: "He's like all the rest of them", and replied: "Good gracious, I'm an old woman and I might never come to that. Besides, there's one condition that must be observed: age must be respected. It must never happen that an elderly woman . . . (mumble) . . . a mere boy. That would be terrible." "I understand perfectly," replied the staff surgeon. Some of the officers, and among them one who had been a suitor of hers in her youth, laughed out loud. The lady then asked to be taken to the Chief Medical Officer, with whom she was*

---

[1] [This was during the 1914–18 War, in which one of her sons was engaged on active service.]

[2] [*'Liebesdienste'* means in the first instance 'services performed for love', i.e. 'unremunerated services'; but it could bear another, less respectable, meaning.]

acquainted, so that the whole matter could be thrashed out; but she found, to her consternation, that she could not recall his name. Nevertheless, the staff surgeon, most politely and respectfully, showed her the way up to the second floor by a very narrow, iron, spiral staircase, which led directly from the room to the upper storeys of the building. As she went up she heard an officer say: "That's a tremendous decision to make—no matter whether a woman's young or old! Splendid of her!" Feeling simply that she was doing her duty, she walked up an interminable staircase.

'The dream was repeated twice in the course of a few weeks, with, as the lady remarked, some quite unimportant and meaningless modifications.'[1]

From its continuous nature, the dream resembles a daytime phantasy: there are few breaks in it, and some of the details of its content could have been explained if they had been enquired into, but that, as you know, was not done. But what is remarkable and interesting from our point of view is that the dream shows several gaps—gaps not in the dreamer's memory of the dream but in the content of the dream itself. At three points the content was, as it were, extinguished; the speeches in which these gaps occurred were interrupted by a mumble. As no analysis was carried out, we have, strictly speaking, no right to say anything about the sense of the dream. Nevertheless there are hints on which conclusions can be based (for instance, in the phrase 'love services'); but above all, the portions of the speeches immediately preceding the mumbles call for the gaps to be filled in, and in an unambiguous manner. If we make the insertions, the content of the phantasy turns out to be that the dreamer is prepared, by way of fulfilling a patriotic duty, to put herself at the disposal of the troops, both officers and other ranks, for the satisfaction of their erotic needs. This is, of course, highly objectionable, the model of a shameless libidinal phantasy—but it does not appear in the dream at all. Precisely at the points at which the context would call for this admission, the manifest dream contains an indistinct mumble: something has been lost or suppressed.

You will, I hope, think it plausible to suppose that it was

[1] [This dream was later (in 1919) added as a footnote to *I. of D.* Cf. the beginning of Chapter IV.]

precisely the objectionable nature of these passages that was the motive for their suppression. Where shall we find a parallel to such an event? You need not look far in these days. Take up any political newspaper and you will find that here and there the text is absent and in its place nothing except the white paper is to be seen. This, as you know, is the work of the press censorship. In these empty places there was something that displeased the higher censorship authorities and for that reason it was removed—a pity, you feel, since no doubt it was the most interesting thing in the paper—the 'best bit'.

On other occasions the censorship has not gone to work on a passage *after* it has already been completed. The author has seen in advance which passages might expect to give rise to objections from the censorship and has on that account toned them down in advance, modified them slightly, or has contented himself with approximations and allusions to what would genuinely have come from his pen. In that case there are no blank places in the paper, but circumlocutions and obscurities of expression appearing at certain points will enable you to guess where regard has been paid to the censorship in advance.

Well, we can keep close to this parallel. It is our view that the omitted pieces of the speeches in the dream which were concealed by a mumble have likewise been sacrificed to a censorship. We speak in so many words of a '*dream-censorship*', to which some share in dream-distortion is to be attributed. Wherever there are gaps in the manifest dream the dream-censorship is responsible for them. We should go further, and regard it as a manifestation of the censorship wherever a dream-element is remembered especially faintly, indefinitely and doubtfully among other elements that are more clearly constructed. But it is only rarely that this censorship manifests itself so undisguisedly—so naïvely, one might say—as in this example of the dream of 'love services'. The censorship takes effect much more frequently according to the second method, by producing softenings, approximations and allusions instead of the genuine thing.

I know of no parallel in the operations of the press-censorship to a third manner of working by the dream-censorship; but I am able to demonstrate it from precisely the one example of a dream which we have analysed so far. You will recall the dream of the 'three bad theatre-tickets for 1 florin 50' [p. 122]. In the latent thoughts of that dream the element 'over-hurriedly, too early' stood in the foreground. Thus: it was absurd to marry so *early*—it was also absurd to take the theatre-tickets so *early*—it was ridiculous of the sister-in-law to part with her money in such a *hurry* to buy jewellery with it. Nothing of this central element of the dream-thoughts passed over into the manifest dream; in it the central position is taken by the 'going to the theatre' and 'taking the tickets'. As a result of this displacement of accent, this fresh grouping of the elements of the content, the manifest dream has become so unlike the latent dream-thoughts that no-one would suspect the presence of the latter behind the former. This displacement of accent is one of the chief instruments of dream-distortion and it is what gives the dream the strangeness on account of which the dreamer himself is not inclined to recognize it as his own production.

Omission, modification, fresh grouping of the material—these, then, are the activities of the dream-censorship and the instruments of dream-distortion. The dream-censorship itself is the originator, or one of the originators, of the dream-distortion which we are now engaged in examining. We are in the habit of combining the concepts of modification and re-arrangement under the term 'displacement'.

After these remarks on the activities of the dream-censorship, we will now turn to its dynamics. I hope you do not take the term too anthropomorphically, and do not picture the 'censor of dreams' as a severe little manikin or a spirit living in a closet in the brain and there discharging his office; but I hope too that you do not take the term in too 'localizing' a sense, and do not think of a 'brain-centre', from which a censoring influence of this kind issues, an influence which would be brought to an end if the 'centre' were damaged or removed. For the time being it is nothing more than a serviceable term for describing a dynamic relation. The word does not prevent our asking by what purposes[1] this influence is exercised and against what purposes it is directed. And we shall not be surprised to learn that we have come up against the dream-censorship once already, though perhaps without recognizing it.

[1] [Or, here and in what follows, 'trends'. Cf. footnote 1, p. 40 above.]

For that is in fact the case. You will recall that when we began to make use of our technique of free association we made a surprising discovery. We became aware that our efforts at proceeding from the dream-element to the unconscious element for which it is a substitute were being met by a *resistance* [p. 116]. This resistance, we said, could be of different magnitudes, sometimes enormous and sometimes quite insignificant. In the latter case we need to pass through only a small number of intermediate links in our work of interpretation; but when the resistance is large we have to traverse long chains of associations from the dream-element, we are led far away from it and on our path we have to overcome all the difficulties which represent themselves as critical objections to the ideas that occur. What we met with as resistance in our work of interpretation must now be introduced into the dream-work in the form of the dream-censorship. The resistance to interpretation is only a putting into effect[1] of the dream-censorship. It also proves to us that the force of the censorship is not exhausted in bringing about the distortion of dreams and thereafter extinguished, but that the censorship persists as a permanent institution which has as its aim the maintenance of the distortion. Moreover, just as the strength of the resistance varies in the interpretation of each element in a dream, so too the magnitude of the distortion introduced by the censorship varies for each element in the same dream. If we compare the manifest and the latent dream, we shall find that some particular latent elements have been completely eliminated, others modified to a greater or less extent, while yet others have been carried over into the manifest content of the dream unaltered or even perhaps strengthened.

But we wanted to enquire what are the purposes which exercise the censorship and against what purposes it is directed. Now this question, which is fundamental for the understanding of dreams and perhaps, indeed, of human life, is easy to answer

---

[1] ['*Objektivierung.*' Literally, 'making objective'. The term is used several times in an early paper of Freud's on hypnotic treatment (1892–93) and again in *Studies on Hysteria* (1895d). Freud himself seems to use the term '*Realisierung*' (realization), as a synonym.]

if we look through the series of dreams which have been interpreted. The purposes which exercise the censorship are those which are acknowledged by the dreamer's waking judgement, those with which he feels himself at one. You may be sure that if you reject an interpretation of one of your own dreams which has been correctly carried out, you are doing so for the same motives for which the dream-censorship has been exercised, the dream-distortion brought about and the interpretation made necessary. Take the dream of our fifty-year-old lady [p. 137]. She thought her dream disgusting without having analysed it, and she would have been still more indignant if Dr. von Hug-Hellmuth had told her anything of its inevitable interpretation; it was precisely because of this condemnation by the dreamer that the objectionable passages in her dream were replaced by a mumble.

The purposes *against* which the dream-censorship is directed must be described in the first instance from the point of view of that agency itself. If so, one can only say that they are invariably of a reprehensible nature, repulsive from the ethical, aesthetic and social point of view—matters of which one does not venture to think at all or thinks only with disgust. These wishes, which are censored and given a distorted expression in dreams, are first and foremost manifestations of an unbridled and ruthless egoism. And, to be sure, the dreamer's own ego appears in every dream and plays the chief part in it, even if it knows quite well how to hide itself so far as the manifest content goes. This '*sacro egoismo*' of dreams is certainly not unrelated to the attitude we adopt when we sleep, which consists in our withdrawing our interest from the whole external world.[1]

The ego, freed from all ethical bonds, also finds itself at one with all the demands of sexual desire, even those which have long been condemned by our aesthetic upbringing and those which contradict all the requirements of moral restraint. The desire for pleasure—the 'libido', as we call it—chooses its objects without inhibition, and by preference, indeed, the forbidden ones: not only other men's wives, but above all incestuous objects, objects sanctified by the common agreement of man-

[1] [In a footnote added in 1925 to Section D of Chapter V of *I. of D*. Freud made some qualification of his statement that dreams are entirely egoistic.]

kind, a man's mother and sister, a woman's father and brother. (The dream of our fifty-year-old lady, too, was incestuous; her libido was unmistakably directed to her son. [Cf. footnote 1, p. 137.]) Lusts which we think of as remote from human nature show themselves strong enough to provoke dreams. Hatred, too, rages without restraint. Wishes for revenge and death directed against those who are nearest and dearest in waking life, against the dreamer's parents, brothers and sisters, husband or wife, and his own children are nothing unusual. These censored wishes appear to rise up out of a positive Hell; after they have been interpreted when we are awake, no censorship of them seems to us too severe.

But you must not blame the dream itself on account of its evil content. Do not forget that it performs the innocent and indeed useful function of preserving sleep from disturbance. This wickedness is not part of the essential nature of dreams. Indeed you know too that there are dreams which can be recognized as the satisfaction of justified wishes and of pressing bodily needs. These, it is true, have no dream-distortion; but they have no need of it, for they can fulfil their function without insulting the ethical and aesthetic purposes[1] of the ego. Bear in mind, too, that dream-distortion is proportionate to two factors. On the one hand it becomes greater the worse the wish that has to be censored; but on the other hand it also becomes greater the more severe the demands of the censorship at the moment. Thus a strictly brought-up and prudish young girl, with a relentless censorship, will distort dream-impulses which we doctors, for instance, would have to regard as permissible, harmless, libidinal wishes, and on which in ten years' time the dreamer herself will make the same judgement.

Furthermore, we have not got nearly far enough yet to be able to feel indignant at this result of our work of interpretation. We do not yet, I think, understand it properly; but our first duty is to defend it against certain aspersions. There is no difficulty in finding a weak point in it. Our dream-interpretations are made on the basis of the premisses which we have already accepted [p. 100 f.]—that dreams in general have a sense, that it is legitimate to carry across from hypnotic to normal sleep the fact of the existence of mental processes which

[1] [See footnote, p. 140 above.]

are at the time unconscious, and that everything that occurs to
the mind is determined. If on the basis of these premises we had
arrived at plausible findings from dream-interpretation, we
should have been justified in concluding that the premises
were valid. But how about it if these findings seem to be as I
have pictured them? We should then be tempted to say: 'These
are impossible, senseless or at the least most improbable findings; so there was something wrong about the premises. Either
dreams are not psychical phenomena, or there is nothing
unconscious in the normal state, or our technique has a flaw in
it. Is it not simpler and more satisfactory to suppose this rather
than accept all the abominations which we are supposed to
have discovered on the basis of our premises?'

Yes, indeed! Both simpler and more satisfactory—but not
necessarily on that account more correct. Let us give ourselves
time: the matter is not yet ripe for judgement. And first, we can
further strengthen the criticism of our dream-interpretations.
The fact that the findings from them are so disagreeable and
repellent need not, perhaps, carry very great weight. A stronger
argument is that the dreamers to whom we are led to attribute
such wishful purposes by the interpretation of their dreams
reject them most emphatically and for good reasons. 'What?'
says one of them, 'you want to convince me from this dream
that I regret the money I have spent on my sister's dowry and
my brother's education? But that cannot be so. I work entirely
for my brothers and sisters; I have no other interest in life but
to fulfil my duties to them, which, as the eldest of the family,
I promised our departed mother I would do.' Or a woman
dreamer would say: 'You think I wish my husband was dead?
That is a shocking piece of nonsense! It is not only that we are
most happily married—you would probably not believe me if
I said that—but his death would rob me of everything I possess
in the world.' Or another man would answer us: 'You say that
I have sensual desires for my sister? That is ridiculous! She
means nothing at all to me. We are on bad terms with each
other and I have not exchanged a word with her for years.' We
might still take it lightly, perhaps, if these dreamers neither
confirmed nor denied the purposes we attribute to them; we
might say that these were just things they did not know about
themselves. But when they feel in themselves the precise con-

trary of the wish we have interpreted to them and when they are able to prove to us by the lives they lead that they are dominated by this contrary wish, it must surely take us aback. Has not the time come to throw aside the whole work we have done on dream-interpretation as something which its findings have reduced *ad absurdum*?

No, not even now. Even this stronger argument collapses if we examine it critically. Granted that there are unconscious purposes in mental life, nothing is proved by showing that purposes opposed to these are dominant in conscious life. Perhaps there is room in the mind for contrary purposes, for contradictions, to exist side by side. Possibly, indeed, the dominance of one impulse is precisely a necessary condition of its contrary being unconscious. We are after all left, then, with the first objections that were raised: the findings of dream-interpretation are not simple and they are very disagreeable. We may reply to the first that all your passion for what is simple will not be able to solve a single one of the problems of dreams. You must get accustomed here to assuming a complicated state of affairs. And we may reply to the second that you are plainly wrong to use a liking or disliking that you may feel as the ground for a scientific judgement. What difference does it make if the findings of dream-interpretation seem disagreeable to you or, indeed, embarrassing and repulsive? '*Ça n'empêche pas d'exister*', as I heard my teacher Charcot say in a similar case when I was a young doctor.[1] One must be humble and hold back one's sympathies and antipathies if one wants to discover what is real in this world. If a physicist were able to prove to you that in a short period organic life on this earth would be brought to an end by freezing, would you venture to make the same reply to him: 'That cannot be so, the prospect is too disagreeable'? You would, I think, be silent, until another physicist came and pointed out to the first one an error in his premisses or calculations. When you reject something that is disagreeable to you, what you are doing is *repeating* the

[1] [Charcot's remark in full was: '*La théorie, c'est bon, mais ça n'empêche pas d'exister.*' ('Theory is good; but it doesn't prevent thing from existing' A favourite quotation of Freud's. See his obituary of Charcot (1893*f*), where the circumstances are described.]

mechanism of constructing dreams rather than understanding it and surmounting it.

You will promise now, perhaps, to disregard the repellent character of the censored dream-wishes and will withdraw upon the argument that after all it is unlikely that such a large space should be given to the evil in the constitution of human beings. But do your own experiences justify your saying this? I will not discuss how you may appear to yourselves; but have you found so much benevolence among your superiors and competitors, so much chivalry among your enemies and so little envy in your social surroundings that you feel it your duty to protest against egoistic evil having a share in human nature? Are you not aware of how uncontrolled and untrustworthy the average person is in everything to do with sexual life? Or do you not know that all the transgressions and excesses of which we dream at night are daily committed in real life by waking men? What does psycho-analysis do here but confirm Plato's old saying that the good are those who are content to dream of what the others, the bad, really do?[1]

And now turn your eyes away from individuals and consider the Great War which is still laying Europe waste. Think of the vast amount of brutality, cruelty and lies which are able to spread over the civilized world. Do you really believe that a handful of ambitious and deluding men without conscience could have succeeded in unleashing all these evil spirits if their millions of followers did not share their guilt? Do you venture, in such circumstances, to break a lance on behalf of the exclusion of evil from the mental constitution of mankind?[2]

You will represent to me that I am giving a one-sided judgement on the War: that it has also brought to light what is finest and noblest in men, their heroism, their self-sacrifice, their social sense. No doubt; but are you not now showing yourselves as accessories to the injustice that has so often been done to psycho-analysis in reproaching it with denying one thing because it has asserted another? It is not our intention to dispute the noble endeavours of human nature, nor have we ever done anything

[1] [Quoted in 'The Moral Sense in Dreams' in *I. of D.,* Chap. I.]
[2] [Freud's strongest impeachment of the destructive side of human nature was made in Chapters V and VI of *Civilization and its Discontents* (1930a), (Norton, 1962).]

to detract from their value. On the contrary; I am exhibiting to you not only the evil dream-wishes which are censored but also the censorship, which suppresses them and makes them unrecognizable. We lay a stronger emphasis on what is evil in men only because other people disavow it and thereby make the human mind, not better, but incomprehensible. If now we give up this one-sided ethical valuation, we shall undoubtedly find a more correct formula for the relation between good and evil in human nature.

There it is, then. We need not give up the findings of our work on the interpretation of dreams even though we cannot but regard them as strange. Perhaps we shall be able to approach an understanding of them later from another direction. For the time being let us hold fast to this: dream-distortion is a result of the censorship which is exercised by recognized purposes of the ego against wishful impulses in any way objectionable that stir within us at night-time during our sleep. Why this should happen particularly at night-time and where these reprehensible wishes come from—these are matters on which, no doubt, much still remains for questioning and research.

But it would be unfair if we neglected at this point to emphasize sufficiently another outcome of our investigations. The dream-wishes which seek to disturb us in our sleep are unknown to us and indeed we only learnt of them through dream-interpretation. They are thus to be described, in the sense we have discussed, as unconscious for the time being. But we must reflect that they are unconscious too for more than the time being. The dreamer also disavows them, as we have seen in so many instances, after he has come to know them through the interpretation of his dream. We are then faced once again with the position we first came across in the 'hiccoughing' slip of the tongue [p. 49], where the proposer of the toast protested indignantly that neither then nor at any earlier time had he become conscious of any disrespectful impulse towards his Chief. Already at the time we felt some doubts about the weight of an assurance of this kind, and suggested instead the hypothesis that the speaker was permanently unaware of the presence of this impulse in him. This situation is repeated now with every interpretation of a strongly distorted dream and consequently gains an increased importance in its bearing on the view we have taken. We are now prepared to assume that there are in the mind processes and purposes of which one knows nothing at all, has known nothing for a long time, and has even perhaps never known anything. With this the unconscious acquires a new sense for us; the characteristic of 'for the time being' or 'temporary' disappears from its essential nature. It can mean *permanently* unconscious and not merely 'latent at the time'. We shall of course have to hear more about this on some other occasion.

SYMBOLISM IN DREAMS[1]

LADIES AND GENTLEMEN,—We have found that the distortion
in dreams, which interferes with our understanding of them, is
the result of a censoring activity which is directed against unacceptable, unconscious wishful impulses. We have not, of
course, maintained that the censorship is the sole factor responsible for the distortion in dreams, and in fact when we study
them further we can discover that other factors play a part in
producing this result. This amounts to our saying that even if
the dream-censorship was out of action we should still not be
in a position to understand dreams, the manifest dream would
still not be identical with the latent dream-thoughts.

We come upon this other factor which prevents dreams from
being lucid, this new contribution to dream-distortion, by
noticing a gap in our technique. I have already admitted to
you [p. 105] that it does sometimes really happen that nothing
occurs to a person under analysis in response to particular
elements of his dreams. It is true that this does not happen as
often as he asserts; in a great many cases, with perseverance,
an idea is extracted from him. But nevertheless there remain
cases in which an association fails to emerge or, if it *is* extracted,
does not give us what we expected from it. If this happens
during a psycho-analytic treatment, it has a peculiar significance with which we are not here concerned.[2] But it also

---

[1] [As Freud tells us in *The Interpretation of Dreams,* it was
relatively late before he realized the full importance of dream-
symbolism, largely under the influence of Wilhelm Stekel (1911).
It was not until the fourth (1914) edition of *The Interpretation
of Dreams* that a special section was devoted to the subject. That
section (Chapter VI, Section E) represents, apart from the present
lecture, Freud's main discussion of symbolism. The topic appears,
of course, in many other places both in *The Interpretation of
Dreams* and in other works throughout Freud's life, and references to these will be found at a few points below. It may be
added, however, that the present lecture has claims to being regarded as the most important of all Freud's writings on symbolism.]

[2] [The reference here is to the blocking of free associations by
unconscious stirring-up of the transference. Cf. 'The Dynamics
of Transference' (1912*b*). See also Lecture XXVII below].

happens in the interpretation of normal people's dreams or in that of our own. If we convince ourselves that in such cases no amount of pressure is of any use, we eventually discover that this unwished-for event regularly occurs in connection with particular dream-elements, and we begin to recognize that a fresh general principle is at work where we had begun by thinking we were only faced by an exceptional failure of technique.

In this way we are tempted to interpret these 'mute' dream-elements ourselves, to set about translating them with our own resources. We are then forced to recognize that whenever we venture on making a replacement of this sort we arrive at a satisfactory sense for the dream, whereas it remains senseless and the chain of thought is interrupted so long as we refrain from intervening in this way. An accumulation of many similar cases eventually gives the necessary certainty to what began as a timid experiment.

I am putting all this in a rather schematic way; but that is permissable, after all, for didactic purposes, nor has it been falsified, but merely simplified.

In this way we obtain constant translations for a number of dream-elements—just as popular 'dream-books' provide them for *everything* that appears in dreams. You will not have forgotten, of course, that when we use our *associative* technique constant replacements of dream-elements never come to light.

You will object at once that this method of interpretation strikes you as far more insecure and open to attack than the earlier one by means of free association. There is, however, something further. For when, with experience, we have collected enough of these constant renderings, the time comes when we realize that we should in fact have been able to deal with these portions of dream-interpretation from our own knowledge, and that they could really be understood without the dreamer's associations. How it is that we must necessarily have known their meaning will become clear in the second half of our present discussion.

A constant relation of this kind between a dream-element and its translation is described by us as a 'symbolic' one, and the dream-element itself as a 'symbol' of the unconscious dream-thought. You will recall that earlier, when we were investigating the relations between dream-elements and the 'genuine' thing behind them, I distinguished three such relations—those of a part to a whole, of allusion and of plastic portrayal. I warned you at the time that there was a fourth, but I did not name it [p. 122]. This fourth relation is the symbolic one which I am now introducing. It gives occasion for some most interesting discussions, and I will turn to them before laying before you the detailed results of our observations of symbolism.

Symbolism is perhaps the most remarkable chapter of the theory of dreams. In the first place, since symbols are stable translations, they realize to some extent the ideal of the ancient as well as of the popular interpretation of dreams, from which, with our technique, we had departed widely. They allow us in certain circumstances to interpret a dream without questioning the dreamer, who indeed would in any case have nothing to tell us about the symbol. If we are acquainted with the ordinary dream-symbols, and in addition with the dreamer's personality, the circumstances in which he lives and the impressions which preceded the occurrence of the dream, we are often in a position to interpret a dream straightaway—to translate it at sight, as it were. A piece of virtuosity of this kind flatters the dream-interpreter and impresses the dreamer; it forms an agreeable contrast to the laborious work of questioning the dreamer. But do not allow yourselves to be led astray by this. It is not our business to perform acts of virtuosity. Interpretation based on a knowledge of symbols is not a technique which can replace or compete with the associative one. It forms a supplement to the latter and yields results which are only of use when introduced into it. And as regards acquaintance with the dreamer's psychical situation, you must bear in mind that the dreams of people you know well are not the only ones you have to analyse, that you are not as a rule familiar with the events of the previous day, which were the instigators of the dream, but that the associations of the person you are analysing will provide you precisely with a knowledge of what we call the psychical situation.

Moreover it is quite specially remarkable—having regard, too, to some considerations which we shall mention later [cf. p. 169]—that the most violent resistances have been expressed once again to the existence of a symbolic relation between dreams and the unconscious. Even people of judgement and reputation, who, apart from this, have gone a long way in agreeing with psycho-analysis, have at this point withheld their support. This behaviour is all the stranger in view, first, of the fact that symbolism is not peculiar to dreams alone and is not characteristic of them, and, secondly, that symbolism in dreams is by no means a discovery of psycho-analysis, however many other surprising discoveries it has made. The philosopher K. A. Scherner (1861) must be described as the discoverer of dream-symbolism, if its beginning is to be placed in modern times at all. Psycho-analysis has confirmed Scherner's findings, though it has made material modifications in them.

You will now want to hear something of the nature of dream-symbolism and to be given some examples of it. I will gladly tell you what I know, though I must confess that our understanding of it does not go as far as we should like.

The essence of this symbolic relation is that it is a comparison, though not a comparison of *any* sort. Special limitations seem to be attached to the comparison, but it is hard to say what these are. Not everything with which we can compare an object or a process appears in dreams as a symbol for it. And on the other hand a dream does not symbolize every possible element of the latent dream-thoughts but only certain definite ones. So there are restrictions here in both directions. We must admit, too, that the concept of a symbol cannot at present be sharply delimited: it shades off into such notions as those of a replacement or representation, and even approaches that of an allusion. With a number of symbols the comparison which underlies them is obvious. But again there are other symbols in regard to which we must ask ourselves where we are to look for the common element, the *tertium comparationis*, of the supposed comparison. On further reflection we may afterwards discover it or it may definitely remain concealed. It is strange, moreover, that if a symbol is a comparison it should not be brought to light by an association, and that the dreamer should not be acquainted with it but should make use of it without knowing about it: more than that, indeed, that the dreamer feels no inclination to acknowledge the comparison even after it has been pointed out to him. You see, then, that a symbolic relation is a comparison of a quite special kind, of which we do not as yet clearly grasp the basis, though perhaps we may later arrive at some indication of it.

The range of things which are given symbolic representation in dreams is not wide: the human body as a whole, parents, children, brothers and sisters, birth, death, nakedness—and something else besides. The one typical—that is regular— representation of the human figure as a whole is a *house*, as was recognized by Scherner, who even wanted to give this symbol a transcendant importance which it does not possess. It may happen in a dream that one finds oneself climbing down the façade of a house, enjoying it at one moment, frightened at another. The houses with smooth walls are men, the ones with projections and balconies that one can hold on to are women [cf. p. 159 below]. One's parents appear in dreams as the *Emperor* and *Empress*, the *King* and *Queen* [loc. cit.] or other honoured personages; so here dreams are displaying much filial piety. They treat children and brothers and sisters less tenderly: these are symbolized as *small animals* or *vermin*. Birth is almost invariably represented by something which has a connection with *water*: one either falls into the water or climbs out of it, one rescues someone from the water or is rescued by someone—that is to say, the relation is one of mother to child [cf. p. 160]. Dying is replaced in dreams by *departure*, by a *train journey* [cf. p. 161], being dead by various obscure and, as it were, timid hints, nakedness by *clothes* and *uniforms*. You see how indistinct the boundaries are here between symbolic and allusive representation.

It is a striking fact that, compared with this scanty enumeration, there is another field in which the objects and topics are represented with an extraordinarily rich symbolism. This field is that of sexual life—the genitals, sexual processes, sexual intercourse. The very great majority of symbols in dreams are sexual symbols. And here a strange disproportion is revealed. The topics I have mentioned are few, but the symbols for them are extremely numerous, so that each of these things can be expressed by numbers of almost equivalent symbols. The outcome, when they are interpreted, gives rise to general objection.

For, in contrast to the multiplicity of the representations in the dream, the interpretations of the symbols are very monotonous, and this displeases everyone who hears of it; but what is there that we can do about it?

Since this is the first time I have spoken of the subject-matter of sexual life in one of these lectures, I owe you some account of the way in which I propose to treat the topic. Psycho-analysis finds no occasion for concealments and hints, it does not think it necessary to be ashamed of dealing with this important material, it believes it is right and proper to call everything by its correct name, and it hopes that this will be the best way of keeping irrelevant thoughts of a disturbing kind at a distance. The fact that these lectures are being given before a mixed audience of both sexes can make no difference to this. Just as there can be no science *in usum Delphini*,[1] there can be none for schoolgirls; and the ladies among you have made it clear by their presence in this lecture-room that they wish to be treated on an equality with men.

The male genitals, then, are represented in dreams in a number of ways that must be called symbolic, where the common element in the comparison is mostly very obvious. To begin with, for the male genitals as a whole the sacred number 3 is of symbolic significance [cf. p. 163 f.]. The more striking and for both sexes the more interesting component of the genitals, the male organ, finds symbolic substitutes in the first instance in things that resemble it in shape—things, accordingly, that are long and up-standing, such as *sticks, umbrellas, posts, trees* and so on; further, in objects which share with the thing they represent the characteristic of penetrating into the body and injuring—thus, sharp *weapons* of every kind, *knives, daggers, spears, sabres,* but also fire-arms, *rifles, pistols* and *revolvers* (particularly suitable owing to their shape). In the anxiety dreams of girls, being followed by a man with a knife or a fire-arm plays a large part. This is perhaps the commonest instance of dream-symbolism and you will now be able to translate it easily. Nor is there any difficulty in understanding how it is that the male organ can be replaced by objects from which water flows—

1 [Cf. footnote 2, p. 102.]

water-taps, *watering-cans*, or *fountains*—or again by other objects which are capable of being lengthened, such as *hanging-lamps*, *extensible pencils*, etc. A no less obvious aspect of the organ explains the fact that *pencils*, *pen-holders*, *nail-files*, *hammers*, and other *instruments* are undoubted male sexual symbols.

The remarkable characteristic of the male organ which enables it to rise up in defiance of the laws of gravity, one of the phenomena of erection, leads to its being represented symbolically by *balloons*, *flying-machines* and most recently by *Zeppelin airships*. But dreams can symbolize erection in yet another, far more expressive manner. They can treat the sexual organ as the essence of the dreamer's whole person and make him himself *fly*. Do not take it to heart if dreams of flying, so familiar and often so delightful, have to be interpreted as dreams of general sexual excitement, as erection-dreams. Among students of psycho-analysis, Paul Federn [1914] has placed this interpretation beyond any doubt; but the same conclusion was reached from his investigations by Mourly Vold [1910–12, **2**, 791], who has been so much praised for his sobriety, who carried out the dream-experiments I have referred to [p. 87] with artificially arranged positions of the arms and legs and who was far removed from psycho-analysis and may have known nothing about it. And do not make an objection out of the fact that women can have the same flying dreams as men. Remember, rather, that our dreams aim at being the fulfilments of wishes and that the wish to be a man is found so frequently, consciously or unconsciously, in women. Nor will anyone with a knowledge of anatomy be bewildered by the fact that it is possible for women to realize this wish through the same sensations as men. Women possess as part of their genitals a small organ similar to the male one; and this small organ, the clitoris, actually plays the same part in childhood and during the years before sexual intercourse as the large organ in men.[1]

Among the less easily understandable male sexual symbols are certain *reptiles* and *fishes*, and above all the famous symbol of the *snake*. It is certainly not easy to guess why *hats* and *overcoats* or *cloaks* are employed in the same way, but their symbolic significance is quite unquestionable [cf. p. 157]. And finally we can ask ourselves whether the replacement of the

[1] [This is further discussed on p. 318 below.]

male limb by another limb, the foot or the hand, should be described as symbolic. We are, I think, compelled to do so by the context and by counterparts in the case of women.

The female genitals are symbolically represented by all such objects as share their characteristic of enclosing a hollow space which can take something into itself: by *pits, cavities* and *hollows,* for instance, by *vessels* and *bottles,* by *receptacles, boxes, trunks, cases, chests, pockets,* and so on. *Ships,* too, fall into this category. Some symbols have more connection with the uterus than with the female genitals: thus, *cupboards, stoves* and, more especially, *rooms.* Here room-symbolism touches on house-symbolism. *Doors* and *gates,* again, are symbols of the genital orifice. Materials, too, are symbols for women [cf. p. 160]: *wood, paper* and objects made of them, like *tables* and *books.* Among animals, *snails* and *mussels* at least are undeniably female symbols; among parts of the body, the *mouth* (as a substitute for the genital orifice); among buildings, *churches* and *chapels.* Not every symbol, as you will observe, is equally intelligible.

The breasts must be reckoned with the genitals, and these, like the larger hemispheres of the female body, are represented by *apples, peaches,* and *fruit* in general. The pubic hair of both sexes is depicted in dreams as *woods* and *bushes.* The complicated topography of the female genital parts makes one understand how it is that they are often represented as *landscapes,* with rocks, woods and water,[1] while the imposing mechanism of the male sexual apparatus explains why all kinds of complicated machinery which is hard to describe serve as symbols for it.

Another symbol of the female genitals which deserves mention is a *jewel-case.*[2] *Jewel* and *treasure* are used in dreams as well as in waking life to describe someone who is loved. *Sweets* frequently represent sexual enjoyment. Satisfaction obtained from a person's own genitals is indicated by all kinds of *playing,* including *piano-playing.* Symbolic representations *par excellence* of masturbation are *gliding* or *sliding* and *pulling off a branch* [cf. p. 164]. The *falling out of a tooth* or the *pulling out of a tooth* is a particularly notable dream-symbol. Its first meaning is

[1] [A dream with a quantity of landscape symbolism is reported below, p. 193.]

[2] [This played a prominent part in the analysis of the first dream in the case history of 'Dora' (1905e).]

undoubtedly castration as a punishment for masturbating [loc. cit.]. We come across special representations of sexual intercourse less often than might be expected from what has been said so far. Rhythmical activities such as *dancing, riding* and *climbing* must be mentioned here, as well as violent experiences such as *being run over;* so, too, certain *manual crafts,* and, of course, *threatening with weapons.*

You must not picture the use or the translation of these symbols as something quite simple. In the course of them all kinds of things happen which are contrary to our expectations. It seems almost incredible, for instance, that in these symbolic representations the differences between the sexes are often not clearly observed. Some symbols signify genitals in general, irrespective of whether they are male or female: for instance, a *small* child, a *small* son or a *small* daughter.[1] Or again, a predominantly male symbol may be used for the female genitals or vice versa. We cannot understand this till we have obtained some insight into the development of sexual ideas in human beings. In some instances the ambiguity of the symbols may only be an apparent one; and the most marked symbols, such as *weapons, pockets* and *chests* are excluded from this bisexual use.

I will now go on to make a survey, starting not from the thing represented but from the symbol, of the fields from which sexual symbols are mostly derived, and I will make a few additional remarks, with special reference to the symbols where the common element in the comparison is not understood. The *hat* is an obscure symbol of this kind—perhaps, too, head-coverings in general—with a male significance as a rule, but also capable of a female one.[2] In the same way an *overcoat* or *cloak* means a man, perhaps not always with a genital reference; it is open to you to ask why.[3] Neckties, which hang down and are not worn

[1] [That is, any one of these three may be used in a dream as a symbol for either the male or the female genitals.]

[2] [Hat-symbolism was discussed by Freud in his short paper 'A Connection between a Symbol and a Symptom' (1916c).]

[3] In *I. of D.,* VI(E), Freud suggests that the explanation may be a verbal assonance between '*Mann* and '*Mantel*' (the German for 'overcoat' or 'cloak'). A further discussion of this symbol occurs in Lecture XXIX of the *New Introductory Lectures* (1933a), p. 488 below.]

by women, are a definitely male symbol. *Underclothing* and *linen* in general are female. *Clothes* and *uniforms*, as we have already seen, are a substitute for nakedness or bodily shapes. *Shoes* and *slippers* are female genitals. *Tables* and *wood* have already been mentioned as puzzling but certainly female symbols. *Ladders*, *steps* and *staircases*, or, more precisely, walking on them, are clear symbols of sexual intercourse. On reflection, it will occur to us that the common element here is the rhythm of walking up them—perhaps, too, the increasing excitement and breathlessness the higher one climbs [cf. p. 164].

We have earlier referred to *landscapes* as representing the female genitals. *Hills* and *rocks* are symbols of the male organ. *Gardens* are common symbols of the female genitals. *Fruit* stands, not for children, but for the breasts. *Wild animals* mean people in an excited sensual state, and further, evil instincts or passions. *Blossoms* and *flowers* indicate women's genitals, or, in particular, virginity. Do not forget that blossoms are actually the genitals of plants.[1]

We are acquainted already with *rooms* as a symbol. The representation can be carried further, for windows, and doors in and out of rooms, take over the meaning of orifices in the body. And the question of the room being *open* or *locked* fits in with this symbolism, and the *key* that opens it is a decidedly male symbol.

Here, then, is material used for symbolism in dreams. It is not complete and could be carried deeper as well as further. But I fancy it will seem to you more than enough and may even have exasperated you. 'Do I really live in the thick of sexual symbols?' you may ask. 'Are all the objects around me, all the clothes I put on, all the things I pick up, all of them sexual symbols and nothing else?' There is really ground enough for raising astonished questions, and, as a first one, we may enquire how we in fact come to know the meaning of these dream-symbols, upon which the dreamer himself gives us insufficient information or none at all.

My reply is that we learn it from very different sources— from fairy tales and myths, from buffoonery and jokes, from

[1] [A dream with a large amount of flower symbolism is reported in Section C of Chapter VI of *I. of D.* See also Section D of that chapter.]

folklore (that is, from knowledge about popular manners and customs, sayings and songs) and from poetic and colloquial linguistic usage. In all these directions we come upon the same symbolism, and in some of them we can understand it without further instruction. If we go into these sources in detail, we shall find so many parallels to dream-symbolism that we cannot fail to be convinced of our interpretations.

According to Scherner, as we have said [p. 153], the human body is often represented in dreams by the symbol of a house. Carrying this representation further, we found that windows, doors and gates stood for openings in the body and that façades of houses were either smooth or provided with balconies and projections to hold on to. But the same symbolism is found in our linguistic usage—when we greet an acquaintance familiarly as an 'altes Haus' ['old house'], when we speak of giving someone 'eins aufs Dachl' [a knock on the head, literally, 'one on the roof'], or when we say of someone else that 'he's not quite right in the upper storey'. In anatomy the orifices of the body are in so many words termed 'Leibespforten' [literally, 'portals of the body'].

It seems surprising at first to find one's parents in dreams as an imperial or royal couple. But it has its parallel in fairy tales. It begins to dawn on us that the many fairy tales which begin 'Once upon a time there were a King and Queen' only mean to say that there were once a father and mother. In a family the children are jokingly called 'princes' and the eldest 'crown prince'. The King himself calls himself the father of his country. We speak of small children jokingly as 'Würmer' ['worms'] and speak sympathetically of a child as 'der arme Wurm' ['the poor worm'].

Let us go back to house-symbolism. When in a dream we make use of the projections on houses for catching hold of, we may be reminded of a common vulgar expression for well-developed breasts: 'She's got something to catch hold of.' There is another popular expression in such cases: 'She's got plenty of wood in front of the house', which seems to confirm our interpretation of wood as a female, maternal symbol.

And, speaking of wood, it is hard to understand how that material came to represent what is maternal and female. But here comparative philology may come to our help. Our German word '*Holz*' seems to come from the same root as the Greek '*ὕλη* [hulē]', meaning 'stuff' 'raw material'. This seems to be an instance of the not uncommon event of the general name of a material eventually coming to be reserved for some particular material. Now there is an island in the Atlantic named 'Madeira'. This name was given to it by the Portuguese when they discovered it, because at that time it was covered all over with woods. For in the Portuguese language '*madeira*' means 'wood'. You will notice, however, that '*madeira*' is only a slightly modified form of the Latin word '*materia*', which once more means 'material' in general. But '*materia*' is derived from '*mater*', 'mother': the material out of which anything is made is, as it were, a mother to it. This ancient view of the thing survives, therefore, in the symbolic use of wood for 'woman' or 'mother'.

Birth is regularly expressed in dreams by some connection with water: one falls into the water or one comes out of the water—one gives birth or one is born. We must not forget that this symbol is able to appeal in two ways to evolutionary truth, Not only are all terrestrial mammals, including man's ancestors. descended from aquatic creatures (this is the more remote of the two facts), but every individual mammal, every human being, spent the first phase of its existence in water—namely as an embryo in the amniotic fluid in its mother's uterus, and came out of that water when it was born. I do not say that the dreamer knows this; on the other hand, I maintain that he need not know it. There is something else that the dreamer probably knows from having been told it in his childhood; and I even maintain of that too that his knowledge of it contributed nothing to the construction of the symbol. He was told in his nursery that the stork brings the babies. But where does it fetch them from? From the pond, or from the stream—once again, then, from the water. One of my patients after he had been given this information—he was a little Count at the time —disappeared for a whole afternoon. He was found at last lying by the edge of the castle pool, with his little face bending over the surface of the water eagerly peering down to try and see the babies at the bottom. [Cf. p. 318 below.]

In myths about the birth of heroes—to which Otto Rank [1909] has devoted a comparative study, the oldest being that of King Sargon of Agade (about 2800 B.C.)—a predominant part is played by exposure in the water and rescue from the water. Rank has perceived that these are representations of birth, analogous to those that are usual in dreams. If one rescues someone from the water in a dream, one is making oneself into his mother, or simply into *a* mother. In myths a person who rescues a baby from the water is admitting that she is the baby's true mother. There is a well-known comic anecdote according to which an intelligent Jewish boy was asked who the mother of Moses was. He replied without hesitation: 'The Princess.' 'No', he was told, 'she only took him out of the water.' 'That's what *she* says', he replied, and so proved that he had found the correct interpretation of the myth.[1]

Departure in dreams means dying. So, too, if a child asks where someone is who has died and whom he misses, it is common nursery usage to reply that he has gone on a journey. Once more I should like to contradict the belief that the dream-symbol is derived from this evasion. The dramatist is using the same symbolic connection when he speaks of the after-life as 'the undiscovered country from whose bourn no *traveller* returns'. Even in ordinary life it is common to speak of 'the last journey'. Every one acquainted with ancient rituals is aware of how seriously (in the religion of Ancient Egypt, for instance) the idea is taken of a journey to the land of the dead. Many copies have survived of *The Book of the Dead*, which was supplied to the mummy like a Baedeker to take with him on the journey. Ever since burial-places have been separated from dwelling-places the dead person's last journey has indeed become a reality.

It is just as little the case that genital symbolism is something that is found only in dreams. Every one of you has probably at one time or another spoken impolitely of a woman as an '*alte Schachtel*' ['old box'], perhaps without knowing that you were using a genital symbol. In the New Testament we find woman referred to as 'the weaker vessel'. The Hebrew scriptures, written in a style that comes close to poetry, are full of sexually symbolic expressions, which have not always been correctly understood and whose exegesis (for instance, in the case of the

---

[1] [Freud used this 'correct interpretation of the myth' as the basis of his last work, *Moses and Monotheism* (1939a).]

Song of Solomon[1]) has led to some misunderstandings. In later Hebrew literature it is very common to find a woman represented by a house, whose door stands for the sexual orifice. A man complains, for instance, in a case of lost virginity, that he has 'found the door open'. So, too, the symbol of a table for a woman in these writings. Thus, a woman says of her husband: 'I laid the table for him, but he turned it round.' Lame children are said to come about through the man's 'turning the table round'. I take these examples from a paper by Dr. L. Levy of Brünn [1914].

The fact that ships, too, in dreams stand for women is made credible by the etymologists, who tell us that '*Schiff* [ship]' was originally the name of an earthenware vessel and is the same word as '*Schaff*' [a dialect word meaning 'tub']. That ovens represent women and the uterus is confirmed by the Greek legend of Periander of Corinth and his wife Melissa. The tyrant, according to Herodotus, conjured up the shade of his wife, whom he had loved passionately but had murdered out of jealousy, to obtain some information from her. The dead woman proved her identity by saying that he (Periander) had '*pushed his bread into a cold oven*', as a disguise for an event which no one else could know of. In the periodical *Anthropophyteia*, edited by F. S. Krauss, an invaluable source of knowledge of sexual anthropology,[2] we learn that in a particular part of Germany they say of a woman who has given birth to a child that '*her oven has come to pieces*'. Kindling fire, and everything to do with it, is intimately interwoven with sexual symbolism. Flame is always a male genital, and the hearth is its female counterpart.

If you may have felt surprised at the frequency with which landscapes are used in dreams to represent the female genitals, you can learn from mythology the part played by *Mother Earth* in the concepts and cults of the peoples of antiquity and how their view of agriculture was determined by this symbolism. You will perhaps be inclined to trace the fact that in dreams a room represents a woman to the common usage in our language by which '*Frau*' is replaced by '*Frauenzimmer*'[3]—the

[1] [Some examples are given in Section D of Chapter VI of *I. of D.*]

[2] [Cf. Freud's appreciative letter to Krauss (1910*f*).]

[3] [Literally 'woman's apartment'. The word is very often used in German as a slightly derogatory synonym for 'woman'.]

human being is replaced by the apartment allotted to her. Similarly we speak of the 'Sublime Porte'[1], meaning the Sultan and his government. So too the title of the Ancient Egyptian ruler, 'Pharaoh', means simply 'Great Courtyard'. (In the Ancient East the courts between the double gateways of a city were public meeting-places like the market-places of the classical world.) This derivation, however, appears to be too superficial. It seems to me more likely that a room became the symbol of a woman as being the space which encloses human beings. We have already found 'house' used in a similar sense; and mythology and poetical language enable us to add 'city', 'citadel', 'castle' and 'fortress' as further symbols for 'woman'. The question could be easily settled from the dreams of people who do not speak or understand German. During the last few years I have mainly treated foreign-speaking patients, and I seem to remember that in their dreams too '*Zimmer*' ['room'] meant '*Frauenzimmer*', though they had no similar usage in their languages. There are other indications that the symbolic relation can go beyond the limits of language—which, incidentally was asserted long ago by an old investigator of dreams, Schubert [1814]. However, none of my dreamers were completely ignorant of German, so the decision must be left to psychoanalysts who can collect data from unilingual people in other countries.

There is scarcely one of the symbolic representations of the male genitals which does not recur in joking, vulgar or poetic usage, especially in the ancient classical dramatists. But here we meet not only the symbols which appear in dreams, but others besides—for instance tools employed in various operations, and particularly the plough. Moreover, the symbolic representation of masculinity leads us to a very extensive and much disputed region, which, on grounds of economy, we shall avoid. I should like, however, to devote a few words to one symbol, which, as it were, falls outside this class—the number 3.[2] Whether this number owes its sacred character to this symbolic connection remains undecided. But what seems certain is that a number of tripartite things that occur in nature—the clover leaf, for

---

[1] [Literally, 'Gateway', the old diplomatic term for the Ottoman Court at Constantinople before 1923, derived *via* the French from the Turkish title.]   [2] [Cf. p. 220 below.]

instance—owe their use for coats of arms and emblems to this symbolic meaning. Similarly, the tripartite lily—the so-called *fleur-de-lis*—and the remarkable heraldic device of two islands so far apart as Sicily and the Isle of Man—the *triskeles* (three bent legs radiating from a centre)—seem to be stylized versions of the male genitals. Likenesses of the male organ were regarded in antiquity as the most powerful *apotropaic* (means of defence) against evil influences, and, in conformity with this, the lucky charms of our own day can all be easily recognized as genital or sexual symbols. Let us consider a collection of such things—as they are worn, for instance, in the form of small silver hanging trinkets: a four-leaved clover, a pig, a mushroom, a horse-shoe, a ladder, a chimney-sweep. The four-leaved clover has taken the place of the three-leaved one which is really suited to be a symbol. The pig is an ancient fertility symbol. The mushroom is an undoubted penis-symbol: there are mushrooms [fungi] which owe their systematic name (*Phallus impudicus*) to their unmistakable resemblance to the male organ. The horseshoe copies the outline of the female genital orifice, while the chimney-sweep, who carries the ladder, appears in this company on account of his activities, with which sexual intercourse is vulgarly compared. (Cf. *Anthropophyteia*.) We have made the acquaintance of his ladder in dreams as a sexual symbol; here German linguistic usage comes to our help and shows us how the word '*steigen*' ['to climb', or 'to mount'] is used in what is *par excellence* a sexual sense. We say '*den Frauen nachsteigen*' ['to run' (literally 'climb') 'after women'], and '*ein alter Steiger*' ['an old rake' (literally 'climber')]. In French, in which the word for steps on a staircase is '*marches*', we find a precisely analogous term '*un vieux marcheur*'. The fact that in many large animals climbing or 'mounting' on the female is a necessary preliminary to sexual intercourse probably fits into this context.[1]

'Pulling off a branch' as a symbolic representation of masturbation is not merely in harmony with vulgar descriptions of the act[2] but has far-reaching mythological parallels. But that masturbation, or rather the punishment for it—castration—, should be represented by the falling out or pulling out of teeth

[1] [This is largely repeated from Freud's Nuremberg Congress paper (1910*d*).]
[2] [Cf. the English 'tossing off'.]

is especially remarkable, since there is a counterpart to it in anthropology which can be known to only a very small number of dreamers. There seems to me no doubt that the circumcision practised by so many peoples is an equivalent and substitute for castration. And we now learn that certain primitive tribes in Australia carry out circumcision as a puberty rite (at the festival to celebrate a boy's attaining sexual maturity), while other tribes, their near neighbours, have replaced this act by the knocking out of a tooth.

Here I bring my account of these specimens to an end. They are only specimens. We know more on the subject; but you may imagine how much richer and more interesting a collection like this would be if it were brought together, not by amateurs like us, but by real professionals in mythology, anthropology, philology and folklore.

A few consequences force themselves on our notice; they cannot be exhaustive, but they offer us food for reflection.

In the first place we are faced by the fact that the dreamer has a symbolic mode of expression at his disposal which he does not know in waking life and does not recognize. This is as extraordinary as if you were to discover that your housemaid understood Sanskrit, though you know that she was born in a Bohemian village and never learnt it. It is not easy to account for this fact by the help of our psychological views. We can only say that the knowledge of symbolism is unconscious[1] to the dreamer, that it belongs to his unconscious mental life. But even with this assumption we do not meet the point. Hitherto it has only been necessary for us to assume the existence of unconscious endeavours—endeavours, that is, of which, temporarily or permanently, we know nothing. Now, however, it is a question of more than this, of unconscious pieces of knowledge, of connections of thought, of comparisons between different objects which result in its being possible for one of them to be regularly put in place of the other. These comparisons are not freshly made on each occasion; they lie ready to hand and are complete, once and for all. This is implied by the fact of their agreeing in the case of different individuals—possibly, indeed, agreeing in spite of differences of language. What can

[1] [Cf. footnote, p. 21.]

be the origin of these symbolic relations? Linguistic usage covers only a small part of them. The multiplicity of parallels in other spheres of knowledge are mostly unknown to the dreamer; we ourselves have been obliged to collect them laboriously.

Secondly, these symbolic relations are not something peculiar to dreamers or to the dream-work through which they come to expression. This same symbolism, as we have seen, is employed by myths and fairy tales, by the people in their sayings and songs, by colloquial linguistic usage and by the poetic imagination. The field of symbolism is immensely wide, and dream-symbolism is only a small part of it: indeed, it serves no useful purpose to attack the whole problem from the direction of dreams. Many symbols which are commonly used elsewhere appear in dreams very seldom or not at all. Some dream-symbols are not to be found in all other fields but only, as you have seen, here and there. One gets an impression that what we are faced with here is an ancient but extinct mode of expression, of which different pieces have survived in different fields, one piece only here, another only there, a third, perhaps, in slightly modified forms in several fields. And here I recall the phantasy of an interesting psychotic patient, who imagined a 'basic language' of which all these symbolic relations would be residues.[1]

Thirdly, it must strike you that the symbolism in the other fields I have mentioned is by no means solely sexual symbolism, whereas in dreams symbols are used almost exclusively for the expression of sexual objects and relations. This is not easily explained either. Are we to suppose that symbols which originally had a sexual significance later acquired another application and that, furthermore, the toning-down of representation by symbols into other kinds of representation may be connected with this? These questions can evidently not be answered so long as we have considered dream-symbolism alone. We can only hold firmly to the suspicion that there is a specially intimate relation between true symbols and sexuality.

In this connection we have been given an important hint

[1] [This was Senatspräsident Schreber, whose case history was analysed by Freud (1911c).]

during the last few years. A philologist, Hans Sperber [1912], of Uppsala, who works independently of psycho-analysis, has put forward the argument that sexual needs have played the biggest part in the origin and development of speech. According to him, the original sounds of speech served for communication, and summoned the speaker's sexual partner; the further development of linguistic roots accompanied the working activities of primal man. These activities, he goes on, were performed in common and were accompanied by rhythmically repeated utterances. In this way a sexual interest became attached to work. Primal man made work acceptable, as it were, by treating it as an equivalent and substitute for sexual activity. The words enunciated during work in common thus had two meanings; they denoted sexual acts as well as the working activity equated with them. As time went on, the words became detached from the sexual meaning and fixed to the work. In later generations the same thing happened with new words, which had a sexual meaning and were applied to new forms of work. In this way a number of verbal roots would have been formed, all of which were of sexual origin and had subsequently lost their sexual meaning. If the hypothesis I have here sketched out is correct, it would give us a possibility of understanding dream-symbolism. We should understand why dreams, which preserve something of the earliest conditions, have such an extraordinarily large number of sexual symbols, and why, in general, weapons and tools always stand for what is male, while materials and things that are worked upon stand for what is female. The symbolic relation would be the residue of an ancient verbal identity; things which were once called by the same name as the genitals could now serve as symbols for them in dreams.

The parallels we have found to dream-symbolism also allow us to form an estimate of the characteristic of psycho-analysis which enables it to attract general interest in a way in which neither psychology nor psychiatry has succeeded in doing. In the work of psycho-analysis links are formed with numbers of other mental sciences, the investigation of which promises results of the greatest value: links with mythology and philology, with folklore, with social psychology and the theory of religion. You will not be surprised to hear that a periodical has grown up on psycho-analytic soil whose sole aim is to foster these links. This periodical is known as *Imago*, founded in 1912 and edited by Hanns Sachs and Otto Rank.[1] In all these links the share of psycho-analysis is in the first instance that of giver and only to a less extent that of receiver. It is true that this brings it an advantage in the fact that its strange findings become more familiar when they are met with again in other fields; but on the whole it is psycho-analysis which provides the technical methods and the points of view whose application in these other fields should prove fruitful. The mental life of human individuals, when subjected to psycho-analytic investigation, offers us the explanations with the help of which we are able to solve a number of riddles in the life of human communities or at least to set them in a true light.

Incidentally, I have said nothing at all to you yet as to the circumstances in which we can obtain our deepest insight into the hypothetical 'primal language' and as to the field in which most of it has survived. Until you know this you cannot form an opinion of its whole significance. For this field is that of the neuroses and its material is the symptoms and other manifestations of neurotic patients, for the explanation and treatment of which psycho-analysis was, indeed, created.

The fourth of my reflections takes us back to the beginning and directs us along our prescribed path. I have said [p. 149] that even if there were no dream-censorship dreams would still not be easily intelligible to us, for we should still be faced with the task of translating the symbolic language of dreams into that of our waking thought. Thus symbolism is a second and independent factor in the distortion of dreams, alongside of the dream-censorship. It is plausible to suppose, however, that the dream-censorship finds it convenient to make use of symbolism, since it leads towards the same end—the strangeness and incomprehensibility of dreams.

It will shortly become clear whether a further study of dreams may not bring us up against yet another factor that contributes to the distortion of dreams. But I should not like to leave the subject of dream-symbolism without once more [p. 152] touch-

[1] [It ceased publication in 1941. A journal with a similar aim, *The American Imago*, was founded by Hanns Sachs in Boston in 1939.]

ing on the problem of how it can meet with such violent resistance in educated people when the wide diffusion of symbolism in myths, religion, art and language is so unquestionable. May it not be that what is responsible is once again its connection with sexuality?

LECTURE XI

THE DREAM-WORK[1]

LADIES AND GENTLEMEN,—When you have thoroughly grasped
the dream-censorship and representation by symbols, you will
not yet, it is true, have completely mastered the distortion in
dreams, but you will nevertheless be in a position to understand
most dreams. In doing so you will make use of both of the two
complementary techniques: calling up ideas that occur to the
dreamer till you have penetrated from the substitute to the
genuine thing and, on the ground of your own knowledge, replacing the symbols by what they mean. Later on we shall discuss some uncertainties that arise in this connection.

We can now take up once more a task that we tried to carry
out previously with inadequate means, when we were studying
the relations between the elements of dreams and the genuine
things they stood for. We laid down four main relations of the
kind [p. 120 ff.]: the relation of a part to a whole, approximation
or allusion, the symbolic relation and the plastic representation
of words. We now propose to undertake the same thing on a
larger scale, by comparing the manifest content of a dream *as a
whole* with the latent dream as it is revealed by interpretation.

I hope you will never again confuse these two things with
each other. If you reach that point, you will probably have gone
further in understanding dreams than most readers of my *Interpretation of Dreams*. And let me remind you once again that the
work which transforms the latent dream into the manifest one
is called the *dream-work*. The work which proceeds in the contrary direction, which endeavours to arrive at the latent dream
from the manifest one, is our *work of interpretation*. This work of
interpretation seeks to undo the dream-work. The dreams of
infantile type which we recognize as obvious fulfilments of
wishes have nevertheless experienced some amount of dream-
work—they have been transformed from a wish into an actual
experience and also, as a rule, from thoughts into visual images.

[1] [The whole of Chapter VI of *I. of D.* (over a third of the entire book)
is devoted to the dream-work.]

170

In their case there is no need for interpretation but only for un-
doing these two transformations. The additional dream-work
that occurs in other dreams is called 'dream-distortion', and
this has to be undone by our work of interpretation.

Having compared the interpretations of numerous dreams, I
am in a position to give you a summary description of what the
dream-work does with the material of the latent dream-
thoughts. I beg you, however, not to try to understand too much
of what I tell you. It will be a piece of description which should
be listened to with quiet attention.

The first achievement of the dream-work is *condensation*.[1] By
that we understand the fact that the manifest dream has a
smaller content than the latent one, and is thus an abbreviated
translation of it. Condensation can on occasion be absent; as a
rule it is present, and very often it is enormous. It is never
changed into the reverse; that is to say, we never find that the
manifest dream is greater in extent or content than the latent
one. Condensation is brought about (1) by the total omission
of certain latent elements, (2) by only a fragment of some complexes in the latent dream passing over into the manifest one
and (3) by latent elements which have something in common
being combined and fused into a single unity in the manifest
dream.

If you prefer it, we can reserve the term 'condensation' for
the last only of these processes. Its results are particularly easy
to demonstrate. You will have no difficulty in recalling instances from your own dreams of different people being condensed into a single one. A composite figure of this kind may
look like A perhaps, but may be dressed like B, may do something that we remember C doing, and at the same time we may
know that he is D. This composite structure is of course emphasizing something that the four people have in common. It is
possible, naturally, to make a composite structure out of things
or places in the same way as out of people, provided that the
various things and places have in common something which is
emphasized by the latent dream. The process is like constructing a new and transitory concept which has this common

[1] [Condensation is discussed, with numerous examples, in Section A of Chapter VI of *I. of D.*]

element as its nucleus. The outcome of this superimposing of the separate elements that have been condensed together is as a rule a blurred and vague image, like what happens if you take several photographs on the same plate.[1]

The production of composite structures like these must be of great importance to the dream-work, since we can show that, where in the first instance the common elements necessary for them were missing, they are deliberately introduced—for instance, through the choice of the words by which a thought is expressed. We have already come across condensations and composite structures of this sort. They played a part in the production of some slips of the tongue. You will recall the young man who offered to '*begleitdigen*' ['*begleiten* (accompany)' + '*beleidigen* (insult)', p. 33] a lady. Moreover, there are jokes of which the technique is based on a condensation like this.[2] But apart from these cases, it may be said that the process is something quite unusual and strange. It is true that counterparts to the construction of these composite figures are to be found in some creations of our imagination, which is ready to combine into a unity components of things that do not belong together in our experience—in the centaurs, for instance, and the fabulous beasts which appear in ancient mythology or in Böcklin's pictures. The 'creative' imagination, indeed, is quite incapable of *inventing* anything; it can only combine components that are strange to one another. But the remarkable thing about the procedure of the dream-work lies in what follows. The material offered to the dream-work consists of thoughts—a few of which may be objectionable and unacceptable, but which are correctly constructed and expressed. The dream-work puts these thoughts into another form, and it is a strange and incomprehensible fact that in making this translation (this rendering, as it were, into another script or language) these methods of merging or combining are brought into use. After all, a translation normally endeavours to preserve the distinctions made in the text and particularly to keep things that are similar separate. The dream-work, quite the contrary, tries to condense

[1] [Freud more than once compared the result of condensation with Francis Galton's 'composite photographs', e.g. Chapter IV of *I of D*.]

[2] [This technique is discussed, with many examples, in the first section of Chapter II of Freud's book on jokes (1905c), (Norton, 1960).]

two different thoughts by seeking out (like a joke) an ambiguous word in which the two thoughts may come together. We need not try to understand this feature all at once, but it may become important for our appreciation of the dream-work.

But although condensation makes dreams obscure, it does not give one the impression of being an effect of the dream-censorship. It seems traceable rather to some mechanical or economic factor, but in any case the censorship profits by it.

The achievements of condensation can be quite extraordinary. It is sometimes possible by its help to combine two quite different latent trains of thought into one manifest dream, so that one can arrive at what appears to be a sufficient interpretation of a dream and yet in doing so can fail to notice a possible 'over-interpretation'.[1]

In regard to the connection between the latent and the manifest dream, condensation results also in no simple relation being left between the elements in the one and the other. A manifest element may correspond simultaneously to several latent ones, and, contrariwise, a latent element may play a part in several manifest ones—there is, as it were, a criss-cross relationship [cf. p. 125]. In interpreting a dream, moreover, we find that the associations to a single manifest element need not emerge in succession: we must often wait till the whole dream has been interpreted.

Thus the dream-work carries out a very unusual kind of transcription of the dream-thoughts: it is not a word-for-word or a sign-for-sign translation; nor is it a selection made according to fixed rules—as though one were to reproduce only the consonants in a word and to leave out the vowels; nor is it what might be described as a representative selection—one element being invariably chosen to take the place of several; it is something different and far more complicated.

The second achievement of the dream-work is *displacement*.[2] Fortunately we have made some preliminary examination of

---

[1] [This is commented on at several points in *I. of D.*, e.g., near the end of Chapter VII, Section A. An example of such a second interpretation will be found in Chapter IV in *I. of D.*]

[2] [Displacement is the subject of Section B of Chapter VI of *I. of D.*, but it comes up for discussion at a great many other places in the book.]

this: for we know that it is entirely the work of the dream-censorship. It manifests itself in two ways: in the first, a latent element is replaced not by a component part of itself but by something more remote—that is, by an allusion; and in the second, the psychical accent is shifted from an important element on to another which is unimportant, so that the dream appears differently centred and strange.

Replacing something by an allusion to it is a process familiar in our waking thought as well, but there is a difference. In waking thought the allusion must be easily intelligible, and the substitute must be related in its subject-matter to the genuine thing it stands for. Jokes, too, often make use of allusion. They drop the precondition of there being an association in subject-matter, and replace it by unusual external[1] associations such as similarity of sound, verbal ambiguity, and so on. But they retain the precondition of intelligibility: a joke would lose all its efficiency if the path back from the allusion to the genuine thing could not be followed easily.[2] The allusions employed for displacement in dreams have set themselves free from both of these restrictions. They are connected with the element they replace by the most external and remote relations and are therefore unintelligible; and when they are undone, their interpretation gives the impression of being a bad joke[3] or of an arbitrary and forced explanation dragged in by the hair of its head. For the dream-censorship only gains its end if it succeeds in making it impossible to find the path back from the allusion to the genuine thing.

Displacement of accent is unheard-of as a method of expressing thoughts. We sometimes make use of it in waking thought in order to produce a comic effect. I can perhaps call up the impression it produces of going astray if I recall an anecdote. There was a blacksmith in a village, who had committed a capital offence. The Court decided that the crime must be

[1] [An 'external' association is one that is based not on the *meaning* of the two associated words, but on superficial connections (such as similarity of sound) or purely accidental ones.]

[2] [An account of the 'allusion' technique of jokes with a number of examples appears in Section II of Chapter II of the book on jokes (1905c), (Norton, 1960). The necessity for their being easily intelligible is discussed ibid., 150.]

[3] [This is further discussed on p. 235 f. below.]

punished; but as the blacksmith was the only one in the village and was indispensable, and as on the other hand there were three tailors living there, one of *them* was hanged instead.[1]

The third achievement of the dream-work is psychologically the most interesting. It consists in transforming thoughts into visual images.[2] Let us keep it clear that this transformation does not affect *everything* in the dream-thoughts; some of them retain their form and appear as thoughts or knowledge in the manifest dream as well; nor are visual images the only form into which thoughts are transformed. Nevertheless they comprise the essence of the formation of dreams; this part of the dream-work is, as we already know, the second most regular one [p. 129], and we have already made the acquaintance of the 'plastic' representation of words in the case of individual dream-elements [p. 121].

It is clear that this achievement is not an easy one. To form some idea of its difficulties, let us suppose that you have undertaken the task of replacing a political leading article in a newspaper by a series of illustrations. You will thus have been thrown back from alphabetic writing to picture writing. In so far as the article mentioned people and concrete objects you will replace them easily and perhaps even advantageously by pictures; but your difficulties will begin when you come to the representation of abstract words and of all those parts of speech which indicate relations between thoughts—such as particles, conjunctions and so on. In the case of abstract words you will be able to help yourselves out by means of a variety of devices. For instance, you will endeavour to give the text of the article a different wording, which may perhaps sound less usual but which will contain more components that are concrete and capable of being represented. You will then recall that most abstract words are 'watered-down' concrete ones, and you will for that reason hark back as often as possible to the original concrete meaning of such words. Thus you will be pleased to find

---

[1] [This was a favourite anecdote of Freud's. He told it ten years earlier than this in his book on jokes (1905c), p. 206, and again eight years later in *The Ego and the Id* (1923b),   (Norton, 1960), p. 45.]

[2] [The main discussion of this is in Section C of Chapter VI of *I. of D.*]

that you can represent the 'possession' of an object by a real, physical sitting down on it.[1] And the dream-work does just the same thing. In such circumstances you will scarcely be able to expect very great accuracy from your representation: similarly, you will forgive the dream-work for replacing an element so hard to put into pictures as, for example, 'adultery' [*'Ehebruch'*, literally, 'breach of marriage'], by another breach—a broken leg [*'Beinbruch'*].[2] And in this way you will succeed to

---

[1] [The German word *'besitzen'* ('to possess') is more obviously connected with sitting than its English equivalent (*'sitzen'* = 'to sit'). An example of 'sitting down on' in a dream with the meaning of 'possession' occurred in one of the dreams of 'Little Hans'. See Section II of his case history (1909*b*), *Standard Ed.*, **10**, 37 and 39.]

[2] While I am correcting the proofs of these pages chance has put into my hands a newspaper cutting which offers an unexpected confirmation of what I have written above:—

'DIVINE PUNISHMENT

'A Broken Arm for a Broken Marriage.

'Frau Anna M., wife of a militiaman, sued Frau Klementine K. for adultery. According to the statement of claim, Frau K. had carried on an illicit relationship with Karl M., while her own husband was at the front and was actually making her an allowance of 70 Kronen [about £3.10 or $17] a month. Frau K. had already received a considerable amount of money from the plaintiff's husband, while she and her child had to live in hunger and poverty. Fellow-soldiers of her husband had informed her that Frau K. had visited taverns with M. and had sat there drinking till far into the night. On one occasion the defendant had asked the plaintiff's husband in the presence of several other soldiers whether he would not get a divorce soon from "his old woman" and set up with her. Frau K.'s caretaker also reported that she had repeatedly seen the plaintiff's husband in the house most incompletely dressed.

'Before a court in the Leopoldstadt [district of Vienna] Frau K. yesterday denied knowing M., so that there could be no question of her having intimate relations with him.

'A witness, Albertine M., stated, however, that she had surprised Frau K. kissing the plaintiff's husband.

'At a previous hearing, M., under examination as a witness, had denied having intimate relations with the defendant. Yesterday the Judge received a letter in which the witness withdrew the statements he had made on the earlier occasion and admitted that he had had a love-affair with Frau K. up till the previous June. He had only denied his relations with the defendant at the former hearing because she had come to him before the hearing and begged him on her knees to save her and say nothing. "Today", the witness wrote, "I feel compelled some extent in compensating for the clumsiness of the picture writing that is supposed to take the place of the alphabetic script.

For representing the parts of speech which indicate relations between thoughts—'because', 'therefore', 'however', etc.—you will have no similar aids at your disposal; those constituents of the text will be lost so far as translation into pictures goes. In the same way, the dream-work reduces the content of the dream-thoughts to its raw material of objects and activities. You will feel pleased if there is a possibility of in some way hinting, through the subtler details of the pictures, at certain relations not in themselves capable of being represented. And just so does the dream-work succeed in expressing some of the content of the latent dream-thoughts by peculiarities in the *form* of the manifest dream—by its clarity or obscurity, by its division into several pieces, and so on. The number of part-dreams into which a dream is divided usually corresponds to the number of main topics or groups of thoughts in the latent dream. A short introductory dream will often stand in the relation of a prelude to a following, more detailed, main dream or may give the motive for it[1]; a subordinate clause in the dream-thoughts will be replaced by the interpolation of a change of scene into the manifest dream, and so on. Thus the form of dreams is far from being without significance and itself calls for interpretation. When several dreams occur during the same night, they often have the same meaning and indicate that an attempt is being made to deal more and more efficiently with a stimulus of increasing insistence. In individual dreams a particularly difficult element may be represented by several symbols —by 'doublets'.[2]

If we make a series of comparisons between the dream-thoughts and the manifest dreams which replace them, we

---

to make a full confession to the Court, for I have broken my left arm and this seems to me to be a divine punishment for my wrong-doing."

'The Judge stated that the penal offence had lapsed under the statute of limitations. The plaintiff then withdrew her claim and the defendant was discharged.'

[1] [This is discussed, with an example, in Section C of Chapter VI of *I. of D.*]

[2] [In philology the term is used of two different words with the same etymology: e.g. 'fashion' and 'faction', both from the Latin '*factio*'.]

shall come upon all kinds of things for which we are unprepared: for instance, that nonsense and absurdity in dreams have
their meaning. At this point, indeed, the contrast between the
medical and the psycho-analytic view of dreams reaches a pitch
of acuteness not met with elsewhere. According to the former,
dreams are senseless because mental activity in dreams has
abandoned all its powers of criticism; according to our view,
on the contrary, dreams become senseless when a piece of criticism included in the dream-thoughts—a judgement that 'this is
absurd'—has to be represented. The dream you are familiar
with of the visit to the theatre ('three tickets for 1 florin 50')
[p. 122] is a good example of this. The judgement it expressed
was: 'it was absurd to marry so early.' [1]

Similarly, in the course of our work of interpretation we
learn what it is that corresponds to the doubts and uncertainties
which the dreamer so often expresses as to whether a particular
element occurred in a dream, whether it was this or whether,
on the contrary, it was something else. There is as a rule nothing in the latent dream-thoughts corresponding to these doubts
and uncertainties; they are entirely due to the activity of the
dream-censorship and are to be equated with an attempt at
elimination which has not quite succeeded. [2]

Among the most surprising findings is the way in which the
dream-work treats contraries that occur in the latent dream.
We know already [p. 171] that conformities in the latent
material are replaced by condensations in the manifest dream.
Well, contraries are treated in the same way as conformities,
and there is a special preference for expressing them by the
same manifest element. Thus an element in the manifest dream
which is capable of having a contrary may equally well be expressing either itself or its contrary or both together: only the
sense can decide which translation is to be chosen. This connects with the further fact that a representation of 'no'—or at
any rate an unambiguous one—is not to be found in dreams.

A welcome analogy to this strange behaviour of the dream-

[1] [Absurdity in dreams is discussed in Section G of Chapter VI
of *I. of D.*]
[2] [Cf. Section A of Chapter VII in *I. of D.* Doubt as a symptom
of obsessional neurosis is discussed in Lecture XVII (p. 259 f. below).]

work is provided for us in the development of language. Some philologists have maintained that in the most ancient languages contraries such as 'strong—weak', 'light—dark', 'big—small' are expressed by the same verbal roots. (What we term 'the antithetical meaning of primal words.') Thus in Ancient Egyptian *'ken'* originally meant 'strong' and 'weak'. In speaking, misunderstanding from the use of such ambivalent words was avoided by differences of intonation and by the accompanying gesture, and in writing, by the addition of what is termed a 'determinative'—a picture which is not itself intended to be spoken. For instance, *'ken'* meaning 'strong' was written with a picture of a little upright man after the alphabetic signs; when *'ken'* stood for 'weak', what followed was the picture of a man squatting down limply. It was only later, by means of slight modifications of the original homologous word, that two distinct representations were arrived at of the contraries included in it. Thus from *'ken'* 'strong—weak' were derived *'ken'* 'strong' and *'kan'* weak'. The remains of this ancient antithetical meaning seem to have been preserved not only in the latest developments of the oldest languages but also in far younger ones and even in some that are still living. Here is some evidence of this, derived from K. Abel (1884).[1]

In Latin, words that remained ambivalent in this way are *'altus'* ('high' and 'deep') and *'sacer'* ('sacred' and 'accursed').

As instances of modifications of the same root I may mention *'clamare'* ('to cry'), *'clam'* ('softly', 'quietly', 'secretly'); *'siccus'* ('dry'), *'succus'* ('juice'). And in German: *'Stimme'* ['voice'], *'stumm'* ['dumb'].

If we compare related languages, there are numerous examples. In English, 'to lock'; in German, *'Loch'* ['hole'] and *'Lücke'* ['gap']. In English, 'to cleave'; in German, *'kleben'* ['to stick'].

The English word 'without' (which is really 'with—without') is used to-day for 'without' alone. 'With', in addition to its combining sense, originally had a removing one; this is still to be seen in the compounds 'withdraw' and 'withhold'. Similarly with the German *'wieder'* ['together with' and *'wider'* 'against'].

---

[1] [Freud wrote a long review of Abel's monograph (1910e), from which much of what he says here is quoted in a condensed form. He returns to the subject in Lecture XV, p. 229 f. below.]

Another characteristic of the dream-work also has its counterpart in the development of language. In Ancient Egyptian, as well as in other, later languages, the order of the sounds in a word can be reversed, while keeping the same meaning. Examples of this in English and German are: '*Topf*' ['pot']— 'pot'; 'boat'—'tub'; 'hurry'—*Ruhe*' ['rest']; '*Balken*' ['beam']— '*Kloben*' ['log'] and 'club'; 'wait'—'*täuwen*' ['tarry']. Similarly in Latin and German: '*capere*'—'*packen*' ['to seize']; '*ren*'—'*Niere*' ['kidney'].

Reversals like this, which occur here with individual words, take place in various ways in the dream-work. We already know reversal of meaning, replacement of something by its opposite [p. 178]. Besides this we find in dreams reversals of situation, of the relation between two people—a 'topsy-turvy' world. Quite often in dreams it is the hare that shoots the sportsman. Or again we find a reversal in the order of events, so that what precedes an event causally comes after it in the dream —like a theatrical production by a third-rate touring company, in which the hero falls down dead and the shot that killed him is not fired in the wings till afterwards. Or there are dreams where the whole order of the elements is reversed, so that to make sense in interpreting it we must take the last one first and the first one last. You will remember too from our study of dream-symbolism that going or falling into the water means the same as coming out of it—that is, giving birth or being born [p. 153], and that climbing up a staircase or a ladder is the same thing as coming down it [p. 158]. It is not hard to see the advantage that dream-distortion can derive from this freedom of representation.

These features of the dream-work may be described as *archaic*. They are equally characteristic of ancient systems of expression by speech and writing and they involve the same difficulties, which we shall have to discuss again later in a critical sense.[1]

And now a few more considerations. In the case of the dream-work it is clearly a matter of transforming the latent thoughts which are expressed in words into sensory images, mostly of a visual sort. Now our thoughts originally arose from sensory images of that kind: their first material and their preliminary

[1] [See Lecture XIII below.]

stages were sense impressions, or, more properly, mnemic images of such impressions. Only later were words attached to them and the words in turn linked up into thoughts. The dream-work thus submits thoughts to a *regressive* treatment[1] and un-does their development; and in the course of the regression everything has to be dropped that had been added as a new acquisition in the course of the development of the mnemic images into thoughts.

Such then, it seems, is the dream-work. As compared with the processes we have come to know in it, interest in the manifest dream must pale into insignificance. But I will devote a few more remarks to the latter, since it is of it alone that we have immediate knowledge.

It is natural that we should lose some of our interest in the manifest dream. It is bound to be a matter of indifference to us whether it is well put together, or is broken up into a series of disconnected separate pictures. Even if it has an apparently sensible exterior, we know that this has only come about through dream-distortion and can have as little organic relation to the internal content of the dream as the façade of an Italian church has to its structure and plan. There are other occasions when this façade of the dream *has* its meaning, and reproduces an important component of the latent dream-thoughts with little or no distortion. But we cannot know this before we have submitted the dream to interpretation and have been able to form a judgement from it as to the amount of distortion that has taken place. A similar doubt arises when two elements in a dream appear to have been brought into a close relation to each other. This may give us a valuable hint that we may bring to-gether what corresponds to these elements in the latent dream as well; but on other occasions we can convince ourselves that what belongs together in the dream-thoughts has been torn apart in the dream.

In general one must avoid seeking to explain one part of the manifest dream by another, as though the dream had been coherently conceived and was a logically arranged narrative. On the contrary, it is as a rule like a piece of breccia, com-posed of various fragments of rock held together by a binding

[1] [The subject of 'regression' is discussed at length in Lecture XXII.]

medium, so that the designs that appear on it do not belong to the original rocks imbedded in it. And there is in fact one part of the dream-work, known as 'secondary revision',[1] whose business it is to make something whole and more or less coherent out of the first products of the dream-work. In the course of this, the material is arranged in what is often a completely misleading sense and, where it seems necessary, interpolations are made in it.

On the other hand, we must not over-estimate the dream-work and attribute too much to it. The achievements I have enumerated exhaust its activity; it can do no more than condense, displace, represent in plastic form and subject the whole to a secondary revision.[2] What appear in the dream as expressions of judgement, of criticism, of astonishment or of inference—none of these are achievements of the dream-work and they are very rarely expressions of afterthoughts about the dream; they are for the most part portions of the latent dream-thoughts which have passed over into the manifest dream with a greater or less amount of modification and adaptation to the context. Nor can the dream-work compose speeches. With a few assignable exceptions, speeches in dreams are copies and combinations of speeches which one has heard or spoken oneself on the day before the dream and which have been included in the latent thoughts either as material or as the instigator of the dream.[3] The dream-work is equally unable to carry out calculations. Such of them as appear in the manifest dream are mostly combinations of numbers, sham calculations which are quite senseless *quâ* calculations and are once again only copies of calculations in the latent dream-thoughts.[4] In these circumstances it is not to be wondered at that the interest which had turned to the dream-work soon tends to move away from it to the latent dream-thoughts, which are revealed, distorted to a greater or less degree, by the manifest dream. But there is no justification for carrying this shift of interest so far that, in looking at the matter theoretically, one replaces the dream entirely

[1] [This is the subject of Section I of Chapter VI of *I. of D.*]

[2] [Elsewhere Freud excluded secondary revision from the dream-work, cf. 'An Evidential Dream' (1913*a*).]

[3] [Cf. *I. of D.*, Last part of Section F of Chapter VI.]

[4] [Cf. *I. of D.*, the discussion of calculations in dreams in Chapter VI(F).]

by the latent dream-thoughts and makes some assertion about the former which only applies to the latter. It is strange that the findings of psycho-analysis could be misused to bring about this confusion. One cannot give the name of 'dream' to anything other than the product of the dream-work—that is to say, the *form* into which the latent thoughts have been transmuted by the dream-work. [Cf. p. 222 ff.]

The dream-work is a process of quite a singular kind, of which the like has not yet become known in mental life. Condensations, displacements, regressive transformations of thoughts into images—such things are novelties whose discovery has already richly rewarded the labours of psycho-analysis. And you can see once more, from the parallels to the dream-work, the connections which have been revealed between psycho-analytic studies and other fields—especially those concerned in the development of speech and thought.[1] You will only be able to form an idea of the further significance of these discoveries when you learn that the mechanism of dream-construction is the model of the manner in which neurotic symptoms arise.

I am also aware that we are not yet able to make a survey of the whole of the new acquisitions which these studies have brought to psychology. I will only point out the fresh proofs they have provided of the existence of unconscious mental acts —for this is what the latent dream-thoughts are—and what an unimaginably broad access to a knowledge of unconscious mental life we are promised by the interpretation of dreams.

But now the time has no doubt come for me to demonstrate to you from a variety of small examples of dreams what I have been preparing you for in the course of these remarks.

[1] [See also some remarks on the construction of jokes on p. 235 f. below.]

LECTURE XII

SOME ANALYSES OF
SAMPLE DREAMS

LADIES AND GENTLEMEN,—You must not be disappointed if I once again put before you fragments of dream-interpretations instead of inviting you to take part in the interpretation of a nice big dream. You will argue that after so many preparations you have a right to it, and you will express your conviction that after so many thousands of dreams have been successfully interpreted, it should have been possible long since to have brought together a collection of excellent sample dreams on which all our assertions about the dream-work and the dream-thoughts could be demonstrated. Just so. But the difficulties that stand in the way of the fulfilment of your wish are too many.

In the first place I must admit that no one carries on the interpretation of dreams as his main occupation. How does it come about, then, that people do interpret them? Occasionally, with no particular end in view, one may interest oneself in the dreams of an acquaintance, or one may work through one's own dreams for a time in order to train oneself in psycho-analytic work; but for the most part what one has to deal with are the dreams of neurotic patients who are under psycho-analytic treatment. These latter dreams are excellent material and are in no way inferior to those of healthy people; but the technique of the treatment necessitates our subordinating dream-interpretation to therapeutic aims, and we have to allow a whole number of dreams to drop after we have extracted something from them that is of service to the treatment.[1] Some dreams that occur during treatment entirely escape any full analysis: since they have arisen out of the great mass of psychical material which is still unknown to us, it is impossible to understand them before the treatment is finished. If I were to report dreams of this kind, it would oblige me to uncover all the

[1] [An account of the reasons for this is given in 'The Handling of Dream-Interpretation in Psycho-Analysis' (1911e).]

secrets of a neurosis as well; and that will not do for us, since it is precisely to prepare us for the study of the neuroses that we have attacked the problem of dreams.

You, however, would be glad to dispense with this material and would prefer to be given an explanation of the dreams of healthy people or of your own dreams. But this cannot be done, on account of their content. It is impossible to submit either oneself or anyone else whose confidence one enjoys to the ruthless exposure that would be involved in a detailed analysis of his dreams, which, as you already know, are concerned with the most intimate part of one's personality. But there is another difficulty in the way apart from that of providing the material. You are aware that dreams present an alien appearance to the dreamer himself, and much more so to anyone who is unacquainted with him personally. Our literature is not poor in good and detailed dream-analyses. I myself have published a few within the framework of case histories.[1] Perhaps the best example of the interpretation of a dream is the one reported by Otto Rank [1910b] consisting of two interrelated dreams dreamt by a young girl, which occupy about two pages of print: but their analysis extends to seventy-six pages. So I should need something like a whole term to conduct you through a piece of work of the sort. If one takes up any comparatively long and much distorted dream, one has to give so many explanations of it, to bring up so much material in the way of associations and memories, to follow up so many by-paths, that a lecture about it would be quite confusing and unsatisfactory. I must therefore ask you to be content with what can be had more easily—an account of small pieces of the dreams of neurotic patients, in which it is possible to recognize this or that point in isolation. What is easiest to demonstrate are dream-symbols and, after them, some characteristics of the regressive representation in dreams. In the case of each of the dreams that follow, I will indicate why it is that I think it worth reporting.[2]

[1] [The main instances of these are the two dreams in the analysis of 'Dora' (1905e) and the childhood dream of the 'Wolf Man' (1918b). The latter case history was not actually published until after the delivery of this lecture, though it had already been written.]

[2] [Only two of the dreams quoted here (Nos. 6 and 7) are to be found elsewhere. Very large numbers of other examples, mainly of Freud's own dreams, are reported and analysed in *I. of D.*]

(1) This dream consisted only of two short pictures: *His uncle was smoking a cigarette although it was a Saturday.—A woman was caressing and fondling him* [the dreamer] *as though he were her child.*

In regard to the first picture the dreamer (a Jew) remarked that his uncle was a pious man who never had done and never could do anything sinful like that. In regard to the woman in the second picture nothing occurred to him except his mother. These two pictures or thoughts must obviously be seen in connection with each other. But how? Since he expressly disputed the reality of his uncle's action, it is plausible to insert an 'if': 'If my uncle, that pious man, were to smoke a cigarette on a Saturday, then I might let myself, too, be cuddled by my mother.' This clearly means that cuddling with his mother was something impermissible, like smoking on a Saturday to a pious Jew. You will recall that I told you [p. 177] that in the course of the dream-work all the relations between the dream-thoughts drop out; these are resolved into their raw material and it is the task of the interpretation to re-insert the omitted relations.

(2) As a result of my publications on dreams I have in a sense become a public consultant on matters relating to them, and for many years I have been receiving communications from the most various sources in which dreams are reported to me or submitted to my judgement. I am of course grateful to anyone who adds enough material to the dream to make an interpretation possible or who gives an interpretation himself. The following dream, dreamt by a medical student in Munich and dating from the year 1910, falls into this category. I am bringing it up in order to show you how impossible it is in general to understand a dream till the dreamer has given us his information about it. For I suspect that at bottom you consider that the ideal method of dream-interpretation is by filling in the meaning of the symbols and that you would like to discard the technique of obtaining associations to the dream; and I am anxious to disabuse you of this damaging mistake.

'July 13, 1910. Towards morning I had this dream: *I was bicycling down the street in Tübingen when a brown dachshund rushed up behind me and seized me by the heel. After a little I got off, sat down on a step, and began to hit at the beast, which had bitten firm hold of me.* (I had no disagreeable feelings either from the bite or from the scene as a whole.) *Some elderly ladies were sitting opposite me and grinning at me. Then I woke up and, as has often happened before, at the moment of transition to waking, the whole dream was clear to me.*'

Symbols are of little help here. But the dreamer reported: 'I have recently fallen in love with a girl, but only from seeing her in the street, and I have had no means of getting in contact with her. The dachshund might have been the pleasantest way of doing so, especially as I am a great animal-lover and I liked this same characteristic in the girl.' He added that he had repeatedly intervened in furious dog-fights with great skill and often to the astonishment of the onlookers. We learn then that the girl he was attracted by was always to be seen in the company of this particular dog. As far as the manifest dream was concerned, however, the girl was omitted and only the dog associated with her was left. The elderly ladies who grinned at him may perhaps have taken the girl's place. His further remarks threw no adequate light on this point. The fact that he was bicycling in the dream is a direct repetition of the remembered situation. He never met the girl with the dog except when he was on his bicycle.

(3) When anyone has lost someone near and dear to him, he produces dreams of a special sort for some time afterwards, in which knowledge of the death arrives at the strangest compromises with the need to bring the dead person to life again. In some of these dreams the person who has died is dead and at the same time still alive, because he does not know he is dead; only if he did know would he die completely. In others, he is half dead and half alive, and each of these states is indicated in a particular way. We must not describe these dreams as simply nonsensical; for being brought to life again is no more inconceivable in dreams than it is, for instance, in fairy tales, in which it occurs as a very usual event. So far as I have been able to analyse such dreams, it has turned out that they are capable of a reasonable solution, but that the pious wish to bring the dead person back to life has been able to operate by the strangest means. I will now put before you a dream of this kind which sounds sufficiently queer and senseless and the analysis of which will show you much for which our theoretical

discussions will have prepared you. It is the dream of a man who had lost his father several years before:

His father was dead but had been exhumed and looked bad. He had been living since then and the dreamer was doing all he could to prevent him noticing it. (The dream then went on to other and apparently very remote matters.)

His father was dead; we know that. His having been exhumed did not correspond to reality; and there was no question of reality in anything that followed. But the dreamer reported that after he had come away from his father's funeral, one of his teeth began to ache. He wanted to treat the tooth according to the precept of Jewish doctrine: 'If thy tooth offend thee, pluck it out!' And he went off to the dentist. But the dentist said: 'One doesn't pluck out a tooth. One must have patience with it. I'll put something into it to kill it; come back in three days and I'll take it out.'

'That "take out",' said the dreamer suddenly, 'that's the exhuming!'

Was the dreamer right about this? It only fits more or less, not completely; for the *tooth* was not taken out, but only something in it that had died. But inaccuracies of this kind can, on the evidence of other experiences, well be attributed to the dream-work. If so, the dreamer had condensed his dead father and the tooth that had been killed but retained; he had fused them into a unity. No wonder, then, that something senseless emerged in the manifest dream, for, after all, not everything that was said about the tooth could fit his father. Where could there possibly be a *tertium comparationis* [p. 152 above] between the tooth and his father, to make the condensation possible?

But no doubt he must have been right, for he went on to say that he knew that if one dreams of a tooth falling out it means that one is going to lose a member of one's family.

This popular interpretation, as we know,[1] is incorrect or at least is correct only in a scurrilous sense. We shall be all the more surprised to find the topic thus touched upon re-appearing behind other portions of the dream's content.

The dreamer now began, without any further encouragement, to talk about his father's illness and death as well as

[1] [See pp. 156 f. and 164 f. above.]

about his own relations with him. His father was ill for a long time, and the nursing and treatment had cost him (the son) a lot of money. Yet it was never too much, he was never impatient, he never wished that after all it might soon come to an end. He was proud of his truly Jewish filial piety towards his father, of his strict obedience to Jewish Law. And here we are struck by a contradiction in the thoughts belonging to the dream. He had identified the tooth and his father. He wanted to proceed with the tooth in accordance with Jewish Law, which commanded him to pluck it out if it caused him pain or offence. He also wanted to proceed with his father, too, in accordance with the precepts of the Law, but in this case it commanded him to spare no expense or trouble, to take every burden on himself and to allow no hostile intention to emerge against the object that was causing him pain. Would not the two attitudes have agreed much more convincingly if he had really developed feelings towards his sick father similar to those towards his sick tooth—that is, if he had wished that an early death would put an end to his unnecessary, painful and costly existence?

I do not doubt that this was really his attitude towards his father during the tedious illness and that his boastful assurances of his filial piety were meant to distract him from these memories. Under such conditions the death-wish against a father is apt to become active and to hide itself under the mask of such sympathetic reflections as that 'it would be a happy release for him'. But please observe that here we have passed a barrier in the latent dream-thoughts themselves. No doubt the first portion of them was unconscious only temporarily—that is, during the construction of the dream; but his hostile impulses against his father must have been permanently unconscious.[1] They may have originated from scenes in his childhood and have occasionally slipped into consciousness, timidly and disguised, during his father's illness. We can assert this with greater certainty of other latent thoughts which have made unmistakable contributions to the content of the dream. Nothing, indeed, is to be discovered in the dream of his hostile impulses towards his father. But if we look for the roots of such hostility to a father in childhood, we shall recall that fear of a father is

[1] [This is carried further at the end of Lecture XIII, p. 212 below.]

set up because, in the very earliest years, he opposes a boy's sexual activities, just as he is bound to do once more from social motives after the age of puberty. This relation to his father applies to our dreamer as well: his love for him included a fair admixture of awe and anxiety, which had their source in his having been early deterred by threats from sexual activity.

The remaining phrases in the manifest dream can be explained now in relation to the masturbation complex. '*He looked bad*' is indeed an allusion to another remark of the dentist's to the effect that it looks bad if one has lost a tooth in that part of the month; but it relates at the same time to the 'looking bad' by which a young man at puberty betrays, or is afraid he betrays, his excessive sexual activity. It was not without relief to his own feelings that in the manifest content the dreamer displaced the 'looking bad' from himself on to his father—one of the kinds of reversal by the dream-work which is familiar to you [p. 180]. '*He had been living since then*' coincides with the wish to bring back to life as well as with the dentist's promise that the tooth would survive. The sentence 'the dreamer was doing all he could *to prevent him* (*his father*) *noticing it*' is very subtly devised to mislead us into thinking that it should be completed by the words 'that he was dead'. The only completion, however, that makes sense comes once more from the masturbation complex; in that connection it is self-evident that the young man did all he could to conceal his sexual life from his father. And finally, remember that we must always interpret what are called 'dreams with a dental stimulus' as relating to masturbation and the dreaded punishment for it. [Cf. footnote, p. 188.]

You can see now how this incomprehensible dream came about. It was done by producing a strange and misleading condensation, by disregarding all the thoughts that were in the centre of the latent thought-process and by creating ambiguous substitutes for the deepest and chronologically most remote of those thoughts.[1]

(4) We have already tried repeatedly to come to understand

[1] [A fragment of a dream very similar to, if not identical with, this one is discussed in *I. of D*. See an example in (II) of Section G in Chapter VI. It is also discussed in 'Formulations on the Two Principles of Mental Functioning' (1911*b*).]

the matter-of-fact and commonplace dreams which have nothing senseless or strange about them but which raise the question of why one should dream about such indifferent stuff.
[Cf. pp. 96–7 and 117.] I will therefore offer you another
example of this kind—three interconnected dreams dreamt by
a young lady in one night.

(a) *She was walking across the hall of her house and struck her head
against a low-hanging chandelier and drew blood.*

No reminiscence, nothing that had really happened. The information she produced in response to it led in quite other
directions. 'You know how badly my hair's falling out. "My
child," my mother said to me yesterday, "if this goes any
further you'll have a head as smooth as a bottom." ' So here
the head stands for the other end of the body. We can understand the chandelier, without any help, as a symbol: all objects
capable of being lengthened are symbols of the male organ
[p. 155]. It was therefore a matter of bleeding at the lower end
of the body, which had arisen from contact with a penis. This
might still be ambiguous. Her further associations showed that
what was in question concerned a belief that menstrual bleeding arises from sexual intercourse with a man—a piece of
sexual theory which counts many faithful believers among
immature girls.

(b) *She saw a deep pit in the vineyard, which she knew had been
caused by a tree being torn out.* She added a remark that the tree
was missing. She meant that she had not seen the tree in her
dream; but the same wording served to express another thought
which made the symbolic interpretation quite certain. The
dream referred to another piece of infantile sexual theory—to
the belief that girls originally had the same genitals as boys and
that their later shape was the result of castration (the tearing
out of a tree).

(c) *She was standing in front of the drawer of her writing-table
which she was so familiar with that she could tell at once if anyone had
been into it.* Like all drawers, chests and cases, the writing-table
drawer stood for the female genitals [p. 156]. She knew that
indications of sexual intercourse (and, as she thought, of touching) could be observed on the genitals and had long feared such
a discovery. In all these three dreams, I think, the accent is to
be placed on *knowledge*. She was recalling the period of her

sexual researches when she was a child, of whose outcome she had been quite proud at the time.[1]

(5) Here is a little more symbolism. But this time I must start with a short preamble on the psychical situation. A gentleman who had passed a night in intercourse with a lady described her as one of those motherly characters in whom the wish for a child breaks irresistibly through in intercourse with a man. The circumstances of this meeting, however, called for a precaution which prevented the fertilizing semen from reaching the woman's uterus. On waking up after this night the woman reported the following dream:

An officer in a red cap was running after her in the street. She fled from him, and ran up the stairs with him still after her. Breathless, she reached her flat, slammed the door behind her and locked it. He stayed outside, and when she looked through the peep-hole, he was sitting on a bench outside and weeping.

You will no doubt recognize the pursuit by the officer in the red cap and the breathless climbing upstairs as representing the sexual act [p. 158]. The fact that it was the dreamer who locked herself up against her pursuer will serve as an example of the reversals that are used so commonly in dreams [p. 180], for it was the man who had avoided the consummation of the sexual act. In the same way, her grief was displaced on to the man, for it was he who wept in the dream—and this was simultaneously a representation of the emission of semen.

I feel sure that you have heard some time or other that it is asserted by psycho-analysis that every dream has a sexual meaning. Well, you yourselves are in a position to form a judgement of the incorrectness of this reproach. You have become acquainted with wishful dreams dealing with the satisfaction of the most obvious needs—hunger and thirst and the longing for freedom—with dreams of convenience and of impatience, and also with purely covetous and egoistic dreams. But at the same time you should bear in mind, as one of the results of psycho-analytic research, that greatly distorted dreams give expression mainly (though, again, not exclusively) to sexual wishes.

[1] [The sexual researches and sexual theories of children are discussed in Lecture XX (p. 317 below).]

(6) I have a particular reason for piling up instances of the use of symbols in dreams. At our first meeting [p. 16 ff.] I lamented the difficulty of providing demonstrations and so of carrying conviction in giving instruction in psycho-analysis. And I have no doubt that you have since come to agree with me. But the different theses of psycho-analysis are so intimately connected that conviction can easily be carried over from a single point to a larger part of the whole. It might be said of psycho-analysis that if anyone holds out a little finger to it it quickly grasps his whole hand. No one, even, who has accepted the explanation of parapraxes can logically withhold his belief in all the rest. A second, equally accessible position is offered by dream-symbolism. Here is the dream of an uneducated woman whose husband was a policeman and who had certainly never heard anything about dream-symbolism or psycho-analysis. Then judge for yourselves whether its explanation by the help of sexual symbols can be called arbitrary and forced:

'. . . *Then someone broke into the house and she was frightened and called out for a policeman. But he had gone into a church, to which a number of steps led up, accompanied amicably by two tramps. Behind the church there was a hill and above it a thick wood. The policeman was dressed in a helmet, gorget and cloak. He had a brown beard. The two tramps, who went along peaceably with the policeman, had sack-like aprons tied round their middles. In front of the church a path led up to the hill; on both sides of it there grew grass and brushwood, which became thicker and thicker and, at the top of the hill, turned into a regular wood.*' [1]

You will have no trouble in recognizing the symbols used. The male genitals are represented by a triad of figures, and the female ones by a landscape with a chapel, hill and wood. Once again you find steps as a symbol for the sexual act. What is called a hill in the dream is also called one in anatomy—the Mons Veneris [the hill of Venus].

(7) And here is yet another dream that must be solved by the insertion of symbols. It is notable and convincing from the fact that the dreamer himself translated all the symbols, though he had no sort of previous theoretical knowledge of

[1] [This dream, originally reported by B. Dattner, appears in *I. of D.* in a very slightly different version. See Example IV in Section E of Chapter VI.]

dream-interpretation. Such an attitude is quite unusual and its determinants are not precisely understood:[1]

'He was going for a walk with his father in a place which must certainly have been the Prater,[2] since he saw the Rotunda, with a small annex in front of it to which a captive balloon was attached, though it looked rather limp. His father asked him what all this was for; he was surprised at his asking, but explained it to him. Then they came into a courtyard which had a large sheet of tin laid out in it. His father wanted to pull off a large piece of it, but first looked around to see if anyone was watching. He told him that he need only tell the foreman and he could take some without any bother. A staircase led down from this yard into a shaft, whose walls were cushioned in some soft material, rather like a leather armchair. At the end of the shaft was a longish platform and then another shaft started. . . .'

The dreamer himself interpreted: 'The Rotunda was my genitals and the captive balloon in front of it was my penis, whose limpness I have reason to complain of.' Going into greater detail, then, we may translate the Rotunda as the bottom (habitually regarded by children as part of the genitals) and the small annex in front of it as the scrotum. His father asked him in the dream what all this was—that is, what was the purpose and function of the genitals. It seemed plausible to reverse this situation and turn the dreamer into the questioner. Since he had in fact never questioned his father in this way, we had to look upon the dream-thought as a wish, or take it as a conditional clause, such as: 'If I had asked my father for sexual enlightenment. . . .' We shall presently find the continuation of this thought in another part of the dream.

The courtyard in which the sheet of tin was spread out is not to be taken symbolically in the first instance. It was derived from the business premises of the dreamer's father. For reasons of discretion I have substituted 'tin' for another material in which his father actually dealt: but I have made no other change in the wording of the dream. The dreamer had entered his father's business and had taken violent objection to the somewhat dubious practices on which the firm's earnings in part depended. Consequently the dream-thought I have just interpreted may have continued in this way: '(If I had asked

---

[1] [Cf. some remarks on this at the beginning of Section E of Chapter VI of *I. of D.*]

[2] [The 'Bois de Boulogne' of Vienna. It includes an amusement park.]

him), he would have deceived me just as he deceives his cus-
tomers.' As regards the 'pulling off' which served to represent
his father's dishonesty in business, the dreamer himself produced
a second explanation—namely that it stood for masturbating.
Not only have we long been familiar with this interpretation
[p. 164], but there was something to confirm it in the fact that
the secret nature of masturbation was represented by its reverse: it might be done openly. Just as we should expect, the
masturbatory activity was once again displaced on to the
dreamer's father, like the questioning in the first scene of the
dream. He promptly interpreted the shaft as a vagina, having
regard to the soft cushioning of its walls. I added on my own
authority [p. 158] that climbing down, like climbing up in
other cases, described sexual intercourse in the vagina.

The dreamer himself gave a biographical explanation of the
further details—that the first shaft was followed by a longish
platform and then by another shaft. He had practised intercourse for a time but had then given it up on account of inhibitions, and he now hoped to be able to resume it by the
help of the treatment.[1]

(8) The two following dreams were dreamt by a foreigner of
a highly polygamous disposition. I repeat them to you as
evidence for my assertion [p. 142] that the dreamer's own ego
appears in every dream even if it is concealed in the manifest
content. The trunks in the dreams were symbols of women:

(a) *He was starting on a journey; his luggage was taken to the
station on a carriage, a number of trunks piled up on it, and among them
two big black ones, like boxes of samples. He said to someone con-
solingly: 'Well, they're only going with me as far as the station.'*

He did in fact travel with a great deal of luggage; but he also
brought a great many stories about women into the treatment.
The two black trunks corresponded to two dark[2] women who
were at the time playing the main part in his life. One of them
had wanted to follow him to Vienna; and on my advice he had
telegraphed to put her off.

(b) A scene at the customs-house: *Another traveller opened his*

---

[1] [This dream and its analysis are reprinted almost exactly from
I. of D. See Example III of Section E in Chapter VI.]
[2] [In German '*schwarz*' ('black').]

box and, coolly smoking a cigarette, said: 'There's nothing in it.' The customs officer seemed to believe him, but felt about once more inside it, and found something quite particularly prohibited. The traveller said in a resigned voice: 'There's nothing to be done about it.'

He himself was the traveller: I was the customs officer. As a rule he was very straightforward in making admissions; but he had intended to keep silent to me about a new connection he had formed with a lady, because he rightly supposed that she was not unknown to me. He displaced the distressing situation of being detected on to a stranger, so that he himself did not seem to appear in the dream.

(9) Here is an example of a symbol which I have not yet mentioned:

He met his sister in the company of two women friends who were themselves sisters. He shook hands with both of them but not with his sister.

No connection with any real occurrence. But his thoughts took him back, rather, to a period in which his observations led him to reflect on how late girls' breasts developed. So the two sisters were breasts; he would have liked to take hold of them with his hand—if only it were not his sister.

(10) Here is an example of death-symbolism in a dream:

He was walking, with two people whose names he knew but had forgotten when he woke up, across a very high, steep iron bridge. Suddenly they had both gone, and he saw a ghost-like man in a cap and linen clothes. He asked him if he was the telegraph-boy. No. Was he the driver? No. Then he walked on further. . . . While he was still dreaming he felt acute anxiety, and after he had woken up he continued the dream with a phantasy that the iron bridge suddenly broke and he fell into the abyss.

People of whom one insists that they are unknown or that one has forgotten their names are mostly people very near to one. The dreamer had a brother and sister; and if he had wished that these two were dead, it would be only fair that in return *he* should be victimized by a fear of death. Of the telegraph-boy he remarked that such people always bring bad news. By his uniform he might equally have been the lamp-lighter; but he puts out the lamps as well, just as the Spirit of Death puts out the torch. The driver made him think of Uhland's poem about King Charles's Voyage, and reminded him of a dangerous sea-voyage with two companions during which he had played the part of the King in the poem.[1] The iron bridge made him think of a recent accident and of the foolish saying: 'Life is a suspension bridge.'[2]

(11) The following dream may count as another representation of death:

An unknown gentleman left a black-edged visiting-card on him.

(12) You will be interested in the following dream in a number of ways, though a neurotic state in the dreamer was one of its preconditions:

He was travelling in a railway-train. The train came to a stop in open country. He thought there was going to be an accident and that he must think of getting away. He went through all the coaches in the train and killed everyone he met—the guard, the engine-driver, and so on.

In connection with this he thought of a story told him by a friend. A lunatic was being conveyed in a compartment on an Italian line, but through carelessness a traveller was allowed in with him. The madman killed the other traveller. Thus he was identifying himself with the madman, and based his right to do so on an obsession by which he was tormented from time to time that he must 'get rid of all accessory witnesses'. But then he himself found a better reason, and this led to the precipitating cause of the dream. At the theatre the night before he had once more seen the girl whom he had wanted to marry but had withdrawn from because she had given him ground for being jealous. In view of the intensity reached by his jealousy he would, he thought, really be 'mad to want to marry her. This meant that he regarded her as so untrustworthy that, in his jealousy, he would have to kill everyone who came his way. We have already come across walking through a series of rooms

---

[1] [In Uhland's poem, *'König Karls Meerfahrt'*, King Charles and his twelve knights are overtaken by a storm on a voyage to the Holy Land. The twelve knights express their uneasiness in turn—but the King sits silently at the helm and steers the ship to safety.]

[2] [This is quoted as an example of a bad joke in a footnote added in 1912 to Freud's book on jokes (1905c), (Norton, 1960), p. 139.]

(here, railway coaches) as a symbol of marriage (a reversal of 'monogamy').[1]

In connection with the train coming to a stop in open country and his being afraid of an accident, he said that once when he was on a railway journey there had been a sudden stop of this kind when they were not in a station. A young lady who was travelling with him had said that there might be going to be a collision and that the safest thing to do was to lift one's legs up high. But this 'lifting the legs high' had also played a part in the many walks and excursions in the country which he had taken with the other girl in the happy early days of their love. This was a fresh argument for thinking he would be mad to marry her now. But my knowledge of the situation made me feel certain that he nevertheless wished he were mad enough to do it.

[1] [This symbol had not been mentioned earlier in these lectures. But in Section E of Chapter VI in *I. of D.*, it is stated that a suite of rooms can stand for a brothel or a harem, or alternatively (by reversal) for a monogamous marriage.]

LECTURE XIII

THE ARCHAIC FEATURES AND INFANTILISM OF DREAMS

LADIES AND GENTLEMEN,—Let us start out once more from the conclusion we arrived at that the dream-work, under the influence of the dream-censorship, transposes the latent dream-thoughts into a different mode of expression. The latent thoughts do not differ from our familiar conscious thoughts of waking life. The new mode of expression is incomprehensible to us owing to many of its features. We have said that it harks back to states of our intellectual development which have long since been superseded—to picture-language, to symbolic connections, to conditions, perhaps, which existed before our thought-language had developed. We have on that account described the mode of expression of the dream-work as *archaic* or *regressive* [p. 180 f.].

You may conclude from this that if we study the dream-work further we must succeed in gaining valuable light on the little-known beginnings of our intellectual development. I hope it will be so; but this work has not so far been started upon. The prehistory into which the dream-work leads us back is of two kinds—on the one hand, into the individual's prehistory, his childhood, and on the other, in so far as each individual somehow recapitulates in an abbreviated form the entire development of the human race, into phylogenetic prehistory too. Shall we succeed in distinguishing which portion of the latent mental processes is derived from the individual prehistoric period and which portion from the phylogenetic one? It is not, I believe, impossible that we shall. It seems to me, for instance, that symbolic connections, which the individual has never acquired by learning, may justly claim to be regarded as a phylogenetic heritage.

This, however, is not the only archaic characteristic of dreams. You are all familiar, of course, from your own experience, with the remarkable amnesia of childhood. I mean the fact that the earliest years of life, up to the age of five, six or eight, have not left behind them traces in our memory like later experiences. Here and there, it is true, we come upon people who can boast of a continuous memory from the first beginnings to the present day; but the other alternative, of gaps in the memory, is by far the more frequent. There has not, in my opinion, been enough astonishment over this fact. By the time a child is two he can speak well, and soon shows that he is at home in complicated mental situations; and he makes remarks which, if they are reported to him many years later, he himself will have forgotten. Moreover, the memory is more efficient at an early age, since it is less overburdened than it is later. Nor is there any reason for regarding the function of memory as a particularly high or difficult mental activity; on the contrary, we can find a good memory in people of very low intellectual standing.[1]

A second remarkable fact to which 1 must draw your attention, and which comes on top of the first one, is that out of the void of memories that covers the earliest years of childhood there stand out a few well-preserved recollections, mostly perceived in plastic form, which cannot justify their survival. Our memory deals with the material of the impressions which impinge on us in later life by making a selection among them. It retains what is of any importance and drops what is unimportant. But this is not true of the childhood memories that have been retained. They do not necessarily correspond to the important experiences of childhood years, nor even to those which must have seemed important from the child's point of view. They are often so commonplace and insignificant that we can only ask ourselves in astonishment why this particular detail has escaped oblivion. I attempted long ago, with the help of analysis, to attack the enigma of childhood amnesia and of the residual memories which interrupt it, and I arrived at the conclusion that even in the case of children it is true in spite of everything that only what is important remains in the memory. But through the processes, already familiar to you, of condensation and more especially of displacement, what is important is replaced in memory by something else which appears unimportant. For this reason I have called these childhood memories

---

[1] [A longer discussion of infantile amnesia will be found in the second of the *Three Essays* (1905d).]

'screen memories', and with a thorough analysis everything that has been forgotten can be extracted from them.[1]

In psycho-analytic treatments we are invariably faced by the task of filling up these gaps in the memory of childhood; and in so far as the treatment is to any extent successful—that is to say, extremely frequently—we also succeed in bringing to light the content of these forgotten years of childhood. Those impressions had never been really forgotten, they were only inaccessible, latent, and had formed part of the unconscious. But it can come about that they emerge from the unconscious spontaneously, and this happens in connection with dreams. It appears that dream-life knows how to find access to these latent, infantile experiences. Excellent examples of this have been reported in the literature and I myself have been able to provide a contribution of the kind. I once dreamt in a certain connection of a person who must have done me a service and whom I saw clearly before me. He was a one-eyed man of small stature, stout, and with his head sunk deep in his shoulders. I concluded from the context that he was a doctor. Luckily I was able to enquire from my mother, who was still alive, what the doctor at my birth-place (which I had left when I was three) had looked like; and I learnt from her that he was one-eyed, short, stout and with his head sunk deep in his shoulders; and I also learnt what the accident was for which he had come to my help and which I myself had forgotten.[2] This fact of dreams having at their disposal the forgotten material of the first years of childhood is thus a further archaic feature.[3]

This same piece of information can be further applied to another of the riddles we have come up against. You recall the amazement which was caused by our discovery that what instigates dreams are actively evil and extravagantly sexual wishes, which have made the censorship and distortion of dreams necessary [p. 142 ff.]. When we have interpreted a

[1] [Screen memories had been discussed by Freud in Chapter IV of *The Psychopathology of Everyday Life* (1901*b*), (Norton, 1965), as well as in a separate paper on the subject published earlier (1899*a*).]

[2] [The dream is described in Chapter I(B) of *I. of D.*, where further references will be found.]

[3] [This fact had been noted by Freud in a letter to Fliess of March 10, 1898 (Freud, 1950*a*, Letter 84).]

dream of this sort to the dreamer and if, to take the most favourable case, he does not actually attack the interpretation, he nevertheless regularly raises the question of where these wishes come from, since they feel alien to him and their opposite is what he is conscious of. We need have no hesitation in pointing out their origin. These evil wishful impulses arise from the past, and often from a past that is not very remote. It can be shown that there was a time when they were familiar and conscious, even if they are no longer so to-day. A woman, whose dream meant that she would like to see her daughter, now seventeen years old, dead before her eyes,[1] found under our guidance that she had indeed at one time harboured this death-wish. The child was the fruit of an unhappy marriage which was soon dissolved. Once, while she still bore her daughter in her womb, in a fit of rage after a violent scene with her husband she had beaten with her fists on her body in order to kill the child inside it. How many mothers, who love their children tenderly, perhaps over-tenderly, to-day, conceived them unwillingly and wished at that time that the living thing within them might not develop further! They may even have expressed that wish in various, fortunately harmless, actions. Thus their death-wish against someone they love, which is later so mysterious, originates from the earliest days of their relationship to that person.

In the same way, a father had a dream which justified the interpretation that he wished for the death of his favourite eldest child. He too was led to remember that there had been a time when this wish was not strange to him. When the child was still an infant in arms, the father, discontented with his choice of a wife, often thought that if the little creature, who meant nothing to him, were to die, he would be free once more and would make better use of his freedom.[2] The same origin can be shown in the case of a great number of similar impulses

[1] [This dream is described at greater length in Chapter IV of *I. of D.* In those passages the girl's age is given three times (in letters) as 'fifteen'. The '17' (in figures) in all the German editions of the present work is perhaps due to a misprint.]

[2] [What appears to be the same story as this is told in much greater detail in connection not with a dream but with a 'bungled action' near the end of Chapter VIII of *The Psychopathology of Everyday Life,* pp. 187–9.]

of hatred; they are recollections of something belonging to the past, which was once conscious and played its part in mental life. You will be inclined to conclude from this that such wishes and such dreams ought not to arise in cases where transformations of this kind in one's relation to someone never occurred, where the relation was of the same kind from the first. I am prepared to admit this; but I must remind you that what you must take into consideration is not the *wording* of the dream but its sense after it has been interpreted. It is possible that a manifest dream of the death of someone loved has merely assumed a horrifying mask and may mean something quite different, or that the loved person is intended as a misleading substitute for someone else.

But the same subject will suggest another and far more serious question. 'Even if,' you will say, 'this death-wish was present at one time and is confirmed by recollection, that is still no explanation. After all, it was superseded long ago, and can only be present to-day in the unconscious as no more than an unemotional memory, not as a powerful impulse. Nothing speaks in favour of this last possibility. Why, then, was it recollected at all in the dream?' This question may justly be raised. An attempt to answer it would lead us too far and would necessitate our taking up a position on one of the most important points in the theory of dreams. But I am obliged to keep within the framework of our discussions and to exercise restraint. So prepare yourselves for a provisional renunciation.[1] Let us content ourselves with the factual evidence that this superseded wish can be shown to be the instigator of the dream, and let us pursue our enquiry whether other evil wishes can be similarly traced back to the past.

We will keep to wishes for getting rid of someone, which may for the most part be attributed to the dreamer's unrestricted egoism. A wish of this kind can very often be pointed to as the constructor of a dream. Whenever anyone in the course of one's life gets in one's way—and how often this must happen in view of the complication of one's relationships in life!—a dream is promptly ready to kill that person, even if it be father or

[1] [Freud returns to this problem at the end of the present lecture (p. 212).]

mother, brother or sister, husband or wife. This wickedness of human nature came as a great surprise to us and we were decidedly disinclined to accept this outcome of dream-interpretation without question. But as soon as we were led to look for the origin of these wishes in the past, we discovered the period of the individual's past in which there was no longer anything strange in such egoism and such wishful impulses, directed even against his closest relatives. It is children, and precisely in those earliest years which are later veiled by amnesia, who often exhibit this egoism to an extremely marked degree and who invariably show clear rudiments or, more correctly speaking, residues of it. Children love themselves first, and it is only later that they learn to love others and to sacrifice something of their own ego to others. Even those people whom a child seems to love from the beginning are loved by him at first because he needs them and cannot do without them—once again from egoistic motives. Not until later does the impulse to love make itself independent of egoism. It is literally true that *his egoism has taught him to love.*

In this connection it will be interesting to compare the child's attitude to his brothers and sisters with that towards his parents. A small child does not necessarily love his brothers and sisters; often he obviously does not. There is no doubt that he hates them as his competitors, and it is a familiar fact that this attitude often persists for long years, till maturity is reached or even later, without interruption. Quite often, it is true, it is succeeded, or let us rather say overlaid, by a more affectionate attitude; but the hostile one seems very generally to be the earlier. This hostile attitude can be observed most easily in children between two and a half and four or five, when a new baby brother or sister appears. It usually meets with a very unfriendly reception. Such remarks as 'I don't like him; the stork can take him away again!' are quite common. After this, every opportunity is taken of disparaging the new arrival and attempts to injure him and even murderous assaults are not unknown. If the difference in age is less, by the time the child's mental activity has awakened to some degree of intensity he finds his competitor already there and adjusts himself to him. If the difference is greater, the new baby may from the first arouse a certain sympathy as an interesting object, a sort of live doll;

and where the difference in age is of eight or more years, solicitous, maternal impulses may already come into play, especially in girls. But, honestly speaking, if one comes upon a wish for the death of a brother or sister behind a dream, there is seldom need to find it puzzling and one can trace its prototype without any trouble in early childhood and often enough in later years of companionship as well.[1]

There is probably no nursery without violent conflicts between its inmates. The motives for these are rivalry for parental love, for common possessions, for living space. The hostile impulses are directed against older as well as against younger members of the family. It was, I believe, Bernard Shaw who remarked: 'As a rule there is only one person an English girl hates more than she hates her mother; and thats her eldest sister.' [2] But there is something in this remark that strikes us as strange. We might at a pinch find hatred and competition with brothers and sisters intelligible. But how can we suppose that feelings of hatred can make their way into the relation between daughter and mother, between parents and children?

This relation is undoubtedly a more favourable one, from the children's point of view as well. That is what our expectations demand; we find an absence of love far more repellent between parents and children than between brothers and sisters. In the former case we have, as it were, made something sacred which in the latter we have left profane. Yet daily observation can show us how frequently the emotional relations between parents and their grown-up children fall behind the ideal set up by society, how much hostility is ready to hand and would be expressed if it were not held back by admixtures of filial piety and affectionate impulses. The motives for this hostility are generally known and their tendency is to divide those of the same sex—the daughter from the mother and the father from the son. The daughter finds in her mother the authority which restricts her will and which is entrusted with the task of imposing on her the renunciation of sexual freedom which society demands; in a few instances she even finds in her a competitor who struggles against being supplanted. The same thing is

---

[1] [The relations between brothers and sisters are discussed with examples in Section D of Chapter V of I. of D.]

[2] [John Tanner in Man and Superman, Act II.]

repeated between the son and his father still more glaringly. In the son's eyes his father embodies every unwillingly tolerated social restraint; his father prevents him from exercising his will, from early sexual pleasure and, where there is common property in the family, from enjoying it. In the case of an heir to the throne this waiting for a father's death reaches an almost tragic height. There seems less danger to the relation between father and daughter or mother and son. This last provides the purest examples of an unchangeable affection, unimpaired by any egoistic considerations.[1]

Why am I speaking of these things, which are after all commonplaces and universally known? Because there is an unmistakable inclination to disavow their importance in life and to make out that the ideal demanded by society is fulfilled far more often than it really is. It is better, however, that the truth should be told by psychologists rather than that the task should be left to cynics. And, incidentally, this disavowal applies only to real life. Narrative and dramatic works of the imagination may freely make play with the themes that arise from a disturbance of this ideal.

There is no need to feel surprised, therefore, if, in a large number of people, dreams disclose their wish to get rid of their parents and especially of the parent of their own sex. We may assume that this wish is also present in waking life and is even conscious sometimes, if it can be masked by some other motive, as was the case with our dreamer in Example 3 [p. 189 above], where it was replaced by pity for his father's useless sufferings. It is rarely that the hostility alone dominates the relationship; far oftener it is in the background of more affectionate impulses by which it is suppressed, and it must wait until a dream isolates it, as it were. What seems to us of enormous size in a dream, on account of this isolation, shrinks up once more when our interpretation has given it its place in the context of real life (Hanns Sachs).[2] But we come upon this dream-wish, too,

[1] [This point is discussed at greater length in Lecture XXXIII of the *New Introductory Lectures,* p. 587.]

[2] [The actual words used by Sachs (1912, 569) were quoted by Freud in a passage which he inserted in 1914 on almost the last page of *I. of D.*]

where it has no relevance in real life, and where the adult need never confess to it in his waking life. The reason for this is that the deepest and most invariable motive for estrangement, especially between two people of the same sex, has already made itself felt in early childhood.

What I have in mind is rivalry in love, with a clear emphasis on the subject's sex. While he is still a small child, a son will already begin to develop a special affection for his mother, whom he regards as belonging to him; he begins to feel his father as a rival who disputes his sole possession. And in the same way a little girl looks on her mother as a person who interferes with her affectionate relation to her father and who occupies a position which she herself could very well fill. Observation shows us to what early years these attitudes go back. We refer to them as the 'Oedipus complex', because the legend of Oedipus realizes, with only a slight softening, the two extreme wishes that arise from the son's situation—to kill his father and take his mother to wife. I do not wish to assert that the Oedipus complex exhausts the relation of children to their parents: it can easily be far more complicated. The Oedipus complex can, moreover, be developed to a greater or less strength, it can even be reversed; but it is a regular and very important factor in a child's mental life, and there is more danger of our under-estimating rather than over-estimating its influence and that of the developments which proceed from it. Incidentally, children often react in their Oedipus attitude to a stimulus coming from their parents, who are frequently led in their preferences by difference of sex, so that the father will choose his daughter and the mother her son as a favourite, or, in case of a cooling-off in the marriage, as a substitute for a love-object that has lost its value.[1]

It cannot be said that the world has shown much gratitude to psycho-analytic research for its revelation of the Oedipus complex. On the contrary, the discovery has provoked the most violent opposition among adults; and those who had neglected to take part in the repudiation of this proscribed and tabooed emotional relationship made up for their fault later by depriving the complex of its value through twisted re-interpreta-

[1] [Freud discusses the Oedipus complex at much greater length in Lecture XXI (p. 329 ff. below).]

tions.[1] It is my unaltered conviction that there is nothing in this to be disavowed or glossed over. We must reconcile ourselves to the fact which was recognized by the Greek legend itself as an inevitable fate. It is once again an interesting fact that the Oedipus complex, which has been rejected from real life, has been left to imaginative writing, has been placed freely, as it were, at its disposal. Otto Rank [1912b] has shown in a careful study how the Oedipus complex has provided dramatic authors with a wealth of themes in endless modifications, softenings and disguises—in distortions, that is to say, of the kind which we are already familiar with as the work of a censorship. We may therefore also ascribe this Oedipus complex to dreamers who have been fortunate enough to escape conflicts with their parents in later life. And, intimately linked with it, we find what we call the 'castration complex',[2] the reaction to the threats against the child aimed at putting a stop to his early sexual activities and attributed to his father.

What we have already learnt from our study of the mental life of children will lead us to expect to find a similar explanation of the other group of forbidden dream-wishes—the excessive sexual impulses. We are thus encouraged to make a study of the development of children's sexual life and from many sources we arrive at what follows.

First and foremost, it is an untenable error to deny that children have a sexual life and to suppose that sexuality only begins at puberty with the maturation of the genitals. On the contrary, from the very first children have a copious sexual life, which differs at many points from what is later regarded as normal. What in adult life is described as 'perverse' differs from the normal in these respects: first, by disregarding the barrier of species (the gulf between men and animals), secondly, by overstepping the barrier against disgust, thirdly that against incest (the prohibition against seeking sexual satisfaction from near blood-relations), fourthly that against members of one's own sex and fifthly the transferring of the part played by the genitals to other organs and areas of the body. None of these

[1] [This is of course an allusion to the secession of Adler and Jung. Cf. footnote, p. 346 below.]

[2] [This is further explained in Lecture XX, p. 317 f. below.]

barriers existed from the beginning; they were only gradually erected in the course of development and education. Small children are free from them. They recognize no frightful gulf between human beings and animals; the arrogance with which men separate themselves from animals does not emerge until later.[1] To begin with, children exhibit no disgust at excreta but acquire this slowly under the pressure of education; they attach no special importance to the distinction between the sexes, but attribute the same conformation of the genitals to both; they direct their first sexual lusts and their curiosity to those who are nearest and for other reasons dearest to them—parents, brothers and sisters, or nurses; and finally, they show (what later on breaks through once again at the climax of a love-relation) that they expect to derive pleasure not only from their sexual organs, but that many other parts of the body lay claim to the same sensitivity, afford them analogous feelings of pleasure and can accordingly play the part of genitals. Children may thus be described as 'polymorphously perverse', and if these impulses only show *traces* of activity, that is because on the one hand they are of less intensity compared with those in later life and on the other hand all a child's sexual manifestations are at once energetically suppressed by education. This suppression is, as it were, extended into theory; for adults endeavour to overlook one portion of the sexual manifestations of children and to disguise another portion by misinterpreting its sexual nature, so that they can then disavow the whole of them. It is often the very same people who in the nursery are furious with any sexual naughtinesses of children and afterwards at their writing-tables defend the sexual purity of the same children. When children are left to themselves, or under the influence of seduction, they often bring about quite considerable achievements in the way of perverse sexual activity. Adults are of course right not to take this too seriously and to regard it as 'childishness', or 'playfulness', for children are not to be condemned as fully capable or fully responsible either before the judgement-seat of morals or before the law; but nonetheless these things exist. They have their importance both as indications of a child's innate constitution and as causes and encouragements of later developments

---

[1] [Freud enlarged on this in a contemporary paper, 'A Difficulty in the Path of Psycho-Analysis' (1917a).]

in him; they give us information on the sexual life of children and so on human sexual life in general. If, therefore, we once more find all these perverse wishful impulses behind our distorted dreams, that only means that in this field too dreams have taken a step backwards into the state of infancy.

Among these forbidden wishes special emphasis deserves to be further laid on the incestuous ones—that is, on those aiming at sexual intercourse with parents and brothers and sisters. You know what horror is felt, or at least professed, in human society at such intercourse, and what stress is laid on the prohibitions directed against it. Tremendous efforts have been made to explain this horror of incest. Some people have supposed that breeding considerations on the part of Nature have found psychical representation in this prohibition, since inbreeding would impair racial characters. Others have maintained that, as a result of living together from early childhood onwards, sexual desire has been diverted from the people in question. In both these cases, it may be remarked, an avoidance of incest would be secured automatically, and it would not be clear why such severe prohibitions were called for, which would point rather to the presence of a strong desire for it. Psycho-analytic researches have shown unmistakably that the choice of an incestuous love-object is, on the contrary, the first and invariable one, and that it is not until later that resistance to it sets in; it is no doubt impossible to trace back this resistance to *individual* psychology.[1]

Let us now bring together what our researches into child-psychology have contributed to our understanding of dreams. We have not only found that the material of the forgotten experiences of childhood is accessible to dreams, but we have also seen that the mental life of children with all its characteristics, its egoism, its incestuous choice of love-objects, and so on, still persists in dreams—that is, in the unconscious, and that dreams carry us back every night to this infantile level. The fact is thus confirmed that *what is unconscious in mental life is also what is infantile*. The strange impression of there being so much evil in people begins to diminish. This frightful evil is simply the

[1] [The whole subject of infantile sexuality is treated again at greater length in Lectures XX and XXI.]

initial, primitive, infantile part of mental life, which we can find in actual operation in children, but which, in part, we overlook in them on account of their small size, and which in part we do not take seriously since we do not expect any high ethical standard from children. Since dreams regress to this level, they give the appearance of having brought to light the evil in us. But this is a deceptive appearance, by which we have allowed ourselves to be scared. We are not so evil as we were inclined to suppose from the interpretation of dreams.

If these evil impulses in dreams are merely infantile phenomena, a return to the beginnings of our ethical development (since dreams simply make us into children once more in our thoughts and feelings), we need not, if we are reasonable, be ashamed of these evil dreams.[1] But what is reasonable is only a *part* of mental life, a number of other things take place in the mind which are not sensible; and so it happens that we *are* ashamed of these dreams in an unreasonable way. We subject them to the dream-censorship, we are ashamed and angry if, as an exception, one of these wishes succeeds in making its way into consciousness in such an undistorted form that we are obliged to recognize it; indeed we are occasionally as ashamed of a *distorted* dream as if we understood it. Only think of the indignant judgement which the excellent elderly lady passed on her uninterpreted dream of the 'love services' [p. 137]. So the problem is not yet cleared up, and it is still possible that further consideration of the evil in dreams may lead us to form another judgement and arrive at another estimate of human nature. [Cf. p. 338 below.]

As the outcome of our whole enquiry, let us grasp two discoveries, though they only signify the beginning of fresh enigmas and fresh doubts. First, the regression of the dream-work is not only a formal but also a material one. It not only translates our thoughts into a primitive form of expression; but it also revives the characteristics of our primitive mental life—the old dominance of the ego, the initial impulses of our sexual life, and even, indeed, our old intellectual endowment, if symbolic connections may be regarded as such. And secondly, all this, which is old

---

[1] [The moral responsibility for the content of dreams was the subject of a special discussion by Freud (Section B of 1925*i*). Cf. also p. 331 below.]

and infantile and was once dominant and alone dominant, must to-day be ascribed to the unconscious, our ideas of which are now becoming altered and extended. 'Unconscious' is no longer the name of what is latent at the moment; the unconscious is a particular realm of the mind with its own wishful impulses, its own mode of expression and its peculiar mental mechanisms which are not in force elsewhere. But the latent dream-thoughts which we have discovered by interpreting dreams do not belong to this realm; they are on the contrary thoughts just as we might have thought them in waking life. Nevertheless, they are unconscious. How, then, is this contradiction to be solved? We begin to suspect that a distinction is to be drawn here. Something which is derived from our conscious life and shares its characteristics—we call it 'the day's residues'—combines with something else coming from the realm of the unconscious in order to construct a dream. The dream-work is accomplished between these two components. The influence exercised upon the day's residues by the addition of the unconscious is no doubt among the determinants of regression. This is the deepest insight that we can reach here into the essential nature of dreams—until we have investigated further regions of the mind. But the time will soon have come to provide another name for the unconscious character of the latent dream-thoughts in order to distinguish it from the unconscious which comes from the realm of the infantile.[1]

We can, of course, raise another question besides: 'What is it that forces psychical activity during sleep to make this regression? Why does it not dispose of the mental stimuli that disturb sleep without doing this? And if, for the purposes of the dream-censorship, it has to make use of disguise by means of the old and now unintelligible mode of expression, what is the point of reviving as well the old mental impulses, wishes and character-traits, which are superseded to-day—of making use of material regression in addition to the formal kind?' The only answer that could satisfy us would be that in this way alone can a dream be constructed, that it is not otherwise dynamically possible to get rid of the stimulus to the dream. But so far we have no right to give such an answer.

[1] [This question is taken up again at the end of Lecture XIV, p. 227.]

LECTURE XIV

WISH-FULFILMENT

LADIES AND GENTLEMEN,—Shall I remind you once more of the ground we have covered so far? Of how, when we began applying our technique, we came up against the distortion in dreams, of how we thought we would begin by evading it and obtained our first decisive information on the essential nature of dreams from the dreams of children? Of how, after that, armed with what we had learnt from that enquiry, we made a direct assault on dream-distortion and, as I hope, overcame it step by step? We are bound to admit, however, that the things we have discovered by the one path and by the other do not entirely correspond. It will be our task to piece the two sets of findings together and reconcile them with each other.

We found from both sources that the dream-work consists essentially in the transformation of thoughts into a hallucinatory experience. How this can happen is sufficiently mysterious; but it is a problem of general psychology with which we are not properly concerned here. We learnt from children's dreams that it is the intention of the dream-work to get rid of a mental stimulus, which is disturbing sleep, by means of the fulfilment of a wish. We were unable to say anything similar of distorted dreams till we found out how to interpret them. But it was from the first our expectation that we should be able to regard distorted dreams in the same light as those of children. The first confirmation of this expectation was brought to us by the discovery that in point of fact *all* dreams are children's dreams, that they work with the same infantile material, with the mental impulses and mechanisms of childhood. Now that we believe we have overcome dream-distortion, we must go on to enquire whether the view of dreams as the fulfilment of wishes is also valid of distorted dreams.

A short time ago we submitted a series of dreams to interpretation, but we left wish-fulfilment completely out of account. I feel sure that you must have repeatedly been driven to ask yourselves: 'But where is the wish-fulfilment, which is supposed

213

to be the aim of the dream-work?' The question is an important one, for it has become the question raised by our lay critics. Human beings, as you know, have an instinctive tendency to fend off intellectual novelties. One of the ways in which this tendency is manifested is by immediately reducing the novelty to the smallest proportions, by compressing it if possible into a single catch-word. 'Wish-fulfilment' has become the catch-word for the new theory of dreams. The layman asks: 'Where is the wish-fulfilment?' And instantly, having heard that dreams are supposed to be wish-fulfilments, and in the very act of asking the question, he answers it with a rejection. He immediately thinks of countless experiences of his own with dreams, in which the dream has been accompanied by feelings ranging from the unpleasurable to severe anxiety, so that the assertion made by the psycho-analytic theory of dreams seems to him most improbable. We have no difficulty in replying that in distorted dreams the wish-fulfilment cannot be obvious but must be looked for, so that it cannot be pointed out until the dream has been interpreted. We know too that the wishes in these distorted dreams are forbidden ones—rejected by the censorship—whose existence was precisely the cause of the dream's distortion, the reason for the intervention of the dream-censorship. But it is difficult to make the lay critic understand that before a dream has been interpreted one cannot enquire about the fulfilment of its wish. He will keep on forgetting this. His rejection of the theory of wish-fulfilment is actually nothing other than a consequence of the dream-censorship, a substitute for the rejection of the censored dream-wishes and an effluence from it.

We too, of course, feel the need to explain to ourselves why there are so many dreams with a distressing content and, especially why there are anxiety-dreams. Here for the first time we come upon the problem of affects in dreams; it would deserve a monograph of its own, but unfortunately we cannot enter into it. If dreams are the fulfilment of wishes, distressing feelings should be impossible in them: the lay critics would appear to be right there. But three kinds of complications must be taken into account which they have not thought of.

[1] Firstly, it may be that the dream-work has not com-

pletely succeeded in creating a wish-fulfilment; so that a portion of the distressing affect in the dream-thoughts has been left over in the manifest dream. In that case analysis would have to show that these dream-thoughts were far more distressing than the dream constructed out of them. That much can always be proved. If so, we must admit that the dream-work has not achieved its aim any more than the dream of drinking, formed in response to the stimulus of thirst, succeeded in quenching the thirst [p. 133 f.]. The dreamer remains thirsty and has to wake up in order to drink. Nevertheless it was a genuine dream, and had lost nothing of a dream's essential nature. We can only say: 'Ut desint vires, tamen est laudanda voluntas.'[1] The intention, at least, which can clearly be recognized, remains praiseworthy. Such instances of failure are no rare event. This is helped by that fact that it is so much harder for the dream-work to alter the sense of a dream's *affects* than of its *content*; affects are sometimes highly resistant. What then happens is that the dream-work transforms the distressing content of the dream-thoughts into the fulfilment of a wish, while the distressing affect persists unaltered. In dreams of this kind the affect is quite inappropriate to the content, and our critics can say that dreams are so far from being wish-fulfilments that even one with a harmless content can be felt as distressing. We can answer this foolish remark by pointing out that it is precisely in dreams like this that the wish-fulfilling purpose of the dream-work appears most clearly, because in isolation. The error arises because those who are unfamiliar with the neuroses picture the link between content and affect as too intimate and therefore cannot imagine the content being altered without a simultaneous alteration of the expression of affect attached to it.[2]

[2] A second factor, which is much more important and far-reaching, but which is equally overlooked by laymen, is the following. No doubt a wish-fulfilment must bring pleasure; but

---

[1] ['Though the strength is lacking, the will deserves to be praised' (Ovid, *Ep. ex Pont.*, 3, 4, 79).]

[2] [The looseness of the connection between ideas and their accompanying affects had been·insisted on by Freud from very early times. See, for instance, his first paper on 'The Neuro-Psychoses of Defence' (1894*a*).]

the question then arises 'To whom?' To the person who has the
wish, of course. But, as we know, a dreamer's relation to his
wishes is a quite peculiar one. He repudiates them and censors
them—he has no liking for them, in short. So that their
fulfilment will give him no pleasure, but just the opposite; and
experience shows that this opposite appears in the form of
anxiety, a fact which has still to be explained. Thus a dreamer
in his relation to his dream-wishes can only be compared to
an amalgamation of two separate people who are linked by
some strong element in common. Instead of enlarging on this,
I will remind you of a familiar fairy tale in which you will find
the same situation repeated. A good fairy promised a poor
married couple to grant them the fulfilment of their first three
wishes. They were delighted, and made up their minds to
choose their three wishes carefully. But a smell of sausages being
fried in the cottage next door tempted the woman to wish for a
couple of them. They were there in a flash; and this was the
first wish-fulfilment. But the man was furious, and in his rage
wished that the sausages were hanging on his wife's nose. This
happened too; and the sausages were not to be dislodged from
their new position. This was the second wish-fulfilment; but
the wish was the man's, and its fulfilment was most disagreeable
for his wife. You know the rest of the story. Since after all they
were in fact one—man and wife—the third wish was bound to
be that the sausages should come away from the woman's nose.
This fairy tale might be used in many other connections; but
here it serves only to illustrate the possibility that if two people
are not at one with each other the fulfilment of a wish of one of
them may bring nothing but unpleasure to the other.[1]

It will not be difficult for us now to reach a still better understanding of anxiety-dreams. We will bring up one more observation and then make up our minds to adopt a hypothesis in
favour of which there is much to be said. The observation is
that anxiety-dreams often have a content entirely devoid of
distortion, a content which has, so to speak, evaded the censorship. An anxiety-dream is often the undisguised fulfilment of a

[1] [The whole of this paragraph was later included by Freud as
a footnote to Section D of Chapter VII in the 1919 edition of
I. of D. The same fairy tale is also quoted, but in quite a different
connection, in Freud's paper on 'The "Uncanny"' (1919h).]

wish—not, of course, of an acceptable wish, but of a repudiated one. The generation of anxiety has taken the place of the censorship. Whereas we can say of an infantile dream that it is the open fulfilment of a permitted wish, and of an ordinary distorted dream that it is the disguised fulfilment of a repressed wish, the only formula which fits an anxiety-dream is that it is the open fulfilment of a repressed wish. The anxiety is a sign that the repressed wish has shown itself stronger than the censorship, that it has put through, or is on the point of putting through, its wish-fulfilment in spite of the censorship. We perceive that what is for it a wish-fulfilment can only be for us, who are on the side of the censorship, an occasion for distressing feelings and for fending the wish off. The anxiety that emerges in the dream is, if you like, anxiety at the strength of these wishes which are normally held down. Why this fending-off appears in the form of anxiety cannot be discovered from the study of dreams alone; anxiety must clearly be studied elsewhere.[1]

We may suppose that what is true of undistorted anxiety-dreams applies also to those which are partly distorted as well as to other unpleasurable dreams, in which the distressing feelings probably correspond to an approach to anxiety. Anxiety-dreams are as a rule also arousal dreams; we usually interrupt our sleep before the repressed wish in the dream has put its fulfilment through completely in spite of the censorship. In that case the function of the dream has failed, but its essential nature is not altered by this. We have compared dreams to the night-watchman or guardian of sleep, who tries to protect our sleep from disturbance [p. 129]. The night-watchman, too, may reach the point of waking the sleeper if he feels he is too weak alone to drive off the disturbance or the danger. Nevertheless we sometimes succeed in holding on to our sleep even when the dream begins to be precarious and to be turning into anxiety. We say to ourselves in our sleep 'after all it's only a dream', and sleep on.

When does it happen that a dream-wish is in a position to overpower the censorship? The condition necessary for this may be fulfilled equally well by the dream-wish or by the dream-censorship. The wish may for an unknown reason be excessively strong on some occasion; but one gets an impression that it is

[1] [It is the subject of Lecture XXV below.]

more often the behaviour of the dream-censorship that is responsible for this displacement of their relative strengths. We have already seen [p. 143] that the censorship acts with varying intensity in each particular case, that it treats each element of a dream with a different degree of severity. We can now add a further hypothesis to the effect that it is in general very variable and does not always employ equal severity to the same objectionable element. If things turn out so that on some occasion it feels itself powerless against a dream-wish which threatens to take it by surprise, instead of distortion, it makes use of its last remaining expedient and abandons the state of sleep, at the same time generating anxiety.

In this connection it strikes us that we are still quite ignorant of why it is that these evil, repudiated wishes become active precisely at night and disturb us during our sleep. The answer is almost bound to lie in some hypothesis going back to the nature of the state of sleep. In day-time the heavy weight of censorship rests on them and as a rule makes it impossible for them to manifest themselves in any activity. At night this censorship, like all the other interests of mental life, is probably withdrawn, or at least greatly reduced, in favour of the single wish to sleep. It is this lowering of the censorship at night that the forbidden wishes have to thank for being able to become active once more. There are some neurotic patients who are unable to sleep and who admit to us that their insomnia was originally intentional. They did not dare to sleep because they were afraid of their dreams—afraid, that is, of the results of the weakening of the censorship. You will easily see, however, that in spite of this the withdrawal of the censorship implies no gross carelessness. The state of sleep paralyses our motive powers. If our evil intentions begin to stir, they can, after all, do nothing more than precisely cause a dream, which is harmless from the practical point of view. It is this soothing consideration that is the basis of the highly sensible remark made by the sleeper—made at night, it is true, but not forming part of dream-life: 'After all it's only a dream. So let us leave it to take its course, and let us sleep on.'

[3] If, in the third place, you will recall our idea that the dreamer fighting against his own wishes is to be compared with

a summation of two separate, though in some way intimately connected, people, you will understand another possibility. For there is a possibility that the fulfilment of a wish may bring about something very far from pleasant—namely, a punishment. Here we can once more use the fairy tale of the three wishes as an illustration. The fried sausages on a plate were the direct fulfilment of the wish of the first person, the woman. The sausages on her nose were the fulfilment of the wish of the second person, the man, but were at the same time a punishment for the woman's foolish wish. (We shall discover in neuroses the motive for the third wish, the last remaining one in the fairy tale.)[1] There are many such punitive trends in the mental life of human beings; they are very powerful, and we may hold them responsible for some of the distressing dreams.[2] Perhaps you will now say that this leaves very little over of the famous wish-fulfilment. But if you look more closely you will admit that you are wrong. Compared with the multiplicity (which I shall mention later) of the things that dreams might be and according to many authorities actually are, our solution—wish-fulfilment, anxiety-fulfilment, punishment-fulfilment—is a very restricted one. We may add that the anxiety is the direct opposite of the wish, that opposites are especially close to one another in associations and that in the unconscious they coalesce [p. 178 ff.]; and further, that the punishment is also the ful-filment of a wish—of the wish of the other, censoring person.

On the whole, therefore, I have made no concession to your objection to the theory of wish-fulfilment. It is our duty, how-ever, to be able to indicate the wish-fulfilment in any distorted dream we may come across, and we shall certainly not evade the task. Let us go back to the dream we have already inter-preted of the three bad theatre-tickets for 1 florin 50 [pp. 122 and 139], from which we have already learnt so much. I hope you still recollect it. A lady, whose husband had told her during the day that her friend Elise, who was only three months her junior, had become engaged, dreamt that she was at the theatre with her husband. One side of the stalls was almost empty. Her husband said to her that Elise and her fiancé had wanted

---

[1] [It is not clear what is intended here.]
[2] [Punishment dreams are discussed in *I. of D.* See the Rosegger dreams in Chapter VI (H) and the discussion of wish-fulfilment in Chapter VII.]

to go to the theatre too but had not been able to, since they had only got bad seats—three for 1 florin 50. She thought it would not really have done any harm if they had. We found that the dream-thoughts related to her anger at having married so early and to her dissatisfaction with her husband. We may be curious to discover how these gloomy thoughts were transformed into the fulfilment of a wish and where any trace of it is to be found in the manifest content of the dream. We already know that the element 'too early, in a hurry' was eliminated from the dream by the censorship [p. 140]. The empty stalls were an allusion to it. The mysterious 'three for 1 florin 50' now becomes more intelligible to us with the help of the symbolism with which we have meanwhile become acquainted. The '3'[1] really means a man [or husband] and the manifest element is easy to translate: buying a husband with her dowry. ('I could have got one ten[2] times better with my dowry.') 'Marrying' is clearly replaced by 'going to the theatre'. 'Taking the theatre tickets too early' is, indeed, an immediate substitute for 'marrying too early'. This substitution is, however, the work of a wish-fulfilment. Our dreamer was not always so dissatisfied with her early marriage as she was on the day when she received the news of her friend's engagement. She had been proud of it at one time and regarded herself as at an advantage over her friend. Simple-minded girls, after becoming engaged, are reputed often to express their joy that they will soon be able to go to the theatre, to all the plays which have hitherto been prohibited, and will be allowed to see everything. The pleasure in looking, or curiosity, which is revealed in this was no doubt originally a sexual desire to look [scopophilia], directed towards sexual happenings and especially on to the girls' parents, and hence it became a powerful motive for urging them to an early marriage. In this way a visit to the theatre became an obvious substitute, by way of allusion, for being married. Thus the dreamer, in her present anger at her early marriage, harked back to the time at which early marriage was the fulfilment of a wish because it satisfied her scopophilia, and, under the lead of

---

[1] I have not mentioned another plausible interpretation of this '3' in a childless woman, since this analysis brought up no material in support of it. [Cf. p. 163 f. above.]

[2] [This is presumably a slip for 'a hundred'. Cf. above, p. 124.]

this old wishful impulse, she replaced marriage by going to the theatre.

I cannot be accused of having specially chosen out the most convenient example as evidence of a concealed wish-fulfilment. The procedure would have had to be the same in the case of other distorted dreams. I cannot demonstrate this to you now, and I will only express my conviction that it could always be successfully accomplished. I will, however, dwell a little longer on this theoretical point. Experience has taught me that it is one of those most exposed to attack in the whole theory of dreams, and that many contradictions and misunderstandings arise from it. Apart from this, you may perhaps still be under the impression that I have already withdrawn part of my assertion in saying that a dream is a fulfilled wish or the opposite of one, or a realized anxiety or punishment; and you may think this is an opportunity of forcing further qualifications out of me. I have also been reproached for putting forward things that seem to me obvious in a manner that is too concise and consequently unconvincing.

When someone has accompanied us so far in the interpretation of dreams and has accepted everything that has been brought forward up to this point, it often happens that he comes to a halt at wish-fulfilment and says: 'Granted that dreams always have a sense, and that that sense can be discovered by the technique of psycho-analysis, why must that sense, all evidence to the contrary, be invariably pushed into the formula of wish-fulfilment? Why should not the sense of this nightly thinking be of as many kinds as that of daytime thinking? Why, that is, should not a dream correspond sometimes to a fulfilled wish, sometimes, as you yourself say, to the opposite of that or to a realized fear, but sometimes express an intention, a warning, a reflection with its "pros" and "cons", or a reproach, a scruple of conscience, an attempt at preparing for a coming task, and so on? Why must it always be only a wish, or at most its opposite?'

It might be thought that a difference of opinion on this point is unimportant, if one is agreed on the rest. It is enough, it might be said, that we have discovered the sense of dreams and the way of recognizing it; it is of less importance if we seem to have defined that sense too narrowly. But that is not so. A misunderstanding on this point affects the essence of our discoveries about dreams and endangers their value for the understanding of the neuroses. Moreover, a compromise of this sort —what is highly thought of in commercial life as being 'accommodating'—is not in place, but detrimental rather, in scientific affairs.

My first answer to the question why dreams should not have a variety of meanings in the sense indicated is as usual in such cases: 'I don't know why they shouldn't. I should have no objection. As far as I'm concerned it could be so. There's only one detail in the way of this broader and more convenient view of dreams—that it isn't so in reality.' My second answer would be that the hypothesis that dreams correspond to a variety of forms of thinking and intellectual operations is not unfamiliar to me myself. I once reported a dream in one of my case histories which appeared on three nights in succession and then no more, and I explained this behaviour by the fact that the dream corresponded to an *intention*, and did not need to be repeated after the intention had been carried out.[1] Later on I published a dream which corresponded to an *admission*.[2] How, then, can I contradict myself and assert that dreams are never anything but a fulfilled wish?

I do it because I will not allow a foolish misunderstanding to pass which may rob us of the fruit of our efforts with dreams —a misunderstanding which confuses the dream with the latent dream-thoughts, and asserts of the former something that applies solely to the latter. For it is quite correct to say that a dream can represent and be replaced by everything you have just enumerated—an intention, a warning, a reflection, a preparation, an attempt at solving a problem, and so on. But if you look properly, you will see that all this only applies to the latent dream-thoughts, which have been transformed into the dream. You learn from interpretations of dreams that people's unconscious thinking is concerned with these intentions, preparations, reflections, and so on, out of which the dream-work then makes the dreams. If at the moment you are not interested

[1] [This was the first dream in the analysis of 'Dora' (1905e).]
[2] [Cf. 'An Evidential Dream' (1913a).]

in the dream-work, but are greatly interested in people's unconscious thought-activity, you then eliminate the dream-work and say of the dream what is in practice quite correct—that it corresponds to a warning, an intention, and so on. What often happens in psycho-analytic activity is that our efforts are chiefly directed only to doing away with the dream-form and inserting in the context instead of it the latent thoughts out of which the dream was made.

Thus, quite incidentally, we learn from our examination of the latent dream-thoughts that all these highly complicated mental acts that we have named can take place unconsciously—a discovery as imposing as it is perplexing!

But to go back, you are only correct so long as you are clearly aware that you have used an abbreviated form of expression and so long as you do not believe that the multiplicity you have been describing is to be related to the essential nature of dreams. When you speak of a 'dream', you must mean either the manifest dream—that is, the product of the dream-work—or, at most, the dream-work itself as well—that is, the psychical process which forms the manifest dream out of the latent dream-thoughts. Any other use of the word is a confusion of ideas and can only lead to mischief.[1] If you are making statements about the latent thoughts behind the dream, do so directly and do not obscure the problem of dreams by the loose manner in which you speak. The latent dream-thoughts are the material which the dream-work transforms into the manifest dream. Why should you want to confuse the material with the activity which forms it? If you do, what advantage have you over those who only knew the product of the activity and could not explain where it came from or how it was made?

The only essential thing about dreams is the dream-work that has influenced the thought-material. We have no right to ignore it in our theory, even though we may disregard it in certain practical situations. Analytic observation shows further that the dream-work never restricts itself to translating these thoughts into the archaic or regressive mode of expression that

[1] [Further discussions on the proper use of the term 'dream' will be found in two footnotes added in 1925 and 1914 respectively to *I. of D.* See the end of Section I in Chapter VI and Section D in Chapter VII and also at the end of Section I of 'Dreams and Telepathy' (1922*a*).]

is familiar to you. In addition, it regularly takes possession of something else, which is not part of the latent thoughts of the previous day, but which is the true motive force for the construction of the dream. This indispensable addition is the equally unconscious wish for the fulfilment of which the content of the dream is given its new form. A dream may thus be any sort of thing in so far as you are only taking into account the thoughts it represents—a warning, an intention, a preparation, and so on; but it is always also the fulfilment of an unconscious wish and, if you are considering it as a product of the dreamwork, it is only that. A dream is therefore never simply an intention, or a warning, but always an intention, etc., translated into the archaic mode of thought by the help of an unconscious wish and transformed to fulfil that wish. [See p. 227, *n.* 2.] The one characteristic, the wish-fulfilment, is the invariable one; the other may vary. It may for its part once more be a wish, in which case the dream will, with the help of an unconscious wish, represent as fulfilled a latent wish of the previous day.

I can understand all this very clearly; but I cannot tell whether I have succeeded in making it intelligible to you as well. And I also have difficulty in proving it to you. That cannot be done without carefully analysing a great many dreams, and on the other hand this most critical and important point in our view of dreams cannot be convincingly represented without referring to what is coming later. It is impossible to suppose that, since everything is intimately interrelated, one can penetrate deeply into the nature of one thing without having concerned oneself with other things of a similar nature. Since we still know nothing of the dream's nearest relatives, neurotic symptoms, we must once more rest content at this point with what we have achieved. I will only give you one more illustrative example and lay before you one fresh consideration.

Let us once again take up the dream we have already so often returned to: the dream of the three theatre-tickets for 1 florin 50. (I can assure you that I originally chose out this example without any special purpose in view.) You know the latent dream-thoughts: anger at having been in such a hurry to get married which arose when she heard the news that her friend had only just become engaged, putting a low value on her husband and the idea that she might have got a better one if only she had waited. We already know the wish which made a dream out of these thoughts: it was the desire to look, to be able to go to the theatre, most probably an offshoot of her old curiosity to discover at long last what really happens when one is married. This curiosity is, as we know, regularly directed by children towards their parents' sexual life; it is an infantile curiosity, and, so far as it still persists later, an instinctual impulse with roots reaching back into infancy. But the news the dreamer had received during the day gave no occasion for awakening this desire to look, but only for awakening anger and regret. This wishful impulse was not in the first instance connected with the latent dream-thoughts; and we were able to include the outcome of the dream-interpretation in the analysis without taking any account of that impulse. But the anger in itself was not capable of creating a dream. A dream could not arise out of the thoughts that 'it was absurd to marry so early' until they had awakened the old wish to see at long last what happens in marriage. This wish then gave the dream-content its form by replacing marriage by going to the theatre, and the form was that of an earlier wish-fulfilment: 'There! now I may go to the theatre and look at everything that's forbidden, and you mayn't! I'm married and you must wait!' In this way the dreamer's present situation was transformed into its opposite, an old triumph was put in the place of her recent defeat. And, incidentally, a satisfaction of her scopophilia was mixed with a satisfaction of her egoistic competitive sense. This satisfaction then determined the manifest content of the dream, in which the position actually was that she was sitting in the theatre while her friend could not gain admission to it. The portions of the content of the dream behind which the latent dream-thoughts still lay concealed were superimposed on this situation of satisfaction as a misplaced and unintelligible modification of it. The dream's interpretation had to disregard everything that served to represent the wish-fulfilment and to re-establish the distressing latent dream-thoughts from these obscure remaining hints.

The fresh consideration I wish to bring before you is to draw your attention to the latent dream-thoughts which have now been put in the foreground. I beg you not to forget that in the first place they are unconscious[1] to the dreamer, and secondly that they are completely rational and coherent so that they can be understood as natural reactions to the precipitating cause of the dream, and thirdly that they can be the equivalent of any mental impulse or intellectual operation. I shall now describe these thoughts more strictly than before as the 'day's residues', whether the dreamer confesses to them or not. I shall now distinguish between the day's residues and the latent dream-thoughts, and, in conformity with our earlier usage, I shall designate as latent dream-thoughts everything we learn in interpreting the dream, whereas the day's residues are only a portion of the latent dream-thoughts. Our view is then that something is added to the day's residues, something that was also part of the unconscious, a powerful but repressed wishful impulse; and it is this alone that makes the construction of the dream possible. The influence of this wishful impulse on the day's residues creates the further portion of the latent dream-thoughts—that which need no longer appear rational and intelligible as being derived from waking life.

I have made use of an analogy for the relation of the day's residues to the unconscious wish, and I can only repeat it here. In every undertaking there must be a capitalist who covers the required outlay and an *entrepreneur* who has the idea and knows how to carry it out. In the construction of dreams, the part of the capitalist is always played by the unconscious wish alone; it provides the psychical energy for the construction of the dream. The *entrepreneur* is the day's residues, which decide how this outlay is to be employed. It is possible, of course, for the capitalist himself to have the idea and the expert knowledge or for the *entrepreneur* himself to possess capital. This simplifies the practical situation but makes its theoretical understanding more difficult. In economics the same person is constantly divided into his two aspects of capitalist and *entrepreneur* and this restores the fundamental situation on which our analogy was based. In dream-construction the same variations occur and I will leave them for you to follow out.[2]

[1] [See footnote p. 21 above.]
[2] [This analogy appeared originally in Section C of Chapter VII of *I. of D.*, where it is illustrated at greater length.]

We cannot advance any further here, for you have probably long been disturbed by a doubt which deserves to be given a hearing. 'Are the day's residues,' you will ask, 'really unconscious in the same sense as the unconscious wish which must be added to them in order to make them capable of producing a dream?' Your suspicion is correct. This is the salient point of the whole business. They are *not* unconscious in the same sense. The dream-wish belongs to a different unconscious—to the one which we have already recognized as being of infantile origin and equipped with peculiar mechanisms [p. 210]. It would be highly opportune to distinguish these two kinds of unconscious by different names. But we would prefer to wait till we have become familiar with the field of phenomena of the neuroses. People consider a single unconscious as something fantastic. What will they say when we confess that we cannot make shift without two of them?[1]

Let us break off here. Once again you have only heard something incomplete. But is it not hopeful to reflect that this knowledge has a continuation, which either we ourselves or other people will bring to light? And have not we ourselves learnt enough that is new and surprising?

---

[1] [The question of the uses of the term 'unconscious' was a crucial one for Freud's theories. He touched on it at several points in the course of these lectures (particularly on pp. 113, 189, 212, 227, 294 ff. and—a last brief mention—on p. 437). But he was evidently already feeling uncomfortable about it and in fact revised his views on the whole subject some years later in *The Ego and the Id* (1923*b*), (Norton, 1960).   A full account of the problem and its history will be found in the Editor's Introduction to that work.   The new solution is also explained in Lecture XXXI of the *New Introductory Lectures* (1933*a*).]

[2] [Page 224, line 14. At the end of this sentence all the German editions have the plural, '*dieser Wünsche* (those wishes)', which would seem to obscure the meaning. An examination of the original manuscript (which is not very clear) appears to show that Freud in fact wrote, or intended to write, the singular, '*dieses Wunsches*'. A shorter, though essentially similar, account of the whole process is given in 'An Evidential Dream' (1913*a*).]

LECTURE XV

UNCERTAINTIES AND CRITICISMS

LADIES AND GENTLEMEN,—We will nevertheless not leave the field of dreams without dealing with the commonest doubts and uncertainties which our novelties and our theories have given rise to so far. Attentive listeners among you will themselves have collected some of the relevant material.

(1) You may have formed an impression that, even though the technique is correctly carried out, the findings of our interpretative work on dreams admit of so many uncertainties as to defeat any secure translation of the manifest dream into the latent dream-thoughts. You will argue in support of this that in the first place one never knows whether a particular element of the dream is to be understood in its actual sense or as a symbol, since the things employed as symbols do not cease on that account to be themselves. If, however, one has no objective clue for deciding this, the interpretation must at that point be left to the arbitrary choice of the interpreter. Furthermore, as a result of the fact that in the dream-work contraries coalesce, it is always left undetermined whether a particular element is to be understood in a positive or negative sense—as itself or as its contrary [p. 178]. Here is a fresh opportunity for the interpreter to exercise an arbitrary choice. Thirdly, in consequence of the reversals of every kind of which dreams are so fond [p. 180], it is open to the interpreter to carry out a reversal like this in connection with any passage in the dream he chooses. And lastly, you will mention having heard that one is never certain whether the interpretation one has found for a dream is the only possible one. We run the risk of overlooking a perfectly admissible 'over-interpretation' of the same dream [p. 173]. In these circumstances, you will conclude, so much room is left to the interpreter's arbitrary decision as to be incompatible with objective certainty in the findings. Or alternatively you may suppose that the fault does not lie with dreams but that the inadequacies of our dream-

228

interpretation are to be attributed to errors in our views and premisses.

All your material is unimpeachable, but it does not, I think, justify your conclusions, and in two respects: namely that the interpretation of dreams is, as you insist, at the mercy of arbitrary choice and that the lack of results throws doubts on the correctness of our procedure. If instead of the interpreter's arbitrary choice you would speak of his skill, his experience and his understanding, I should agree with you. We cannot, of course, do without a personal factor of that kind, especially in the more difficult problems of dream-interpretation. But the position is no different in other scientific occupations. There is no means of preventing one person from handling a particular technique worse than another, or one person from making better use of it than another. What in other ways gives an impression of arbitrariness—in, for instance, the interpretation of symbols—is done away with by the fact that as a rule the interconnection between the dream-thoughts, or the connection between the dream and the dreamer's life, or the whole psychical situation in which the dream occurs, selects a single one from among the possible determinations presented and dismisses the rest as unserviceable. The conclusion that because of the imperfections of dream-interpretation our hypotheses are incorrect is invalidated by pointing out that on the contrary ambiguity or indefiniteness is a characteristic of dreams which was necessarily to be anticipated.

Let us recall that we have said that the dream-work makes a translation of the dream-thoughts into a primitive mode of expression similar to picture-writing [p. 175 ff.]. All such primitive systems of expression, however, are characterized by indefiniteness and ambiguity of this sort, without justifying us in casting doubts on their serviceability. The coalescence of contraries in the dream-work is, as you know, analogous to the so-called 'antithetical meaning of primal words' in the most ancient languages. Indeed, Abel (1884), the philologist to whom we owe this line of thought, implores us not to suppose that communications made by one person to another with the help of such ambivalent words were on that account ambiguous. On the contrary, intonation and gesture must have made it quite certain in the context of the speech which of the two contraries the speaker intended to convey. In writing, where gesture is absent, its place was taken by an additional pictograph which was not intended to be spoken—for instance by a picture of a little man, limply squatting or stiffly erect, according to whether the ambiguous hieroglyph '*ken*' was to mean 'weak' or 'strong'. In this way, in spite of the ambiguity of the sounds and signs, misunderstanding was avoided. [Cf. above, p. 179.]

The old systems of expression—for instance, the scripts of the most ancient languages—betray vagueness in a variety of ways which we would not tolerate in our writing to-day. Thus in some Semitic scripts only the consonants in the words are indicated. The reader has to insert the omitted vowels according to his knowledge and the context. The hieroglyphic script behaves very similarly, though not precisely in the same way; and for that reason the pronunciation of Ancient Egyptian remains unknown to us. The sacred script of the Egyptians is indefinite in yet other ways. For instance, it is left to the arbitrary decision of the scribe whether he arranges the pictures from right to left or from left to right. In order to be able to read it one must obey the rule of reading towards the faces of the figures, birds, and so on. But the scribe might also arrange the pictographs in *vertical* columns, and in making inscriptions on comparatively small objects he allowed considerations of decorativeness and space to influence him in altering the sequence of the signs in yet other ways. The most disturbing thing about the hieroglyphic script is, no doubt, that it makes no separation between words. The pictures are placed across the page at equal distances apart; and in general it is impossible to tell whether a sign is still part of the preceding word or forms the beginning of a new word. In Persian cuneiform script, on the other hand, an oblique wedge serves to separate words.

An extremely ancient language and script, which however is still used by four hundred million people, is the Chinese. You must not suppose that I at all understand it; I only obtained some information about it because I hoped to find analogies in it to the indefiniteness of dreams. Nor has my expectation been disappointed. The Chinese language is full of instances of indefiniteness which might fill us with alarm. As is well known, it consists of a number of syllabic sounds, which are spoken either singly or combined into pairs. One of the principal dialects has some four hundred such sounds. Since, however, the vocabulary of this dialect is reckoned at about four thousand words, it follows that each sound has on an average ten different meanings—some fewer but some correspondingly more. There are quite a number of methods of avoiding ambiguity, since one cannot infer from the context alone which of the ten meanings of the syllabic sound the speaker intends to evoke in the hearer. Among these methods are those of combining two sounds into a compound word and of using four different 'tones' in the pronunciation of the syllables. It is even more interesting from the point of view of our comparison to learn that this language has practically no grammar. It is impossible to tell of any of the monosyllabic words whether it is a noun or a verb or an adjective; and there are no verbal inflections by which one could recognize gender, number, termination, tense or mood. Thus the language consists, one might say, solely of the raw material, just as our thought-language is resolved by the dream-work into its raw material, and any expression of relations is omitted. In Chinese the decision in all cases of indefiniteness is left to the hearer's understanding and this is guided by the context. I have made a note of an example of a Chinese proverb which, literally translated, runs:

'Little what see much what wonderful.'

This is not hard to understand. It may mean: 'The less someone has seen, the more he finds to wonder at'; or: 'There is much to wonder at for him who has seen little.' There is, of course, no question of distinguishing between these two translations, which only differ grammatically. In spite of this indefiniteness, we have been assured that the Chinese language is a quite excellent vehicle for the expression of thought. So indefiniteness need not necessarily lead to ambiguity.

It must, of course, be admitted that the system of expression by dreams occupies a far more unfavourable position than any of these ancient languages and scripts. For after all they are fundamentally intended for communication: that is to say, they are always, by whatever method and with whatever assistance, meant to be understood. But precisely this characteristic is absent in dreams. A dream does not want to say anything to anyone. It is not a vehicle for communication; on the contrary, it is meant to remain ununderstood. For that reason we must

not be surprised or at a loss if it turns out that a number of
ambiguities and obscurities in dreams remain undecided. The
one certain gain we have derived from our comparison is the
discovery that these points of uncertainty which people have
tried to use as objections to the soundness of our dream-interpretations are on the contrary regular characteristics of all
primitive systems of expression.

The question of how far the intelligibility of dreams in fact
extends can only be answered by practice and experience.[1] Very
far, I believe; and my view is confirmed if we compare the results produced by correctly trained analysts. The lay public,
including the scientific lay public, are well known to enjoy
making a parade of scepticism when faced by the difficulties
and uncertainties of a scientific achievement. I think they are
wrong in this. You are perhaps not all aware that a similar
situation arose in the history of the deciphering of the Baby-
lonian–Assyrian inscriptions. There was a time when public
opinion was very much inclined to regard the decipherers of
cuneiform as visionaries and the whole of their researches as a
'swindle'. But in 1857 the Royal Asiatic Society made a decisive experiment. It requested four of the most highly respected
experts in cuneiform, Rawlinson, Hincks, Fox Talbot and
Oppert, to send it, in sealed envelopes, independent translations of a newly discovered inscription; and, after a comparison
between the four productions, it was able to announce that the
agreement between these experts went far enough to justify a
belief in what had so far been achieved and confidence in
further advances. The derision on the part of the learned lay
world gradually diminished after this, and since then certainty
in reading cuneiform documents has increased enormously.

(2) A second group of doubts is closely connected with the
impression, which no doubt you yourselves have not escaped,
that a number of the solutions to which we find ourselves
driven in interpreting dreams seem to be forced, artificial,
dragged in by the hair of their head—arbitrary, that is, or even
comic and facetious. Remarks to this effect are so frequent that

[1] [Cf. a later paper on 'The Limits to the Possibility of Interpretation',
Section A of 'Some Additional Notes on Dream-Interpretation as a
Whole' (1925*i*).]

I will choose at random the last that has been reported to me. So listen to this. In free Switzerland the head of a training-college was recently removed from his post on account of his interest in psycho-analysis. He entered a protest, and a Berne newspaper published the report of the school authorities on his appeal. I will select a few sentences dealing with psycho-analysis from this document: 'Moreover we are surprised at the far-fetched and artificial character of many of the examples, which are also to be found in the volume by Dr. Pfister of Zurich which is quoted. . . . It is really surprising, therefore, that the head of a training-college should accept all these assertions and pretended proofs without criticism.' These sentences are represented as a decision reached by someone 'making a calm judgement'. It is rather this calmness, I think, which is 'artificial'. Let us examine these remarks more closely, in the expectation that a little reflection and a little expert knowledge can be of no disadvantage even to a calm judgement.

It is truly refreshing to see how swiftly and unerringly a person can arrive at a judgement on some delicate problem of depth-psychology after his first impression of it. The interpretations seem to him far-fetched and forced and he does not like them; so they are false and all this business of interpretation is worthless. Not even a fleeting thought is given to the other possibility—that there are good reasons why these interpretations are bound to have this appearance; after which the further question would follow of what these good reasons are.

The matter under consideration relates in essence to the results of displacement, which you have become acquainted with as the most powerful instrument of the dream-censorship. With the help of displacement the dream-censorship creates substitutive structures which we have described as allusions. But they are allusions which are not easily recognizable as such, from which the path back to the genuine thing is not easily traced, and which are connected with the genuine thing by the strangest, most unusual, external associations.[1] In all these cases it is a question, however, of things which are *meant* to be hidden, which are condemned to concealment, for that is what the dream-censorship is aiming at. But we must not expect that a

[1] [See footnote 1, p. 174 above.]

thing which has been hidden will be found in its own place, in its proper position. The frontier-control commissions which are operating to-day are more cunning in this respect than the Swiss school authorities. In their search for documents and plans they are not content with examining brief-cases and portfolios, but they consider the possibility that spies and smugglers may have these forbidden things in the most secret portions of their clothing where they decidedly do not belong—for instance, between the double soles of their boots. If the hidden things are there, it will certainly be possible to call them 'far-fetched', but it is also true that a great deal will have been found.[1]

If we recognize that the links between a latent dream-element and its manifest substitute can be of the most out-of-the-way and peculiar nature, sometimes appearing comic and sometimes resembling a joke, we are basing ourselves on copious experience of examples which, as a rule, we have not solved ourselves. It is often impossible to give such interpretations on our own account: no sensible person could guess at the connection. The dreamer gives us the translation either all at once by a direct association—*he* is able to, since it was he who produced the substitute—or else he brings up so much material that the solution no longer calls for any particular acumen, but presents itself, so to speak, as a matter of course. If the dreamer fails to assist in one or other of these two ways, the manifest element in question will for ever remain unintelligible to us. I will, if I may, give you an example which occurred to me recently. One of my women patients lost her father in the course of the treatment. Since then she has taken every opportunity of bringing him to life in her dreams. In one of these her father appeared (in a particular connection of no further relevance) and said: '*It's a quarter past eleven, it's half-past eleven, it's a quarter to twelve.*' By way of interpretation of this oddity all that occurred to her was that her father liked his grown-up children to appear punctually at the family meals. No doubt this was connected with the dream-element, but it threw no light on its origin. There was a suspicion, based on the immediate situation in the treatment, that a carefully suppressed critical revolt against her beloved and honoured father played some part in the dream. In the further course of her associations, apparently remote

---

[1] [There is some untranslatable punning here in the original.]

from the dream, she told how the day before there had been a lot of talk about psychology in her presence, and a relative of hers had remarked: 'The *Urmensch* [primal man] survives in all of us.' This seemed to provide us with the explanation. It had given her an excellent opportunity of bringing her dead father to life once again. She made him in the dream into an '*Uhrmensch*' ['clock-man'] by making him announce the quarter-hours at midday.

You will not be able to escape the resemblance of this example to a joke; and it has in fact often happened that a joke of the dreamer's has been regarded as a joke of the interpreter's. There are other instances in which it has been far from easy to decide whether what we are dealing with is a joke or a dream. But you will recall that the same doubt arose in the case of some parapraxes—slips of the tongue [p. 43 f.]. A man reported as a dream of his that his uncle had given him a kiss while they were sitting in his *auto*(mobile).[1] He himself very quickly added the interpretation: it meant '*auto-erotism*' (a term from the theory of the libido, indicating satisfaction obtained without any outside object). Had the man set out, then, to have some fun with us and was he passing off a joke that had occurred to him as a dream? I think not; I believe he really dreamt it. But what is the origin of this puzzling similarity? This question once led me temporarily aside from my path by compelling me to make jokes themselves the subject of a detailed investigation.[2] It was there shown how jokes originate: a preconscious[3] train of thought is abandoned for a moment to be worked over in the unconscious, and from this it emerges as a joke. Under the influence of the unconscious it is subjected to the effects of the mechanisms that hold sway there—condensation and displacement—the same processes that we have found concerned in the dream-work; and it is to this common feature that is to be ascribed the similarity, when it occurs, between jokes and dreams. But the unintended 'dream-joke' brings none of the

[1] [This dream is reported in *I of D.*, in Chapter VI in Section (F).]
[2] *Jokes and their Relation to the Unconscious*(1905c),(Norton, 1960). Freud relates in *I. of D.*, VI(A), how he was led into writing that work by a critic (Wilhelm Fliess) who complained that the dreams he reported were too full of jokes. See also a passage on this point in the book on jokes itself, (p. 173).]
[3] [This term is explained in Lecture XIX, p. 296 below.]

yield of pleasure of a true joke. You can learn why if you go more deeply into the study of jokes. A 'dream-joke' strikes us as a bad joke; it does not make us laugh, it leaves us cold.[1]

In this, however, we are treading in the footsteps of the dream-interpretation of antiquity, which, along with much that is unserviceable, has left us some good examples of dream-interpretation, which we ourselves could not better. I will repeat to you a dream which was of historic importance and which is reported of Alexander the Great, with slight variations, by Plutarch and Artemidorus of Daldis [cf. p. 86 above]. When the king was laying siege to the obstinately defended city of Tyre (322 B.C.), he once dreamt that he saw a dancing satyr. Aristander, the dream-interpreter, who was present with the army, interpreted the dream by dividing the word 'Satyros' into σὰ Τύρος [sa Turos] (thine is Tyre), and therefore promised that he would triumph over the city. Alexander was led by this interpretation to continue the siege and eventually captured Tyre. The interpretation, which has a sufficiently artificial appearance, was undoubtedly the right one.[2]

[3] I can well imagine that you will be especially impressed when you hear that objections to our view of dreams have even been made by people who have themselves, as psycho-analysts, been engaged for a considerable time in interpreting dreams. It would have been too much to expect that such an abundant encouragement to fresh errors as this theory offers should have been neglected; and so, as a result of conceptual confusions and unjustified generalizations, assertions have been made which are not far behind the medical view of dreams in their incorrectness. You know one of them already. It tells us that dreams are concerned with attempts at adaptation to present conditions and with attempts at solving future problems—that they have a 'prospective purpose' (Maeder [1912]). We have already shown [p. 222] that this assertion is based on a confusion between the dream and the latent dream-thoughts and is therefore based on disregarding the dream-work. As a characteriza-

---

[1] [See the end of Chapter VI of the book on jokes. The point has already been mentioned above on p. 174.]

[2] [This is also reported in Chapter II of I. of D., n.]

tion of the unconscious intellectual activity of which the latent dream-thoughts form part, it is on the one hand no novelty and on the other not exhaustive, since unconscious intellectual activity is occupied with many other things besides preparing for the future.[1] A far worse confusion seems to underlie the assurance that the idea of death will be found behind every dream [Stekel, 1911, 34]. I am not clear exactly what is meant by this formula. But I suspect that it conceals a confusion between the dream and the dreamer's whole personality. [Cf. *I. of D.*, 5, 397.]

An unjustifiable generalization, based on a few good examples, is involved in the statement that every dream allows of two interpretations—one which agrees with our account, a 'psycho-analytic' one, and another, an 'anagogic' one, which disregards the instinctual impulses and aims at representing the higher functions of the mind (Silberer [1914]).[2] There are dreams of this kind, but you will try in vain to extend this view even to a majority of dreams. Again, after all that I have said to you, you will find quite incomprehensible an assertion that all dreams are to be interpreted bisexually, as a confluence of two currents described as a masculine and a feminine one (Adler [1910]). [Cf. *I. of D.*, 5, 397.] There are, of course, a few dreams of this kind too; and you may learn later that they are constructed like certain hysterical symptoms. The reason why I have mentioned all these discoveries of fresh universal characteristics of dreams is in order to warn you against them or at least to leave you in no doubt as to what I think of them.

(4) One day the objective value of research into dreams seemed to be put in question by an observation that patients under analytic treatment arrange the content of their dreams in accordance with the favourite theories of their physicians— some dreaming predominantly of sexual instinctual impulses, others of the struggle for power and yet others even of

---

[1] [This theory of Maeder's was dealt with at length by Freud in two footnotes to *I. of D.,* See the end of Section I of Chapter VI and Section D of Chapter VII.]

[2] [This was fully discussed in Section A of Chapter VII in *I. of D.,* as well as in 'Dreams and Telepathy' (1922*a*), and in a footnote to 'A Metapyschological Supplement to the Theory of Dreams' (1917*d*).]

rebirth (Stekel). The weight of this observation was, however, diminished by the reflection that human beings had dreams before there was any psycho-analytic treatment which could give those dreams a direction, and that people who are now under treatment used also to dream during the period before the treatment started. What was true about this novelty could soon be seen to be self-evident and of no relevance to the theory of dreams. The day's residues which instigate dreams are left over from powerful interests in waking life. When the remarks made by the physician and the hints he gives become of significance to the patient, they enter the circle of the day's residues and can provide psychical stimuli for the construction of dreams like any other emotionally coloured interests of the previous day which have not been dealt with, and they then operate like somatic stimuli which impinge on the sleeper during his sleep. The trains of thought set going by the physician can, like these other instigators of dreams, appear in the manifest content of a dream or be discovered in its latent content. Indeed, we know that a dream can be experimentally produced, or, to put it more correctly, a part of the dream-material can be introduced into the dream. In producing these effects on his patients, an analyst is thus playing a part no different from an experimenter who, like Mourly Vold, gives particular postures to the limbs of the subjects of his experiments. [Cf. p. 87 above.]

It is often possible to influence dreamers as to what they shall dream *about*, but never as to *what* they shall dream. The mechanism of the dream-work and the unconscious dream-wish are exempt from any outside influence. In considering dreams with a somatic stimulus, we have already found [p. 96 f.] that the characteristic nature and independence of dream-life are shown in the reaction with which dreams respond to the somatic or mental stimuli that are brought to bear. The thesis which we have been discussing, and which seeks to throw doubt on the objectivity of research into dreams, is thus once again based on a confusion—this time between the dream and the dream-material.[1]

[1] [For a further discussion of this, see Section VII of 'Remarks on the Theory and Practice of Dream-Interpretation' (1923c).]

This then, Ladies and Gentlemen, is what I wanted to tell you about the problems of dreams. As you will guess, there is much that I have had to pass over, and you will have been aware that on almost every point what I have said has necessarily been incomplete. That, however, is due to the connection between the phenomena of dreaming and those of the neuroses. We have studied dreams as an introduction to the theory of the neuroses, and this was certainly a more correct procedure than if we had done the opposite. But just as dreams prepare the way to an understanding of the neuroses, so, on the other hand, a true appreciation of dreams can only be achieved after a knowledge of neurotic phenomena.[1]

I cannot tell what you will think of it, but I must assure you that I do not regret having claimed so much of your interest and of the time available to us for the problems of dreams. There is nothing else from which one can so quickly arrive at a conviction of the correctness of the theses by which psychoanalysis stands or falls. Exacting work over many months and even years is called for to show that the symptoms of a case of neurotic illness have a sense, serve a purpose and arise out of the patient's experiences in life. On the other hand, only a few hours' effort may be enough to prove that the same thing is true of a dream which is, to start with, confused to the point of being unintelligible, and thus to confirm all the premises of psycho-analysis—the unconscious nature of mental processes, the peculiar mechanisms which they obey and the instinctual forces which are expressed in them. And when we bear in mind the sweeping analogy between the structure of dreams and that of neurotic symptoms and at the same time consider the rapidity of the transformation which makes a dreamer into a waking and reasonable man, we arrive at a certainty that neuroses too are based only on an alteration in the play of forces between the powers of mental life.[2]

[1] [There is a reference back to dreams near the end of the last lecture of the present series, p. 456 below.]

[2] [Freud dealt with the subject of dreams again in the first of his *New Introductory Lectures,* p. 471 below.]

PART III
GENERAL THEORY
OF THE NEUROSES
(1917 [1916–17])

PSYCHO-ANALYSIS AND PSYCHIATRY

LADIES AND GENTLEMEN,—I am delighted to see you again, at the beginning of a new academic year, for a resumption of our discussions. Last year I spoke to you of the way in which psycho-analysis deals with parapraxes and dreams. This year I should like to introduce you to an understanding of the phenomena of neurosis, which, as you will soon learn, have a great deal in common with both of the others. But I must warn you in advance that I shall not be able to offer you the same position in relation to me this year as I did last year. At that time I set great store on never taking a step without remaining in agreement with your judgement; I discussed a great deal with you and gave way to your objections—in fact I recognized you and your 'common sense' as a deciding factor. But this is no longer possible and for a simple reason. Parapraxes and dreams were not unfamiliar to you as phenomena; we might say that you had as much experience or could easily obtain as much experience of them as I had. The region of the phenomena of neurosis is, however, strange to you; in so far as you are not doctors yourselves, you have no other access to them than through what I have to tell you; and of what help is the best judgement if it is not accompanied by familiarity with the material that is to be judged?

But you must not take this warning of mine to mean that I propose to give you dogmatic lectures and to insist on your unqualified belief. Such a misunderstanding would do me a grave injustice. I do not wish to arouse conviction; I wish to stimulate thought and to upset prejudices. If as a result of lack of knowledge of the material you are not in a position to form a judgement, you should neither believe nor reject. You should listen and allow what I tell you to work on you. It is not so easy to arrive at convictions, or, if they are reached easily, they soon turn out to be worthless and incapable of resistance. The only person who has a right to a conviction is someone who, like me, has worked for many years at the same material and who, in doing so, has himself had the same new and surprising experiences. What is the good, then, in the sphere of the intellect, of these sudden convictions, these lightning-like conversions, these instantaneous rejections? Is it not clear that the 'coup de foudre', love at first sight, is derived from quite another sphere, from that of the emotions? We do not even require of our *patients* that they should bring a conviction of the truth of psycho-analysis into the treatment or be adherents of it. Such an attitude often raises our suspicions. The attitude that we find the most desirable in them is a benevolent scepticism. So you too should endeavour to allow the psycho-analytic view to grow up quietly in you alongside of the popular or psychiatric one, till opportunities arise for the two to influence each other, to compete with each other and to unite in leading to a conclusion.

On the other hand, you should not for a moment suppose that what I put before you as the psycho-analytic view is a speculative system. It is on the contrary empirical—either a direct expression of observations or the outcome of a process of working them over. Whether this working-over has been carried out in an adequate and justifiable manner will appear in the course of the further advance of the science, and indeed I may assert without boasting, after a lapse of nearly twenty-five years, and having reached a fairly advanced age,[1] that these observations are the result of particularly hard, concentrated and deep-going work. I have often had an impression that our opponents were unwilling to take any account of this origin of our theses, as though they thought what was in question were merely subjectively determined notions to which someone else might oppose others of his own choice. This behaviour of our opponents is not entirely intelligible to me. It may perhaps be due to the fact that, as a doctor, one usually makes so little contact with neurotic patients and pays so little attention to what they say that one cannot imagine the possibility that anything valuable could be derived from their communications—the possibility, that is, of carrying out any thorough observations upon them. I take this opportunity of assuring you that in the course of these lectures I shall indulge in very little controversy, especially with individuals. I have never been able to convince myself of

[1] [Freud was about 60 at this time.]

the truth of the maxim that strife is the father of all things. I believe it is derived from the Greek sophists and is at fault, like them, through overvaluing dialectics. It seems to me, on the contrary, that what is known as scientific controversy is on the whole quite unproductive, apart from the fact that it is almost always conducted on highly personal lines. Up to a few years ago I was able to boast that I had only once engaged in a regular scientific dispute—with one single worker (Löwenfeld of Munich).[1] It ended in our becoming friends and we have remained so to this day. But I did not repeat the experiment for a long time, as I did not feel sure that the outcome would be the same.[2]

Now you will no doubt conclude that a rejection such as this of all written discussion argues a high degree of inaccessibility to objections, of obstinacy, or, to use the polite colloquial scientific term, of pig-headedness [Verranntheit]. I should like to say in reply that when once, after such hard work, one has arrived at a conviction, one has at the same time acquired a certain right to retain that conviction with some tenacity. I may also urge that in the course of my work I have modified my views on a few important points, changed them and replaced them by fresh ones—and in each case, of course, I have made this publicly known. And the outcome of this frankness? Some people have taken no notice whatever of my self-corrections and continue to this day to criticize me for hypotheses which have long ceased to have the same meaning for me. Others reproach me precisely for these changes and regard me as untrustworthy on their account. Of course! a person who has occasionally changed his opinions is deserving of no belief at all, since he has made it all too likely that his latest assertions may also be mistaken; but a person who has unflinchingly maintained what he once asserted, or who cannot be quickly enough persuaded to give it up, must naturally be pig-headed or stubborn! What

[1] [This was on the subject of Freud's early theories on anxiety. His second paper on the question (1895f) was entirely concerned with Löwenfeld's criticisms. Löwenfeld himself, though never an adherent to Freud's views, ultimately became much more favourable to them.]

[2] [There is an allusion in this to Freud's much more recent controversies with Adler and Jung, especially in his 'History of the Psycho-Analytic Movement' (1914d), (Norton, 1966).]

can one do, in the face of these contradictory objections by the critics, but remain as one is and behave in accordance with one's own judgement? I am resolved to do that, and I shall not be deterred from modifying or withdrawing any of my theories, as my advancing experience may require. In regard to *fundamental* discoveries I have hitherto found nothing to alter, and I hope this will remain true in the future.[1]

I am to put before you, then, the psycho-analytic view of the phenomena of neurosis. In doing so, the best plan would seem to be to make a start in connection with the phenomena we have already dealt with, for the sake both of analogy and contrast; and I will begin with a symptomatic action [p. 61] which I have seen many people perform during my consulting hours. We analysts cannot do much for the people who come to us in our consulting-room to lay before us in a quarter of an hour the miseries of a long lifetime. Our deeper knowledge makes it difficult for us to give the kind of opinion another doctor would—'There's nothing wrong with you'—with the added advice: 'You should arrange for a mild hydropathic treatment.' One of my colleagues who was asked what he did with his consultation patients shrugged his shoulders and replied: 'I fine them so-and-so many *Kronen* for a frivolous waste of time.' So you will not be surprised to hear that even in the case of busy psycho-analysts their consulting hours are not apt to be very lively. I have had the ordinary door between my waiting-room and my consulting- and treatment-room doubled

---

[1] [Perhaps the chief change in Freud's views up to the time of this lecture had been his abandonment of the purely traumatic causation of the neuroses and his insistence instead on the importance of the innate instinctual forces and on the great part played by phantasies. On this see his paper on the part played by sexuality in the neuroses (1906a). Later on there were, of course, to be further important changes in his views—for instance on the nature of anxiety in *Inhibitions, Symptoms and Anxiety* (1926d), and on the sexual development of women in the Editor's Note to 'Some Psychical Consequences of the Anatomical Distinction between the Sexes' (1925j). But what lay ahead above all were a revision of the theory of the instincts in *Beyond the Pleasure Principle* (1920g) and a new structural picture of the mind in *The Ego and the Id* (1923b), (Norton, 1960). All these changes were to be discussed fifteen years later in the *New Introductory Lectures*.]

and given a baize lining. There can be no doubt about the purpose of this arrangement. Now it constantly happens that a person whom I have brought in from the waiting-room omits to shut the door behind him and almost always he leaves *both* doors open. As soon as I notice this I insist in a rather unfriendly tone on his or her going back and making good the omission— even if the person concerned is a well-dressed gentleman or a fashionable lady. This makes an impression of uncalled-for pedantry. Occasionally, too, I have put myself in a foolish position by making this request when it has turned out to be a person who cannot touch a door-handle himself and is glad if someone with him spares him the necessity. But in the majority of cases I have been right; for anyone who behaves like this and leaves the door open between a doctor's waiting-room and consulting-room is ill-mannered and deserves an unfriendly reception. But do not take sides over this till you have heard the sequel. For this carelessness on the part of the patient only occurs when he has been alone in the waiting-room and has therefore left an empty room behind him; it never happens if other people, strangers to him, have been waiting with him. In this latter case he knows quite well that it is in his interest not to be overheard while he is talking to the doctor, and he never fails to shut both the doors carefully.

Thus the patient's omission is neither accidentally nor senselessly determined; and indeed it is not unimportant, for, as we shall see, it throws light on the newcomer's attitude to the doctor. The patient is one of the great multitude who have a craving for mundane authority, who wish to be dazzled and intimidated. He may have enquired on the telephone as to the hour at which he could most easily get an appointment; he had formed a picture of a crowd of people seeking for help, like the crowd outside one of Julius Meinl's branches.[1] He now comes into an empty, and moreover extremely modestly furnished, waiting-room, and is shocked. He has to make the doctor pay for the superfluous respect which he had intended to offer him: so—he omits to shut the door between the waiting-room and the consulting-room. What he means to say to the doctor by his conduct is: 'Ah, so there's no one here and no one's likely to

[1] [The war-time queue outside one of the popular Austrian grocery chain-stores.]

come while I'm here.' He would behave equally impolitely and disrespectfully during the consultation if his arrogance were not given a sharp reprimand at the very beginning.

The analysis of this small symptomatic action tells you nothing you did not know before: the thesis that it was not a matter of chance but had a motive, a sense and an intention, that it had a place in an assignable mental context and that it provided information, by a small indication, of a more important mental process. But, more than anything else, it tells you that the process thus indicated was unknown to the consciousness of the person who carried out the action, since none of the patients who left the two doors open would have been able to admit that by this omission he wanted to give evidence of his contempt. Some of them would probably have been aware of a sense of disappointment when they entered the empty waiting-room; but the connection between this impression and the symptomatic action which followed certainly remained unknown to their consciousness.

Beside this small analysis of a symptomatic action we will now place an observation on a patient. I choose this one because it is fresh in my memory, but also because it can be reported comparatively briefly. A certain amount of detail is indispensable in any such account.

A young officer, home on short leave, asked me to undertake the treatment of his mother-in-law, who, though in the happiest circumstances, was embittering her own life and the lives of her relatives through an absurd idea. In this way I made the acquaintance of a well-preserved lady of fifty-three, friendly and simple in her nature, who told me the following story without any reluctance. She lived in the country, most happily married, with her husband, who was at the head of a large factory. She could not give enough praise to her husband's affectionate solicitude. It had been a love-match thirty years ago, and since then there had never been any trouble, discord or cause for jealousy. Her two children were happily married; her husband (and their father), out of a sense of duty, was not yet willing to retire. A year before, she had received an anonymous letter accusing her excellent husband of a love affair with a young girl; and the incredible—and to herself unintelligible

—result was that she immediately believed it, and since then her happiness had been destroyed. The course of events, in greater detail, was something like this. She had a housemaid with whom she used, perhaps too often, to have intimate talks. This girl pursued another one with a positively malicious hostility because she had done so much better for herself in life, though she was of no higher origin. Instead of going into service, this other girl had managed to get a commercial training, had entered the factory and, as a result of shortness of personnel, owing to members of the staff being called up for military service, she was promoted to a good position. She now lived in the factory itself, had social relations with all the gentlemen and was actually addressed as 'Fräulein'. The girl who had made less of a success in life was of course ready to repeat all kinds of bad things of her former schoolmate. One day our lady had a conversation with the housemaid about a gentleman who had been staying with them, who was well known not to be living with his wife but to be having an affair with another woman. She did not know how it happened, but she suddenly said: 'The most dreadful thing that could happen to me would be if I were to learn that my dear husband was having an affair too.' The next day she received an anonymous letter by post which, as though by magic, gave her this very information, written in a disguised hand. She decided, probably rightly, that the letter was the work of the malicious housemaid, since it specified as her husband's mistress the girl whom the servant pursued with her hatred. But although she at once saw through the intrigue and had seen enough instances where she lived of how little credence such cowardly denunciations deserved, what happened was that the letter instantly prostrated her. She became terribly excited, sent for her husband at once and reproached him violently. Her husband laughed the accusation off and did the best possible thing. He brought in the family doctor (who was also the factory doctor) who made efforts to soothe the unfortunate lady. The further conduct of both of them was also entirely sensible. The housemaid was dismissed, but the alleged rival was not. Since then the patient had repeatedly been pacified to the point of no longer believing the content of the anonymous letter, but never thoroughly and never for long. It was enough for her to hear the young lady's name mentioned or to meet her in the street and a fresh attack of distrust, pain and reproaches would burst out in her.

This, then, is the case history of this excellent woman. Not much psychiatric experience was needed to understand that, in contrast to other neurotics, she was giving too mild an account of her case—that she was, as we say, dissimulating—and that she had never really got over her belief in the accusation contained in the anonymous letter.

What attitude, then, will a psychiatrist adopt in a case of illness like this? We know already how he would behave to the symptomatic action of the patient who fails to shut the consulting-room door. He pronounces it to be a chance event of no psychological interest with which he has no further concern. But this procedure cannot be carried over to the illness of the jealous woman. The symptomatic action seems to be a matter of indifference; but the symptom forces itself on our attention as a matter of importance. It is accompanied by intense subjective suffering and, as an objective fact, it threatens the communal life of a family; it is thus an undeniable subject of psychiatric interest. The psychiatrist will start by endeavouring to characterize the symptom by some essential feature. The idea with which the woman torments herself cannot in itself be called absurd; it does, indeed, happen that elderly gentlemen have love affairs with young girls. But there is something else about it which *is* absurd and hard to understand. The patient had no other reason at all for believing that her affectionate and loyal husband belonged to this otherwise not so rare class of husbands except what was asserted in the anonymous letter. She knew that this document had no evidential value and she was able to give a satisfying explanation of its origin. She ought therefore to have been able to tell herself that she had no ground whatever for her jealousy, and she did tell herself so. But in spite of this she suffered as much as if she regarded this jealousy as completely justified. Ideas of this kind, which are inaccessible to logical arguments based on reality, are by general agreement described as *delusions*. The good lady, then, was suffering from *delusions of jealousy*. This is no doubt the essential feature of this case of illness.

After this first point has been established our psychiatric interest will become even livelier. If a delusion is not to be got rid of by a reference to reality, no doubt it did not originate from reality either. Where else did it originate? There are delusions of the most varied content: why in our case is the content of the delusion jealousy in particular? In what kind of people do delusions, and especially delusions of jealousy, come about? We should like to hear what the psychiatrist has to say about this; but at this point he leaves us in the lurch. He enters into only a single one of our enquiries. He will investigate the woman's family history and will *perhaps* give us this reply: 'Delusions come about in people in whose families similar and other psychical disorders have repeatedly occurred.' In other words, if this woman developed a delusion she was predisposed to it by hereditary transmission. No doubt that is something; but is it all we want to know? Was this the only thing that contributed to the causation of the illness? Must we be content to suppose that it is a matter of indifference or caprice or is inexplicable whether a delusion of jealousy arises rather than any other sort? And ought we to understand the assertion of the predominance of the hereditary influence in a negative sense as well—that no matter what experiences this woman's mind encountered she was destined some time or other to produce a delusion? You will want to know why it is that scientific psychiatry will give us no further information. But my reply to you is: 'he is a rogue who gives more than he has.' The psychiatrist knows no way of throwing more light on a case like this one. He must content himself with a diagnosis and a prognosis—uncertain in spite of a wealth of experience—of its future course.

But can psycho-analysis do more here? Yes, it actually can. I hope to be able to show you that, even in a case so hard of access as this, it can discover something which makes a first understanding possible. And to begin with I would draw your attention to the inconspicuous detail that the patient herself positively provoked the anonymous letter, which now gave support to her delusion, by informing the scheming housemaid on the previous day that it would cause her the greatest unhappiness if her husband had a love affair with a young girl. In this way she first put the notion of sending the anonymous letter into the housemaid's head. Thus the delusion acquires a certain independence of the letter; it had been present already in the patient as a fear—or was it as a wish? Let us now add to this the small further indications yielded by only two analytic sessions. The patient, indeed, behaved in a very unco-operative way when, after telling me her story, she was asked for her further thoughts, ideas and memories. She said that nothing occurred to her, that she had told me everything already, and after two sessions the experiment with me had in fact to be broken off because she announced that she already felt well and that she was sure the pathological idea would not come back. She only said this, of course, from resistance and from dread of the continuation of the analysis. Nevertheless, during these two sessions she let fall a few remarks which allowed of, and indeed necessitated, a particular interpretation; and this interpretation threw a clear light on the genesis of her delusion of jealousy. She herself was intensely in love with a young man, with the same son-in-law who had persuaded her to come to me as a patient. She herself knew nothing, or perhaps only a very little, of this love; in the family relationship that existed between them it was easy for this passionate liking to disguise itself as innocent affection. After all our experiences elsewhere, it is not hard for us to feel our way into the mental life of this upright wife and worthy mother, of the age of fifty-three. Being in love like this, a monstrous and impossible thing, could not become conscious; but it remained in existence and, even though it was unconscious, it exercised a severe pressure. Something had to become of it, some relief had to be looked for; and the easiest mitigation was offered, no doubt, by the mechanism of displacement which plays a part so regularly in the generating of delusional jealousy. If not only were she, the old woman, in love with a young man, but if also her old husband were having a love affair with a young girl, then her conscience would be relieved of the weight of her unfaithfulness. The phantasy of her husband's unfaithfulness thus acted as a cooling compress on her burning wound. Her own love had not become conscious to her, but its mirror-reflection, which brought her such an advantage, now became conscious as an obsession and delusion. No arguments against it could, of course, have any effect, for they were only directed against the mirror-image and not against the original which gave the other its strength and which lay hidden, inviolable, in the unconscious.

Let us now bring together what this effort at a psycho-analysis, short and impeded as it was, has brought to light for an understanding of this case—assuming, of course, that our enquiries were correctly carried out, which I cannot here submit to your judgement. Firstly, the delusion has ceased to be absurd or unintelligible; it had a sense, it had good motives and it fitted into the context of an emotional experience of the patient's. Secondly, the delusion was necessary, as a reaction to an unconscious mental process which we have inferred from other indications, and it was precisely to this connection that it owed its delusional character and its resistance to every logical and realistic attack. It itself was something desired, a kind of consolation. Thirdly, the fact that the delusion turned out to be precisely a jealous one and not one of another kind was unambiguously determined by the experience that lay behind the illness.[1] You recall of course that, the day before, she had told the scheming maid that the most dreadful thing that could happen to her would be her husband's unfaithfulness. Nor will you have overlooked the two important analogies between this case and the symptomatic action which we analysed—the explanation of its sense or intention and its relation to something unconscious that was involved in the situation.

Naturally this does not answer all the questions that we might ask in connection with this case. On the contrary, the case bristles with further problems—some that have in general not yet become soluble and others which could not be solved owing to the particular circumstances being unfavourable. For instance, why did this lady who was happily married fall in love with her son-in-law? and why did the relief, which might have been possible in other ways, take the form of this mirror-image, this projection of her state on to her husband? You must not think it is otiose or frivolous to raise such questions. We already have some material at our disposal which might possibly serve to answer them. The lady was at a critical age, at which sexual needs in women suffer a sudden and undesired increase; that alone might account for the event. Or it may further have been that her excellent and faithful husband had for some years no longer enjoyed the sexual capacity which the well-preserved woman required for her satisfaction. Experience has shown us

---

[1] [This sentence occurs in a less clear form in some of the earlier German editions.]

that it is precisely men in this position, whose faithfulness can consequently be taken for granted, who are distinguished by treating their wives with unusual tenderness, and by showing particular forbearance for their nervous troubles. Or, again, it may not be without significance that the object of this pathogenic love was precisely the young husband of one of her daughters. A powerful erotic tie with a daughter, which goes back in the last resort to the mother's sexual constitution, often finds a way of persisting in a transformation of this sort. In this connection I may perhaps remind you that the relation between mother-in-law and son-in-law has been regarded from the earliest times of the human race as a particularly awkward one and that among primitive people it has given rise to very powerful taboo regulations and 'avoidances'.[1] The relation is frequently excessive by civilized standards both in a positive and negative direction. Which of these three factors became operative in our case, or whether two of them or perhaps all three came together, I cannot, it is true, tell you; but that is only because I was not permitted to continue the analysis of the case for more than two sessions.

I notice now, Gentlemen, that I have been talking to you about a number of things which you are not yet prepared to understand. I did so in order to carry out the comparison between psychiatry and psycho-analysis. But there is one thing that I can ask you now. Have you observed any sign of a contradiction between them? Psychiatry does not employ the technical methods of psycho-analysis; it omits to make any inferences from the *content* of the delusion, and, in pointing to heredity, it gives us a very general and remote aetiology instead of indicating first the more special and proximate causes. But is there a contradiction, an opposition in this? Is it not rather a case of one supplementing the other? Does the hereditary factor contradict the importance of experience? Do not the two things rather combine in the most effective manner? You will grant that there is nothing in the nature of psychiatric work which could be opposed to psycho-analytic research. What is opposed to psycho-analysis is not psychiatry but psychiatrists. Psycho-

[1] [See first essay of *Totem and Taboo* (1912–13) (Norton, 1952.)]

analysis is related to psychiatry approximately as histology is to anatomy: the one studies the external forms of the organs, the other studies their construction out of tissues and cells. It is not easy to imagine a contradiction between these two species of study, of which one is a continuation of the other. To-day, as you know, anatomy is regarded by us as the foundation of scientific medicine. But there was a time when it was as much forbidden to dissect the human cadaver in order to discover the internal structure of the body as it now seems to be to practise psycho-analysis in order to learn about the internal mechanism of the mind. It is to be expected that in the not too distant future it will be realized that a scientifically based psychiatry is not possible without a sound knowledge of the deeper-lying unconscious processes in mental life.

Perhaps, however, the much-abused psycho-analysis has friends among you who will be pleased if it can be justified from another direction—from the therapeutic side. As you know, our psychiatric therapy is not hitherto able to influence delusions. Is it possible, perhaps, that psycho-analysis can do so, thanks to its insight into the mechanism of these symptoms? No, Gentlemen, it cannot. It is as powerless (for the time being at least) against these ailments as any other form of therapy. *We* can understand, indeed, what has happened in the patient, but we have no means of making the patient himself understand it. You have heard how I was unable to pursue the analysis of this delusion beyond a first beginning. Will you be inclined to maintain on that account that an analysis of such cases is to be rejected because it is fruitless? I think not. We have a right, or rather a duty, to carry on our research without consideration of any immediate beneficial effect. In the end—we cannot tell where or when—every little fragment of knowledge will be transformed into power, and into therapeutic power as well. Even if psycho-analysis showed itself as unsuccessful in every other form of nervous and psychical disease as it does in delusions, it would still remain completely justified as an irreplaceable instrument of scientific research. It is true that in that case we should not be in a position to practise it. The human material on which we seek to learn, which lives, has its own will and needs its motives for co-operating in our work, would hold back from us. Let me therefore end my remarks to-day by

informing you that there are extensive groups of nervous disorders in which the transformation of our better understanding
into therapeutic power has actually taken place, and that in
these illnesses, which are difficult of access by other means, we
achieve, under favourable conditions, successes which are
second to no others in the field of internal medicine.[1]

[1] [Psycho-analysis as a method of psychotherapy is the subject of the
last lecture of the series (XXVIII).]

LECTURE XVII

THE SENSE OF SYMPTOMS

LADIES AND GENTLEMEN,—In the last lecture I explained to you that clinical psychiatry takes little notice of the outward form or content of individual symptoms, but that psycho-analysis takes matters up at precisely that point and has established in the first place the fact that symptoms have a sense and are related to the patient's experiences. The sense of neurotic symptoms was first discovered by Josef Breuer from his study and successful cure (between 1880 and 1882) of a case of hysteria which has since become famous. It is true that Pierre Janet brought forward the same evidence independently; indeed, the French worker can claim priority of publication, for it was only a decade later (in 1893 and 1895), while he was collaborating with me, that Breuer published his observation. In any case it may seem a matter of some indifference who made the discovery, for, as you know, every discovery is made more than once and none is made all at once. And, apart from this, success does not always go along with merit: America is not named after Columbus. The great psychiatrist Leuret[1] gave it as his opinion, before Breuer and Janet, that even the delusional ideas of the insane would certainly be found to have a sense if only we understood how to translate them. I must admit that for a long time I was prepared to give Janet very great credit for throwing light on neurotic symptoms, because he regarded them as expressions of *idées inconscientes* which dominated the patients.[2] But since then he has expressed himself with exaggerated reserve, as if he wanted to admit that the unconscious had been nothing more to him than a form of words, a makeshift, *une façon de parler*—that he had meant nothing real by it.[3] Since then I have ceased to understand Janet's writings; but I think he has unnecessarily forfeited much credit.

Thus neurotic symptoms have a sense, like parapraxes and

---

[1] [François Leuret (1797–1851). (Leuret, 1834, 131.)]
[2] [See, for example, Janet, 1888.]
[3] [For the gist of this see Janet, 1913, 39.]

dreams, and, like them, have a connection with the life of those who produce them. I should now like to make this important discovery plainer to you by a few examples. I can indeed only assert, I cannot prove, that it is always and in every instance so. Anyone who looks for experiences himself, will find convincing evidence. But for certain reasons I shall choose these examples from cases not of hysteria but of another, highly remarkable neurosis which is fundamentally very much akin to it and about which I have a few introductory remarks to make.

This neurosis, known as 'obsessional neurosis', is not so popular as the universally familiar hysteria. It is not, if I may express myself thus, so obtrusively noisy, it behaves more like a private affair of the patient's, it dispenses almost entirely with somatic phenomena, and creates all its symptoms in the mental sphere. Obsessional neurosis and hysteria are the forms of neurotic illness upon the study of which psycho-analysis was first built, and in the treatment of which, too, our therapy celebrates its triumphs. But obsessional neurosis, in which the puzzling leap from the mental to the physical plays no part, has actually, through the efforts of psycho-analysis, become more perspicuous and familiar to us than hysteria, and we have learnt that it displays certain extreme characteristics of the nature of neurosis far more glaringly.

Obsessional neurosis is shown in the patient's being occupied with thoughts in which he is in fact not interested, in his being aware of impulses in himself which appear very strange to him and in his being led to actions the performance of which give him no enjoyment, but which it is quite impossible for him to omit. The thoughts (obsessions) may be senseless in themselves, or merely a matter of indifference to the subject; often they are completely silly, and invariably they are the starting-point of a strenuous mental activity, which exhausts the patient and to which he only surrenders himself most unwillingly. He is obliged against his will to brood and speculate as though it were a question of his most important vital problems. The impulses which the patient is aware of in himself may also make a childish and senseless impression; but as a rule they have a content of the most frightful kind, tempting him, for instance, to commit serious crimes, so that he not merely disavows them as alien to himself, but flies from them in horror and protects himself from carrying them out by prohibitions, renunciations and restrictions upon his freedom. At the same time, these impulses never—literally never—force their way through to performance; the outcome lies always in victory for the flight and the precautions. What the patient actually carries out—his so-called obsessional actions—are very harmless and certainly trivial things, for the most part repetitions or ceremonial elaborations of the activities of ordinary life. But these necessary activities (such as going to bed, washing, dressing or going for a walk) become extremely tedious and almost insoluble tasks. In different forms and cases of obsessional neurosis the pathological ideas, impulses and actions are not combined in equal proportions; it is the rule, rather, that one or other of these factors dominates the picture and gives its name to the illness, but the common element in all these forms is sufficiently unmistakable.

Certainly this is a crazy illness. The most extravagant psychiatric imagination would not, I think, have succeeded in constructing anything like it; and if one did not see it before one every day one would never bring oneself to believe in it. Do not suppose, however, that you will help the patient in the least by calling on him to take a new line, to cease to occupy himself with such foolish thoughts and to do something sensible instead of his childish pranks. He would like to do so himself, for he is completely clear in his head, shares your opinion of his obsessional symptoms and even puts it forward to you spontaneously. Only he cannot help himself. What is carried into action in an obsessional neurosis is sustained by an energy to which we probably know nothing comparable in normal mental life. There is only one thing he can do: he can make displacements, and exchanges, he can replace one foolish idea by another somewhat milder, he can proceed from one precaution or prohibition to another, instead of one ceremonial he can perform another. He can displace the obsession but not remove it. The ability to displace any symptom into something far removed from its original conformation is a main characteristic of his illness. Moreover it is a striking fact that in his condition the contradictions (polarities) with which mental life is interlaced [cf. p. 301 below] emerge especially sharply differentiated. Alongside of obsessions with a positive and negative content, *doubt* makes itself felt in the intellectual field and little by little it begins to gnaw even at what is usually most certain. The whole position ends up in an ever-increasing degree of indecision, loss of energy and restriction of freedom. At the same time, the obsessional neurotic starts off with a very energetic disposition, he is often extraordinarily self-willed and as a rule he has intellectual gifts above the average. He has usually reached a satisfactorily high level of ethical development; he exhibits over-conscientiousness, and is more than ordinarily correct in his behaviour. You can imagine that no small amount of work is needed before one can make one's way any distance into this contradictory hotchpotch of character-traits and symptoms. And to begin with we aim at nothing whatever else than understanding a few of the symptoms and being able to interpret them.

Perhaps you would like to know in advance, having in mind our earlier talks, what attitude contemporary psychiatry adopts towards the problems of obsessional neurosis. But it is a meagre chapter. Psychiatry gives names to the different obsessions but says nothing further about them. On the other hand it insists that those who suffer from these symptoms are 'degenerates'. This gives small satisfaction; in fact it is a judgement of value— a condemnation instead of an explanation. We are supposed to think that every possible sort of eccentricity may arise in degenerates. Well, it is true that we must regard those who develop such symptoms as somewhat different in their nature from other people. But we may ask: are they more 'degenerate' than other neurotics—than hysterical patients, for instance, or those who fall ill of psychoses? Once again, the characterization is evidently too general. Indeed, we may doubt whether there is any justification for it at all, when we learn that such symptoms occur too in distinguished people of particularly high capacities, capacities important for the world at large. It is true that, thanks to their own discretion and to the untruthfulness of their biographers, we learn little that is intimate about the great men who are our models; but it may nevertheless happen that one of them, like Émile Zola, may be a fanatic for the truth, and we then learn from him of the many strange obsessional habits to which he was a life-long victim.[1]

Psychiatry has found a way out by speaking of '*dégénérés*

[1] E. Toulouse, *Émile Zola, enquête médico-psychologique*, Paris, 1896.

supérieurs'. Very nice. But we have found from psycho-analysis that it is possible to get permanently rid of these strange obsessional symptoms, just as of other complaints and just as in people who are not degenerate. I myself have succeeded repeatedly in this.[1]

I shall give you only two examples of the analysis of an obsessional symptom: one an old observation which I cannot find a better one to replace, and another recently met with. I limit myself to this small number, because it is impossible in such reports to avoid being very diffuse and entering into every detail.

A lady, nearly thirty years of age, who suffered from the most severe obsessional manifestations and whom I might perhaps have helped if a malicious chance had not brought my work to nothing—I may be able to tell you more about this later on—performed (among others) the following remarkable obsessional action many times a day. She ran from her room into another neighbouring one, took up a particular position there beside a table that stood in the middle, rang the bell for her housemaid, sent her on some indifferent errand or let her go without one, and then ran back into her own room. This was certainly not a very distressing symptom, but was nevertheless calculated to excite curiosity. The explanation was reached in the most unequivocal and unobjectionable manner, free from any possible contribution on the doctor's part. I cannot see how I could possibly have formed any suspicion of the sense of this obsessional action or could have offered any suggestion on how it was to be interpreted. Whenever I asked the patient 'Why do you do that? What sense has it?' she answered: 'I don't know.' But one day, after I had succeeded in defeating a major, fundamental doubt of hers, she suddenly knew the answer and told me what it was that was connected with the obsessional action. More than ten years before, she had married a man very much older than herself, and on the wedding-night he was impotent.

[1] [Freud probably discussed obsessional neurosis more often than any other disorder—from the beginning of his career almost to the end of it. A list of some of the more important references will be found in an Appendix to his 'Notes upon a Case of Obsessional Neurosis' (1909*d*).]

Many times during the night he had come running from his room into hers to try once more, but every time without success. Next morning he had said angrily: 'I should feel ashamed in front of the housemaid when she makes the bed,' took up a bottle of red ink that happened to be in the room and poured its contents over the sheet, but not on the exact place where a stain would have been appropriate. I could not understand at first what this recollection had to do with the obsessional action in question; the only resemblance I could find was in the repeated running from one room into the other, and perhaps also in the entrance of the housemaid. My patient then led me up to the table in the second room and showed me a big stain on the tablecloth. She further explained that she took up her position in relation to the table in such a way that the maid who had been sent for could not fail to see the stain. There could no longer be any doubt of the intimate connection between the scene on her wedding-night and her present obsessional action, though all kinds of other things remained to be learnt.

It was clear, in the first place, that the patient was identifying herself with her husband; she was playing his part by imitating his running from one room into the other. Further, to carry on the analogy, we must agree that the bed and the sheet were replaced by the table and the tablecloth. This might seem arbitrary, but surely we have not studied dream-symbolism to no purpose. In dreams too we often find a table which has to be interpreted as a bed. Table and bed[1] together stand for marriage, so that the one can easily take the place of the other.

It already seems proved that the obsessional action had a sense; it appears to have been a representation, a repetition, of the significant scene. But we are not obliged to come to a halt here. If we examine the relation between the two more closely, we shall probably obtain information about something that goes further—about the intention of the obsessional action. Its kernel was obviously the summoning of the housemaid, before whose eyes the patient displayed the stain, in contrast to her husband's remark that he would feel ashamed in front of the maid. Thus he, whose part she was playing, did not feel ashamed in front of the maid; accordingly the stain was in the

[1] [The English phrase is 'bed and board', which is itself a translation of a law-Latin term for marriage.]

right place. We see, therefore, that she was not simply repeating
the scene, she was continuing and at the same time correcting
it; she was putting it right. But by this she was also correcting
the other thing, which had been so distressing that night and
had made the expedient with the red ink necessary—his impotence. So the obsessional action was saying: 'No, it's not true.
He had no need to feel ashamed in front of the housemaid; he
was not impotent.' It represented this wish, in the manner of a
dream, as fulfilled in a present-day action; it served the purpose
of making her husband superior to his past mishap.

Everything I could tell you about this woman fits in with
this. Or, more correctly speaking, everything else we know
about her points the way to this interpretation of what was in
itself an unintelligible obsessional action. The woman had been
living apart from her husband for years and was struggling with
an intention to obtain a legal divorce. But there was no question
of her being free of him; she was forced to remain faithful to
him; she withdrew from the world so as not to be tempted; she
exculpated and magnified his nature in her imagination. Indeed, the deepest secret of her illness was that by means of it
she protected her husband from malicious gossip, justified her
separation from him and enabled him to lead a comfortable
separate life. Thus the analysis of a harmless obsessional action
led directly to the inmost core of an illness, but at the same
time betrayed to us no small part of the secret of obsessional
neurosis in general. I am glad to let you dwell a little on this
example because it combines conditions which we could not
fairly expect to find in every case. Here the interpretation of the
symptom was discovered by the patient herself at a single blow,
without any prompting or intervention on the analyst's part;
and it resulted from a connection with an event which did not
(as is usually the case) belong to a forgotten period of childhood, but which had happened in the patient's adult life and
had remained undimmed in her memory. All the objections
which criticism is normally in the habit of raising against our
interpretation of symptoms fall to the ground in this particular
case. We cannot hope always to have such good luck.[1]

[1] [Freud had given a shorter account of this case, though with
some further details, in his paper on 'Obsessive Actions and Religious Practices' (1907b).]

And one thing more. Were you not struck by the way in which this unobtrusive obsessional action has led us into the intimacies of the patient's life? A woman cannot have anything much more intimate to tell than the story of her wedding-night. Is it a matter of chance and of no further significance that we have arrived precisely at the intimacies of sexual life? No doubt it might be the result of the choice I have made on this occasion. Do not let us be too hasty in forming our judgement, and let us turn to my second example, which is of quite a different kind— a sample of a very common species, a sleep-ceremonial.

A nineteen-year-old girl, well developed and gifted, was the only child of parents to whom she was superior in education and intellectual liveliness. As a child she had been wild and high-spirited, and in the course of the last few years had changed, without any visible cause, into a neurotic. She was very irritable, particularly towards her mother, always dissatisfied and depressed, and inclined to indecisiveness and doubt; finally she admitted that she was no longer able to walk by herself across squares or along comparatively wide streets. We will not concern ourselves much with her complicated illness, which called for at least two diagnoses—agoraphobia and obsessional neurosis—but will dwell only on the fact that she also developed a sleep-ceremonial, with which she tormented her parents. In a certain sense it may be said that every normal person has his sleep-ceremonial or that he has established certain necessary conditions the non-fulfilment of which interferes with his going to sleep; he has imposed certain forms on the transition from the waking to the sleeping state and repeats them in the same manner every evening. But everything that a healthy person requires as a necessary condition for sleep can be understood rationally, and if external circumstances call for a change he will comply easily and without waste of time. A pathological ceremonial, however, is unyielding and insists on being carried through, even at the cost of great sacrifices; it too is screened by having a rational basis and at a superficial glance seems to diverge from the normal only by a certain exaggerated meticulousness. On closer examination, nevertheless, we can see that the screen is insufficient, that the ceremonial comprises some stipulations which go far beyond its rational basis and others which positively run counter to it. Our present patient put forward as a pretext for her nightly precautions that she needed quiet in order to sleep and must exclude every source of noise. With that end in view she did two kinds of things. The big clock in her room was stopped, all the other clocks or watches in the room were removed, and her tiny wrist-watch was not allowed even to be inside her bedside table. Flower-pots and vases were collected on the writing-table so that they might not fall over in the night and break, and disturb her in her sleep. She was aware that these measures could find only an *ostensible* justification in the rule in favour of quiet: the ticking of the little watch would not have been audible even if it had been left lying on the top of the bedside table, and we have all had experience of the fact that the regular ticking of a pendulum-clock never disturbs sleep but acts, rather, as a soporific. She admitted too that her fear that flower-pots and vases, if they were left in their places, might fall over and break of their own accord lacked all plausibility. In the case of other stipulations made by the ceremonial the need for quiet was dropped as a basis. Indeed, the requirement that the door between her room and her parents' bedroom should stay half-open—the fulfilment of which she ensured by placing various objects in the open doorway—seemed on the contrary to act as a source of disturbing noises. But the most important stipulations related to the bed itself. The pillow at the top end of the bed must not touch the wooden back of the bedstead. The small top-pillow must lie on this large pillow in one specific way only —namely, so as to form a diamond shape. Her head had then to lie exactly along the long diameter of the diamond. The eiderdown (or '*Duchent*' as we call it in Austria[1]) had to be shaken before being laid on the bed so that its bottom end became very thick; afterwards, however, she never failed to even out this accumulation of feathers by pressing them apart.

With your leave I will pass over the remaining, often very trivial, details of the ceremonial; they would teach us nothing new, and would lead us too far afield from our aims. But you

[1] [Elsewhere in Germany the French word '*duvet*' is usual. This object is normally an undivided bag of feathers, not, as in England, quilted into a number of separate compartments.]

must not overlook the fact that all this was not carried out smoothly. There was always an apprehension that things might not have been done properly. Everything must be checked and repeated, doubts assailed first one and then another of the safety measures, and the result was that one or two hours were spent, during which the girl herself could not sleep and would not allow her intimidated parents to sleep either.

The analysis of these torments did not proceed so simply as that of our earlier patient's obsessional action. I was obliged to give the girl hints and propose interpretations, which were always rejected with a decided 'no' or accepted with contemptuous doubt. But after this first reaction of rejection there followed a time during which she occupied herself with the possibilities put before her, collected associations to them, produced recollections and made connections, until by her own work she had accepted all the interpretations. In proportion as this happened, she relaxed the performance of her obsessional measures, and even before the end of the treatment she had given up the whole ceremonial. You must understand, too, that the work of analysis as we carry it out to-day quite excludes the systematic treatment of any individual symptom till it has been entirely cleared up. We are, on the contrary, obliged to keep on leaving any particular topic, in the certain expectation of coming back to it again in other connections. The interpretation of her symptoms which I am about to give you is accordingly a synthesis of findings which were arrived at, interrupted by other work, over a period of weeks and months.

Our patient gradually came to learn that it was as symbols of the female genitals that clocks were banished from her equipment for the night. Clocks and watches—though elsewhere we have found other symbolic interpretations for them[1]—have arrived at a genital role owing to their relation to periodic processes and equal intervals of time. A woman may boast that her menstruation behaves with the regularity of clockwork. Our patient's anxiety, however, was directed in particular against being disturbed in her sleep by the ticking of a clock. The ticking of a clock may be compared with the knocking or throbbing

[1] [Another reason for the dislike of clocks and watches felt by obsessional neurotics is mentioned in the 'Rat Man' analysis (1909d).]

in the clitoris during sexual excitement.[1] She had in fact been repeatedly woken from her sleep by this sensation, which had now become distressing to her; and she gave expression to this fear of an erection in the rule that all clocks and watches that were going should be removed from her neighbourhood at night. Flower-pots and vases, like all vessels [p. 156], are also female symbols. Taking precautions against their falling and being broken at night was thus not without its good sense. We know the widespread custom of breaking a vessel or plate at betrothal ceremonies. Each man present gets hold of a fragment, and we may regard this as a sign of his resigning the claims he had upon the bride in virtue of a marriage-regulation dating from before the establishment of monogamy.[2] In connection with this part of her ceremonial the girl produced a recollection and several associations. Once when she was a child she had fallen down while she was carrying a glass or china vase and had cut her finger and bled profusely. When she grew up and came to know the facts about sexual intercourse she formed an anxious idea that on her wedding-night she would not bleed and would thus fail to show that she was a virgin. Her precautions against vases being broken thus meant a repudiation of the whole complex concerned with virginity and bleeding at the first intercourse—a repudiation equally of the fear of bleeding and of the contrary fear of not bleeding. These precautions, which she subsumed under her avoidance of noise, had only a remote connection with it.

She found out the central meaning of her ceremonial one day when she suddenly understood the meaning of the rule that the pillow must not touch the back of the bedstead. The pillow, she said, had always been a woman to her and the upright wooden back a man. Thus she wanted—by magic, we must interpolate—to keep the man and woman apart—that is, to separate her parents from each other, not to allow them to have sexual intercourse. In earlier years, before she had established the ceremonial, she had tried to achieve the same aim in a more

---

[1] [Freud had reported a similar connection in his paper on a case of paranoia (1915f).]

[2] [Cf. a reference to 'group marriage' in *Totem and Taboo* (1912-13), (Norton, 1952), and a discussion in 'The Taboo of Virginity' (1918a).]

direct way. She had simulated fear (or had exploited a tendency to fear which was already present) in order that the connecting doors between her parents' bedroom and the nursery should not be shut. This rule had, indeed, been retained in her present ceremonial. In that way she gave herself the opportunity of listening to her parents, but in making use of it she brought on an insomnia which lasted for months. Not satisfied with disturbing her parents by this means, she contrived to be allowed from time to time to sleep in her parents' bed between them. The 'pillow' and the 'wooden back' were thus really unable to come together. Finally, when she was so big that it became physically uncomfortable for her to find room in the bed between her parents, she managed, by a conscious simulation of anxiety, to arrange for her mother to exchange places with her for the night and to leave her own place so that the patient could sleep beside her father. This situation no doubt became the starting-point of phantasies whose after-effect was to be seen in the ceremonial.

If a pillow was a woman, then the shaking of the eiderdown till all the feathers were at the bottom and caused a swelling there had a sense as well. It meant making a woman pregnant; but she never failed to smooth away the pregnancy again, for she had for years been afraid that her parents' intercourse would result in another child and so present her with a competitor. On the other hand, if the big pillow was a woman, the mother, then the small top-pillow could only stand for the daughter. Why did this pillow have to be placed diamond-wise and her head precisely along its centre line? It was easy to recall to her that this diamond shape is the inscription scribbled on every wall to represent the open female genitals. If so, she herself was playing the man and replacing the male organ by her head. (Cf. the symbolism of beheading for castrating.)[1]

Wild thoughts, you will say, to be running through an unmarried girl's head. I admit that is so. But you must not forget that I did not make these things but only interpreted them. A sleep-ceremonial like this is a strange thing too,[2] and you will

[1] [See Freud's paper on this subject (1916c), which includes a short reference to the present case.]

[2] [An almost equally elaborate sleep-ceremonial had been reported by Freud long before, in his second paper on the neuro-psychoses of defence (1896b).]

not fail to see how the ceremonial corresponds to the phantasies which are revealed by the interpretation. But I attach more importance to your noticing that what was seen in the ceremonial was a precipitate not of a *single* phantasy but of a number of them, though they had a nodal point somewhere, and, further, that the rules laid down by the ceremonial reproduced the patient's sexual wishes at one point positively and at another negatively—in part they represented them, but in part they served as a defence against them.

More could be made, too, of the analysis of this ceremonial if it could be properly linked up with the patient's other symptoms. But our path does not lead in that direction. You must be content with a hint that the girl was in the grip of an erotic attachment to her father whose beginnings went back to her childhood. Perhaps that was why she behaved in such an unfriendly way to her mother [p. 264]. Nor can we overlook the fact that the analysis of this symptom has once again taken us back to a patient's sexual life. We shall perhaps be less surprised at this the more often we gain an insight into the sense and intention of neurotic symptoms.

I have shown you, then, on the basis of two chosen examples, that neurotic symptoms have a sense, like parapraxes and dreams, and that they have an intimate connection with the patient's experiences. Can I expect you to believe this extremely important thesis on the evidence of two examples? No. But can you require me to go on giving you further examples till you declare yourselves convinced? No, once more. For, in view of the detailed fashion in which I deal with each single case, I should have to devote a five-hour course of lectures to settling this one point in the theory of the neuroses. So I must be content with having given you a trial proof of my assertion and, for the rest, I refer you to the reports given in the literature of the subject—to the classical interpretations of symptoms in Breuer's first case (of hysteria),[1] to the striking light thrown upon the most obscure symptoms of what is known as dementia praecox by C. G. Jung [1907], at a time when he was merely a psycho-analyst and had not yet aspired to be a prophet, and all the other papers that have since than filled our periodicals.

[1] [Included in *Studies on Hysteria* (1895d), the Case of Anna O.]

There has been no lack of investigations precisely on these lines. The analysis, interpretation and translation of neurotic symptoms proved so attractive to psycho-analysts that for a time they neglected the other problems of neurosis.

If any of you undertakes exertions of this kind, he will certainly gain a powerful impression of the wealth of evidential material. But he will also come up against a difficulty. The sense of a symptom lies, as we have found, in some connection with the patient's experience. The more individual is the form of the symptom the more reason we shall have for expecting to be able to establish this connection. The task is then simply to discover, in respect to a senseless idea and a pointless action, the past situation in which the idea was justified and the action served a purpose. The obsessional action of our patient who ran to the table and rang for the housemaid is a perfect model of this kind of symptom. But there are—and they are very frequent—symptoms of quite another character. They must be described as 'typical' symptoms of an illness; they are approximately the same in all cases, individual distinctions disappear in them or at least shrink up to such an extent that it is difficult to bring them into connection with the patients' individual experience and to relate them to particular situations they have experienced. Let us look once more at obsessional neurosis. The sleep-ceremonial of our second patient already has much that is typical about it, though at the same time it has enough individual traits to make what I might call a 'historical' interpretation possible. But all these obsessional patients have a tendency to repeat, to make their performances rhythmical and to keep them isolated from other actions. The majority of them wash too much. Patients who suffer from agoraphobia (topophobia or fear of spaces), which we no longer regard as obsessional neurosis but describe as 'anxiety hysteria', often repeat the same features in their symptoms with wearisome monotony: they are afraid of enclosed spaces, of large open squares, of lengthy roads and streets. They feel protected if they are accompanied by an acquaintance or followed by a vehicle, and so on. On this similar background, however, different patients nevertheless display their individual requirements—whims, one is inclined to say—which in some cases contradict one another directly. One patient avoids only narrow streets and another only wide ones; one can go out only if there are few people in the street, another only if there are many. In the same way, hysteria, in spite of its wealth of individual traits, has a superfluity of common, typical symptoms, which seem to resist any easy historical derivation. And we must not forget that it is these typical symptoms, indeed, which give us our bearings when we make our diagnosis. Suppose, in a case of hysteria, we have really traced a typical symptom back to an experience or a chain of similar experiences—a case of hysterical vomiting, for instance, to a series of disgusting impressions—then we are at a loss when the analysis in a similar case of vomiting reveals a series of a quite different kind of ostensibly effective experiences. It looks, then, as though for unknown reasons hysterical patients are bound to produce vomiting and as though the historical precipitating causes revealed by analysis were only pretexts which, if they happen to be there, are exploited by this internal necessity.

So we are now faced by the depressing discovery that, though we can give a satisfactory explanation of the individual neurotic symptoms by their connection with experiences, our skill leaves us in the lurch when we come to the far more frequent typical symptoms. Furthermore, I am far from having made you acquainted with all the difficulties that arise when consistently pursuing the historical interpretation of symptoms. Nor do I intend to do so; for, though it is my intention not to gloss things over to you or conceal them, I cannot throw you into perplexity and confusion at the very beginning of our common studies. It is true that we have only made a beginning with our efforts at understanding the significance of symptoms; but we will hold fast to what we have achieved and pursue our way step by step to a mastery of what we have not yet understood. I will try to console you, therefore, with the reflection that any fundamental distinction between one kind of symptom and the other is scarcely to be assumed. If the individual symptoms are so unmistakably dependent on the patient's experience, it remains possible that the typical symptoms may go back to an experience which is in itself typical—common to all human beings. Other features which recur regularly in neuroses may be general reactions which are imposed on the patients by the nature of their pathological change, like the repetitions or doubts in obsessional neurosis. In short, we have no grounds for premature despair; we shall see what remains to be seen.

A quite similar difficulty faces us in the theory of dreams. I could not deal with it in our earlier discussions on dreams. The manifest content of dreams is of the greatest diversity and individual variety, and we have shown in detail what one derives from this content by means of analysis. But alongside of these there are dreams which equally deserve to be called 'typical', which happen in everyone in the same way, dreams with a uniform content, which offer the same difficulties to interpretation. They are dreams of falling, flying, floating, swimming, of being inhibited, of being naked and certain other anxiety-dreams—which lead, in different people, now to this and now to that interpretation, without any light being thrown on their monotony and typical occurrence. But in these dreams too we observe that this common background is enlivened by additions that vary individually; and it is probable that, with a widening of our knowledge, it will be possible, without constraint, to include these dreams too in the understanding of dream-life which we have acquired from other dreams.[1]

[1] [See the section on 'typical' dreams in *The Interpretation of Dreams* (1900a), Chapter V (D).]

LECTURE XVIII

FIXATION TO TRAUMAS—
THE UNCONSCIOUS

LADIES AND GENTLEMEN,—In my last lecture I expressed a desire that our work should go forward on the basis not of our doubts but of our discoveries. We have not yet had any discussion of two of the most interesting implications that follow from our two sample analyses.

To take the first of these. Both patients give us an impression of having been 'fixated' to a particular portion of their past, as though they could not manage to free themselves from it and were for that reason alienated from the present and the future. They then remained lodged in their illness in the sort of way in which in earlier days people retreated into a monastery in order to bear the burden there of their ill-fated lives. What had brought this fate upon our first patient was the marriage which she had in real life abandoned. By means of her symptoms she continued to carry on her dealings with her husband. We learnt to understand the voices that pleaded for him, that excused him, that put him on a pedestal and that lamented his loss. Although she was young and desirable to other men, she had taken every precaution, real and imaginary (magical), to remain faithful to him. She did not show herself to strangers and she neglected her personal appearance; furthermore, once she had sat down in a chair she was unable to get out of it quickly,[1] she refused to sign her name, and she could not make any presents, on the ground that no one ought to receive anything from her.

The same effect was produced on the life of our second patient, the young girl, by an erotic attachment to her father which had started during the years before her puberty. The conclusion she herself drew was that she could not marry as long as she was so ill. We, however, may suspect that she had become so ill in order not to have to marry and in order to remain with her father.

[1] [This symptom is further described and explained in Freud's other account of the case (1907b).]

We cannot dismiss the question of why, in what way and for what motive a person can arrive at such a remarkable attitude to life and one that is so inexpedient—assuming that this attitude is a general characteristic of neuroses and not a special peculiarity of these two patients. And in fact it is a general feature, of great practical importance, in every neurosis. Breuer's first hysterical patient [p. 257 above] was similarly fixated to the period when she was nursing her father in a serious illness. In spite of her recovery, in a certain respect she remained cut off from life; she remained healthy and efficient but avoided the normal course of a woman's life.[1] In every one of our patients, analysis shows us that they have been carried back to some particular period of their past by the symptoms of their illness or their consequences. In the majority of cases, indeed, a very early phase of life is chosen for the purpose—a period of their childhood or even, laughable as this may sound, of their existence as an infant at the breast.

The closest analogy to this behaviour of our neurotics is afforded by illnesses which are being produced with special frequency precisely at the present time by the war—what are described as traumatic neuroses. Similar cases, of course, appeared before the war as well, after railway collisions and other alarming accidents involving fatal risks. Traumatic neuroses are not in their essence the same thing as the spontaneous neuroses which we are in the habit of investigating and treating by analysis; nor have we yet succeeded in bringing them into harmony with our views, and I hope I shall be able at some time to explain to you the reason for this limitation.[2] But in one respect we may insist that there is a complete agreement between them. The traumatic neuroses give a clear indication that a fixation to the moment of the traumatic accident lies at their root. These patients regularly repeat the traumatic situation in their dreams;[3] where hysteriform attacks occur that admit of an analysis, we find that the attack corresponds to a

---

[1] [Anna O. was never married. See Jones, 1953.]

[2] [Traumatic neuroses are mentioned again on p. 381 below. Freud was later able to throw more light on the war neuroses (1919d).]

[3] [This particular point played a part in Freud's first discussion of the 'compulsion to repeat' a few years later. See *Beyond the Pleasure Principle* (1920g).]

complete transplanting of the patient into the traumatic situation.[1] It is as though these patients had not finished with the traumatic situation, as though they were still faced by it as an immediate task which has not been dealt with; and we take this view quite seriously. It shows us the way to what we may call an *economic* view of mental processes.[2] Indeed, the term 'traumatic' has no other sense than an economic one. We apply it to an experience which within a short period of time presents the mind with an increase of stimulus too powerful to be dealt with or worked off in the normal way, and this must result in permanent disturbances of the manner in which the energy operates.

This analogy is bound to tempt us to describe as traumatic those experiences too to which our neurotic patients seem to be fixated. This would promise to offer us a simple determinant for the onset of neurosis. Neurosis could then be equated with a traumatic illness and would come about owing to inability to deal with an experience whose affective colouring was excessively powerful. And this indeed was actually the first formula in which (in 1893 and 1895) Breuer and I accounted theoretically for our new observations.[3] A case like that of the first of the two patients in my last lecture—the young married woman separated from her husband—fits in very well with this view. She had not got over the failure of her marriage and remained attached to that trauma. But our second case—that of the girl with a fixation upon her father—shows us already that the formula is not sufficiently comprehensive. On the one hand, a little girl's being in love like this with her father is something so common and so frequently surmounted that the term 'traumatic' applied to it would lose all its meaning; and, on the other hand, the patient's history showed us that in the first instance her erotic fixation appeared to have passed off without doing any damage, and it was only several years later that it reappeared in the symptoms of the obsessional neurosis. Here,

[1] [This was already recognized in Section IV of the Breuer and Freud 'Preliminary Communication' (1893a).]

[2] [Freud returns to this later (p. 356).]

[3] [See, for instance, Section II of the Breuer and Freud 'Preliminary Communication' (1893a), and in particular its last two paragraphs.]

then, we foresee complications, a greater wealth of determinants for the onset of illness; but we may also suspect that there is no need to abandon the traumatic line of approach as being erroneous: it must be possible to fit it in and subsume it somewhere else.

Here once more, then, we must break off the course we have started on. For the moment it leads no further and we shall have to learn all kinds of other things before we can find its proper continuation.[1] But on the subject of fixation to a particular phase in the past we may add that such behaviour is far more widespread than neurosis. Every neurosis includes a fixation of that kind, but not every fixation leads to a neurosis, coincides with a neurosis or arises owing to a neurosis. A perfect model of an affective fixation to something that is past is provided by mourning, which actually involves the most complete alienation from the present and the future. But even the judgement of a layman will distinguish sharply between mourning and neurosis. There are, on the other hand, neuroses which may be described as a pathological form of mourning.[2]

It may happen, too, that a person is brought so completely to a stop by a traumatic event which shatters the foundations of his life that he abandons all interest in the present and future and remains permanently absorbed in mental concentration upon the past. But an unfortunate such as this need not on that account become a neurotic. We will not attach too much value to this one feature, therefore, in characterizing neurosis, however regularly present and however important it may usually be.

Let us turn now to the second of the discoveries which follow from our analyses; in its case we need not fear having to make a subsequent qualification of our views. I have described to you how our first patient carried out a senseless obsessional action and how she reported an intimate memory from her past life as having some connection with it: and how afterwards I

[1] [The subject is taken up again in Lecture XXII.]
[2] [See on this Freud's metapsychological paper 'Mourning and Melancholia' (1917e), actually published after the delivery of this lecture, though written two years earlier. A short reference to melancholia appears in Lecture XXVI, p. 427 f. below.]

examined the connection between the two and discovered the intention of the obsessional action from its relation to the memory. But there is one factor which I have entirely neglected, though it deserves our fullest attention. However often the patient repeated her obsessional action, she knew nothing of its being derived from the experience she had had. The connection between the two was hidden from her; she could only quite truthfully reply that she did not know what it was that was making her carry out her action. Then suddenly one day, under the influence of the treatment, she succeeded in discovering the connection and reported it to me. But she still knew nothing of the intention with which she was performing the obsessional action—the intention of correcting a distressing portion of the past and of putting her beloved husband in a better light. It took a fairly long time and called for much labour before she understood and admitted to me that such a motive alone could have been the driving force of her obsessional action.

The link with the scene after her unhappy wedding-night and the patient's affectionate motive constituted, taken together, what we have called the 'sense' of the obsessional action. But while she was carrying out the obsessional action this sense had been unknown to her in both directions—both its 'whence' and its 'whither'. [Cf. p. 284 below.] Mental processes had therefore been at work in her and the obsessional action was the effect of them; she had been aware of this effect in a normal mental fashion, but none of the mental predeterminants of this effect came to the knowledge of her consciousness. She behaved in precisely the same way as a hypnotized subject whom Bernheim had ordered to open an umbrella in the hospital ward five minutes after he woke up. The man carried out this instruction when he was awake, but he could produce no motive for his action.[1] It is a state of affairs of this sort that we have before our eyes when we speak of the existence of *unconscious mental processes*. We can challenge anyone in the world to give a more correct scientific account of this state of affairs, and if he does we will gladly renounce our hypothesis of unconscious mental processes. Till that happens, however, we will hold fast to the

[1] [Freud gave a much fuller account of this episode, at which he himself was present, in his last, unfinished, paper 'Some Elementary Lessons in Psycho-Analysis' (1940*b* [1938]). See also above, p. 103.]

hypothesis; and if someone objects that here the unconscious is nothing real in a scientific sense, is a makeshift, *une façon de parler*, we can only shrug our shoulders resignedly and dismiss what he says as unintelligible. Something not real, which produces effects of such tangible reality as an obsessional action![1]

And we meet with what is in essence the same thing in our second patient. She had made a rule that the pillow must not touch the back of the bedstead, and she had to obey this rule though she did not know where it came from, what it meant or to what motives it owed its power. Whether she herself regarded the rule as a matter of indifference, or whether she struggled against it or raged against it or decided to transgress it—none of this made any difference to her carrying it out. It had to be obeyed, and she asked herself vainly why. We must recognize, however, that these symptoms of obsessional neurosis, these ideas and impulses which emerge one knows not whence, which prove so resistant to every influence from an otherwise normal mind, which give the patient himself the impression of being all-powerful guests from an alien world, immortal beings intruding into the turmoil of mortal life—these symptoms offer the plainest indication of there being a special region of the mind, shut off from the rest. They lead, by a path that cannot be missed, to a conviction of the existence of the unconscious in the mind; and that is precisely why clinical psychiatry, which is acquainted only with a psychology of consciousness, can deal with these symptoms in no other way than by declaring them to be signs of a special sort of degeneracy. Obsessional ideas and obsessional impulses are not, of course, themselves unconscious, any more than the performance of obsessional actions escapes conscious perception. They would not have become symptoms if they had not forced their way into consciousness. But their psychical predeterminants which we infer by means of analysis, the connections into which we insert them by interpretation, are unconscious, at least until we have made them conscious to the patient by the work of analysis.

If, now, you consider further that the state of affairs which we have established in our two cases is confirmed for every symptom of every neurotic illness—that always and every-

[1] [Cf. above, p. 257.]

where the sense of the symptoms is unknown to the patient and that analysis regularly shows that these symptoms are derivatives of unconscious processes but can, subject to a variety of favourable circumstances, be made conscious—if you consider this, you will understand that in psycho-analysis we cannot do without what is at the same time unconscious and mental, and are accustomed to operate with it as though it were something palpable to the senses. But you will understand as well, perhaps, how incapable of forming a judgement on this question are all those other people, who are only acquainted with the unconscious as a concept, who have never carried out an analysis and have never interpreted dreams or found a sense and intention in neurotic symptoms. To say it for our ends once again: the possibility of giving a sense to neurotic symptoms by analytic interpretation is an unshakeable proof of the existence—or, if you prefer it, of the necessity for the hypothesis—of unconscious mental processes.

But that is not all. Thanks to a second discovery of Breuer's, which seems to me even more significant than the other [p. 257] and which he shared with no one, we learn still more of the connection between neurotic symptoms and the unconscious. Not only is the sense of the symptoms regularly unconscious, but there is an inseparable relation between this fact of the symptoms being unconscious and the possibility of their existing. You will understand me in a moment. I follow Breuer in asserting that every time we come upon a symptom we can infer that there are certain definite unconscious processes in the patient which contain the sense of the symptom. But it is also necessary for that sense to be unconscious in order that the symptom can come about. Symptoms are never constructed from conscious processes; as soon as the unconscious processes concerned have become conscious, the symptom must disappear. Here you will at once perceive a means of approach to therapy, a way of making symptoms disappear. And in this way Breuer did in fact restore his hysterical patient—that is, freed her from her symptoms; he found a technique for bringing to her consciousness the unconscious processes which contained the sense of the symptoms, and the symptoms disappeared.

This discovery of Breuer's was not the result of speculation but of a fortunate observation made possible by the patient's co-operation.[1] Nor should you torment yourselves with attempts at understanding it by tracing it back to something already known; you should recognize in it a new fundamental fact, by whose help much else will become explicable. Allow me, therefore, to repeat the same thing to you in another way.

The construction of a symptom is a substitute for something else that did not happen. Some particular mental processes should normally have developed to a point at which consciousness received information of them. This, however, did not take place, and instead—out of the interrupted processes, which had been somehow disturbed and were obliged to remain unconscious—the symptom emerged. Thus something in the nature of an exchange has taken place; if this can be reversed the therapy of the neurotic symptoms will have achieved its task.

This discovery of Breuer's is still the foundation of psychoanalytic therapy. The thesis that symptoms disappear when we have made their unconscious predeterminants conscious has been confirmed by all subsequent research, although we meet with the strangest and most unexpected complications when we attempt to carry it through in practice. Our therapy works by transforming what is unconscious into what is conscious, and it works only in so far as it is in a position to effect that transformation.

And now I must quickly make a short digression, to avoid the risk of your imagining that this therapeutic work is accomplished too easily. From what I have so far said a neurosis would seem to be the result of a kind of ignorance—a not knowing about mental events that one ought to know of. This would be a close approximation to some well-known Socratic doctrines, according to which even vices are based on ignorance. Now it would as a rule be very easy for a doctor experienced in analysis to guess what mental impulses had remained unconscious in a particular patient. So it ought not to be very difficult, either, for him to restore the patient by communicating his knowledge to him and so remedying his ignorance. One part at least of the symptom's unconscious sense could be easily dealt with in this way, though it is true that the doctor cannot guess much about the other part—the connection between the

[1] [Breuer's description of the occurrence will be found in his case history of Anna O. in *Studies on Hysteria* (1895d).]

symptoms and the patient's experiences—, since he himself does not know those experiences but must wait till the patient remembers them and tells them to him. But even for this a substitute can in some instances be found. One can make enquiries about these experiences from the patient's relatives and they will often be able to recognize which of them had a traumatic effect, and they can even sometimes report experiences of which the patient himself knows nothing because they occurred at a very early period of his life. Thus, by combining these two methods, we should have a prospect of relieving the patient of his pathogenic ignorance with little expense of time or trouble.

If only that was how things happened! We came upon discoveries in this connection for which we were at first unprepared. Knowledge is not always the same as knowledge: there are different sorts of knowledge, which are far from equivalent psychologically. 'Il y a fagots et fagots', as Molière has said.[1] The doctor's knowledge is not the same as the patient's and cannot produce the same effects. If the doctor transfers his knowledge to the patient as a piece of information, it has no result. No, it would be wrong to say that. It does not have the result of removing the symptoms, but it has another one—of setting the analysis in motion, of which the first signs are often expressions of denial. The patient knows after this what he did not know before—the sense of his symptom; yet he knows it just as little as he did. Thus we learn that there is more than one kind of ignorance. We shall need to have a somewhat deeper understanding of psychology to show us in what these differences consist.[2] But our thesis that the symptoms vanish when their sense is known remains true in spite of this. All we have to add is that the knowledge must rest on an internal change in the patient such as can only be brought about by a piece of psychical work with a particular aim. We are faced here by problems which will presently be brought together into the *dynamics* of the construction of symptoms.

I must ask now, Gentlemen, whether what I am saying to you is not too obscure and complicated. Am I not confusing you by so often taking back what I have said or qualifying it—by starting up trains of thought and then dropping them? I

[1] [*Le médecin malgré lui*, I, 6.]
[2] [Freud returns to this question in Lecture XXVII, p. 436 below.]

should be sorry if that were so. But I have a strong dislike of simplifying things at the expense of truthfulness. I have no objection to your receiving the full impact of the many-sidedness and complexity of our subject; and I think, too, that it does no harm if I tell you more on every point than you can at the moment make use of. I am aware, after all, that every listener or reader puts what is presented to him into shape in his mind, shortens it and simplifies it, and selects from it what he would like to retain. Up to a certain point it is no doubt true that the more there is at one's disposal the more one is left with. Permit me to hope that, in spite of all the trimmings, you have clearly grasped the essential part of what I have told you—about the sense of symptoms, about the unconscious and about the relation between them. No doubt you have also understood that our further efforts will lead in two directions: first towards discovering how people fall ill and how they can come to adopt the neurotic attitude to life—which is a clinical problem; and secondly towards learning how the pathological symptoms develop from the determinants of the neurosis—which remains a problem of mental dynamics. There must moreover be a point somewhere at which the two problems converge.

I will not go into this any further to-day. But since we still have some time to spare, I should like to direct your attention to another characteristic of our two analyses, which, once again, it will only be possible to appreciate fully later on—to the gaps in the patients' memories, their amnesias. As you have heard [p. 201], the task of a psycho-analytic treatment can be expressed in this formula: its task is to make conscious everything that is pathogenically unconscious. You will perhaps be surprised to learn, then, that this formula can be replaced by another one: its task is to fill up all the gaps in the patient's memory, to remove his amnesias. This would amount to the same thing. We are thus implying that the amnesias of neurotic patients have an important connection with the origin of their symptoms. If, however, you consider the case of our first analysis you will not find this view of amnesia justified. The patient had *not* forgotten the scene from which her obsessive action was derived; on the contrary, she had a vivid recollection of it; nor did anything else forgotten play a part in the origin of the symptom. The position with our second patient (the girl with the obsessional ceremonial), though less clear, was on the whole analogous. She had not really forgotten her behaviour in earlier years—the fact that she had insisted on the door between her parents' bedroom and her own being left open and that she had driven her mother out of her place in her parents' bed; she remembered this very plainly, even though with hesitation and unwillingly. The only thing we can consider striking is that the first patient, in carrying out her obsessional action on countless occasions, had never *once* noticed its resemblance to her experience on her wedding-night, and that the memory of it did not occur to her when she was directly asked to look for the motives of her obsessional action. And the same thing applies to the girl, whose ceremonial and its causes were moreover connected with a situation which was identically repeated every evening.[1] In both these cases there was no true amnesia, no missing memory; but a connection had been broken which ought to have led to the reproduction or re-emergence of the memory.

A disturbance of memory of this kind is enough for obsessional neurosis; but the case is different with hysteria. As a rule the latter neurosis is marked by amnesias on a really large scale. In analysing each separate hysterical symptom one is usually led to a whole chain of impressions of events, which, when they recur, are expressly described by the patient as having been till then forgotten. On the one hand, this chain reaches back to the earliest years of life, so that the hysterical amnesia can be recognized as an immediate continuation of the infantile amnesia which, for us normal people, conceals the beginnings of our mental life. [Cf. p. 199 f. above.] On the other hand, we learn with astonishment that even the patient's most recent experiences can be subject to forgetting, and that the occasions which precipitated the outbreak of the illness or led to its intensification are in particular encroached upon, if not completely swallowed up, by amnesia. It regularly happens that important details have disappeared from the total picture of a recent recollection of this sort or that they have been replaced by falsifications of memory. Indeed it happens with

[1] [I.e. her father and mother sleeping together.]

almost equal regularity that certain memories of recent experiences only emerge shortly before the end of an analysis—
memories which had been held back till that late moment and
had left perceptible gaps in the continuity of the case.

Such restrictions upon the faculty of memory are, as I have
said, characteristic of hysteria, in which, indeed, states also
arise as symptoms—hysterical attacks—which need leave no
trace behind them in the memory . If things are different in
obsessional neurosis, you may conclude that what we are dealing with in these amnesias is a psychological characteristic of
the change that occurs in hysteria and is not a universal
feature of neuroses in general. The importance of this distinction is reduced by the following consideration. We have
comprised two things as the 'sense' of a symptom: its 'whence'
and its 'whither' or 'what for' [p. 277]—that is, the impressions and experiences from which it arose and the intentions
which it serves. Thus the 'whence' of a symptom resolves itself
into impressions which came from outside, which were necessarily once conscious and may have since become unconscious
through forgetting. The 'whither' of a symptom, its purpose, is
invariably, however, an endopsychic process, which may possibly have been conscious at first but may equally well never
have been conscious and may have remained in the unconscious from the very start. Thus it is not of great importance
whether the amnesia has laid hold on the 'whence' as well—the
experiences on which the symptom is supported—as happens
in hysteria; it is on the 'whither', the purpose of the symptom,
which may have been unconscious from the beginning, that its
dependence on the unconscious is founded—and no less firmly
in obsessional neurosis than in hysteria.

But in thus emphasizing the unconscious in mental life we
have conjured up the most evil spirits of criticism against
psycho-analysis. Do not be surprised at this, and do not suppose
that the resistance to us rests only on the understandable
difficulty of the unconscious or the relative inaccessibility of the
experiences which provide evidence of it. Its source, I think, lies
deeper. In the course of centuries the *naïve* self-love of men has
had to submit to two major blows at the hands of science. The
first was when they learnt that our earth was not the centre of

the universe but only a tiny fragment of a cosmic system of scarcely imaginable vastness. This is associated in our minds with the name of Copernicus, though something similar had already been asserted by Alexandrian science. The second blow fell when biological research destroyed man's supposedly privileged place in creation and proved his descent from the animal kingdom and his ineradicable animal nature. This revaluation has been accomplished in our own days by Darwin, Wallace and their predecessors, though not without the most violent contemporary opposition. But human megalomania will have suffered its third and most wounding blow from the psychological research of the present time which seeks to prove to the ego that it is not even master in its own house, but must content itself with scanty information of what is going on unconsciously in its mind. We psycho-analysts were not the first and not the only ones to utter this call to introspection; but it seems to be our fate to give it its most forcible expression and to support it with empirical material which affects every individual. Hence arises the general revolt against our science, the disregard of all considerations of academic civility and the releasing of the opposition from every restraint of impartial logic.[1] And beyond all this we have yet to disturb the peace of this world in still another way, as you will shortly hear.

[1] [Freud had developed this theme at greater length in a paper on 'A Difficulty in the Path of Psycho-Analysis' (1917a).]

LECTURE XIX

RESISTANCE AND REPRESSION[1]

LADIES AND GENTLEMEN,—Before we can make any further progress in our understanding of the neuroses, we stand in need of some fresh observations. Here we have two such, both of which are very remarkable and at the time when they were made were very surprising. Our discussions of last year will, it is true, have prepared you for both of them.[2]

In the first place, then, when we undertake to restore a patient to health, to relieve him of the symptoms of his illness, he meets us with a violent and tenacious resistance, which persists throughout the whole length of the treatment. This is such a strange fact that we cannot expect it to find much credence. It is best to say nothing about it to the patient's relatives, for they invariably regard it as an excuse on our part for the length or failure of our treatment. The patient, too, produces all the phenomena of this resistance without recognizing it as such, and if we can induce him to take our view of it and to reckon with its existence, that already counts as a great success. Only think of it! The patient, who is suffering so much from his symptoms and is causing those about him to share his sufferings, who is ready to undertake so many sacrifices in time, money, effort and self-discipline in order to be freed from those symptoms— we are to believe that this same patient puts up a struggle in the interest of his illness against the person who is helping him. How

[1] [The essence of Freud's views on repression is already given in his contribution to *Studies on Hysteria* (1895d). He gave a similar description of his discovery in the first section of his history of the psycho-analytic movement (1914d), (Norton, 1966). An account of the development of Freud's theory of repression will be found in the Editor's Note to his metapsychological paper on the subject (1915d)—a paper which, together with Section IV of the paper on 'The Unconscious' (1915e), contains Freud's deepest reflections on the question.]

[2] [The concept of resistance had been introduced in Lecture VII, p. 116 above. The second observation is described on p. 298 below.]

improbable such an assertion must sound! Yet it is true; and when its improbability is pointed out to us, we need only reply that it is not without analogies. A man who has gone to the dentist because of an unbearable toothache will nevertheless try to hold the dentist back when he approaches the sick tooth with a pair of forceps.

The patient's resistance is of very many sorts, extremely subtle and often hard to detect; and it exhibits protean changes in the forms in which it manifests itself. The doctor must be distrustful and remain on his guard against it.

In psycho-analytic therapy we make use of the same technique that is familiar to you from dream-interpretation. We instruct the patient to put himself into a state of quiet, unreflecting self-observation, and to report to us whatever internal perceptions he is able to make—feelings, thoughts, memories—in the order in which they occur to him. At the same time we warn him expressly against giving way to any motive which would lead him to make a selection among these associations or to exclude any of them, whether on the ground that it is too *disagreeable* or too *indiscreet* to say, or that it is too *unimportant* or *irrelevant*, or that it is *nonsensical* and need not be said. We urge him always to follow only the surface of his consciousness and to leave aside any criticism of what he finds, whatever shape that criticism may take; and we assure him that the success of the treatment, and above all its duration, depends on the conscientiousness with which he obeys this fundamental technical rule of analysis.[1] We already know from the technique of

[1] [Freud had already stated the rule in connection with the interpreting of dreams in Lecture VII, p. 115 above. He first laid it down in Chapter II of *The Interpretation of Dreams* (1900a) and again in his contribution to Löwenfeld's book on obsessional phenomena (Freud, 1904a [1903]). The actual term 'fundamental rule' was first used in the technical paper on 'The Dynamics of Transference' (1912b), where an Editor's footnote gives some other early references. Perhaps the fullest account is in another technical paper, 'On Beginning the Treatment' (1913c). Among later mentions may be noted a passage near the beginning of Chapter IV of the *Autobiographical Study* (1925d), (Norton, 1963), and an interesting allusion to the deeper reasons for the obstacles to obeying the rule, towards the end of Chapter VI of *Inhibitions, Symptoms and Anxiety* (1926d). In the latter passage, in the course of a discussion of the part

dream-interpretation that the associations giving rise to the doubts and objections I have just enumerated are precisely the ones that invariably contain the material which leads to the uncovering of the unconscious.   [Cf. Lecture VII, p. 116.]

The first thing we achieve by setting up this fundamental technical rule is that it becomes the target for the attacks of the resistance. The patient endeavours in every sort of way to extricate himself from its provisions. At one moment he declares that nothing occurs to him, at the next that so many things are crowding in on him that he cannot get hold of anything. Presently we observe with pained astonishment that he has given way first to one and then to another critical objection: he betrays this to us by the long pauses that he introduces into his remarks. He then admits that there is something he really cannot say—he would be ashamed to; and he allows this reason to prevail against his promise. Or he says that something has occurred to him, but it concerns another person and not himself and is therefore exempt from being reported. Or, what has now occurred to him is really too unimportant, too silly and senseless: I cannot possibly have meant him to enter into thoughts like that. So it goes on in innumerable variations, and one can only reply that 'to say everything' really does mean 'to say everything'.

One hardly comes across a single patient who does not make an attempt at reserving some region or other for himself so as to prevent the treatment from having access to it. A man, whom I can only describe as of the highest intelligence, kept silence in this way for weeks on end about an intimate love-affair, and, when he was called to account for having broken the sacred rule, defended himself with the argument that he thought this particular story was his private business. Analytic treatment does not, of course, recognize any such right of asylum. Suppose that in a town like Vienna the experiment was made of treating a square such as the Hohe Markt, or a church like St. Stephen's, as places where no arrests might be made, and suppose we then wanted to catch a particular criminal. We could be quite sure of finding him in the sanctuary. I once decided to allow a man, on whose efficiency much depended in the external world, the

played by the defensive process of 'isolation' in ordinary directed thinking, Freud mentions especially the difficulties felt by obsessional neurotics in this connection. See below, p. 289.]

right to make an exception of this kind because he was bound under his oath of office not to make communications about certain things to another person. He, it is true, was satisfied with the outcome; but I was not. I determined not to repeat an attempt under such conditions.

Obsessional neurotics understand perfectly how to make the technical rule almost useless by applying their over-conscientiousness and doubts to it.[1] Patients suffering from anxiety hysteria occasionally succeed in carrying the rule *ad absurdum* by producing only associations which are so remote from what we are in search of that they contribute nothing to the analysis. But it is not my intention to induct you into the handling of these technical difficulties. It is enough to say that in the end, through resolution and perseverance, we succeed in extorting a certain amount of obedience to the fundamental technical rule from the resistance—which thereupon jumps over to another sphere.

It now appears as an *intellectual* resistance, it fights by means of arguments and exploits all the difficulties and improbabilities which normal but uninstructed thinking finds in the theories of analysis. It is now our fate to hear from this single voice all the criticisms and objections which assail our ears in a chorus in the scientific literature of the subject. And for this reason none of the shouts that reach us from outside sound unfamiliar. It is a regular storm in a tea-cup. But the patient is willing to be argued with; he is anxious to get us to instruct him, teach him, contradict him, introduce him to the literature, so that he can find further instruction. He is quite ready to become an adherent of psycho-analysis—on condition that analysis spares him personally. But we recognize this curiosity as a resistance, as a diversion from our particular tasks, and we repel it. In the case of an obsessional neurotic we have to expect special tactics of resistance. He will often allow the analysis to proceed on its way uninhibited, so that it is able to shed an ever-increasing light upon the riddle of his illness. We begin to wonder in the end, however, why this enlightenment is accompanied by no practical advance, no diminution of the symptoms. We are then able to realize that resistance has withdrawn on to the doubt belonging to the obsessional neurosis and from that position is successfully defying us. It is as though the

[1] [Cf. the end of the last footnote.]

patient were saying: 'Yes, that's all very nice and interesting, and I'll be very glad to go on with it further. It would change my illness a lot if it were true. But I don't in the least believe that it *is* true; and, so long as I don't believe it, it makes no difference to my illness.' Things can proceed like this for a long time, till finally one comes up against this uncommitted attitude itself, and the decisive struggle then breaks out.[1]

Intellectual resistances are not the worst: one always remains superior to them. But the patient also knows how to put up resistances, without going outside the framework of the analysis, the overcoming of which is among the most difficult of technical problems. Instead of remembering, he *repeats* attitudes and emotional impulses from his early life which can be used as a resistance against the doctor and the treatment by means of what is known as 'transference'.[2] If the patient is a man, he usually extracts this material from his relation to his father, into whose place he fits the doctor, and in that way he makes resistances out of his efforts to become independent in himself and in his judgements, out of his ambition, the first aim of which was to do things as well as his father or to get the better of him, or out of his unwillingness to burden himself for the second time in his life with a load of gratitude. Thus at times one has an impression that the patient has entirely replaced his better intention of making an end to his illness by the alternative one of putting the doctor in the wrong, of making him realize his impotence and of triumphing over him. Women have a masterly gift for exploiting an affectionate, erotically tinged transference to the doctor for the purposes of resistance. If this attachment reaches a certain height, all their interest in the immediate situation in the treatment and all the obligations they undertook at its commencement vanish; their jealousy, which is never absent, and their exasperation at their inevitable rejection, however considerately expressed, are bound to have a damaging effect on their personal understanding with the

---

[1] [The part played by doubt in cases of obsessional neurosis is referred to above in Lecture XVII, p. 259. The necessity for special technical methods in dealing with such cases was mentioned by Freud a little later in his Budapest Congress paper (1919*a*).]

[2] [Lecture XXVII, p. 431 below, is devoted to a full discussion of this phenomenon.]

doctor and so to put out of operation one of the most powerful motive forces of the analysis.

Resistances of this kind should not be one-sidedly condemned. They include so much of the most important material from the patient's past and bring it back in so convincing a fashion that they become some of the best supports of the analysis if a skilful technique knows how to give them the right turn. Nevertheless, it remains a remarkable fact that this material is always in the service of the resistance to begin with and brings to the fore a *façade* that is hostile to the treatment. It may also be said that what is being mobilized for fighting against the alterations we are striving for are character-traits, attitudes of the ego. In this connection we discover that these character-traits were formed in relation to the determinants of the neurosis and in reaction against its demands, and we come upon traits which cannot normally emerge, or not to the same extent, and which may be described as latent. Nor must you get an impression that we regard the appearance of these resistances as an unforeseen risk to analytic influence. No, we are aware that these resistances are bound to come to light; in fact we are dissatisfied if we cannot provoke them clearly enough and are unable to demonstrate them to the patient. Indeed we come finally to understand that the overcoming of these resistances is the essential function of analysis[1] and is the only part of our work which gives us an assurance that we have achieved something with the patient.

If you further consider that the patient makes all the chance events that occur during his analysis into interferences with it, that he uses as reasons for slackening his efforts every diversion outside the analysis, every comment by a person of authority in his environment who is hostile to analysis, any chance organic illness or any that complicates his neurosis and, even, indeed, every improvement in his condition—if you consider all this, you will have obtained an approximate, though still incomplete, picture of the forms and methods of the resistance, the struggle against which accompanies every analysis.[2]

[1] [That this was a relatively late development in analytic technique is shown, for instance, by a paragraph in Freud's Nuremberg Congress paper (1910*d*).]

[2] [The present description of the forms taken by resistance in general is as full as any by Freud. But the special case of transference-resistance is discussed in greater detail in his paper on 'The Dynamics of Transference' (1912*b*).]

I have treated this point in such great detail because I must now inform you that this experience of ours with the resistance of neurotics to the removal of their symptoms became the basis of our dynamic view of the neuroses. Originally Breuer and I myself carried out psychotherapy by means of hypnosis; Breuer's first patient[1] was treated throughout under hypnotic influence, and to begin with I followed him in this. I admit that at that period the work proceeded more easily and pleasantly, and also in a much shorter time. But results were capricious and not lasting; and for that reason I finally dropped hypnosis.[2] And I then understood that an insight into the dynamics of these illnesses had not been possible so long as hypnosis was employed.[3] That state was precisely able to withhold the existence of the resistance from the doctor's perception. It pushed the resistance back, making a certain area free for analytic work, and dammed it up at the frontiers of that area in such a way as to be impenetrable, just as doubt does in obsessional neurosis. For that reason I have been able to say that psycho-analysis proper began when I dispensed with the help of hypnosis.[4]

If, however, the recognition of resistance has become so important, we should do well to find room for a cautious doubt whether we have not been too light-heartedly assuming resistances. Perhaps there really are cases of neurosis in which associations fail for other reasons, perhaps the arguments against our hypotheses really deserve to have their content examined, and perhaps we are doing patients an injustice in so conveniently setting aside their intellectual criticisms as resistance. But, Gentlemen, we did not arrive at this judgement

is as full as any by Freud. But the special case of transference-resistance is discussed in greater detail in his paper on 'The Dynamics of Transference' (1912b).]

[1] [See Lecture XVIII, p. 279 f. above.]

[2] [Fairly exact dates for Freud's use of hypnotism (1887–1896) will be found in an Editor's footnote to the case of Lucy R. in *Studies on Hysteria* (1895d).]

[3] [Freud tells us that he first realized the great importance of resistance during his analysis of Elisabeth von R. He was at that time using the 'pressure' technique, without hypnosis. See *Studies on Hysteria* (1895d).]

[4] [Cf. Freud's statement in very similar words in the first section of his history of the psycho-analytic movement (1914d), (Norton, 1966). Earlier he had not been inclined to draw such a clear-cut line.]

lightly. We have had occasion to observe all these critical patients at the moment of the emergence of a resistance and after its disappearance. For resistance is constantly altering its intensity during the course of a treatment; it always increases when we are approaching a new topic, it is at its most intense while we are at the climax of dealing with that topic, and it dies away when the topic has been disposed of. Nor do we ever, unless we have been guilty of special clumsiness in our technique, have to meet the full amount of resistance of which a patient is capable. We have therefore been able to convince ourselves that on countless occasions in the course of his analysis the same man will abandon his critical attitude and then take it up again. If we are on the point of bringing a specially distressing piece of unconscious material to his consciousness, he is extremely critical; he may previously have understood and accepted a great deal, but now it is just as though those acquisitions have been swept away; in his efforts for opposition at any price, he may offer a complete picture of someone who is an emotional imbecile. But if we succeed in helping him to overcome this new resistance, he recovers his insight and understanding. Thus his critical faculty is not an independent function, to be respected as such, it is the tool of his emotional attitudes and is directed by his resistance. If there is something he does not like, he can put up a shrewd fight against it and appear highly critical; but if something suits his book, he can, on the contrary, show himself most credulous. Perhaps none of us are very different; a man who is being analysed only reveals this dependence of the intellect upon emotional life so clearly because in analysis we are putting such great pressure on him.

How, then, do we account for our observation that the patient fights with such energy against the removal of his symptoms and the setting of his mental processes on a normal course? We tell ourselves that we have succeeded in discovering powerful forces here which oppose any alteration of the patient's condition; they must be the same ones which in the past brought this condition about. During the construction of his symptoms something must have taken place which we can now reconstruct from our experiences during the *resolution* of his symptoms. We already know from Breuer's observation that there is a precondition for the existence of a symptom: some mental process must not have been brought to an end normally —so that it could become conscious. The symptom is a substitute for what did not happen at that point [p. 280 above]. We now know the point at which we must locate the operation of the force which we have surmised. A violent opposition must have started against the entry into consciousness of the questionable mental process, and for that reason it remained unconscious. As being something unconscious, it had the power to construct a symptom. This same opposition, during psychoanalytic treatment, sets itself up once more against our effort to transform what is unconscious into what is conscious. This is what we perceive as resistance. We have proposed to give the pathogenic process which is demonstrated by the resistance the name of *repression.*

We must now form more definite ideas about this process of repression. It is the precondition for the construction of symptoms; but it is also something to which we know nothing similar. Let us take as our model an impulse, a mental process that endeavours to turn itself into an action. We know that it can be repelled by what we term a rejection or condemnation. When this happens, the energy at its disposal is withdrawn from it; it becomes powerless, though it can persist as a memory. The whole process of coming to a decision about it runs its course within the knowledge of the ego. It is a very different matter if we suppose that the same impulse is subjected to repression. In that case it would retain its energy and no memory of it would remain behind; moreover the process of repression would be accomplished unnoticed by the ego. This comparison, therefore, brings us no nearer to the essential nature of repression.

I will put before you the only theoretical ideas which have proved of service for giving a more definite shape to the concept of repression. It is above all essential for this purpose that we should proceed from the purely descriptive meaning of the word 'unconscious' to the systematic meaning of the same word.[1] That is, we will decide to say that the fact of a psychical

---

[1] [See footnote 1, p. 227 above. The spatial analogy to resistance and repression, which follows here, is similar to the one in the second of his *Five Lectures* (1910a).]

process being conscious or unconscious is only one of its attributes and not necessarily an unambiguous one. If a process of this kind has remained unconscious, its being kept away from consciousness may perhaps only be an indication of some vicissitude it has gone through, and not that vicissitude itself. In order to form a picture of this vicissitude, let us assume that every mental process—we must admit one exception, which we shall mention at a later stage[1]—exists to begin with in an unconscious stage or phase and that it is only from there that the process passes over into the conscious phase, just as a photographic picture begins as a negative and only becomes a picture after being turned into a positive. Not every negative, however, necessarily becomes a positive; nor is it necessary that every unconscious mental process should turn into a conscious one. This may be advantageously expressed by saying that an individual process belongs to begin with to the system of the unconscious and can then, in certain circumstances, pass over into the system of the conscious.

The crudest idea of these systems is the most convenient for us—a spatial one. Let us therefore compare the system of the unconscious to a large entrance hall, in which the mental impulses jostle one another like separate individuals. Adjoining this entrance hall there is a second, narrower, room—a kind of drawing-room—in which consciousness, too, resides. But on the threshold between these two rooms a watchman performs his function: he examines the different mental impulses, acts as a censor, and will not admit them into the drawing-room if they displease him. You will see at once that it does not make much difference if the watchman turns away a particular impulse at the threshold itself or if he pushes it back across the threshold after it has entered the drawing-room. This is merely a question of the degree of his watchfulness and of how early he carries out his act of recognition. If we keep to this picture, we shall be able to extend our nomenclature further. The impulses in the entrance hall of the unconscious are out of sight of the conscious, which is in the other room; to begin with they must remain unconscious. If they have already pushed their way forward to the threshold and have been turned back by the watchman,

[1] [The exception, which seems to have escaped mention, must no doubt be the case of external perception.]

then they are inadmissible to consciousness;[1] we speak of them as *repressed*. But even the impulses which the watchman has allowed to cross the threshold are not on that account necessarily conscious as well; they can only become so if they succeed in catching the eye of consciousness. We are therefore justified in calling this second room the system of the *preconscious*. In that case becoming conscious retains its purely descriptive sense. For any particular impulse, however, the vicissitude of repression consists in its not being allowed by the watchman to pass from the system of the unconscious into that of the preconscious. It is the same watchman whom we get to know as resistance when we try to lift the repression by means of the analytic treatment.

Now I know you will say that these ideas are both crude and fantastic and quite impermissible in a scientific account. I know that they are crude: and, more than that, I know that they are incorrect, and, if I am not very much mistaken, I already have something better to take their place.[2] Whether it will seem to you equally fantastic I cannot tell. They are preliminary working hypotheses, like Ampère's manikin swimming in the electric current,[3] and they are not to be despised in so far as they are of service in making our observations intelligible. I should like to assure you that these crude hypotheses of the two rooms, the watchman at the threshold between them and consciousness as a spectator at the end of the second room, must nevertheless be very far-reaching approximations to the real facts. And I should like to hear you admit that our terms, 'unconscious', 'preconscious' and 'conscious', prejudge things far less and are far easier to justify than others which have been proposed or are in use, such as 'subconscious', 'paraconscious', 'intraconscious' and the like.[4]

---

[1] ['*Bewusstseinsunfähig.*' The term is due to Breuer, who constructed it on the model of '*hoffähig*' ('admissible to Court', 'having the *entrée*'). See Section 5 of his contribution to *Studies on Hysteria* (1895*d*).

[2] [What Freud had in mind is not obvious.]

[3] [A.-M. Ampère (1775–1836), one of the founders of the science of electro-magnetism, made use of a magnetic metal manikin in one of his early experiments establishing the relation between electricity and magnetism.]

[4] [Freud gives an explanation of his objection to the term 'sub-

It will therefore be of greater importance to me if you warn me that an arrangement of the mental apparatus, such as I have here assumed in order to explain neurotic symptoms, must necessarily claim general validity and must give us information about normal functioning as well. You will, of course, be quite right in this. At the moment we cannot pursue this implication further; but our interest in the psychology of the forming of symptoms cannot but be increased to an extraordinary extent if there is a prospect, through the study of pathological conditions, of obtaining access to the normal mental events which are so well concealed.

Perhaps you recognize, moreover, what it is that supports our hypotheses of the two systems, and their relation to each other and to consciousness? After all, the watchman between the unconscious and the preconscious is nothing else than the *censorship*, to which, as we found, the form taken by the manifest dream is subject. [Cf. Lecture IX, p. 139 above.] The day's residues, which we recognized as the instigators of the dream, were preconscious material which, at night-time and in the state of sleep, had been under the influence of unconscious and repressed wishful impulses; they had been able, in combination with those impulses and thanks to their energy, to construct the latent dream. Under the dominance of the unconscious system this material had been worked over (by condensation and displacement) in a manner which is unknown or only exceptionally permissible in normal mental life—that is, in the preconscious system. We came to regard this difference in their manner of operating as what characterizes the two systems; the relation which the preconscious has to consciousness was regarded by us merely as an indication of its belonging to one of the two systems.[1] Dreams are not pathological phenomena; they can appear in any healthy person under the conditions of a state of sleep. Our hypothesis about the structure of the mental apparatus, which allows us to understand the formation alike of dreams and of neurotic symptoms, has an incontrovertible

conscious' near the end of Chapter II of his work on lay analysis (1926*e*), (Norton, 1950). See also an Editor's footnote to Section I of 'The Unconscious' (1915*e*).

[1] [Cf. the discussions at the end of Lectures XIII and XIV, pp. 212 and 227.]

claim to being taken into account in regard to normal mental life as well.

That much is what we have to say for the moment about repression. But it is only the *precondition* for the construction of symptoms. Symptoms, as we know, are a substitute for something that is held back by repression. It is a long step further, however, from repression to an understanding of this substitutive structure. On this other side of the problem, these questions arise out of our observation of repression: what kind of mental impulses are subject to repression? by what forces is it accomplished? and for what motives? So far we have only one piece of information on these points. In investigating resistance we have learnt that it emanates from forces of the ego, from known and latent character traits [p. 291 above]. It is these too, therefore, that are responsible for repression, or at any rate they have a share in it. We know nothing more at present.

At this point the second of the two observations which I mentioned to you earlier [at the opening of this Lecture] comes to our help. It is quite generally the case that analysis allows us to arrive at the intention of neurotic symptoms. This again will be nothing new to you. I have already demonstrated it to you in two cases of neurosis.[1] But, after all, what do two cases amount to? You are right to insist on its being demonstrated to you in two hundred cases—in countless cases. The only trouble is that I cannot do that. Once again, your own experience must serve instead, or your belief, which on this point can appeal to the unanimous reports of all psycho-analysts.

You will recollect that, in the two cases whose symptoms we submitted to a detailed investigation, the analysis initiated us into these patients' most intimate sexual life. In the first case we further recognized with particular clarity the intention or purpose of the symptom we were examining; in the second case this was perhaps somewhat concealed by a factor which will be mentioned later [p. 300 below]. Well, every other case that we submit to analysis would show us the same thing that we have found in these two examples. In every instance we should be introduced by the analysis into the patient's sexual experiences and wishes; and in every instance we should be bound to see

[1] [In Lecture XVII, p. 261 ff. above.]

that the symptoms served the same intention. We find that this intention is the satisfaction of sexual wishes; the symptoms serve for the patients' sexual satisfaction; they are a substitute for satisfaction of this kind, which the patients are without in their lives.

Think of our first patient's obsessional action. The woman was without her husband, whom she loved intensely but with whom she could not share her life on account of his deficiencies and weaknesses. She had to remain faithful to him; she could not put anyone else in his place. Her obsessional symptom gave her what she longed for, set her husband on a pedestal, denied and corrected his weaknesses and above all his impotence. This symptom was fundamentally a wish-fulfilment, just like a dream—and moreover, what is not always true of a dream, an *erotic* wish-fulfilment. In the case of our second patient you could at least gather that her ceremonial sought to obstruct intercourse between her parents or prevent it from producing a new baby. You will also probably have guessed that it was at bottom endeavouring to put her herself in her mother's place. Once again, therefore, a setting-aside of interferences with sexual satisfaction and a fulfilment of the patient's own sexual wishes. I shall soon come to the complication I have hinted at.

I should like to anticipate, Gentlemen, the qualifications which I shall have to make later in the universal validity of these statements. I will therefore point out to you that all I have said here about repression and the formation and meaning of symptoms was derived from three forms of neurosis—anxiety hysteria, conversion hysteria and obsessional neurosis—and that in the first instance it is also valid only for these forms. These three disorders, which we are accustomed to group together as '*transference neuroses*',[1] also circumscribe the region in which psycho-analytic therapy can function. The other neuroses have been far less thoroughly studied by psycho-analysis; in one group of them the impossibility of therapeutic influence has been a reason for this neglect. Nor should you forget that psycho-analysis is still a very young science, that preparing for it costs much trouble and time, and that not at all long ago it

[1] [The explanation of this term is given in a later lecture, p. 445 below.]

was being practised single-handed. Nevertheless, we are every-where on the point of penetrating to an understanding of these other disorders which are not transference neuroses. I hope later to be able to introduce you to the extensions of our hypotheses and findings which result from adaptation to this new material, and to show you that these further studies have not led to contradictions but to the establishment of higher unities.[1] If, then, everything I am saying here applies to the transference neuroses, let me first increase the value of symptoms by a new piece of information. For a comparative study of the determining causes of falling ill leads to a result which can be expressed in a formula: these people fall ill in one way or another of *frustration*, when reality prevents them from satisfying their sexual wishes.[2] You see how excellently these two findings tally with each other. It is only thus that symptoms can be properly viewed as substitutive satisfactions for what is missed in life.

No doubt all kinds of objections can still be raised to the assertion that neurotic symptoms are substitutes for sexual satisfactions. I will mention two of them to-day. When you yourselves have carried out analytic examinations of a considerable number of neurotics, you will perhaps tell me, shaking your head, that in a lot of cases my assertion is simply not true; the symptoms seem rather to have the contrary purpose of excluding or of stopping sexual satisfaction. I will not dispute the correctness of your interpretation. The facts in psycho-analysis have a habit of being rather more complicated than we like. If they were as simple as all that, perhaps it might not have needed psycho-analysis to bring them to light. Indeed, some of the features of our second patient's ceremonial show signs of this ascetic character with its hostility to sexual satisfaction: when, for instance, she got rid of the clocks and watches [p. 265], which had the magical meaning of avoiding erections during the night [p. 267], or when she tried to guard against flower-pots falling and breaking [p. 265], which was equivalent to protecting her virginity [p. 267]. In some other cases of bed-ceremonials, which I have been able to analyse, this negative character was far more outspoken; the ceremonial might con-

---

[1] [See the discussion of narcissism in Lecture XXVI.]

[2] [This is discussed in greater detail in Lecture XXII, p. 344 ff. below.]

sist exclusively of defensive measures against sexual memories and temptations. However, we have already found often enough that in psycho-analysis opposites imply no contradiction.[1] We might extend our thesis and say that symptoms aim either at a sexual satisfaction or at fending it off, and that on the whole the positive, wish-fulfilling character prevails in hysteria and the negative, ascetic one in obsessional neurosis. If symptoms can serve the purpose both of sexual satisfaction and of its opposite, there is an excellent basis for this double-sidedness or polarity in a part of their mechanism which I have so far not been able to mention. For, as we shall hear, they are the products of a compromise and arise from the mutual interference between two opposing currents; they represent not only the repressed but also the repressing force which had a share in their origin. One side or the other may be more strongly represented; but it is rarely that one influence is entirely absent. In hysteria a convergence of both intentions in the same symptom is usually achieved. In obsessional neurosis the two portions are often separated; the symptom then becomes diphasic [falls into two stages] and consists in two actions, one after the other, which cancel each other out.[2]

We shall not be able to dismiss a second objection so easily. If you survey a fairly long series of interpretations of symptoms, you will probably start by judging that the concept of a substitutive sexual satisfaction has been stretched to its extreme limits in them. You will not fail to emphasize the fact that these symptoms offer nothing real in the way of satisfaction, that often enough they are restricted to the revival of a sensation or the representation of a phantasy derived from a sexual complex. And you will further point out that these supposed sexual satisfactions often take on a childish and discreditable form, approximate to an act of masturbation perhaps, or recall dirty kinds of naughtiness which are forbidden even to children—habits of which they have been broken. And, going on from this, you will also express surprise that we are representing as a sexual satisfaction what would rather have to be described as the

---

[1] [E.g. in Lecture XI, p. 178 above.]
[2] [Examples of this will be found, with a discussion, in Section E of Part I of the 'Rat Man' case history (1909d).]

satisfaction of lusts that are cruel or horrible or would even have to be called unnatural. We shall come to no agreement, Gentlemen, on this latter point till we have made a thorough investigation of the sexual life of human beings and till, in doing so, we have decided what it is that we are justified in calling 'sexual'.

LECTURE XX

THE SEXUAL LIFE OF HUMAN BEINGS[1]

LADIES AND GENTLEMEN,—One would certainly have supposed that there could be no doubt as to what is to be understood by 'sexual'. First and foremost, what is sexual is something improper, something one ought not to talk about. I have been told that the pupils of a celebrated psychiatrist made an attempt once to convince their teacher of how frequently the symptoms of hysterical patients represent sexual things. For this purpose they took him to the bedside of a female hysteric, whose attacks were an unmistakable imitation of the process of childbirth. But with a shake of his head he remarked: 'Well, there's nothing sexual about childbirth.' Quite right. Childbirth need not in every case be something improper.

I see that you take offence at my joking about such serious things. But it is not altogether a joke. Seriously, it is not easy to decide what is covered by the concept 'sexual'. Perhaps the only suitable definition would be 'everything that is related to the distinction between the two sexes'. But you will regard that as colourless and too comprehensive. If you take the fact of the sexual act as the central point, you will perhaps define as sexual everything which, with a view to obtaining pleasure, is concerned with the body, and in particular with the sexual organs, of someone of the opposite sex, and which in the last resort aims at the union of the genitals and the performance of the sexual act. But if so you will really not be very far from the equation of what is sexual with what is improper, and childbirth will really not be anything sexual. If, on the other hand, you take the reproductive function as the nucleus of sexuality, you risk excluding a whole number of things which are not aimed at

[1] [Freud's principal work on this subject was, of course, his *Three Essays on the Theory of Sexuality* (1905d), to which he made a large number of additions and corrections in a succession of editions over the subsequent twenty years. A list of his chief other contributions to the subject is given in an appendix to that work. The material in this and the following lecture is mainly derived from the *Three Essays*.]

303

reproduction but which are certainly sexual, such as masturbation and perhaps even kissing. But we are already prepared to find that attempts at a definition always lead to difficulties; so let us renounce the idea of doing better in this particular case. We may suspect that in the course of the development of the concept 'sexual' something has happened which has resulted in what Silberer has aptly called an 'error of superimposition'.[1]

On the whole, indeed, when we come to think of it, we are not quite at a loss in regard to what it is that people call sexual. Something which combines a reference to the contrast between the sexes, to the search for pleasure, to the reproductive function and to the characteristic of something that is improper and must be kept secret—some such combination will serve for all practical purposes in everyday life. But for science that is not enough. By means of careful investigations (only made possible, indeed, by disinterested self-discipline) we have come to know groups of individuals whose 'sexual life' deviates in the most striking way from the usual picture of the average. Some of these 'perverse' people have, we might say, struck the distinction between the sexes off their programme. Only members of their own sex can rouse their sexual wishes; those of the other sex, and especially their sexual parts, are not a sexual object for them at all, and in extreme cases are an object of disgust. This implies, of course, that they have abandoned any share in reproduction. We call such people homosexuals or inverts. They are men and women who are often, though not always, irreproachably fashioned in other respects, of high intellectual and ethical development, the victims only of this one fatal deviation. Through the mouth of their scientific spokesmen they represent themselves as a special variety of the human species—a 'third sex' which has a right to stand on an equal footing beside the other two. We shall perhaps have an opportunity of examining their claims critically. [Cf. p. 307 f. below.] Of course they are not, as they also like to assert, an '*élite*' of man-

---

[1] ['*Überdeckungsfehler.*' See Silberer, 1914, 161. What Silberer seems to have in mind is mistakenly thinking that you are looking at a single thing, when in fact you are looking at two different things superimposed on each other.]

kind; there are at least as many inferior and useless individuals among them as there are among those of a different sexual kind.

This class of perverts at any rate behave to their sexual objects in approximately the same way as normal people do to theirs. But we now come to a long series of abnormal people whose sexual activity diverges more and more widely from what seems desirable to a sensible person. In their multiplicity and strangeness they can only be compared to the grotesque monsters painted by Breughel for the temptation of St. Anthony or to the long procession of vanished gods and believers which Flaubert leads past, before the eyes of his pious penitent.[1] Such a medley calls for some kind of arrangement if it is not to confuse our senses. We accordingly divide them into those in whom, like the homosexuals, the sexual *object* has been changed, and others in whom the sexual *aim* is what has primarily been altered. The first group includes those who have renounced the union of the two genitals and who replace the genitals of one of the couple engaged in the sexual act by some other part or region of the body; in this they disregard the lack of suitable organic arrangements as well as any impediment offered by feelings of disgust. (They replace the vulva, for instance, by the mouth or anus.) Others follow, who, it is true, still retain the genitals as an object—not, however, on account of their sexual function but of other functions in which the genital plays a part either for anatomical reasons or because of its propinquity. We find from them that the excretory functions, which have been put aside as improper during the upbringing of children, retain the ability to attract the whole of sexual interest. Then come others again, who have abandoned the genital as an object altogether, and have taken some other part of the body as the object they desire—a woman's breast, a foot or a plait of hair. After them come others for whom parts of the body are of no importance but whose every wish is satisfied by a piece of clothing, a shoe, a piece of underclothing—the fetishists. Later in the procession come people who require the whole object indeed, but make quite definite demands of it—strange or horrible—even that it must have become a defenceless corpse,

[1] [Flaubert's *La tentation de Saint Antoine*, Part V of the final version (1874).]

and who, using criminal violence, make it into one so that they may enjoy it. But enough of this kind of horror!

The second group is led by perverts who have made what is normally only an introductory or preparatory act into the aim of their sexual wishes. They are people whose desire it is to look at the other person or to feel him or to watch him in the performance of his intimate actions, or who expose parts of their own bodies which should be covered, in the obscure expectation that they may be rewarded by a corresponding action in return. Next come the sadists, puzzling people whose tender endeavours have no other aim than to cause pain and torment to their object, ranging from humiliation to severe physical injuries; and, as though to counterbalance them, their counterparts, the masochists, whose only pleasure it is to suffer humiliations and torments of every kind from their loved object either symbolically or in reality. There are still others in whom several of these abnormal preconditions are united and intertwined; and lastly, we must learn that each of these groups is to be found in two forms: alongside of those who seek their sexual satisfaction in reality are those who are content merely to *imagine* that satisfaction, who need no real object at all, but can replace it by their phantasies.

Now there cannot be the slightest doubt that all these crazy, eccentric and horrible things really constitute the sexual activity of these people. Not only do they themselves regard them as such and are aware that they are substitutes for each other, but we must admit that they play the same part in their lives as normal sexual satisfaction does in ours; they make the same, often excessive sacrifices for them, and we can trace both in the rough and in finer detail the points at which these abnormalities are based on what is normal and the points at which they diverge from it. Nor can you fail to notice that here once again you find the characteristic of being improper, which clings to sexual activity, though here it is for the most part intensified to the point of being abominable.

Well, Ladies and Gentlemen, what attitude are we to adopt to these unusual kinds of sexual satisfaction? Indignation, an expression of our personal repugnance and an assurance that we ourselves do not share these lusts will obviously be of no help. Indeed, that is not what we have been asked for. When all is said and done, what we have here is a field of phenomena like any other. A denial in the form of an evasive suggestion that after all these are only rarities and curiosities would be easy to refute. On the contrary, we are dealing with quite common and widespread phenomena. If, however, it is argued that we need not allow our views of sexual life to be misled by them because they are one and all aberrations and deviations of the sexual instinct, a serious answer is called for. Unless we can understand these pathological forms of sexuality and can co-ordinate them with normal sexual life, we cannot understand normal sexuality either. In short, it remains an unavoidable task to give a complete theoretical account of how it is that these perversions can occur and of their connection with what is described as normal sexuality.

We shall be helped in this by a piece of information and two fresh observations. We owe the former to Iwan Bloch [1902–3]. It corrects the view that all these perversions are 'signs of degeneracy' by showing that aberrations of this kind from the sexual aim, loosenings like these of the tie with the sexual object, have occurred from time immemorial, in all periods known to us, among all peoples, the most primitive and the most civilized, and have occasionally obtained toleration and general recognition. The two observations were derived from the psycho-analytic investigation of neurotics; they are bound to have a decisive influence on our view of the sexual perversions.

I have said that neurotic symptoms are substitutes for sexual satisfaction [p. 299], and I indicated to you that the confirmation of this assertion by the analysis of symptoms would come up against a number of difficulties. For it can only be justified if under 'sexual satisfaction' we include the satisfaction of what are called perverse sexual needs, since an interpretation of symptoms of that kind is forced upon us with surprising frequency. The claim made by homosexuals or inverts to being exceptions collapses at once when we learn that homosexual impulses are invariably discovered in every single neurotic, and that a fair number of symptoms give expression to this latent inversion. Those who call themselves homosexuals are only the conscious and manifest inverts, whose number is nothing compared to that of the *latent* homosexuals. We are compelled, however, to regard choice of an object of one's own sex as a divergence in erotic life which is of positively habitual occurrence, and we are learning more and more to ascribe an especially high importance to it. No doubt this does not do away with the differences between manifest homosexuality and a normal attitude; their practical significance remains, but their theoretical value is greatly diminished. We have even found that a particular disease, paranoia, which is not to be counted among the transference neuroses, regularly arises from an attempt to fend off excessively strong homosexual impulses.[1] You will perhaps recall that one of our patients (p. 262) behaved in her obsessional action like a man, her own husband whom she had left; neurotic women very commonly produce symptoms in this way in the character of a man. Even if this is not actually to be regarded as homosexuality, it is closely related to its preconditions.

As you probably know, the hysterical neurosis can produce its symptoms in any system of organs and so disturb any function. Analysis shows that in this way all the so-called perverse impulses which seek to replace the genital by some other organ manifest themselves: these organs are then behaving like substitutive genitals. The symptoms of hysteria have actually led us to the view that the bodily organs, besides the functional part they play, must be recognized as having a sexual (erotogenic) significance, and that the execution of the first of these tasks is disturbed if the second of them makes too many claims.[2] Countless sensations and innervations which we come across as symptoms of hysteria in organs that have no apparent connection with sexuality are in this way revealed to us as being in the nature of fulfilments of perverse sexual impulses in relation to which other organs have acquired the significance of the sexual parts. We learn too to what a large extent the organs for the intake of nourishment and for excretion can in particular become the vehicles of sexual excitation. Here, then, we have the same thing that we were shown by the perversions; only in their case it was visible easily and unmistakably, whereas in

[1] [Paranoia is further discussed in Lecture XXVI, p. 423 ff. below.]

[2] [This point is discussed at greater length in a paper on psychogenic disturbance of vision (1910*i*).]

hysteria we have to take a circuitous path by way of the interpretation of symptoms, and do not then ascribe the perverse sexual impulses concerned to the subject's consciousness but locate them in his unconscious.

Of the many symptomatic pictures in which obsessional neurosis appears, the most important turn out to be those provoked by the pressure of excessively strong sadistic sexual impulses (perverse, therefore, in their aim). The symptoms, indeed, in accordance with the structure of an obsessional neurosis, serve predominantly as a *defence* against these wishes or give expression to the struggle between satisfaction and defence. But satisfaction does not come off too badly either; it succeeds in roundabout ways in putting itself into effect in the patients' behaviour and is preferably directed against themselves and makes them into self-tormentors. Other forms of the neurosis, the brooding kinds, correspond to an excessive sexualization of actions which ordinarily have their place on the path to normal sexual satisfaction—an excessive sexualization of wanting to look or to touch or to explore. Here we have the explanation of the great importance of the fear of touching and of the obsession for washing. An unsuspectedly large proportion of obsessional actions may be traced back to masturbation, of which they are disguised repetitions and modifications;[1] it is a familiar fact that masturbation, though a single and uniform action, accompanies the most various forms of sexual phantasying.

I should not have much difficulty in giving you a far more intimate picture of the relations between perversion and neurosis; but I think what I have already said will serve our purpose. We must however guard against being misled by what I have told you of the meaning of symptoms into over-estimating the frequency and intensity of people's perverse inclinations. It is possible, as you have heard [p. 300], to fall ill of a neurosis as a result of a frustration of normal sexual satisfaction. But when a real frustration like this occurs, the need moves over on to abnormal methods of sexual excitation. You will later learn the way in which this happens [p. 344 ff.]. But in any case you

[1] [The mechanism of the development of obsessional actions is described in detail in the paper on obsessions and religion (1907b).]

will realize that as a result of this 'collateral' damming-back [of the normal sexual current] the perverse impulses must emerge more strongly than they would have if normal sexual satisfaction had met with no obstacle in the real world.[1] Moreover a similar influence is to be recognized also as affecting the *manifest* perversions. In some cases they are provoked or made active if the normal satisfaction of the sexual instinct encounters too great difficulties for temporary reasons or because of permanent social regulations.[2] In other cases, it is true, the inclination to perversions is quite independent of such favouring conditions; they are, we might say, the normal species of sexual life for those particular individuals.

For the moment, perhaps, you may have an impression that I have confused rather than explained the relation between normal and perverse sexuality. But you must bear the following consideration in mind. If it is true that increased difficulty in obtaining normal sexual satisfaction in real life, or deprivation of that satisfaction, brings out perverse inclinations in people who had not shown any previously, we must suppose that there was something in these people which came half-way to meet the perversions; or, if you prefer it, the perversions must have been present in them in a latent form.

And this brings us to the second novelty that I announced to you [p. 307].[3] For psycho-analytic research has had to concern itself, too, with the sexual life of children, and this is because the memories and associations arising during the analysis of symptoms [in adults] regularly led back to the early years of childhood. What we inferred from these analyses was later confirmed point by point by direct observations of children.[4] And it then

---

[1] [This analogy of a collateral flow through intercommunicating channels is more clearly explained in Section 6 of the first of Freud's *Three Essays on Sexuality* (1905d). Cf. also below, p. 345.]

[2] [This last point is discussed at length in Freud's paper on ' "Civilized" Sexual Morality and Modern Nervous Illness' (1908d).]

[3] [The first was the important part played in the neuroses by perverse sexuality. What follows was touched on more briefly in Lecture XIII, p. 208 ff. above.]

[4] [The earliest of these direct observations were made in the case of 'Little Hans' (1909b).]

turned out that all these inclinations to perversion had their roots in childhood, that children have a predisposition to all of them and carry them out to an extent corresponding to their immaturity—in short, that perverse sexuality is nothing else than a magnified infantile sexuality split up into its separate impulses.

At all events you will now see the perversions in a new light and no longer fail to realize their connection with the sexual life of human beings: but at the price of what surprises and of what feelings of distress over these incongruities! No doubt you will feel inclined at first to deny the whole business: the fact that children have anything that can be described as sexual life, the correctness of our observations and the justification for finding any kinship between the behaviour of children and what is later condemned as perversion. So allow me to begin by explaining to you the motives for your opposition, and then to present you with the sum of our observations. To suppose that children have no sexual life—sexual excitations and needs and a kind of satisfaction—but suddenly acquire it between the ages of twelve and fourteen, would (quite apart from any observations) be as improbable, and indeed senseless, biologically as to suppose that they brought no genitals with them into the world and only grew them at the time of puberty. What *does* awaken in them at this time is the reproductive function, which makes use for its purposes of physical and mental material already present. You are committing the error of confusing sexuality and reproduction and by doing so you are blocking your path to an understanding of sexuality, the perversions and the neuroses. This error is, however, a tendentious one. Strangely enough, it has its source in the fact that you yourselves were once children and, while you were children, came under the influence of education. For society must undertake as one of its most important educative tasks to tame and restrict the sexual instinct when it breaks out as an urge to reproduction, and to subject it to an individual will which is identical with the bidding of society. It is also concerned to postpone the full development of the instinct till the child shall have reached a certain degree of intellectual maturity, for, with the complete irruption of the sexual instinct, educability is for practical purposes at an end. Otherwise, the instinct would break down every dam and wash away the laboriously erected work of civilization. Nor is the task of taming it ever an easy one; its success is sometimes too small, sometimes too great. The motive of human society is in the last resort an economic one; since it does not possess enough provisions to keep its members alive unless they work, it must restrict the number of its members and divert their energies from sexual activity to work. It is faced, in short, by the eternal, primaeval exigencies of life, which are with us to this day.[1]

Experience must no doubt have taught the educators that the task of making the sexual will of the new generation tractable could only be carried out if they began to exercise their influence very early, if they did not wait for the storm of puberty but intervened already in the sexual life of children which is preparatory to it. For this reason almost all infantile sexual activities were forbidden to children and frowned upon; an ideal was set up of making the life of children asexual, and in course of time things came to the point at which people really believed they were asexual and thereafter science pronounced this as its doctrine. To avoid contradicting their belief and their intentions, people since then overlook the sexual activities of children (no mean achievement) or are content in science to take a different view of them. Children are pure and innocent, and anyone who describes them otherwise can be charged with being an infamous blasphemer against the tender and sacred feelings of mankind.

Children are alone in not falling in with these conventions. They assert their animal rights with complete *naïveté* and give constant evidence that they have still to travel the road to purity. Strangely enough, the people who deny the existence of sexuality in children do not on that account become milder in their educational efforts but pursue the manifestations of what they deny exists with the utmost severity—describing them as 'childish naughtinesses'. It is also of the highest theoretical interest that the period of life which contradicts the prejudice of an asexual childhood most glaringly—the years of a child's life up to the age of five or six—is afterwards covered in most people by the veil of amnesia which is only completely torn away by an analytic enquiry, though it has been per-

[1] [See p. 22 f. above.]

meable earlier for the construction of a few dreams. [Cf. p. 201 above.]

I will now set out before you what is most definitely known about the sexual life of children. Let me at the same time, for convenience sake, introduce the concept of 'libido'. On the exact analogy of 'hunger', we use 'libido' as the name of the force (in this case that of the sexual instinct, as in the case of hunger that of the nutritive instinct) by which the instinct manifests itself. Other concepts, such as sexual 'excitation' and 'satisfaction', call for no explanation. You yourselves will easily perceive that the sexual activities of infants in arms are mostly a matter of interpretation, or you will probably use that as a ground of objection. These interpretations are arrived at on the basis of analytic examinations made by tracing from the symptoms backwards. In an infant the first impulses of sexuality make their appearance attached to other vital functions. His main interest is, as you know, directed to the intake of nourishment; when children fall asleep after being sated at the breast, they show an expression of blissful satisfaction which will be repeated later in life after the experience of a sexual orgasm. This would be too little on which to base an inference. But we observe how an infant will repeat the action of taking in nourishment without making a demand for further food; here, then, he is not actuated by hunger. We describe this as sensual sucking,[1] and the fact that in doing this he falls asleep once more with a blissful expression shows us that the act of sensual sucking has in itself alone brought him satisfaction. Soon, as we know, things come to a point at which he cannot go to sleep without having sucked. A paediatrician in Budapest, Dr. Lindner [1879], was the first to point out long ago the sexual nature of this activity. Those who are in charge of children, and who have no theoretical views on the subject, seem to form a similar judgement of sucking. They have no doubt of its only purpose being to obtain pleasure, class it as one of a child's 'naughtinesses' and compel him to abandon it by causing him distress, if he will not give it up of his own accord. Thus we learn that infants perform actions which have no purpose other

[1] [The German nursery terms here used are 'lutschen' or 'ludeln', for which there is no obvious English equivalent.]

than obtaining pleasure. It is our belief that they first experience this pleasure in connection with taking nourishment but that they soon learn to separate it from that accompanying condition. We can only refer this pleasure to an excitation of the areas of the mouth and lips; we call those parts of the body 'erotogenic zones' and describe the pleasure derived from sucking as a sexual one. We shall no doubt have to discuss further whether this description is justifiable.

If an infant could speak, he would no doubt pronounce the act of sucking at his mother's breast by far the most important in his life. He is not far wrong in this, for in this single act he is satisfying at once the two great vital needs. We are therefore not surprised to learn from psycho-analysis how much psychical importance the act retains all through life. Sucking at the mother's breast is the starting-point of the whole of sexual life, the unmatched prototype of every later sexual satisfaction, to which phantasy often enough recurs in times of need. This sucking involves making the mother's breast the first object of the sexual instinct. I can give you no idea of the important bearing of this first object upon the choice of every later object, of the profound effects it has in its transformations and substitutions in even the remotest regions of our sexual life. But at first the infant, in his sucking activity, gives up this object and replaces it by a part of his own body. He begins to suck his thumbs or his own tongue. In this way he makes himself independent of the consent of the external world as regards gaining pleasure, and besides this he increases it by adding the excitation of a second area of his body. The erotogenic zones are not all equally generous in yielding pleasure; it is therefore an important experience when the infant, as Lindner reports, discovers, in the course of feeling around, the specially excitable regions afforded by his genitals and so finds his way from sucking to masturbation.

In forming this opinion of sensual sucking we have already become acquainted with two decisive characteristics of infantile sexuality. It makes its appearance attached to the satisfaction of the major organic needs, and it behaves *auto-erotically* —that is, it seeks and finds its objects in the infant's own body. What has been shown most clearly in connection with the intake of nourishment is repeated in part with the excretions.

We conclude that infants have feelings of pleasure in the process of evacuating urine and faeces and that they soon contrive to arrange those actions in such a way as to bring them the greatest possible yield of pleasure through the corresponding excitations of the erotogenic zones of the mucous membrane. It is here for the first time (as Lou Andreas-Salomé [1916] has subtly perceived) that they encounter the external world as an inhibiting power, hostile to their desire for pleasure, and have a glimpse of later conflicts both external and internal. An infant must not produce his excreta at whatever moment he chooses, but when other people decide that he shall. In order to induce him to forgo these sources of pleasure, he is told that everything that has to do with these functions is improper and must be kept secret. This is where he is first obliged to exchange pleasure for social respectability. To begin with, his attitude to his excreta themselves is quite different. He feels no disgust at his faeces, values them as a portion of his own body with which he will not readily part, and makes use of them as his first 'gift', to distinguish people whom he values especially highly. Even after education has succeeded in its aim of making these inclinations alien to him, he carries on his high valuation of faeces in his estimate of 'gifts' and 'money'. On the other hand he seems to regard his achievements in urinating with peculiar pride.[1]

I know you have been wanting for a long time to interrupt me and exclaim: 'Enough of these atrocities! You tell us that defaecating is a source of sexual satisfaction, and already exploited in infancy! that faeces is a valuable substance and that the anus is a kind of genital! We don't believe all that—but we do understand why paediatricians and educationists have given a wide berth to psycho-analysis and its findings.' No, Gentlemen. You have merely forgotten that I have been trying to introduce the facts of infantile sexual life to you in connection with the facts of the sexual perversions. Why should you

[1] [The relations between faeces and money were discussed by Freud in a paper on 'Character and Anal Erotism' (1908b) and in a later one, almost contemporary with the present lecture, 'On Transformations of Instinct as Exemplified in Anal Erotism' (1917c). The connection between micturition and pride had been shown in a dream-analysis in The Interpretation of Dreams (1900a). See example IV of Section H in Chapter VI.]

not be aware that for a large number of adults, homosexual and heterosexual alike, the anus does really take over the role of the vagina in sexual intercourse? And that there are many people who retain a voluptuous feeling in defaecating all through their lives and describe it as being far from small? As regards interest in the act of defaecation and enjoyment in watching someone else defaecating, you can get children themselves to confirm the fact when they are a few years older and able to tell you about it. Of course, you must not have systematically intimidated them beforehand, or they will quite understand that they must be silent on the subject. And as to the other things that you are anxious not to believe, I will refer you to the findings of analysis and of the direct observation of children and will add that it calls for real ingenuity not to see all this or to see it differently. Nor do I complain if you find the kinship between infantile sexual activity and sexual perversions something very striking. But it is in fact self-evident: if a child has a sexual life at all it is bound to be of a perverse kind; for, except for a few obscure hints, children are without what makes sexuality into the reproductive function. On the other hand, the abandonment of the reproductive function is the common feature of all perversions. We actually describe a sexual activity as perverse if it has given up the aim of reproduction and pursues the attainment of pleasure as an aim independent of it. So, as you will see, the breach and turning-point in the development of sexual life lies in its becoming subordinate to the purposes of reproduction. Everything that happens before this turn of events and equally everything that disregards it and that aims solely at obtaining pleasure is given the uncomplimentary name of 'perverse' and as such is proscribed.

Allow me, therefore, to proceed with my brief account of infantile sexuality. What I have already reported of two systems of organs [nutritional and excretory] might be confirmed in reference to the others. A child's sexual life is indeed made up entirely of the activities of a number of component instincts which seek, independently of one another, to obtain pleasure, in part from the subject's own body and in part already from an external object. Among these organs the genitals come into prominence very soon. There are people in whom obtaining pleasure from their own genitals, without the assistance of any other genitals or of an object, continues uninterruptedly from infantile masturbation to the unavoidable masturbation[1] of puberty and persists for an indefinite length of time afterwards. Incidentally, the topic of masturbation is not one that can be so easily disposed of: it is something that calls for examination from many angles.[2]

Though I am anxious to cut short this discussion still further, I must nevertheless tell you a little about the sexual researches of children: they are too characteristic of infantile sexuality and of too great significance for the symptomatology of the neuroses to be passed over.[3] Infantile sexual researches begin very early, sometimes before the third year of life. They do not relate to the distinction between the sexes,[4] for this means nothing to children, since they (or at any rate boys) attribute the same male genital to both sexes. If, afterwards, a boy makes the discovery of the vagina from seeing his little sister or a girl playmate, he tries, to begin with, to disavow the evidence of his senses, for he cannot imagine a human creature like himself who is without such a precious portion. Later on, he takes fright at the possibility thus presented to him; and any threats that may have been made to him earlier, because he took too intense an interest in his little organ, now produce a deferred effect. He comes under the sway of the castration complex,[5] the

---

[1] ['*Notonanie.*' Literally, masturbation by necessity, i.e. forced on the subject by circumstances.]

[2] Freud's fullest remarks on the subject are in his 'Contribution to a Discussion on Masturbation' (1912*f*), where an Editor's Note gives further references.]

[3] [See 'On the Sexual Theories of Children' (1908*c*).]

[4] [This statement and the related one at the beginning of the next paragraph were corrected by Freud later, in a footnote to his paper on the anatomical distinction between the sexes (1925*j*). He there argues that the problem of sex-distinction came first and that of the origin of babies afterwards, at any rate in girls.]

[5] [This has already been mentioned above (on p. 208), and appears again below (on p. 368 ff.). The first published discussions on the castration complex appeared in Freud's case history of 'Little Hans' (1909*b*), though it had been referred to in an earlier paper on the sexual theories of children (1908*c*). Its relation to the Oedipus complex was fully examined in later years, more particularly in Freud's papers on 'The Dissolution of the Oedipus Complex' (1924*d*) and on the anatomical distinction between the sexes (1925*j*).]

form taken by which plays a great part in the construction of his character if he remains normal, in his neurosis if he falls ill, and in his resistances if he comes into analytic treatment. As regards little girls, we can say of them that they feel greatly at a disadvantage owing to their lack of a big, visible penis, that they envy boys for possessing one and that, in the main for this reason, they develop a wish to be a man—a wish that re-emerges later on, in any neurosis that may arise if they meet with a mishap in playing a feminine part. In her childhood, moreover, a girl's clitoris takes on the role of a penis entirely: it is characterized by special excitability and is the area in which auto-erotic satisfaction is obtained. The process of a girl's becoming a woman depends very much on the clitoris passing on this sensitivity to the vaginal orifice in good time and completely. In cases of what is known as sexual anaesthesia in women the clitoris has obstinately retained its sensitivity.

The sexual interest of children begins by turning, rather, to the problem of where babies come from[1]—the same problem which underlies the question put by the Theban Sphinx—and it is most often raised by egoistic fears on the arrival of a new baby. The reply which is ready to hand in the nursery, that babies are brought by the stork [p. 160], comes up against disbelief on the part even of small children far oftener than we are aware. The sense of being defrauded of the truth by the grown-ups contributes much to making children feel lonely and to developing their independence. But a child is not in a position to solve this problem by his own means. His undeveloped sexual constitution sets definite limits to his power of perception. He begins by supposing that babies come from people taking in something special in their food, nor does he know that only women can have babies. Later he becomes aware of this limitation and ceases to regard eating as the origin of babies—though the theory persists in fairy tales. When the child has grown bigger, he soon notices that his father must play some part in getting babies, but he cannot guess what. If he happens to witness a sexual act, he regards it as an attempt at subjugation, a struggle, and this is the sadistic misunderstanding of coition. But at first he does not connect this act with the coming into being of a baby. So, too, if he finds traces of blood on his

[1] [See the last footnote but one.]

mother's bed or on her underclothes, he takes it as a sign that she has been injured by his father. Still later in childhood, he no doubt suspects that the man's sexual organ has an essential share in producing babies, but the only function he can attribute to that part of the body is micturition.

From the very first, children are at one in thinking that babies must be born through the bowel; they must make their appearance like lumps of faeces. This theory is not abandoned until all anal interests have been deprived of their value, and it is then replaced by the hypothesis that the navel comes open or that the area of the breast between the nipples is where birth takes place. In this way the child in the course of his researches comes nearer to the facts about sex, or, feeling at a loss owing to his ignorance, he passes them by till, usually in the years before puberty, he is given what is as a rule a depreciatory and incomplete explanation, which often produces traumatic effects.

You will no doubt have heard, Gentlemen, that in psycho-analysis the concept of what is sexual has been unduly extended in order to support the theses of the sexual causation of the neuroses and the sexual meaning of symptoms. You are now in a position to judge for yourselves whether this extension is unjustified. We have only extended the concept of sexuality far enough to be able to comprise the sexual life of perverts and of children. We have, that is to say, given it back its true compass. What is called sexuality outside psycho-analysis relates only to a restricted sexual life, which serves the purpose of reproduction and is described as normal.

LECTURE XXI

THE DEVELOPMENT OF THE LIBIDO AND THE SEXUAL ORGANIZATIONS

GENTLEMEN,—I am under the impression that I have not succeeded in bringing home to you quite convincingly the importance of the perversions for our view of sexuality, and I should therefore like so far as I can to improve and supplement what I have said.

It is not the case that the perversions alone would have obliged us to make the change in the concept of sexuality which has brought such violent contradictions down on us. The study of infantile sexuality had even more to do with it and it was the concurrence of the two which was decisive for us. But the manifestations of infantile sexuality, however unmistakable they may be in later childhood, seem to melt into indefiniteness towards their beginnings. Anyone who chooses to disregard the history of their development and their analytic context will deny that they are of a sexual character and will attribute some undifferentiated character to them instead. You must not forget that at the moment we are not in possession of any generally recognized criterion of the sexual nature of a process, apart, once again, from a connection with the reproductive function which we must reject as being too narrow-minded. The biological criteria, such as the periodicities of twenty-three and twenty-eight days postulated by Wilhelm Fliess [1906], are still highly debatable; the chemical characteristics of the sexual process, which we may suspect, are still awaiting discovery. On the other hand, the sexual perversions of adults are something tangible and unambiguous. As is already shown by the name by which they are universally known, they are unquestionably sexual. Whether they are described as indications of degeneracy or in any other way, no one has yet had the courage to class them as anything but phenomena of sexual life. On their account alone we are justified in asserting that sexuality and reproduction do not coincide, for it is obvious that all of them disavow the aim of reproduction.

320

I find a parallel here which is not uninteresting. Whereas for most people 'conscious' and 'psychical' are the same, we have been obliged to extend the concept of 'psychical' and to recognize something 'psychical' that is not 'conscious'. And in just the same way, whereas other people declare that 'sexual' and 'connected with reproduction' (or, if you prefer to put it more shortly, 'genital') are identical, we cannot avoid postulating something 'sexual' that is not 'genital'—has nothing to do with reproduction. The similarity here is only a formal one, but it is not without a deeper foundation.

But if the existence of sexual perversions is such a decisive argument in this question, why has it not long since had its effect and settled the matter? I really cannot say. I think it is connected with the fact that these sexual perversions are subject to a quite special ban, which has even affected theory and has stood in the way of the scientific consideration of them. It is as though no one could forget that they are not only something disgusting but also something monstrous and dangerous—as though people felt them as seductive, and had at bottom to fight down a secret envy of those who were enjoying them. One is reminded of the admission made by the condemnatory Landgraf in the famous *Tannhäuser* parody:

'Im Venusberg vergass er Ehr und Pflicht!
—Merkwürdig, unser einem passiert
                    so etwas nicht.'[1]

In reality perverts are poor wretches, rather, who have to pay extremely dear for their hard-won satisfaction.

What makes the activity of perverts so unmistakably sexual in spite of all the strangeness of its objects and aims is the fact that as a rule an act of perverse satisfaction nevertheless ends in complete orgasm and voidance of the genital products. This is of course only the result of the people concerned being adults. In children orgasm and genital excretion are scarcely possible; their place is taken by hints which are once more not recognized as being clearly sexual.

[1] ['The Venusberg made him forget
   Honour and Duty thus!—
   Strange how these things don't happen
   To people such as us.'—By Nestroy (cf. p. 352*n*.).]

There is something else that I must add in order to complete our view of sexual perversions. However infamous they may be, however sharply they may be contrasted with normal sexual activity, quiet consideration will show that some perverse trait or other is seldom absent from the sexual life of normal people. Even a kiss can claim to be described as a perverse act, since it consists in the bringing together of two oral erotogenic zones instead of the two genitals. Yet no one rejects it as perverse; on the contrary, it is permitted in theatrical performances as a softened hint at the sexual act. But precisely kissing can easily turn into a complete perversion—if, that is to say, it becomes so intense that a genital discharge and orgasm follow upon it directly, an event that is far from rare. We can learn, too, that for one person feeling and looking at the object are indispensable preconditions of sexual enjoyment, that another person will pinch or bite at the climax of sexual excitation, that the highest pitch of excitement in lovers is not always provoked by the genitals but by some other region of the object's body, and any number of similar things besides. There is no sense in excluding people with individual traits of this kind from the class of the normal and putting them among the perverts. On the contrary, we shall recognize more and more clearly that the essence of the perversions lies not in the extension of the sexual aim, not in the replacement of the genitals, not even always in the variant choice of the object, but solely in the exclusiveness with which these deviations are carried out and as a result of which the sexual act serving the purpose of reproduction is put on one side. In so far as the perverse actions are inserted in the performance of the normal sexual act as preparatory or intensifying contributions, they are in reality not perversions at all. The gulf between normal and perverse sexuality is of course very much narrowed by facts of this kind. It is an easy conclusion that normal sexuality has emerged out of something that was in existence before it, by weeding out certain features of that material as unserviceable and collecting together the rest in order to subordinate them to a new aim, that of reproduction.

Before we make use of our familiarity with the perversions to plunge once again into the study of infantile sexuality on the basis of clearer premisses, I must draw your attention to an important difference between them. Perverse sexuality is as a rule excellently centred: all its actions are directed to an aim—usually to a single one; one component instinct has gained the upper hand in it and is either the only one observable or has subjected the others to its purposes. In that respect there is no distinction between perverse and normal sexuality other than the fact that their dominating component instincts and consequently their sexual aims are different. In both of them, one might say, a well-organized tyranny has been established, but in each of the two a different family has seized the reins of power. Infantile sexuality, on the other hand, lacks, speaking generally, any such centring and organization; its separate component instincts have equal rights, each of them goes its own way to obtaining pleasure. Both the absence and the presence of centring harmonize well, of course, with the fact that both perverse and normal sexuality have arisen out of infantile sexuality. Incidentally, there are also cases of perverse sexuality which have a much greater resemblance to the infantile kind, since in them numerous component instincts have put through (or, more correctly, have persisted in) their aims independently of one another. It is better in such cases to speak of infantilism in sexual life rather than of a perversion.

Thus forearmed we can proceed to the consideration of a suggestion which we shall certainly not be spared. 'Why', we shall be asked, 'are you so obstinate in describing as being already sexuality what on your own evidence are indefinable manifestations in childhood out of which sexual life will later develop? Why should you not be content instead with giving them a physiological description and simply say that in an infant at the breast we already observe activities, such as sensual sucking or holding back the excreta, which show us that he is striving for "organ-pleasure"?[1] In that way you would have avoided the hypothesis, so repugnant to every feeling, of the smallest babies having a sexual life.'—Indeed, Gentlemen, I have no objection at all to organ-pleasure. I know that even the supreme pleasure

---

[1] ['*Organlust.*' The term occurs in 'Instincts and their Vicissitudes' (1915c), where Freud seems to have used it for the first time. He uses it again below in the *New Introductory Lectures*, p. 562. The *concept*, of course, is familiar from the time of the *Three Essays* (1905d), Essay II.]

of sexual union is only an organ-pleasure attached to the activity of the genitals. But can you tell me when this originally indifferent organ-pleasure acquires the sexual character which it undoubtedly possesses in the later phases of development? Do we know any more about 'organ-pleasure' than about sexuality? You will reply that it gains its sexual character precisely when the genitals begin to play their part; 'sexual' coincides with 'genital'. You will even reject the objection raised by the perversions by pointing out to me that in the majority of perversions a genital orgasm is after all aimed at, even if it is arrived at by a method other than the union of the genitals. You are certainly taking up a much stronger position in determining the characteristics of what is sexual if you knock out of it the relation to reproduction which is made untenable by the perversions and put genital activity in its place. But, if so, we are no longer far apart: it is only a question of the genital organs versus the other organs. What are you going to do, however, about the numerous experiences which show you that the genitals can be represented as regards their yield of pleasure by other organs, as in the case of kissing or of the perverse practices of voluptuaries or of the symptoms of hysteria? In that neurosis it is quite usual for signs of stimulation, sensations and innervations, and even the processes of erection, which belong properly to the genitals, to be displaced on to other, remote regions of the body—as, for instance, by transposition upwards, to the head and face. Being thus convinced that you have nothing to catch hold of for your characterization of what is sexual, you will no doubt have to make up your minds to follow my example and extend the description of being 'sexual' to the activities of early childhood, too, which strive for organ-pleasure.

And now, for my justification, there are two other considerations which I must ask you to take into account. As you know, we call the dubious and indefinable pleasurable activities of earliest childhood sexual because, in the course of analysis, we arrive at them from the symptoms after passing through indisputably sexual material. They need not necessarily themselves be sexual on that account—agreed! But take an analogous case. Suppose we had no means of observing the development from their seed of two dicotyledonous plants, the apple-tree and the bean, but that it was possible in both cases for us to trace their development backwards from the fully developed individual plant to the first seedling with two seed-leaves. The two seed-leaves have a neutral appearance; they are just alike in both cases. Am I then to suppose that they are really alike, and that the specific difference between an apple-tree and a bean is only introduced into the plants later? Or is it biologically more correct to believe that this difference is already there in the seedling, although I cannot observe any distinction in the seed-leaves? But we are doing the same thing when we call the pleasure in the activities of an infant-in-arms a sexual one. I cannot discuss here whether each and every organ-pleasure should be called a sexual one or whether, alongside of the sexual one, there is another which does not deserve to be so called. I know too little about organ-pleasure and its determinants; and, in view of the retrogressive character of analysis in general, I cannot feel surprised if at the very end I arrive at what are for the time being indefinable factors.

And one thing more! On the whole you will have gained very little for what you want to assert—the sexual purity of children —even if you succeed in convincing me that it would be better to regard the activities of infants-in-arms as non-sexual. For the sexual life of children is already free from all these doubts from the third year of life onwards: at about that time the genitals already begin to stir, a period of infantile masturbation—of genital satisfaction, therefore—sets in, regularly perhaps. The mental and social phenomena of sexual life need no longer be absent; the choice of an object, an affectionate preference for particular people, a decision, even, in favour of one of the two sexes, jealousy—all these have been established by impartial observations made independently of psycho-analysis and before its time, and they can be confirmed by any observer who cares to see them. You will object that you have never doubted the early awakening of affection; you have only doubted whether this affection bears a 'sexual' character. It is true that children have already learnt to conceal this between the ages of three and eight. But if you are attentive you will be able nevertheless to collect enough evidence of the 'sensual' aims of this affection, and whatever you still lack after that can easily be supplied in plenty by the investigations of analysis. The sexual aims at this period of life are intimately connected with the child's contemporary sexual researches, of which I have given you some instances [p. 317]. The perverse character of some of these aims is of course dependent on the child's constitutional immaturity, for he has not yet discovered the aim that consists in the act of copulation.

From about the sixth to the eighth year of life onwards, we can observe a halt and retrogression in sexual development, which, in cases where it is most propitious culturally, deserves to be called a period of latency. The latency period may also be absent: it need not bring with it any interruption of sexual activity and sexual interests along the whole line. The majority of experiences and mental impulses before the start of the latency period now fall victim to infantile amnesia—the forgetting (already discussed by us [p. 199 ff.]) which veils our earliest youth from us and makes us strangers to it. The task is set us in every psycho-analysis of bringing this forgotten period back into memory. It is impossible to avoid a suspicion that the beginnings of sexual life which are included in that period have provided the motive for its being forgotten—that this forgetting, in fact, is an outcome of repression.

From the third year of life a child's sexual life shows much agreement with an adult's. It differs from the latter, as we already know, in lacking a firm organization under the primacy of the genitals, in its inevitable traits of perversion and also, of course, in the far lesser intensity of the whole trend. But from the point of view of theory the most interesting phases of sexual, or, as we will say, of libidinal, development lie earlier than this point of time. This course of development takes place so rapidly that we should probably never have succeeded in getting a firm hold of its fleeting pictures by direct observation. It was only with the help of the psycho-analytic investigation of the neuroses that it became possible to discern the still earlier phases of the development of the libido. These are nothing but constructions, to be sure, but, if you carry out psycho-analyses in practice, you will find that they are necessary and useful constructions. You will soon learn how it comes about that pathology can here put us in possession of conditions which we should inevitably overlook in a normal subject.

Accordingly, I can now describe to you the form taken by a child's sexual life before the establishment of the primacy of the genitals, preparations for which are made in the first period of infancy preceding the latency period and which is permanently organized from puberty onwards. A kind of loose organization which may be called 'pregenital' exists during this early period. During this phase what stand in the forefront are not the genital component instincts but the sadistic and anal ones. The contrast between 'masculine' and 'feminine' plays no part here as yet. Its place is taken by the contrast between 'active' and 'passive', which may be described as a precursor of the sexual polarity and which later on is soldered to that polarity. What appears to us as masculine in the activities of this phase, when we look at it from the point of view of the genital phase, turns out to be an expression of an instinct for mastery which easily passes over into cruelty. Trends with a passive aim are attached to the erotogenic zone of the anal orifice, which is very important at this period. The instincts for looking and for gaining knowledge [the scopophilic and epistemophilic instincts] are powerfully at work; the genitals actually play a part in sexual life only as organs for the excretion of urine. The component instincts of this phase are not without objects, but those objects do not necessarily converge into a single object. The sadistic-anal organization is the immediate forerunner of the phase of genital primacy. Detailed study shows how much of it is retained in the later definitive shape of things and shows too the way in which its component instincts are compelled to take their place in the new genital organization.[1] Behind the sadistic-anal phase of libidinal development we get a glimpse of a still earlier and more primitive stage of organization, in which the erotogenic zone of the mouth plays the chief part. As you will guess, the sexual activity of sensual sucking [p. 313] belongs to it. We must admire the understanding of the Ancient Egyptians who, in their art, represented children, including the God Horus, with a finger in their mouth. Only recently Abraham [1916] has given examples of the traces which this primitive oral phase leaves behind it in later sexual life.

I can well suppose, Gentlemen, that this last account of the

[1] [Freud afterwards interposed a 'phallic' phase between the sadistic-anal and genital organizations (Freud, 1923e).]

sexual organizations has obstructed rather than instructed you, and it may be that I have once more entered too much into details. But you must have patience. What you have just heard will derive increased value for you from its later application. For the present you should keep firmly in mind that sexual life (or, as we put it, the libidinal function) does not emerge as something ready-made and does not even develop further in its own likeness, but passes through a series of successive phases which do not resemble one another; its development is thus several times repeated—like that of a caterpillar into a butterfly. The turning-point of this development is the subordination of all the component sexual instincts under the primacy of the genitals and along with this the subjection of sexuality to the reproductive function. This is preceded by a sexual life that might be described as distracted—the independent activity of the different component instincts striving for organ-pleasure. This anarchy is mitigated by abortive beginnings of 'pregenital' organizations—a sadistic-anal phase preceded by an oral one, which is perhaps the most primitive. In addition, there are the various, still incompletely known, processes which lead one stage of organization over to the subsequent and next higher one. We shall learn later[1] what an important light is thrown on the neuroses by the fact that the libido passes through such a long course of development and one which has so many breaks in it.

To-day we will follow yet another side of this development—namely the relation of the component sexual instincts to their object. Or rather, we will make a hasty survey of this development and dwell somewhat longer on one of its rather late consequences. A few of the components of the sexual instinct, then, have an object from the first and hold fast to it—for instance, the instinct for mastery (sadism) and the scopophilic and epistemophilic instincts. Others, more definitely linked to particular erotogenic zones of the body, have one to begin with only, so long as they are still attached to the non-sexual functions [cf. p. 313 above], and give it up when they become separated from them. Thus the first object of the oral component of the sexual instinct is the mother's breast which satisfies the infant's

[1] [Actually in the next lecture.]

need for nourishment. The erotic component, which is satisfied simultaneously during the [nutritive] sucking, makes itself independent with the act of *sensual* sucking [*lutschen*]; it gives up the outside object and replaces it by an area of the subject's own body. The oral instinct becomes *auto-erotic*, as are the anal and other erotogenic instincts from the first. Further development, to put the matter as concisely as possible, has two aims: firstly, the abandonment of auto-erotism, the replacement of the subject's own body once more by an outside object, and secondly, the unification of the various objects of the separate instincts and their replacement by a single object. This can, of course, only be achieved if the object is again a whole body, similar to the subject's own. Nor can it be effected unless a number of the auto-erotic instinctual impulses are left behind as being unserviceable.

The processes of finding an object are fairly complex and no comprehensive account has hitherto been given of them. For our purposes it may be specially pointed out that when, in the years of childhood before puberty, the process has in some respects reached a conclusion, the object that has been found turns out to be almost identical with the first object of the oral pleasure-instinct, which was reached by attachment [to the nutritional instinct].[1] Though it is not actually the mother's breast, at least it is the mother. We call the mother the first *love-object*. For we speak of love when we bring the mental side of the sexual trends into the foreground and want to force back the underlying physical or 'sensual' instinctual demands or to forget them for a moment. At the time at which the child's mother becomes his love-object the psychical work of repression has already begun in him, which is withdrawing from his knowledge awareness of a part of his sexual aims. To his choice of his mother as a love-object everything becomes attached which, under the name of the 'Oedipus complex', has attained so much importance in the psycho-analytic explanation of the neuroses and has played no less a part, perhaps, in the resistance to psycho-analysis. [Cf. p. 207 above.][2]

[1] [This is further explained in Lecture XXVI, p. 426 below.]
[2] [Freud's first published account of the Oedipus complex was given in Section D of Chapter V in *The Interpretation of Dreams* (1900a), though he had put it forward earlier in a letter to Fliess

Listen to this episode which occurred in the course of the present war. One of the stout disciples of psycho-analysis was stationed as medical officer on the German front somewhere in Poland. He attracted his colleagues' attention by the fact that he occasionally exercised an unexpected influence on a patient. When he was questioned, he acknowledged that he was employing the methods of psycho-analysis and declared his readiness to convey his knowledge to his colleagues. Every evening thereafter the medical officers of the corps, his colleagues and his superiors, came together in order to learn the secret doctrines of analysis. All went well for a while; but when he spoke to his audience about the Oedipus complex, one of his superiors rose, declared he did not believe it, that it was a vile act on the part of the lecturer to speak of such things to them, honest men who were fighting for their country and fathers of a family, and that he forbade the continuance of the lectures. That was the end of the matter. The analyst got himself transferred to another part of the front. It seems to me a bad thing, however, if a German victory requires that science shall be 'organized' in this way, and German science will not respond well to organization of such a kind.

And now you will be eager to hear what this terrible Oedipus complex contains. Its name tells you. You all know the Greek legend of King Oedipus, who was destined by fate to kill his father and take his mother to wife, who did everything possible to escape the oracle's decree and punished himself by blinding when he learned that he had none the less unwittingly committed both these crimes. I hope many of you may yourselves have felt the shattering effect of the tragedy in which Sophocles has treated the story. The work of the Athenian dramatist exhibits the way in which the long-past deed of Oedipus is gradually brought to light by an investigation ingeniously protracted and fanned into life by ever fresh relays of evidence. To this extent it has a certain resemblance to the progress of a psychoanalysis. In the course of the dialogue Jocasta, the deluded mother and wife, declares herself opposed to the continuance of

of October 15, 1897 (Freud, 1950a, Letter 71). The actual term 'Oedipus complex' was first introduced much later, in a paper on a special type of object-choice (1910h).]

the enquiry. She appeals to the fact that many people have dreamt of lying with their mothers, but that dreams should be despised. We do not despise dreams—least of all, typical dreams which occur to many people; and we do not doubt that the dream referred to by Jocasta has an intimate connection with the strange and terrifying content of the legend.

It is a surprising thing that the tragedy of Sophocles does not call up indignant repudiation in his audience—a reaction similar to that of our simple-minded army doctor but far better justified. For fundamentally it is an amoral work: it absolves men from moral responsibility, exhibits the gods as promoters of crime and shows the impotence of the moral impulses of men which struggle against crime. It might easily be supposed that the material of the legend had in view an indictment of the gods and of fate; and in the hands of Euripides, the critic and enemy of the gods, it would probably have become such an indictment. But with the devout Sophocles there is no question of an application of that kind. The difficulty is overcome by the pious sophistry that to bow to the will of the gods is the highest morality even when it promotes crime. I cannot think that this morality is a strong point of the play, but it has no influence on its effect. It is not to it that the auditor reacts but to the secret sense and content of the legend. He reacts as though by self-analysis he had recognized the Oedipus complex in himself and had unveiled the will of the gods and the oracle as exalted disguises of his own unconscious. It is as though he was obliged to remember the two wishes—to do away with his father and in place of him to take his mother to wife—and to be horrified at them. And he understands the dramatist's voice as though it were saying to him: 'You are struggling in vain against your responsibility and are protesting in vain of what you have done in opposition to these criminal intentions. You are guilty, for you have not been able to destroy them; they still persist in you unconsciously.' And there is psychological truth contained in this. Even if a man has repressed his evil impulses into the unconscious and would like to tell himself afterwards that he is not responsible for them, he is nevertheless bound to be aware of this responsibility as a sense of guilt whose basis is unknown to him.[1]

There can be no doubt that the Oedipus complex may be

[1] [Cf. a paragraph near the end of Lecture XIII, p. 211 above.]

looked upon as one of the most important sources of the sense of guilt by which neurotics are so often tormented. But more than this: in a study of the beginnings of human religion and morality which I published in 1913 under the title of *Totem and Taboo* [Freud, 1912–13] I put forward a suggestion that mankind as a whole may have acquired its sense of guilt, the ultimate source of religion and morality, at the beginning of its history, in connection with the Oedipus complex. I should be very glad to tell you more about this, but I had better leave it on one side. Once one has begun on that topic it is hard to break off; and we must go back to individual psychology.

What, then, can be gathered about the Oedipus complex from the direct observation of children at the time of their making their choice of an object before the latency period? Well, it is easy to see that the little man wants to have his mother all to himself, that he feels the presence of his father as a nuisance, that he is resentful if his father indulges in any signs of affection towards his mother and that he shows satisfaction when his father has gone on a journey or is absent. He will often express his feelings directly in words and promise his mother to marry her. It will be thought that this amounts to little compared to the deeds of Oedipus; but in fact it is enough, it is the same thing at root. Observation is often obscured by the circumstance that on other occasions the same child will simultaneously give evidence of great affection for his father. But contrary—or, as it is better to say, 'ambivalent'[1]—emotional attitudes, which in adults would lead to a conflict, remain compatible with each other for a long time in children, just as later they find a permanent place beside each other in the unconscious. It will also be objected that the little boy's conduct arises from egoistic motives and gives no grounds for postulating an erotic complex: the child's mother attends to all his needs, so that he has an interest in preventing her from looking after anyone else. This also is true; but it will soon become clear that in this situation as in similar ones the egoistic interest[2] is merely affording a point of support to which the erotic

---

[1] [See below, p. 427 f.]

[2] [This term recurs many times in Lecture XXVI, where some editorial comment is made on it (p. 414).]

trend is attached. The little boy may show the most undisguised sexual curiosity about his mother, he may insist upon sleeping beside her at night, he may force his presence on her while she is dressing or may even make actual attempts at seducing her, as his mother will often notice and report with amusement—all of which puts beyond doubt the erotic nature of his tie with his mother. Nor must it be forgotten that the mother devotes the same attention to a little daughter without producing the same result[1] and that the father often competes with her in looking after the boy and yet fails to gain the same significance as she does. In short, the factor of sexual preference cannot be eliminated from the situation by any criticism. From the standpoint of egoistic interest it would be simply foolish of the little man not to prefer to put up with having two people in his service rather than only one of them.

As you see, I have only described the relation of a *boy* to his father and mother. Things happen in just the same way with little girls, with the necessary changes:[2] an affectionate attachment to her father, a need to get rid of her mother as superfluous and to take her place, a coquetry which already employs the methods of later womanhood—these offer a charming picture, especially in small girls, which makes us forget the possibly grave consequences lying behind this infantile situation. We must not omit to add that the parents themselves often exercise a determining influence on the awakening of a child's Oedipus attitude by themselves obeying the pull of sexual attraction, and that where there are several children the father will give the plainest evidence of his greater affection for his little daughter and the mother for her son. But the spontaneous nature of the Oedipus complex in children cannot be seriously shaken even by this factor.

When other children appear on the scene the Oedipus complex is enlarged into a family complex. This, with fresh support

---

[1] [See, however, the next footnote.]

[2] [It was not till many years later that Freud became fully aware of the lack of symmetry in the Oedipus relations of the two sexes. This emerged in his paper on 'Some Psychical Consequences of the Anatomical Distinction between the Sexes' (1925*j*) and was elaborated in the later one on 'Female Sexuality' (1931*b*). He discusses the question again in Lecture XXXIII of the *New Introductory Lectures,* p. 576 ff., and lastly in Chapter VII of his posthumous *Outline of Psycho-Analysis* (1940*a* [1938]), (Norton, 1949).]

from the egoistic sense of injury, gives grounds for receiving the new brothers or sisters with repugnance and for unhesitatingly getting rid of them by a wish. It is even true that as a rule children are far readier to give verbal expression to *these* feelings of hate than to those arising from the parental complex. If a wish of this kind is fulfilled and the undesired addition to the family is removed again shortly afterwards by death, we can discover from a later analysis what an important experience this death has been to the child, even though it need not have remained fixed in his memory. A child who has been put into second place by the birth of a brother or sister, and who is now for the first time almost isolated from his mother, does not easily forgive her this loss of place; feelings which in an adult would be described as greatly embittered arise in him and are often the basis of a permanent estrangement. We have already mentioned [p. 318] that the child's sexual researches, with all their consequences, usually follow from this vital experience of his. As these brothers and sisters grow up, the boy's attitude to them undergoes very significant transformations. He may take his sister as a love-object by way of substitute for his faithless mother. Where there are several brothers, all of them courting a younger sister, situations of hostile rivalry, which are so important for later life, arise already in the nursery. A little girl may find in her elder brother a substitute for her father who no longer takes an affectionate interest in her as he did in her earliest years. Or she may take a younger sister as a substitute for the baby she has vainly wished for from her father.

This and very much else of a similar nature will be shown to you by the direct observation of children and by the consideration of clearly retained memories from childhood uninfluenced by analysis. From this you will conclude among other things that the position of a child in the family order is a factor of extreme importance in determining the shape of his later life and should deserve consideration in every life-history. But, what is more important, in view of this information which can be so easily obtained, you will not be able to recall without a smile the pronouncements of science in explanation of the prohibition of incest. [Cf. p. 210 above.] There is no end to what has been invented on the subject. It has been said that sexual inclination is diverted from members of the same family who are of the opposite sex by the fact of having lived together from child-hood; or, again, that a biological purpose of avoiding inbreed-ing is represented psychically by an innate horror of incest. In all this the fact is entirely overlooked that such an inexorable prohibition of it in law and custom would not be needed if there were any reliable natural barriers against the temptation to in-cest. The truth is just the opposite. A human being's first choice of an object is regularly an incestuous one, aimed, in the case of the male, at his mother and sister; and it calls for the severest prohibitions to deter this persistent infantile tendency from realization. Among the primitive races still living to-day, among savages, the prohibitions against incest are even very much stricter than among ourselves, and Theodor Reik has only recently shown in a brilliant work [Reik, 1915–16] that the puberty rites of savages, which represent a re-birth, have the sense of releasing the boy from his incestuous bond with his mother and of reconciling him with his father.

Mythology will teach you that incest, which is supposed to be so much detested by humans, is unhesitatingly allowed to the gods. And you may learn from ancient history that incestuous sister-marriage was a sanctified injunction upon the person of the Ruler (among the Egyptian Pharaohs and the Incas of Peru). What was in question was thus a privilege forbidden to the common herd.

Mother-incest was one of the crimes of Oedipus, parricide was the other. It may be remarked in passing that they are also the two great crimes proscribed by totemism, the first socio-religious institution of mankind.[1]

But let us now turn from the direct observation of children to the analytic examination of adults who have become neurotic. What help does analysis give towards a further knowledge of the Oedipus complex? That can be answered in a word. Analysis confirms all that the legend describes. It shows that each of these neurotics has himself been an Oedipus or, what comes to the same thing, has, as a reaction to the complex, become a Hamlet.[2] The analytic account of the Oedipus complex is, of

[1] [Cf. Freud's *Totem and Taboo* (1912–13), (Norton, 1952).]

[2] [Freud's earliest published commentary on *Hamlet* (as well as on *Oedipus Rex*) appeared in *The Interpretation of Dreams* (1900a), Chapter V(D).]

course, a magnification and coarsening of the infantile sketch. The hatred of the father, the death-wishes against him, are no longer hinted at timidly, the affection for the mother admits that its aim is to possess her as a woman. Should we really attribute such blatant and extreme emotional impulses to the tender years of childhood, or is analysis deceiving us by an admixture of some new factor? It is not hard to find one. Whenever someone gives an account of a past event, even if he is a historian, we must take into account what he unintentionally puts back into the past from the present or from some intermediate time, thus falsifying his picture of it. In the case of a neurotic it is even a question whether this putting back is an entirely unintentional one; later on we shall have to discover reasons for this and have to do justice in general to the fact of 'retrospective phantasying'.[1] We can easily see, too, that hatred of the father is reinforced by a number of factors arising from later times and circumstances and that the sexual desires towards the mother are cast into forms which must have been alien as yet to a child. But it would be a vain effort to seek to explain the whole Oedipus complex by retrospective phantasying and to attach it to later times. Its infantile core and more or less of its accessories remain as they were confirmed by the direct observation of children.

The clinical fact which meets us behind the form of the Oedipus complex as it is established by analysis is of the highest practical significance. We learn that at puberty, when the sexual instinct first makes its demands in full strength, the old familiar incestuous objects are taken up again and freshly cathected[2] with libido. The infantile object-choice was only a feeble one, but it was a prelude, pointing the direction for the object-choice at puberty. At this point, then, very intense emotional processes come into play, following the direction of the Oedipus complex or reacting against it, processes which, however, since their premises have become intolerable, must

---

[1] [See the latter part of Lecture XXIII.]

[2] ['*Besetzt*', charged with energy. The concept of '*Besetzungen*' (cathexes), charges of psychical energy, is fundamental to Freud's theories. A discussion of it will be found in an Editor's Appendix to Freud's early paper on *The Neuro-Psychoses of Defense*, (1894a). The term reappears frequently below.]

to a large extent remain apart from consciousness. From this time onwards, the human individual has to devote himself to the great task of detaching himself from his parents, and not until that task is achieved can he cease to be a child and become a member of the social community. For the son this task consists in detaching his libidinal wishes from his mother and employing them for the choice of a real outside love-object, and in reconciling himself with his father if he has remained in opposition to him, or in freeing himself from his pressure if, as a reaction to his infantile rebelliousness, he has become subservient to him. These tasks are set to everyone; and it is remarkable how seldom they are dealt with in an ideal manner —that is, in one which is correct both psychologically and socially. By neurotics, however, no solution at all is arrived at: the son remains all his life bowed beneath his father's authority and he is unable to transfer his libido to an outside sexual object. With the relationship changed round, the same fate can await the daughter. In this sense the Oedipus complex may justly be regarded as the nucleus of the neuroses.[1]

As you may imagine, Gentlemen, I have passed very cursorily over a great number of considerations of both practical and theoretical importance connected with the Oedipus complex. Nor shall I enter into its variations or its possible reversal.[2] Among its remoter connections I will only give you a further hint that it has turned out to have a highly important effect on literary production. In a valuable work Otto Rank [1912b] has shown that dramatists of every period have chosen their material in the main from the Oedipus and incest complex and its variations and disguises. Nor should it be allowed to pass unnoticed that the two criminal wishes of the Oedipus complex were recognized as the true representatives of the uninhibited life of the instincts long before the time of psycho-analysis. Among the writings of the Encyclopaedist Diderot you will find a celebrated dialogue, *Le neveu de Rameau*, which was rendered

---

[1] [Freud had been using this phrase frequently for several years previously. It appears already in a footnote to Section G of his 'Rat Man' case history (1909d).]

[2] [This last point is most fully dealt with in Chapter III of *The Ego and the Id* (1923b), (Norton, 1960).]

into German by no less a person than Goethe. There you may read this remarkable sentence: 'Si le petit sauvage était aban-donné à lui-même, qu'il conservât toute son imbécillité, et qu'il réunît au peu de raison de l'enfant au berceau la violence des passions de l'homme de trente ans, il tordrait le col à son père et coucherait avec sa mère.'[1]

But there is something else that I cannot pass by. The re-minder of dreams given to us by the mother and wife of Oedipus must not be allowed to remain fruitless. Do you recall the out-come of our dream-analyses—how the wishes that construct dreams are so often of a perverse or incestuous nature or reveal an unsuspected hostility to those who are nearest and dearest to the dreamer? At that time [p. 142] we gave no explanation of the origin of these evil impulses. Now you can find it for yourselves. They are allocations of the libido and object-cathexes[2] which date from early infancy and have long since been abandoned as far as conscious life is concerned, but which prove still to be present at night-time and to be capable of func-tioning in a certain sense. Since, however, everyone, and not only neurotics, experiences these perverse, incestuous and mur-derous dreams, we may conclude that people who are normal to-day have passed along a path of development that has led through the perversions and object-cathexes of the Oedipus complex, that that is the path of normal development and that neurotics merely exhibit to us in a magnified and coarsened form what the analysis of dreams reveals to us in healthy people as well. And this is one of the reasons why I dealt with the study of dreams before that of neurotic symptoms.

[1] ['If the little savage were left to himself, preserving all his foolishness and adding to the small sense of a child in the cradle the violent passions of a man of thirty, he would strangle his father and lie with his mother.' Freud quoted this passage again (in Goethe's German version) in his note on 'The Expert Opinion in the Halsmann Case' (1931d) and again (in French) at the end of Part II of his posthumous Outline of Psycho-Analysis (1940a [1938]), (Norton, 1949).]

[2] [I.e. charges of psychical energy concentrated upon objects. See footnote 2, p. 336 above.]

LECTURE XXII

SOME THOUGHTS ON DEVELOPMENT
AND REGRESSION—AETIOLOGY

LADIES AND GENTLEMEN,—You have heard that the libidinal function goes through a lengthy development before it can, in what is described as the normal manner, be enlisted in the service of reproduction. I should now like to bring to your attention the significance of this fact in the causation of the neuroses.

We are, I think, in agreement with the theories of general pathology in assuming that a development of this kind involves two dangers—first, of *inhibition*, and secondly, of *regression*. That is to say, in view of the general tendency of biological processes to variation, it is bound to be the case that not every preparatory phase will be passed through with equal success and completely superseded: portions of the function will be permanently held back at these early stages, and the total picture of development will be qualified by some amount of developmental inhibition.

Let us look for some analogies to these processes in other fields of knowledge. When, as often happened at early periods of human history, a whole people left their place of domicile and sought a new one, we may be certain that the whole of them did not arrive at the new location. Apart from other losses, it must regularly have happened that small groups or bands of the migrants halted on the way and settled at these stopping-places while the main body went further. Or, as you know, to turn to a nearer comparison, in the highest mammals the male sex-glands, which are originally situated deep in the abdominal cavity, start upon a migration at a particular stage of intra-uterine life, which brings them almost directly under the skin of the pelvic extremity. As a consequence of this migration, we find in a number of male individuals that one of these paired organs has remained behind in the pelvic cavity, or that it has become permanently lodged in what is known as the inguinal canal, through which both organs must pass in the course of their migration, or at least that this canal has remained open,

339

though it should normally close up after the sex-glands have completed their change of situation. Or again, when as a young student I was engaged under von Brücke's direction on my first piece of scientific work, I was concerned with the origin of the posterior nerve-roots in the spinal cord of a small fish of very archaic structure;[1] I found that the nerve-fibres of these roots have their origin in large cells in the posterior horn of the grey matter, which is no longer the case in other vertebrates. But I also discovered soon afterwards that nerve-cells of this kind are present outside the grey matter the whole way to what is known as the spinal ganglion of the posterior root; and from this I inferred that the cells of these masses of ganglia had migrated from the spinal cord along the roots of the nerves. This is also shown by their evolutionary history. But in this small fish the whole path of their migration was demonstrated by the cells that had remained behind.[2]

If you go into the matter more closely, you will have no difficulty in detecting the weak points in these comparisons. I will therefore declare without more ado that I regard it as possible in the case of every particular sexual trend that some portions of it have stayed behind at earlier stages of its development, even though other portions may have reached their final goal. You will recognize here that we are picturing every such trend as a current which has been continuous since the beginning of life but which we have divided up, to some extent artificially, into separate successive advances. Your impression that these ideas stand in need of greater clarification is justified; but to attempt it would take us too far afield. Let me further make it clear that we propose to describe the lagging behind of a part trend at an earlier stage as a *fixation*—a fixation, that is, of the instinct.

The second danger in a development by stages of this sort lies in the fact that the portions which have proceeded further may also easily return retrogressively to one of these earlier stages—what we describe as a *regression*. The trend will find itself led into a regression of this kind if the exercise of its function—

[1] [The larval form of the brook lamprey.]
[2] [This is a summary of the findings of two of Freud's very first papers (1877a and 1878a). Cf. his own earlier abstracts of them (1897b, Nos. II and III).]

that is, the attainment of its aim of satisfaction—is met, in its later or more highly developed form, by powerful external obstacles. It is plausible to suppose that fixation and regression are not independent of each other. The stronger the fixations on its path of development, the more readily will the function evade external difficulties by regressing to the fixations—the more incapable, therefore, does the developed function turn out to be of resisting external obstacles in its course. Consider that, if a people which is in movement has left strong detachments behind at the stopping-places on its migration, it is likely that the more advanced parties will be inclined to retreat to these stopping-places if they have been defeated or have come up against a superior enemy. But they will also be in the greater danger of being defeated the more of their number they have left behind on their migration.

It is important for your understanding of the neuroses that you should not leave this relation between fixation and regression out of sight. This will give you a firmer footing in facing the question of how the neuroses are caused—the question of the aetiology of the neuroses which we shall shortly have to meet.

For the moment we will dwell a little longer on regression. After what you have learnt of the development of the libidinal function, you will be prepared to hear that there are regressions of two sorts: a return to the objects first cathected by the libido, which, as we know, are of an incestuous nature, and a return of the sexual organization as a whole to earlier stages. Both sorts are found in the transference neuroses [p. 299] and play a great part in their mechanism. In particular, a return to the first incestuous objects of the libido is a feature that is found in neurotics with positively fatiguing regularity. There is much more to be said about regressions of the libido itself when we take into account as well another group of neuroses, the narcissistic ones, which for the time being we do not intend to do.[1] These disorders give us access to other developmental processes of the libidinal function which we have not yet mentioned, and show us correspondingly new sorts of regression as well. But above all I think I ought to warn you now not to confuse *regression* with *repression* and help you to form a clear idea

[1] [They are discussed in Lecture XXVI.]

of the relations between the two processes.[1] Repression, as you will recall [p. 294 ff.], is the process by which an act which is admissible to consciousness, one, therefore, which belongs to the system *Pcs.*, is made unconscious—is pushed back, therefore, into the system *Ucs.*[2] And we equally speak of repression if the unconscious mental act is altogether forbidden access to the neighbouring preconscious system and is turned back at the threshold by the censorship. Thus the concept of repression involves no relation to sexuality: I must ask you to take special note of that. It indicates a purely psychological process, which we can characterize still better if we call it a 'topographical' one. By this we intend to say that it is concerned with the psychical regions which we have assumed to exist, or, if we drop this clumsy working hypothesis, with the construction of the mental apparatus out of distinct psychical systems.

The comparison we have proposed has drawn our attention for the first time to the fact that we have not hitherto been using the word 'regression' in its general sense but in a quite special one. If we give it its general sense—of a return from a higher to a lower stage of development—then repression too can be subsumed under the concept of regression, for it too can be described as a return to an earlier and deeper stage in the development of a psychical act. In the case of repression, however, this retrogressive movement does not concern us, since we also speak of repression, in the *dynamic* sense, when a psychical act is held back at the lower, unconscious, stage. The fact is that repression is a topographico-dynamic concept, while regression is a purely descriptive one. What we have hitherto spoken of as regression, however, and have related to fixation, has meant exclusively a return of the libido to earlier stopping-places in its development—something, that is, entirely different in its nature from repression and entirely independent of it. Nor can we call regression of the libido a purely psychical process and we cannot tell where we should localize it in the

---

[1] [The extremely close resemblance of the two words to each other is an added misfortune peculiar to English. In German no such similarity exists between '*Regression*' and '*Verdrängung*'.]

[2] ['*Pcs.*' and '*Ucs.*' are the abbreviations first introduced by Freud in the seventh chapter of *The Interpretation of Dreams* (1900*a*), for the preconscious and unconscious mental systems.]

mental apparatus. And though it is true that it exercises the most powerful influence on mental life, yet the most prominent factor in it is the organic one.

Discussions like this, Gentlemen, are bound to become somewhat arid. So let us turn to clinical material in order to find applications of it that will be a little more impressive. Hysteria and obsessional neurosis are, as you know, the two chief representatives of the group of transference neuroses. Now it is true that in hysteria there is a regression of the libido to the primary incestuous sexual objects and that this occurs quite regularly; but there is as good as no regression to an earlier stage of the sexual organization. To offset this, the chief part in the mechanism of hysteria is played by repression. If I might venture to complete what we already know for certain about this neurosis by making a construction, I might explain the position thus. The unification of the component instincts under the primacy of the genitals has been accomplished; but its results come up against the resistance of the preconscious system which is linked with consciousness. Thus the genital organization holds good for the unconscious, but not in the same way for the preconscious; and this rejection on the part of the preconscious brings about a picture which has certain resemblances to the state of things before genital primacy. But it is nevertheless something quite different.

Of the two kinds of regression of the libido, that to an earlier phase of the sexual organization is by far the more striking. Since this is absent in hysteria, and since our whole view of the neuroses is still far too much under the influence of the study of hysteria, which was chronologically the first, the significance of libidinal regression also became clear to us far later than that of repression. We must be prepared to find that our views will be subjected to still further extensions and revaluations when we are able to take into consideration not only hysteria and obsessional neurosis but also the other, narcissistic neuroses.

In obsessional neurosis, on the contrary, it is the regression of the libido to the preliminary stage of the sadistic-anal organization that is the most striking fact and the one which is decisive for what is manifested in symptoms. The love-impulse is obliged, when this has happened, to disguise itself as a sadistic impulse. The obsessional idea 'I should like to kill you', when it has been freed from certain additions which are not a matter of chance but are indispensable, means at bottom nothing other than 'I should like to enjoy you in love'. If you consider further that there has been a simultaneous regression in regard to the object, so that these impulses apply only to those who are nearest and dearest to the patient, you can form some idea of the horror which these obsessions arouse in him and at the same time of the alien appearance which they present to his conscious perception. But repression, too, plays a great part in the mechanism of these neuroses, though in a cursory introduction like ours this is not easily demonstrated. A regression of the libido without repression would never produce a neurosis but would lead to a perversion. From this you can see that repression is the process which is most peculiar to neuroses and is most characteristic of them. Perhaps I may have an opportunity later of telling you what we know of the mechanism of the perversions, and you will see that in their case too things are not so simple as we should be glad to make them out.[1]

I think, Gentlemen, that you will best come to terms with what you have just been told about fixation and regression of the libido if you will regard it as a preparation for research into the aetiology of the neuroses. Hitherto I have only given you one piece of information about this: namely that people fall ill of a neurosis if they are deprived of the possibility of satisfying their libido—that they fall ill owing to 'frustration', as I put it —and that their symptoms are precisely a substitute for their frustrated satisfaction. [Cf. p. 300.] This is not supposed to mean, of course, that every frustration of a libidinal satisfaction makes the person it affects neurotic, but merely that the factor of frustration could be discerned in every case of neurosis that has been examined. Thus [as logicians would say] the proposition is not convertible. No doubt, too, you will have understood that this assertion does not claim to reveal the whole secret of the aetiology of neuroses but is only bringing into prominence one important and indispensable determinant.

In further pursuing the discussion of this thesis, are we to

[1] [This seems to be one of the points to which, as he remarks at the end of these lectures (p. 463), he had no opportunity of returning.]

consider the nature of the frustration or the peculiar character of those who are affected by it? It is extremely seldom, after all, that frustration is universal and absolute. In order to operate pathogenically it must no doubt affect the mode of satisfaction which alone the subject desires, of which alone he is capable. There are in general very many ways of tolerating deprivation of libidinal satisfaction without falling ill as a result. In the first place, we know people who are able to put up with a deprivation of this kind without being injured: they are not happy, they suffer from longing, but they do not fall ill. Next, we must bear in mind that the sexual instinctual impulses in particular are extraordinarily *plastic*, if I may so express it. One of them can take the place of another, one of them can take over another's intensity; if the satisfaction of one of them is frustrated by reality, the satisfaction of another can afford complete compensation. They are related to one another like a network of intercommunicating channels filled with a liquid;[1] and this is so in spite of their being subject to the primacy of the genitals —a state of affairs that is not at all easily combined in a single picture. Further, the component instincts of sexuality, as well as the sexual current which is compounded from them, exhibit a large capacity for changing their object, for taking another in its place—and one, therefore, that is more easily attainable. This displaceability and readiness to accept a substitute must operate powerfully against the pathogenic effect of a frustration. Among these protective processes against falling ill owing to deprivation there is one which has gained special cultural significance. It consists in the sexual trend abandoning its aim of obtaining a component or a reproductive pleasure and taking on another which is related genetically to the abandoned one but is itself no longer sexual and must be described as social. We call this process 'sublimation', in accordance with the general estimate that places social aims higher than the sexual ones, which are at bottom self-interested. Sublimation is, incidentally, only a special case of the way in which sexual trends are attached to other, non-sexual ones [cf. p. 313]. We shall have to discuss it again in another connection.[2]

You may now have an impression that deprivation has been

---

[1] [Cf. footnote 1 above, p. 310.]

[2] [See the end of the next lecture, p. 376.]

reduced to insignificance owing to all these methods of tolerating it. But no, it retains its pathogenic power. The countermeasures are on the whole insufficient. There is a limit to the amount of unsatisfied libido that human beings on the average can put up with. The plasticity or free mobility of the libido is by no means fully preserved in everyone, and sublimation is never able to deal with more than a certain fraction of libido, quite apart from the fact that many people are gifted with only a small amount of capacity to sublimate. The most important of these limitations is evidently that upon the mobility of the libido, since it makes a person's satisfaction depend on the attainment of only a very small number of aims and objects. You have only to recall that an imperfect development of the libido leaves behind it very fertile and perhaps, too, very numerous libidinal fixations to early phases of the organization and of the finding of objects, which are for the most part incapable of real satisfaction, and you will recognize in libidinal fixation the second powerful factor which combines with frustration as the cause of illness. You can declare, as a schematic abbreviation, that libidinal fixation represents the predisposing, internal factor in the aetiology of the neuroses, while frustration represents the accidental, external one.

I take the opportunity here of warning you against taking sides in a quite unnecessary dispute. In scientific matters people are very fond of selecting one portion of the truth, putting it in the place of the whole and of then disputing the rest, which is no less true, in favour of this one portion. In just this way a number of schools of opinion have already split off from the psycho-analytic movement, some of which recognize the egoistic instincts while disavowing the sexual ones, and others attribute importance to the influence of the real tasks of life while overlooking the individual's past[1]—and others besides. Now here we have a similar occasion for pointing a contrast and starting a controversy. Are neuroses *exogenous* or *endogenous* illnesses? Are they the inevitable result of a particular constitution or the product of certain detrimental (traumatic) experiences in life? More particularly, are they brought about by fixation of the

[1] [The schools of Adler and Jung had been discussed at some length by Freud in Section III of his 'History of the Psycho-Analytic Movement' (1914d), (Norton, 1966).]

libido (and the other features of the sexual constitution) or by the pressure of frustration? This dilemma seems to me no more sensible on the whole than another that I might put to you: does a baby come about through being begotten by its father or conceived by its mother? Both determinants are equally indispensable, as you will justly reply. In the matter of the causation of the neuroses the relation, if not precisely the same, is very similar. As regards their causation, instances of neurotic illness fall into a series within which the two factors—sexual constitution and experience, or, if you prefer it, fixation of the libido and frustration—are represented in such a manner that if there is more of the one there is less of the other. At one end of the series are the extreme cases of which you could say with conviction: these people, in consequence of the singular development of their libido, would have fallen ill in any case, whatever they had experienced and however carefully their lives had been sheltered. At the other end there are the cases, as to which, on the contrary, you would have had to judge that they would certainly have escaped falling ill if their lives had not brought them into this or that situation. In the cases lying within the series a greater or lesser amount of predisposition in the sexual constitution is combined with a lesser or greater amount of detrimental experience in their lives. Their sexual constitution would not have led them into a neurosis if they had not had these experiences, and these experiences would not have had a traumatic effect on them if their libido had been otherwise disposed. In this series I can perhaps allow a certain preponderance in significance to the predisposing factors; but even that admission depends on how far you choose to extend the frontiers of neurotic illness.

I propose, Gentlemen, that we should name a series of this kind a 'complemental series', and I forewarn you that we shall have occasion to construct others of the same kind.[1]

[1] [This seems to be Freud's first use of the actual term 'complemental series'. The concept goes back a long way. It appears in a somewhat different form as an 'aetiological equation' in the second paper on anxiety neurosis (1895*f*), where some discussion of the history of the notion will be found in an Editor's Note. It reappears at two points below (pp. 362 and 364), and turns up again in the *New Introductory Lectures,* p. 590, and in Essay III, Part I (C), of *Moses and Monotheism* (1939*a*).]

The tenacity with which the libido adheres to particular trends and objects—what may be described as the 'adhesiveness' of the libido—makes its appearance as an independent factor, varying from individual to individual, whose determinants are quite unknown to us, but whose significance for the aetiology of the neuroses we shall certainly no longer underestimate.[1] We should not, on the other hand, over-estimate the intimacy of this connection. For a similar 'adhesiveness' of the libido occurs (for unknown reasons) under numerous conditions in normal people, and it is found as a determining factor in people who are in one sense the contrary of neurotics—in perverts. It was known even before the days of psycho-analysis (cf. Binet [1888]) that in the anamnesis of perverts a very early impression of an abnormal instinctual trend or choice of object was quite often found, to which the subject's libido remained attached all through his life. It is often impossible to say what it is that enabled this impression to exercise such an intense attraction on the libido. I will describe a case of this sort which I myself observed.

The subject was a man who is to-day quite indifferent to the genitals and other attractions of women, but who can be plunged into irresistible sexual excitement only by a foot of a particular form wearing a shoe. He can recall an event from his sixth year which was decisive for the fixation of his libido. He was sitting on a stool beside the governess who was to give him lessons in English. The governess, who was an elderly, dried-up, plain-looking spinster, with pale-blue eyes and a snub nose, had something wrong with her foot that day, and on that account kept it, wearing a velvet slipper, stretched out on a cushion. Her leg itself was most decently concealed. A thin, scraggy foot, like the one he had then seen belonging to his governess, thereupon became (after a timid attempt at normal sexual activity at puberty) his only sexual object; and the man was irresistibly attracted if a foot of this kind was associated with other features besides which recalled the type of the English governess. This fixation of his libido, however, made him, not

---

[1] [This factor, under various names, was discussed by Freud at least as early as in the first edition of the *Three Essays* (1905d). A number of references are given in an Editor's footnote to the paper on a case of paranoia (1915f).]

into a neurotic, but into a pervert—what we call a foot-fetishist.[1] You see, then, that although an excessive, and moreover premature, fixation of the libido is indispensable for the causation of neuroses, the area of its effects extends far beyond the field of the neuroses. This determinant, too, is as little decisive in itself as is the frustration which we have already talked about.

Thus the problem of the causation of the neuroses seems to grow more complicated. In fact, psycho-analytic investigation makes us acquainted with a fresh factor, which is not taken into account in our aetiological series and which we can recognize easiest in cases in which what has hitherto been a healthy condition is suddenly disturbed by an onset of neurotic illness. In such people we regularly find indications of a contention between wishful impulses or, as we are in the habit of saying, a psychical conflict. One part of the personality champions certain wishes while another part opposes them and fends them off. Without such a conflict there is no neurosis. There would not seem to be anything peculiar in this. Our mental life is, as you know, perpetually agitated by conflicts which we have to settle. No doubt, therefore, special conditions must be fulfilled if such a conflict is to become pathogenic. We must ask what these conditions are, between what mental powers these pathogenic conflicts are played out, and what the relation is between the conflict and the other causative factors.

I hope to be able to give you adequate replies to these questions, even though the replies may be reduced to schematic dimensions. The conflict is conjured up by frustration, as a result of which the libido, deprived of satisfaction, is driven to look for other objects and paths. The necessary precondition of the conflict is that these other paths and objects arouse displeasure in one part of the personality, so that a veto is imposed which makes the new method of satisfaction impossible as it stands. From this point the construction of symptoms pursues

[1] [Two or three years earlier Freud had read a paper to the Vienna Psycho-Analytical Society on a similar case—possibly, even, the same one. The paper has not yet been published, but is summarized by Ernest Jones in the second volume of his Freud biography (1955, 342–3). An account of Freud's many discussions of fetishism is given in the Editor's Note to the paper bearing that title (1927e).]

its course, which we shall follow later.[1] The repudiated libidinal trends nevertheless succeed in getting their way by certain roundabout paths, though not, it is true, without taking the objection into account by submitting to some distortions and mitigations. The roundabout paths are those taken by the construction of symptoms; the symptoms are the fresh or substitute satisfaction which has become necessary owing to the fact of frustration.

The meaning of psychical conflict can be adequately expressed in another way by saying that for an *external* frustration to become pathogenic an *internal* frustration must be added to it. In that case, of course, the external and internal frustration relate to different paths and objects. The external frustration removes one possibility of satisfaction and the internal frustration seeks to exclude *another* possibility, about which the conflict then breaks out. I prefer this way of representing the matter because it has a secret content. For it hints at the probability that the internal impediments arose from real external obstacles during the prehistoric periods of human development.[2]

But what are the powers from which the objection to the libidinal trend arises? What is the other party to the pathogenic conflict? These powers, to put it quite generally, are the non-sexual instinctual forces. We class them together as the 'ego-instincts'.[3] The psycho-analysis of the transference-neuroses gives us no easy access to a further dissecting of them; at most we come to know them to some extent by the resistances which oppose analysis. The pathogenic conflict is thus one between the ego-instincts and the sexual instincts. In a whole number of cases, it looks as though there might also be a conflict between different purely sexual trends. But in essence that is the same thing; for, of the two sexual trends that are in conflict, one is always, as we might say, 'ego-syntonic',[4] while the other provokes the ego's defence. It therefore still remains a conflict between the ego and sexuality.

[1] [In the following lecture.]

[2] [Cf. p. 371 below. The whole question of frustration as a cause of neurosis was discussed by Freud in a paper on 'Types of Onset of Neurosis' (1912c).]

[3] [An account of Freud's use of this term is given in the Editor's Note to 'Instincts and their Vicissitudes' (1915c).]

[4] ['*Ichgerecht*', i.e. in consonance with the ego.]

Over and over again, Gentlemen, when psycho-analysis has claimed that some mental event is the product of the sexual instincts, it has been angrily pointed out to it by way of defence that human beings do not consist only of sexuality, that there are instincts and interests in mental life other than sexual ones, that it ought not to derive 'everything' from sexuality, and so on. Well, it is most gratifying for once in a way to find ourselves in agreement with our opponents. Psycho-analysis has never forgotten that there are instinctual forces as well which are not sexual. It was based on a sharp distinction between the sexual instincts and the ego-instincts, and, in spite of all objections, it has maintained not that the neuroses are derived from sexuality but that their origin is due to a conflict between the ego and sexuality. Nor has it any conceivable reason for disputing the existence or significance of the ego-instincts while it pursues the part played by the sexual instincts in illness and in ordinary life. It has simply been its fate to begin by concerning itself with the sexual instincts because the transference neuroses made them the most easily accessible to examination and because it was incumbent on it to study what other people had neglected.

Nor is it a fact that psycho-analysis has paid no attention whatever to the non-sexual part of the personality. It is precisely the distinction between the ego and sexuality which has enabled us to recognize with special clarity that the ego-instincts pass through an important process of development— a development which is neither completely independent of the libido nor without a counter-effect upon it. Nevertheless, we are far less well acquainted with the development of the ego than of the libido, since it is only the study of the narcissistic neuroses[1] that promises to give us an insight into the structure of the ego. We already have before us, however, a notable attempt by Ferenczi [1913] to make a theoretical construction of the stages of development of the ego, and there are at least two points at which we have a solid basis for judging that development. It is not our belief that a person's libidinal interests are from the first in opposition to his self-preservative interests; on the contrary, the ego endeavours at every stage to remain in harmony with its sexual organization as it is at the time and to fit itself into it. The succession of the different phases of libidinal

[1] [Discussed in Lecture XXVI.]

development probably follows a prescribed programme. But the possibility cannot be rejected that this course of events can be influenced by the ego, and we may expect equally to find a certain parallelism, a certain correspondence, between the developmental phases of the ego and the libido; indeed a disturbance of that correspondence might provide a pathogenic factor. We are now faced by the important consideration of how the ego behaves if its libido leaves a strong fixation behind at some point in its (the libido's) development. The ego may accept this and consequently become to that extent perverse or, what is the same thing, infantile. It may, however, adopt a non-compliant attitude to the libido's settling down in this position, in which case the ego experiences a *repression* where the libido has experienced a *fixation*.

Thus we discover that the third factor in the aetiology of the neuroses, the *tendency to conflict*, is as much dependent on the development of the ego as on that of the libido. Our insight into the causation of the neuroses is thus made more complete. First there is the most general precondition—frustration; next, fixation of the libido which forces it into particular directions; and thirdly, the tendency to conflict, arising from the development of the ego, which rejects these libidinal impulses. The situation, then, is not so very confused and hard to penetrate as it probably seemed to you during the course of my remarks. It is true, however, that we shall find we have not yet finished with it. There is something new to be added and something already familiar to be further examined.

In order to demonstrate to you the influence which the development of the ego has upon the construction of conflicts and upon the causation of neuroses, I should like to put an example before you—one which, it is true, is a complete invention but which is nowhere divorced from probability. I shall describe it (on the basis of the title of one of Nestroy's farces[1]) as 'In the Basement and on the First Floor'. The caretaker of the house inhabits the basement and its landlord, a

[1] [Johann Nestroy (1801–62), famous in Vienna for his comedies and farces. The literal translation of Nestroy's title would be 'On the Ground Floor and on the First Floor': the difference in the social habits of nineteenth-century Vienna and London calls for the alteration.]

wealthy and respectable gentleman, the first floor. Both have
children, and we may suppose that the landlord's little daughter
is allowed to play, without any supervision, with the proletarian
girl. It might very easily happen, then, that the children's
games would take on a 'naughty'—that is to say, a sexual—
character, that they would play at 'father and mother', that
they would watch each other at their most private business
and excite each other's genitals. The caretaker's girl, though
only five or six years old, would have had an opportunity of
observing a good deal of adult sexuality, and she might well
play the part of seductress in all this. These experiences, even
if they were not continued over a long period, would be enough
to set certain sexual impulses to work in the two children; and,
after their games together had ceased, these impulses would for
several years afterwards find expression in masturbation. So
much for their experiences in common; the final outcome in
the two children will be very different. The caretaker's daughter
will continue her masturbation, perhaps, till her menstrual
periods begin and she will then give it up with no difficulty.
A few years later she will find a lover and perhaps have a baby.
She will take up some occupation or other, possibly become a
popular figure on the stage and end up as an aristocrat. Her
career is more likely to be less brilliant, but in any case she will
go through her life undamaged by the early exercise of her
sexuality and free from neurosis. With the landlord's little girl
things will be different. At an early stage and while she is still
a child she will get an idea that she has done something wrong;
after a short time, but perhaps only after a severe struggle,
she will give up her masturbatory satisfaction, but she will
nevertheless still have some sense of oppression about her. When
in her later girlhood she is in a position to learn something of
human sexual intercourse, she will turn away from it with
unexplained disgust and prefer to remain in ignorance. And
now she will probably be subject to a fresh emergence of an
irresistible pressure to masturbate of which she will not dare to
complain. During the years in which she should exercise a
feminine attraction upon some man, a neurosis breaks out in
her which cheats her of marriage and her hopes in life. If after
this an analysis succeeds in gaining an insight into her neurosis,
it will turn out that the well-brought-up, intelligent and

high-minded girl has completely repressed her sexual impulses, but that these, unconscious to her, are still attached to her petty experiences with her childhood friend.

The difference between the lives of these two, in spite of their having had the same experience, rests on the fact that the ego of one of them underwent a development with which the other never met. Sexual activity seemed to the caretaker's daughter just as natural and harmless in later life as it had in childhood. The landlord's daughter came under the influence of education and accepted its demands. From the suggestions offered to it, her ego constructed ideals of feminine purity and abstinence which are incompatible with sexual activity; her intellectual education reduced her interest in the feminine part which she was destined to play. Owing to this higher moral and intellectual development of her ego she came into conflict with the demands of her sexuality.

I will dwell for a little to-day on yet another point in ego-development, partly because I have some remoter aims in view, but also because what follows is precisely calculated to justify the sharp separation between the ego-instincts and the sexual instincts which we favour but which is not self-evident. In forming our judgement of the two courses of development—both of the ego and of the libido—we must lay emphasis on a consideration which has not often hitherto been taken into account. For both of them are at bottom heritages, abbreviated recapitulations of the development which all mankind has passed through from its primaeval days over long periods of time. In the case of the development of the libido, this *phylogenetic* origin is, I venture to think, immediately obvious. Consider how in one class of animals the genital apparatus is brought into the closest relation to the mouth, while in another it cannot be distinguished from the excretory apparatus, and in yet others it is linked to the motor organs—all of which you will find attractively set out in W. Bölsche's valuable book [1911–13]. Among animals one can find, so to speak in petrified form, every species of perversion of the sexual organization. In the case of human beings, however, this phylogenetic point of view is partly veiled by the fact that what is at bottom inherited is nevertheless freshly acquired in the development of the individual,[1] probably because the same conditions which originally necessitated its acquisition persist and continue to operate upon each individual. I should like to add that originally the operation of these conditions was creative but that it is now evocative. Besides this, there is no doubt that the prescribed course of development can be disturbed and altered in each individual by recent external influences. But we know the power which forced a development of this kind upon humanity and maintains its pressure in the same direction to-day. It is, once again, frustration by reality, or, if we are to give it its true, grand name, the pressure of vital needs—Necessity ('Ανάγκη [Ananke]). She has been a strict educator and has made much out of us. The neurotics are among those of her children to whom her strictness has brought evil results; but that is a risk with all education. This appreciation of the necessities of life need not, incidentally, weigh against the importance of 'internal developmental trends', if such can be shown to be present.

Now it is a very noteworthy fact that the sexual instincts and the self-preservative instincts do not behave in the same way towards real necessity.[2] The self-preservative instincts, and everything to do with them, are much easier to educate: they learn early to comply with necessity and to arrange their developments in accordance with the instructions of reality. This is intelligible, since they could not obtain the objects they need in any other way; and without those objects the individual would inevitably perish. The sexual instincts are harder to educate, for at first they have no need of an object. Since they are attached like parasites, as it were, to the other bodily functions, and find their satisfaction auto-erotically on the subject's own body, they are to begin with withdrawn from the educative influence of real necessity, and they retain this characteristic of being self-willed and inaccessible to influence (what we

[1] [This is an echo of a couplet from Goethe's *Faust,* which was a favourite quotation of Freud's. See, for instance, *Totem and Taboo* (1912–13), (Norton, 1952), p. 158, and the closing sentences of his unfinished *Outline of Psycho-Analysis* (1940a [1938]), (Norton, 1949).]

[2] ['*Reale Not*', i.e. the exigencies imposed by reality. For what follows, cf. paragraph (3) of 'Formulations on the Two Principles of Mental Functioning' (1911b).]

describe as being 'unreasonable') in most people in some respect all through their lives. Moreover, as a rule the educability of a youthful individual is at an end when his sexual needs arise in their full strength. Educators are aware of this and act accordingly; but the findings of psycho-analysis may perhaps also induce them to shift the main impact of education on to the earliest years of childhood, from infancy onwards. The little creature is often completed by the fourth or fifth year of life, and after that merely brings gradually to light what is already within him.

In order to appreciate the full significance of the difference which I have pointed out between the two groups of instincts, we shall have to go back a long way and introduce one of those considerations which deserve to be described as *economic* [p. 275 above]. This leads us to one of the most important, but unluckily also one of the most obscure, regions of psychoanalysis. We may ask whether in the operation of our mental apparatus a main purpose can be detected, and we may reply as a first approximation that that purpose is directed to obtaining pleasure. It seems as though our total mental activity is directed towards achieving pleasure and avoiding unpleasure —that it is automatically regulated by the *pleasure principle*.[1] We should of all things like to know, then, what determines the generation of pleasure and unpleasure; but that is just what we are ignorant of. We can only venture to say this much: that pleasure is *in some way* connected with the diminution, reduction or extinction of the amounts of stimulus prevailing in the mental apparatus, and that similarly unpleasure is connected with their increase. An examination of the most intense pleasure which is accessible to human beings, the pleasure of accomplishing the sexual act, leaves little doubt on this point. Since in such processes related to pleasure it is a question of what happens to *quantities* of mental excitation or energy, we call considerations of this kind economic. It will be noticed that we can describe the tasks and achievements of the mental apparatus in another and more general way than by stressing the acquisition of pleasure. We can say that the mental apparatus serves the purpose of mastering and disposing of the amounts of stimulus and sums of excitation that impinge on it from outside and

[1] [See the next footnote.]

inside.[1] It is immediately obvious that the sexual instincts, from beginning to end of their development, work towards obtaining pleasure; they retain their original function unaltered. The other instincts, the ego-instincts, have the same aim to start with. But under the influence of the instructress Necessity, they soon learn to replace the pleasure principle by a modification of it. For them the task of avoiding unpleasure turns out to be almost as important as that of obtaining pleasure. The ego discovers that it is inevitable for it to renounce immediate satisfaction, to postpone the obtaining of pleasure, to put up with a little unpleasure and to abandon certain sources of pleasure altogether. An ego thus educated has become 'reasonable'; it no longer lets itself be governed by the pleasure principle, but obeys the *reality principle*,[2] which also at bottom seeks to obtain pleasure, but pleasure which is assured through taking account of reality, even though it is pleasure postponed and diminished.

The transition from the pleasure principle to the reality principle is one of the most important steps forward in the ego's development. We know already that it is only late and unwillingly that the sexual instincts join in this piece of development, and we shall hear later the consequences for human beings of the fact that their sexuality is content with such a loose connection with external reality. And now in conclusion one last remark on this subject. If man's ego has its process of development like the libido, you will not be surprised to hear that there are also 'regressions of the ego', and you will be anxious to know too what part may be played in neurotic illnesses by this return of the ego to earlier phases of its development.[3]

[1] [This is sometimes referred to as the 'principle of constancy'. It, and the related 'pleasure principle', are discussed in an Editor's Appendix to Freud's first paper on the neuro-psychoses of defence (1894a). See also the footnote on p. 375 below.]

[2] [The term appears first in 'Formulations on the Two Principles of Mental Functioning' (1911b), the Editor's Note to which traces the origin of the concept.]

[3] [Some account of the development of Freud's views on regression and of his various uses of the term will be found in an Editor's note at the end of Part I of the 'Project' of 1895.]

LECTURE XXIII

THE PATHS TO THE FORMATION OF SYMPTOMS

LADIES AND GENTLEMEN,—For laymen the symptoms constitute the essence of a disease and its cure consists in the removal of the symptoms. Physicians attach importance to distinguishing the symptoms from the disease and declare that getting rid of the symptoms does not amount to curing the disease. But the only tangible thing left of the disease after the symptoms have been got rid of is the capacity to form new symptoms. For that reason we will for the moment adopt the layman's position and assume that to unravel the symptoms means the same thing as to understand the disease.

Symptoms—and of course we are dealing now with psychical (or psychogenic) symptoms and psychical illness—are acts detrimental, or at least useless, to the subject's life as a whole, often complained of by him as unwelcome and bringing unpleasure or suffering to him. The main damage they do resides in the mental expenditure which they themselves involve and in the further expenditure that becomes necessary for fighting against them. Where there is an extensive formation of symptoms, these two sorts of expenditure can result in an extraordinary impoverishment of the subject in regard to the mental energy available to him and so in paralysing him for all the important tasks of life. Since this outcome depends mainly on the *quantity* of the energy which is thus absorbed, you will easily see that 'being ill' is in its essence a practical concept. But if you take up a theoretical point of view and disregard this matter of quantity, you may quite well say that we are *all* ill—that is, neurotic—since the preconditions for the formation of symptoms can also be observed in normal people.

We already know that neurotic symptoms are the outcome of a conflict which arises over a new method of satisfying the libido [p. 349]. The two forces which have fallen out meet once again in the symptom and are reconciled, as it were, by the compromise of the symptom that has been constructed. It is for that reason, too, that the symptom is so resistant: it is supported from both sides. We also know that one of the two partners to the conflict is the unsatisfied libido which has been repulsed by reality and must now seek for other paths to its satisfaction. If reality remains relentless even though the libido is ready to take another object in place of the one that has been refused to it, then it will finally be compelled to take the path of regression and strive to find satisfaction either in one of the organizations which it has already outgrown or from one of the objects which it has earlier abandoned. The libido is lured into the path of regression by the fixation which it has left behind it at these points in its development.

The path to perversion branches off sharply from that to neurosis. If these regressions rouse no objection from the ego, no neurosis will come about either; and the libido will arrive at some real, even though no longer normal, satisfaction. But if the ego, which has under its control not only consciousness but also the approaches to motor innervation and accordingly to the realization of mental desires, does not agree with these regressions, conflict will follow. The libido is, as it were, cut off and must try to escape in some direction where, in accordance with the requirements of the pleasure principle, it can find a discharge for its cathexis of energy. It must withdraw from the ego. An escape of this kind is offered it by the fixations on the path of its development which it has now entered on regressively—fixations from which the ego had protected itself in the past by repressions. By cathecting these repressed positions as it flows backward, the libido has withdrawn from the ego and its laws, and has at the same time renounced all the education it has acquired under the ego's influence. It was docile so long as satisfaction beckoned to it; but under the double pressure of external and internal frustration it becomes refractory, and recalls earlier and better times. Such is the libido's fundamentally unchangeable character. The ideas to which it now transfers its energy as a cathexis belong to the system of the unconscious and are subject to the processes which are possible there, particularly to condensation and displacement. In this way conditions are established which completely resemble those in dream-construction. The dream proper, which has been completed in the unconscious and is the fulfilment of an unconscious wishful phantasy, is brought up against a portion of (pre)conscious activity which exercises the office of censorship and which, when it has been indemnified, permits the formation of the manifest dream as a compromise. In the same way, what represents[1] the libido in the unconscious has to reckon with the power of the preconscious ego. The opposition which had been raised against it in the ego pursues it as an 'anticathexis'[2] and compels it to choose a form of expression which can at the same time become an expression of the opposition itself. Thus the symptom emerges as a many-times-distorted derivative of the unconscious libidinal wish-fulfilment, an ingeniously chosen piece of ambiguity with two meanings in complete mutual contradiction. In this last respect, however, there is a distinction between the construction of a dream and of a symptom. For in dream-formation the preconscious purpose is merely concerned to preserve sleep, to allow nothing that would disturb it to make its way into consciousness; it does not insist upon calling out sharply 'No! on the contrary!' to the unconscious wishful impulse. It can afford to be more tolerant because the situation of someone sleeping is less perilous. The state of sleep in itself bars any outlet into reality.

You see, then, that the libido's escape under conditions of conflict is made possible by the presence of fixations. The regressive cathexis of these fixations leads to the circumvention of the repression and to a discharge (or satisfaction) of the libido, subject to the conditions of a compromise being observed. By the roundabout path *viâ* the unconscious and the old fixations, the libido finally succeeds in forcing its way through to real satisfaction—though to one which is extremely restricted and scarcely recognizable as such. Let me add two comments to this conclusion. First, I should like you to notice how closely here the libido and the unconscious on one side and the ego, consciousness and reality on the other are shown to be inter-

[1] ['*Vertretung*', i.e. the representative in psychical terms of the libido regarded as something somatic. A fuller discussion of this notion will be found in the Editor's Note to 'Instincts and their Vicissitudes' (1915c).]

[2] [That is, a force acting in a sense contrary to the primary instinctual energy. See Section IV of 'The Unconscious' (1915e).]

linked, although to begin with they did not belong together at all. And secondly, I must ask you to bear in mind that everything I have said about this and what is still to follow relates only to the formation of symptoms in the neurosis of hysteria.

Where, then, does the libido find the fixations which it requires in order to break through the repressions? In the activities and experiences of infantile sexuality, in the abandoned component trends, in the objects of childhood which have been given up. It is to them, accordingly, that the libido returns. The significance of this period of childhood is twofold: on the one hand, during it the instinctual trends which the child has inherited with his innate disposition first become manifest, and secondly, others of his instincts are for the first time awakened and made active by external impressions and accidental experiences. There is no doubt, I think, that we are justified in making this twofold division. The manifestation of the innate disposition is indeed not open to any critical doubts, but analytic experience actually compels us to assume that purely chance experiences in childhood are able to leave fixations of the libido behind them. Nor do I see any theoretical difficulty in this. Constitutional dispositions are also undoubtedly after-effects of experiences by ancestors in the past; they too were once acquired. Without such acquisition there would be no heredity. And is it conceivable that acquisition such as this, leading to inheritance, would come to an end precisely with the generation we are considering? The significance of infantile experiences should not be totally neglected, as people like doing, in comparison with the experiences of the subject's ancestors and of his own maturity; on the contrary, they call for particular consideration. They are all the more momentous because they occur in times of incomplete development and are for that very reason liable to have traumatic effects. The studies on developmental mechanics by Roux[1] and others have shown that the prick of a needle into an embryonic germinal layer in the act of cell-division results in a severe disturbance of development. The same injury inflicted on a larval or fully grown animal would do no damage.

---

[1] [Wilhelm Roux (1850–1924) was one of the founders of experimental embryology.]

Thus fixation of the libido in the adult, which we introduced into the aetiological equation of neurosis as representing the constitutional factor [p. 346], now falls, for our purposes, into two further parts: the inherited constitution and the disposition acquired in early childhood. As we all know, a diagram is certain of a sympathetic reception from students. So I will summarize the position diagrammatically:[1]

Causation of Neurosis = Disposition due + Accidental [Adult]
                         to Fixation of   Experience
                         Libido   (Traumatic)

Sexual Constitution   Infantile Experience
(Prehistoric Experience)

The hereditary sexual constitution presents us with a great variety of dispositions, according as one component instinct or another, alone or in combination with others, is inherited in particular strength. The sexual constitution forms once again, together with the factor of infantile experience, a 'complemental series' exactly similar to the one we first came to know between disposition and the accidental experience of the adult [p. 347]. In both of them we find the same extreme cases and the same relations between the two factors concerned. And here the question suggests itself of whether the most striking kinds of libidinal regressions—those to earlier stages of the sexual organization—may not be predominantly determined by the hereditary constitutional factor. But it is best to postpone answering this question till we have been able to take a wider range of forms of neurotic illness into account.

Let us dwell now on the fact that analytic research shows the libido of neurotics tied to their infantile sexual experiences. It

---

[1] [Readers may find this diagram easier to follow in the form of a genealogical tree:

Sexual Constitution   + Infantile Experience
(Prehistoric Experience)

                 Disposition due to + Accidental [Adult]
                 Fixation of Libido   Experience (Traumatic)

                          [Neurosis]

thus lends these the appearance of an enormous importance for the life and illness of human beings. They retain this importance undiminished so far as the work of therapeutics is concerned. But if we turn away from that task we can nevertheless easily see that there is a danger here of a misunderstanding which might mislead us into basing our view of life too one-sidedly on the neurotic situation. We must after all subtract from the importance of infantile experiences the fact that the libido has returned to them *regressively*, after being driven out of its later positions. In that case the contrary conclusion becomes very tempting—that these libidinal experiences had no importance at all at the time they occurred but only acquired it regressively. You will recall that we have already considered a similar alternative in our discussion of the Oedipus complex [p. 336].

Once again we shall not find it hard to reach a decision. The assertion that the libidinal cathexis (and therefore the pathogenic significance) of the infantile experiences has been largely intensified by the regression of the libido is undoubtedly correct, but it would lead to error if we were to regard it alone as decisive. Other considerations must be allowed weight as well.

In the first place observation shows, in a manner that excludes all doubt, that the infantile experiences have an importance of their own and give evidence of it already in childhood. Children too have their neuroses, in which the factor of displacement backwards in time is necessarily very much reduced or is even completely absent, since the onset of the illness follows the traumatic experiences immediately. The study of these infantile neuroses protects us from more than one dangerous misunderstanding of the neuroses of adults, just as the dreams of children gave us the key to an understanding of adult dreams.[1] Children's neuroses are very common, much commoner than is supposed. They are often overlooked, regarded as signs of a bad or naughty child, often, too, kept under by the nursery authorities; but they can always be easily recognized in retrospect. They usually appear in the form of *anxiety*

---

[1] [See Lecture VIII. Freud was no doubt thinking here of his analysis of the 'Wolf Man', which he had already completed though it was not yet published: 'From the History of an Infantile Neurosis' (1918*b*).]

hysteria. We shall learn on a later occasion what that means [p. 400 below]. If a neurosis breaks out in later life, analysis regularly reveals it as a direct continuation of the infantile illness which may have emerged as no more than a veiled hint. As I have said, however, there are cases in which these signs of neurosis in childhood proceed uninterruptedly into a lifelong illness. We have been able to analyse a few examples of these children's neuroses in childhood itself—when they were actually present;[1] but far more often we have had to be content with someone who has fallen ill in adult life enabling us to obtain a deferred insight into his childhood neurosis. In such cases we must not fail to make certain corrections and take certain precautions.

In the second place, we must reflect that it would be inconceivable for the libido to regress so regularly to the period of childhood unless there were something there to exercise an attraction on it. The fixation which we have supposed to be present at particular points in the course of development can only have a meaning if we regard it as consisting in the retention of a certain quota of libidinal energy. And finally I may point out to you that between the intensity and pathogenic importance of infantile and of later experiences a complemental relationship exists similar to the series we have already discussed. There are cases in which the whole weight of causation falls on the sexual experiences of childhood, cases in which those impressions exert a definitely traumatic effect and call for no other support than can be afforded them by an average sexual constitution and the fact of its incomplete development. Alongside of these cases there are others in which the whole accent lies on the later conflicts and the emphasis we find in the analysis laid on the impressions of childhood appears entirely as the work of regression. Thus we have extremes of 'developmental inhibition' and 'regression' and between them every degree of co-operation between the two factors.

These facts have a certain interest from the point of view of education, which plans the prevention of neuroses by intervening at an early stage in children's sexual development. So long as one focuses attention principally on infantile sexual experiences, one must suppose that one has done everything for the

---

[1] [Cf. the case history of 'Little Hans' (1909*b*).]

prophylaxis of nervous illnesses by taking care that the child's development is delayed and that it is spared experiences of the sort. We already know, however, that the preconditions for the causation of neuroses are complex and cannot be influenced in general if we take account of only a single factor. Strict protection of the young loses value because it is powerless against the constitutional factor. Besides, it is more difficult to carry out than educationists imagine and it brings with it two fresh dangers which must not be underestimated: the fact that it may achieve too much—that it may encourage an excess of sexual repression, with damaging results, and the fact that it may send the child out into life without any defence against the onrush of sexual demands that is to be looked for at puberty.[1] Thus it remains extremely doubtful how far prophylaxis in childhood can be carried with advantage and whether an altered attitude to the immediate situation may not offer a better angle of approach for the prevention of neuroses.

Let us now go back to the symptoms. They create a substitute, then, for the frustrated satisfaction by means of a regression of the libido to earlier times, with which a return to earlier stages of object-choice or of the organization is inseparably bound up. We discovered some time ago that neurotics are anchored somewhere in their past;[2] we know now that it is at a period of their past in which their libido did not lack satisfaction, in which they were happy. They search about in the history of their life till they find a period of that sort, even if they have to go back as far as the time when they were infants in arms—as they remember it or as they imagine it from later hints. In some way the symptom repeats this early infantile kind of satisfaction, distorted by the censorship arising from the conflict, turned as a rule to a feeling of suffering, and mingled with elements from the precipitating cause of the illness. The kind of satisfaction which the symptom brings has much that is strange about it.

We may disregard the fact that it is unrecognizable to the subject, who, on the contrary, feels the alleged satisfaction as

[1] [Freud elaborated this difficulty in Lecture XXXIV of the *New Introductory Lectures,* p. 613.]

[2] [See for instance the beginning of Lecture XVIII, p. 273 above.]

suffering and complains of it. This transformation is a function of the psychical conflict under pressure of which the symptom had to be formed. What was once a satisfaction to the subject is, indeed, bound to arouse his resistance or his disgust to-day. We are familiar with a trivial but instructive model of this change of mind. The same child who once eagerly sucked the milk from his mother's breast is likely a few years later to display a strong dislike to drinking milk, which his upbringing has difficulties in overcoming. This dislike increases to disgust if a skin forms on the milk or the drink containing it. We cannot exclude the possibility, perhaps, that the skin conjures up a memory of the mother's breast, once so ardently desired. Between the two situations, however, there lies the experience of weaning, with its traumatic effects.

It is something else besides that makes symptoms seem strange to us and incomprehensible as a means of libidinal satisfaction. They do not remind us in the very least of anything from which we are in the habit of normally expecting satisfaction. Usually they disregard objects and in so doing abandon their relation to external reality. We can see that this is a consequence of turning away from the reality principle and of returning to the pleasure principle. But it is also a return to a kind of extended auto-erotism, of the sort that offered the sexual instinct its first satisfactions. In place of a change in the external world these substitute a change in the subject's own body: they set an internal act in place of an external one, an adaptation in place of an action—once again, something that corresponds, phylogenetically, to a highly significant regression. We shall only understand this in connection with something new that we have still to learn from the analytic researches into the formation of symptoms. We must further remember that the same processes belonging to the unconscious play a part in the formation of symptoms as in the formation of dreams— namely, condensation and displacement. A symptom, like a dream, represents something as fulfilled: a satisfaction in the infantile manner. But by means of extreme condensation that satisfaction can be compressed into a single sensation or inner- vation, and by means of extreme displacement it can be restric- ted to one small detail of the entire libidinal complex. It is not to be wondered at if we, too, often have difficulty in recognizing

in a symptom the libidinal satisfaction whose presence we suspect and which is invariably confirmed.

I have warned you that we still have something new to learn;
it is indeed something surprising and perplexing. By means of
analysis, as you know, starting from the symptoms, we arrive
at a knowledge of the infantile experiences to which the libido
is fixated and out of which the symptoms are made. Well, the
surprise lies in the fact that these scenes from infancy are not
always true. Indeed, they are not true in the majority of cases,
and in a few of them they are the direct opposite of the historical truth. As you will see, this discovery is calculated more
than any other to discredit either analysis, which has led to this
result, or the patients, on whose statements the analysis and our
whole understanding of the neuroses are founded. But there is
something else remarkably perplexing about it. If the infantile
experiences brought to light by analysis were invariably real,
we should feel that we were standing on firm ground; if they
were regularly falsified and revealed as inventions, as phantasies of the patient, we should be obliged to abandon this
shaky ground and look for salvation elsewhere. But neither of
these things is the case: the position can be shown to be that the
childhood experiences constructed or remembered in analysis
are sometimes indisputably false and sometimes equally certainly correct, and in most cases compounded of truth and
falsehood. Sometimes, then, symptoms represent events which
really took place and to which we may attribute an influence on
the fixation of the libido, and sometimes they represent phantasies of the patient's which are not, of course, suited to playing
an aetiological role. It is difficult to find one's way about in
this. We can make a first start, perhaps, with a similar discovery—namely, that the isolated childhood memories that
people have possessed consciously from time immemorial and
before there was any such thing as analysis [p. 200 above] may
equally be falsified or at least may combine truth and falsehood
in plenty. In their case there is seldom any difficulty in showing
their incorrectness; so we at least have the reassurance of knowing that the responsibility for this unexpected disappointment
lies, not with analysis, but in some way with the patients.
After a little reflection we shall easily understand what it is

about this state of things that perplexes us so much. It is the low valuation of reality, the neglect of the distinction between it and phantasy. We are tempted to feel offended at the patient's having taken up our time with invented stories. Reality seems to us something worlds apart from invention, and we set a very different value on it. Moreover the patient, too, looks at things in this light in his normal thinking. When he brings up the material which leads from behind his symptoms to the wishful situations modelled on his infantile experiences, we are in doubt to begin with whether we are dealing with reality or phantasies. Later, we are enabled by certain indications to come to a decision and we are faced by the task of conveying it to the patient. This, however, invariably gives rise to difficulties. If we begin by telling him straight away that he is now engaged in bringing to light the phantasies with which he has disguised the history of his childhood (just as every nation disguises its forgotten prehistory by constructing legends), we observe that his interest in pursuing the subject further suddenly diminishes in an undesirable fashion. He too wants to experience realities and despises everything that is merely 'imaginary'. If, however, we leave him, till this piece of work is finished, in the belief that we are occupied in investigating the real events of his childhood, we run the risk of his later on accusing us of being mistaken and laughing at us for our apparent credulity. It will be a long time before he can take in our proposal that we should equate phantasy and reality and not bother to begin with whether the childhood experiences under examination are the one or the other. Yet this is clearly the only correct attitude to adopt towards these mental productions. They too possess a reality of a sort. It remains a fact that the patient has created these phantasies for himself, and this fact is of scarcely less importance for his neurosis than if he had really experienced what the phantasies contain. The phantasies possess *psychical* as contrasted with *material* reality, and we gradually learn to understand that *in the world of the neuroses it is psychical reality which is the decisive kind.*

Among the occurrences which recur again and again in the youthful history of neurotics—which are scarcely ever absent —there are a few of particular importance, which also deserve on that account, I think, to be brought into greater prominence than the rest. As specimens of this class I will enumerate these: observation of parental intercourse, seduction by an adult and threat of being castrated. It would be a mistake to suppose that they are never characterized by material reality; on the contrary, this is often established incontestably through enquiries from older members of the patient's family. It is by no means a rare thing, for instance, for a little boy, who is beginning to play with his penis in a naughty way and is not yet aware that one must conceal such activities, to be threatened by a parent or nurse with having his penis or his sinful hand cut off. Parents will often admit this when they are asked, since they think they have done something useful in making such a threat; a number of people have a correct conscious memory of such a threat, especially if it was made at a somewhat later period. If the threat is delivered by the mother or some other female she usually shifts its performance on to the father—or the doctor. In *Struwwelpeter*, the famous work of the Frankfurt paediatrician Hoffmann (which owes its popularity precisely to an understanding of the sexual and other complexes of childhood), you will find castration softened into a cutting-off of the thumbs as a punishment for obstinate sucking. But it is highly improbable that children are threatened with castration as often as it appears in the analyses of neurotics. We shall be satisfied by realizing that the child puts a threat of this kind together in his imagination on the basis of hints, helped out by a knowledge that auto-erotic satisfaction is forbidden and under the impression of his discovery of the female genitals. [Cf. p. 317 above.] Nor is it only in proletarian families that it is perfectly possible for a child, while he is not yet credited with possessing an understanding or a memory, to be a witness of the sexual act between his parents or other grown-up people; and the possibility cannot be rejected that he will be able to understand and react to the impression *in retrospect*. If, however, the intercourse is described with the most minute details, which would be difficult to observe, or if, as happens most frequently, it turns out to have been intercourse from behind, *more ferarum* [in the manner of animals], there can be no remaining doubt that the phantasy is based on an observation of intercourse between animals (such as dogs) and that its motive was the child's unsatisfied scopophilia during puberty. The extreme achievement on these lines is a phantasy of observing parental intercourse while one is still an unborn baby in the womb. Phantasies of being seduced are of particular interest, because so often they are not phantasies but real memories. Fortunately, however, they are nevertheless not real as often as seemed at first to be shown by the findings of analysis. Seduction by an older child or by one of the same age is even more frequent than by an adult; and if in the case of girls who produce such an event in the story of their childhood their father figures fairly regularly as the seducer, there can be no doubt either of the imaginary nature of the accusation or of the motive that has led to it.[1] A phantasy of being seduced when no seduction has occurred is usually employed by a child to screen the auto-erotic period of his sexual activity. He spares himself shame about masturbation by retrospectively phantasying a desired object into these earliest times. You must not suppose, however, that sexual abuse of a child by its nearest male relatives belongs entirely to the realm of phantasy. Most analysts will have treated cases in which such events were real and could be unimpeachably established; but even so they related to the later years of childhood and had been transposed into earlier times.

The only impression we gain is that these events of childhood are somehow demanded as a necessity, that they are among the essential elements of a neurosis. If they have occurred in reality, so much to the good; but if they have been withheld by reality, they are put together from hints and supplemented by phantasy. The outcome is the same, and up to the present we have not succeeded in pointing to any difference in the consequences, whether phantasy or reality has had the greater share in these events of childhood. Here we simply have once again one of the complemental relations that I have so often mentioned; moreover it is the strangest of all we have met with. Whence comes the need for these phantasies and the material for them? There can be no doubt that their sources lie in the instincts; but it has still to be explained why the same phantasies with the same content are created on every occasion. I am prepared with an

[1] [Cf. a later reference to this, with a further explanation, in Section III of Freud's paper on 'Female Sexuality' (1931b). A full history of Freud's views on this subject is given in an Editor's footnote to the New Introductory Lectures, pp. 584–5.]

answer which I know will seem daring to you. I believe these *primal phantasies*, as I should like to call them, and no doubt a few others as well, are a phylogenetic endowment. In them the individual reaches beyond his own experience into primaeval experience at points where his own experience has been too rudimentary. It seems to me quite possible that all the things that are told to us to-day in analysis as phantasy—the seduction of children, the inflaming of sexual excitement by observing parental intercourse, the threat of castration (or rather castration itself)—were once real occurrences in the primaeval times of the human family, and that children in their phantasies are simply filling in the gaps in individual truth with prehistoric truth. I have repeatedly been led to suspect that the psychology of the neuroses has stored up in it more of the antiquities of human development than any other source.[1]

The things I have just been discussing, Gentlemen, compel me to enter more closely into the origin and significance of the mental activity which is described as 'phantasy' [or 'imagination'].[2] As you are aware, it enjoys a universally high reputation, without its position in mental life having become clear. I have the following remarks to make about it. The human ego is, as you know, slowly educated by the pressure of external necessity to appreciate reality and obey the reality principle; in the course of this process it is obliged to renounce, temporarily or permanently, a variety of the objects and aims at which its striving for pleasure, and not only for sexual pleasure, is directed. But men have always found it hard to renounce pleasure; they cannot bring themselves to do it without some kind of compensation. They have therefore retained a mental

[1] [This discussion of 'primal phantasies' and the possibility of their being inherited was based to a considerable extent on Freud's findings in his 'Wolf Man' case history (1918*b*), which he had completed two or three years earlier. When he came to publish it (in the year following that in which this lecture was delivered), he added two long passages to his original draft, referring back to the present discussion. Cf. Chapters V and VIII of *An Infantile Neurosis.*]

[2] [Freud's main earlier discussions of phantasy will be found in 'Creative Writers and Day-Dreaming' (1908*e*) and 'Hysterical Phantasies and their Relation to Bisexuality' (1908*a*).]

activity in which all these abandoned sources of pleasure and methods of achieving pleasure are granted a further existence —a form of existence in which they are left free from the claims of reality and of what we call 'reality-testing'.[1] Every desire takes before long the form of picturing its own fulfilment; there is no doubt that dwelling upon imaginary wish-fulfilments brings satisfaction with it, although it does not interfere with a knowledge that what is concerned is not real. Thus in the activity of phantasy human beings continue to enjoy the freedom from external compulsion which they have long since renounced in reality. They have contrived to alternate between remaining an animal of pleasure and being once more a creature of reason. Indeed, they cannot subsist on the scanty satisfaction which they can extort from reality. 'We cannot do without auxiliary constructions', as Theodor Fontane once said.[2] The creation of the mental realm of phantasy finds a perfect parallel in the establishment of 'reservations' or 'nature reserves' in places where the requirements of agriculture, communications and industry threaten to bring about changes in the original face of the earth which will quickly make it unrecognizable. A nature reserve preserves its original state which everywhere else has to our regret been sacrificed to necessity. Everything, including what is useless and even what is noxious, can grow and proliferate there as it pleases. The mental realm of phantasy is just such a reservation withdrawn from the reality principle.

The best-known productions of phantasy are the so-called 'day-dreams', which we have already come across [p. 98], imagined satisfactions of ambitious, megalomanic, erotic wishes, which flourish all the more exuberantly the more reality counsels modesty and restraint. The essence of the happiness of phantasy—making the obtaining of pleasure free once more from the assent of reality—is shown in them unmistakably. We know that such day-dreams are the nucleus and prototype of

[1] [I.e. the process of judging whether things are real or not. The deeper implications of this are discussed in Freud's metapsychological paper on dreams (1917d); for full references see the Editor's Note to that paper.]

[2] [Freud quoted this again in a similar connection in Chapter II of *Civilization and its Discontents* (1930a), (Norton, 1962).]

night-dreams. A night-dream is at bottom nothing other than a day-dream that has been made utilizable owing to the liberation of the instinctual impulses at night, and that has been distorted by the form assumed by mental activity at night. We have already become familiar with the idea that even a day-dream is not necessarily conscious—that there are unconscious day-dreams, as well [p. 368]. Such unconscious day-dreams are thus the source not only of night-dreams but also of neurotic symptoms.[1]

The importance of the part played by phantasy in the formation of symptoms will be made clear to you by what I have to tell you. I have explained [p. 359] how in the case of frustration the libido cathects regressively the positions which it has given up but to which some quotas of it have remained adhering. I shall not withdraw this or correct it, but I have to insert a connecting link. How does the libido find its way to these points of fixation? All the objects and trends which the libido has given up have not yet been given up in every sense. They or their derivatives are still retained with a certain intensity in phantasies. Thus the libido need only withdraw on to phantasies in order to find the path open to every repressed fixation. These phantasies have enjoyed a certain amount of toleration: they have not come into conflict with the ego, however sharp the contrasts between them may have been, so long as a particular condition is observed. This condition is of a *quantitative* nature and it is now upset by the backward flow of libido on to the phantasies. As a result of this surplus, the energic cathexis of the phantasies is so much increased that they begin to raise claims, that they develop a pressure in the direction of becoming realized. But this makes a conflict between them and the ego inevitable. Whether they were previously preconscious or conscious, they are now subjected to repression from the direction of the ego and are at the mercy of attraction from the direction of the unconscious. From what are now unconscious phantasies the libido travels back to their origins in the unconscious—to its own points of fixation.

The libido's retreat to phantasy is an intermediate stage on the path to the formation of symptoms and it seems to call for a

[1] [Cf. a long footnote added by Freud in 1920 to the third of his *Three Essays* (1905d).]

special name. C. G. Jung coined the very appropriate one of 'introversion', but then most inexpediently gave it another meaning as well.[1] We will continue to take it that introversion denotes the turning away of the libido from the possibilities of real satisfaction and the hypercathexis[2] of phantasies which have hitherto been tolerated as innocent. An introvert is not yet a neurotic, but he is in an unstable situation: he is sure to develop symptoms at the next shift of forces, unless he finds some other outlets for his dammed-up libido. The unreal character of neurotic satisfaction and the neglect of the distinction between phantasy and reality are on the other hand already determined by the fact of lingering at the stage of introversion.

You will no doubt have observed that in these last discussions I have introduced a fresh factor into the structure of the aetiological chain—namely the quantity, the magnitude, of the energies concerned. We have still to take this factor into account everywhere. A purely qualitative analysis of the aetiological determinants is not enough. Or, to put it another way, a merely *dynamic* view of these mental processes is insufficient; an *economic* line of approach is also needed. We must tell ourselves that the conflict between two trends does not break out till certain intensities of cathexis have been reached, even though the determinants for it have long been present so far as their subject-matter is concerned. In the same way, the pathogenic significance of the constitutional factors must be weighed according to how much *more* of one component instinct than of another is present in the inherited disposition. It may even be

[1] [This had been discussed by Freud earlier, in a footnote to his paper on 'The Dynamics of Transference' (1912*b*), in which he stated that Jung seemed to be applying the term 'introversion' exclusively to dementia praecox. In that footnote further references are given.]

[2] [I.e. charging with an extra amount of psychical energy. Freud generally used the term in this sense: e.g. in 'The Unconscious' (1915*e*), *Beyond the Pleasure Principle* (1920*g*), and 'Humour' (1927*d*). On the other hand he sometimes applied it more specially to the distinction between unconscious and preconscious ideas: once more in Chapter VI of 'The Unconscious', and in Chapter IV of the *Outline* (1940*a* [1938]), (Norton, 1949). Cf. also Part III, Section 1, of the 'Project' of 1895 (Freud, 1950*a*).]

supposed that the disposition of all human beings is qualitatively alike and that they differ only owing to these quantitative conditions. The quantitative factor is no less decisive as regards capacity to resist neurotic illness. It is a matter of *what quota* of unemployed libido a person is able to hold in suspension and of *how large a fraction* of his libido he is able to divert from sexual to sublimated aims. The ultimate aim of mental activity, which may be described qualitatively as an endeavour to obtain pleasure and avoid unpleasure, emerges, looked at from the economic point of view, as the task of mastering the amounts of excitation (mass of stimuli) operating in the mental apparatus and of keeping down their accumulation which creates unpleasure.[1]

This, then, is what I wanted to tell you about the formation of symptoms in the neuroses. But I must not fail to lay emphasis expressly once again on the fact that everything I have said here applies only to the formation of symptoms in hysteria. Even in obsessional neurosis there is much—apart from fundamentals, which remain unaltered—that will be found different. The anticathexes opposing the demands of the instincts (which we have already spoken of in the case of hysteria as well [p. 360]) become prominent in obsessional neurosis and dominate the clinical picture in the form of what are known as 'reaction-formations'. We discover similar and even more far-reaching divergences in the other neuroses, where our researches into the mechanisms of symptom-formation are not yet concluded at any point.

Before I let you go to-day, however, I should like to direct your attention a little longer to a side of the life of phantasy which deserves the most general interest. For there is a path that leads back from phantasy to reality—the path, that is, of

---

[1] [Here Freud appears to be equating the 'pleasure principle' and 'the principle of constancy', though in the earlier passage above (p. 356*f*.), where this subject is touched on, there is a hint at a doubt about this. At a later date he drew a clear distinction between the two: (see Freud), *The Economic Problem of Masochism* (1924*c*). A full discussion of the development of Freud's views on these principles is given in an Editor's footnote to 'Instincts and their Vicissitudes' (1915*c*).]

art. An artist is once more in rudiments an introvert, not far removed from neurosis. He is oppressed by excessively powerful instinctual needs. He desires to win honour, power, wealth, fame and the love of women; but he lacks the means for achieving these satisfactions. Consequently, like any other unsatisfied man, he turns away from reality and transfers all his interest, and his libido too, to the wishful constructions of his life of phantasy, whence the path might lead to neurosis. There must be, no doubt, a convergence of all kinds of things if this is not to be the complete outcome of his development; it is well known, indeed, how often artists in particular suffer from a partial inhibition of their efficiency owing to neurosis. Their constitution probably includes a strong capacity for sublimation and a certain degree of laxity in the repressions which are decisive for a conflict. An artist, however, finds a path back to reality in the following manner. To be sure, he is not the only one who leads a life of phantasy. Access to the half-way region of phantasy is permitted by the universal assent of mankind, and everyone suffering from privation expects to derive alleviation and consolation from it. But for those who are not artists the yield of pleasure to be derived from the sources of phantasy is very limited. The ruthlessness of their repressions forces them to be content with such meagre day-dreams as are allowed to become conscious. A man who is a true artist has more at his disposal. In the first place, he understands how to work over his day-dreams in such a way as to make them lose what is too personal about them and repels strangers, and to make it possible for others to share in the enjoyment of them. He understands, too, how to tone them down so that they do not easily betray their origin from proscribed sources. Furthermore, he possesses the mysterious power of shaping some particular material until it has become a faithful image of his phantasy; and he knows, moreover, how to link so large a yield of pleasure to this representation of his unconscious phantasy that, for the time being at least, repressions are outweighed and lifted by it. If he is able to accomplish all this, he makes it possible for other people once more to derive consolation and alleviation from their own sources of pleasure in their unconscious which have become inaccessible to them; he earns their gratitude and admiration and he has thus achieved *through* his phantasy what originally he had achieved only *in* his phantasy—honour, power and the love of women.[1]

[1] [Cf. 'Creative Writers and Day-Dreaming' (1908*e*), the fifth of Freud's *Five Lectures* (1910*a*), 'Two Principles of Mental Functioning' (1911*b*), and Section II (F) of his contribution to *Scientia* (1913*j*).]

LECTURE XXIV

THE COMMON NEUROTIC STATE

LADIES AND GENTLEMEN,—Now that we have disposed of such a difficult piece of work in our last discussions, I propose for a time to leave the subject and turn to you yourselves.

For I am aware that you are dissatisfied. You pictured an 'Introduction to Psycho-Analysis' [1] very differently. What you expected to hear were lively examples, not theory. On one occasion, you say, when I told you the parable of 'In the Basement and on the First Floor' [p. 352], you grasped something of the way in which neuroses are caused; the observations should have been real ones, however, and not made-up stories. Or when at the start I described two symptoms to you (not invented ones this time, let us hope) and described their solution and their relation to the patients' lives [p. 261], the 'sense' of symptoms dawned on you. You hoped I should go on along those lines. But instead I gave you long-winded theories, hard to grasp, which were never complete but were always having something fresh added to them; I worked with concepts which I had not yet explained to you; I went from a descriptive account of things to a dynamic one and from that to what I called an 'economic' one; I made it hard for you to understand how many of the technical terms I used meant the same thing and were merely being interchanged for reasons of euphony; I brought up such far-reaching conceptions as those of the pleasure and reality principles and of phylogenetically inherited endowments; and, far from introducing you to anything, I paraded something before your eyes which constantly grew more and more remote from you.

Why did I not begin my introduction to the theory of neuroses with what you yourselves know of the neurotic state and what has long aroused your interest—with the peculiar characteristics of neurotic people, their incomprehensible reactions to human intercourse and external influences, their irritability, their incalculable and inexpedient behaviour? Why

[1] [See p. 9 above.]
378

did I not lead you step by step from an understanding of the simpler, everyday forms of the neurotic state to the problems of its enigmatic, extreme manifestations?

Indeed, Gentlemen, I cannot even disagree with you. I am not so enamoured of my skill in exposition that I can declare each of its artistic faults to be a peculiar charm. I think myself that it might have been more to your advantage if I had proceeded otherwise; and that was, indeed, my intention. But one cannot always carry out one's reasonable intentions. There is often something in the material itself which takes charge of one and diverts one from one's first intentions. Even such a trivial achievement as the arrangement of a familiar piece of material is not entirely subject to an author's own choice; it takes what line it likes and all one can do is to ask oneself after the event why it has happened in this way and no other.

One reason is probably that the title 'Introduction to Psycho-Analysis' is no longer applicable to the present section, which is supposed to deal with the neuroses. An introduction to psycho-analysis is provided by the study of parapraxes and dreams; the theory of the neuroses is psycho-analysis itself. It would not, I believe, have been possible to give you a knowledge of the subject-matter of the theory of the neuroses in so short a time except in this concentrated form. It was a question of presenting you with a connected account of the sense and significance of symptoms and of the external and internal determinants and mechanism of their formation. That is what I have tried to do; it is more or less the nucleus of what psycho-analysis has to teach to-day. It involved saying a great deal about the libido and its development and a little, too, about that of the ego. Our introduction had already prepared you in advance for the premises of our technique and for the major considerations of the unconscious and of repression (of resistance). You will discover from one of the next lectures [Lecture XXVI] the points from which the work of psycho-analysis makes its further organic advance. For the time being I have made no secret of the fact that everything I have said is derived from the study of a single group of nervous disorders— what are termed the 'transference neuroses'. Indeed, I have traced the mechanism of symptom-formation in the case only of the hysterical neurosis. Even if you have acquired no thorough knowledge and have not retained every detail, yet I hope that you have formed some picture of the methods by which psycho-analysis works, of the problems which it attacks and of the results at which it has arrived.

I have credited you with a wish that I might have started my description of the neuroses from the behaviour of neurotic people, from an account of the manner in which they suffer under their neurosis, of how they defend themselves against it and how they come to terms with it. No doubt that is an interesting topic, worth investigating; nor would it be very difficult to handle. But it would be of debatable wisdom to start with it. There would be a risk of not discovering the unconscious and at the same time of overlooking the great importance of the libido and of judging everything as it appears to the ego of the neurotic subject. It is obvious that this ego is not a trustworthy or impartial agency. The ego is indeed the power which disavows the unconscious and has degraded it into being repressed; so how can we trust it to be fair to the unconscious? The most prominent elements in what is thus repressed are the repudiated demands of sexuality, and it is quite self-evident that we should never be able to guess their extent and importance from the ego's conceptions. From the moment the notion of repression dawns on us, we are warned against making one of the two contesting parties (and the victorious one, at that) into being judge in the dispute. We are prepared to find that the ego's assertions will lead us astray. If we are to believe the ego, it was active at every point and itself willed and created its symptoms. But we know that it puts up with a good amount of passivity, which it afterwards tries to disguise and gloss over. It is true that it does not always venture on such an attempt; in the symptoms of obsessional neurosis it is obliged to admit that there is something alien which is confronting it and against which it can only defend itself with difficulty.

Anyone whom these warnings do not deter from taking the ego's counterfeits as sterling coin will have an easy time of it and will avoid all the resistances which oppose the psycho-analytic emphasis upon the unconscious, sexuality and the passivity of the ego. He will be able to declare like Alfred Adler that the 'neurotic character'[1] is the cause of neuroses instead of their consequence; but neither will he be in a position to explain a single detail of symptom-formation or a single dream.

You will ask whether it may not be possible, however, to do justice to the part played by the ego in neurotic states and in the formation of symptoms without at the same time grossly neglecting the factors revealed by psycho-analysis. My reply is that that must certainly be possible and will sooner or later be done; but the road followed by the work of psycho-analysis does not admit of actually *beginning* with this. It is of course possible to foresee when psycho-analysis will be confronted by this task. There are neuroses in which the ego plays a far more intensive part than in those we have studied hitherto; we call them the 'narcissistic' neuroses. The investigation of these disorders will enable us to form an impartial and trustworthy judgement of the share taken by the ego in the onset of neuroses.[2]

One of the ways in which the ego is related to its neuroses is, however, so obvious that it was possible to take it into account from the first. It seems never to be absent; but it is most clearly recognizable in a disorder which we are even to-day far from understanding—*traumatic neurosis*. For you must know that the same factors always come into operation in the causation and mechanism of every possible form of neurosis; but the chief importance in the construction of the symptoms falls now upon one and now upon another of these factors. The position is like that among the members of a theatrical company. Each of them is regularly cast for his own stock role—hero, confidant, villain, and so on; but each of them will choose a different piece for his benefit performance. In the same way phantasies which turn into symptoms are nowhere more obvious than in hysteria; the anticathexes or reaction-formations of the ego dominate the picture in obsessional neurosis; what in the case of dreams we have termed 'secondary revision' [p. 182] stands in the fore-front in paranoia in the shape of delusions, and so on.

[1] [*Über den nervösen Charakter* (1912) was the title of one of Adler's earlier works. The title of its English translation is *The Neurotic Constitution*.]

[2] [Freud deals further with this in Lecture XXVI below.]

Thus in traumatic neuroses, and particularly in those brought about by the horrors of war, we are unmistakably presented with a self-interested motive on the part of the ego, seeking for protection and advantage—a motive which cannot, perhaps, create the illness by itself but which assents to it and maintains it when once it has come about. This motive tries to preserve the ego from the dangers the threat of which was the precipitating cause of the illness and it will not allow recovery to occur until a repetition of these dangers seems no longer possible or until compensation has been received for the danger that has been endured.[1]

The ego takes a similar interest, however, in the development and maintenance of the neurosis in every other case. I have already shown [p. 359] that symptoms are supported by the ego, too, because they have a side with which they offer satisfaction to the repressing purpose of the ego. Moreover, settling the conflict by constructing a symptom is the most convenient way out and the one most agreeable to the pleasure principle: it unquestionably spares the ego a large amount of internal work which is felt as distressing. Indeed there are cases in which even the physician must admit that for a conflict to end in neurosis is the most harmless and socially tolerable solution. You must not be surprised to hear that even the physician may occasionally take the side of the illness he is combating. It is not his business to restrict himself in every situation in life to being a fanatic in favour of health. He knows that there is not only neurotic misery in the world but real, irremovable suffering as well, that necessity may even require a person to sacrifice his health; and he learns that a sacrifice of this kind made by a single person can prevent immeasurable unhappiness for many others. If we may say, then, that whenever a neurotic is faced by a conflict he takes flight into illness,[2] yet we must allow that in some cases that flight is fully justified, and a physician who has recognized how the situation lies will silently and solicitously withdraw.

[1] [Cf. Freud's studies on the war neuroses (1919d and 1955c [1920]).]

[2] [This phrase appeared first in Freud's paper on hysterical attacks (1909a), where some further references will be found.]

But let us disregard these exceptional cases and proceed with our discussion. In average circumstances we recognize that by escaping into a neurosis the ego obtains a certain internal 'gain from illness'. In some circumstances of life this is further accompanied by an appreciable *external* advantage bearing a greater or less real value. Consider the commonest example of this sort. A woman who is roughly treated and ruthlessly exploited by her husband will fairly regularly find a way out in neurosis, if her constitution makes it possible, if she is too cowardly or too moral to console herself secretly with another man, if she is not strong enough to separate from her husband in the face of every external deterrent, if she has no prospect of supporting herself or obtaining a better husband and if in addition she is still attached to this brutal husband by her sexual feelings. Her illness now becomes a weapon in her battle with her dominating husband —a weapon which she can use for her defence and misuse for her revenge. To complain of her illness is allowable, though to lament her marriage was probably not. She finds a helper in her doctor, she forces her usually inconsiderate husband to look after her, to spend money on her, to allow her at times to be away from home and so free from her married oppression. When an external or accidental gain from illness like this is really considerable and no real substitute for it is available, you must not reckon very high the chances of influencing the neurosis by your treatment.

You will now protest that what I have told you about the gain from illness argues entirely in favour of the view I have rejected—that the ego itself wills and creates the neurosis [p. 380]. Not too fast, Gentlemen! It may perhaps mean nothing more than that the ego puts up with the neurosis, which it cannot, after all, prevent, and that it makes the best of it, if anything can be made of it at all. That is only one side of the business, the pleasant side, it is true. So far as the neurosis has advantages the ego no doubt accepts it; but it does not only have advantages. As a rule it soon turns out that the ego has made a bad bargain by letting itself in for the neurosis. It has paid too dearly for an alleviation of the conflict, and the sufferings attached to the symptoms are perhaps an equivalent substitute for the torments of the conflict, but they probably involve an increase in unpleasure. The ego would like to free itself from this unpleasure of the symptoms without giving up the gain from illness, and this is just what it cannot achieve. This shows, then, that it was not so entirely active as it thought it was; and we shall bear this well in mind.

In your contact as doctors with neurotics, Gentlemen, you will soon give up expecting that the ones who raise the most lamentations and complaints about their illness will be the most eager to co-operate and will offer you the least resistance. It is rather the opposite. But of course you will easily realize that everything that contributes to the gain from illness will intensify the resistance due to repression and will increase the therapeutic difficulties. But to the portion of gain from illness which is, so to say, born with the illness we have to add another portion which arises later. When a psychical organization like an illness has lasted for some time, it behaves eventually like an independent organism; it manifests something like a self-preservative instinct; it establishes a kind of *modus vivendi* between itself and other parts of the mind, even with those which are at bottom hostile to it; and there can scarcely fail to be occasions when it proves once again useful and expedient and acquires, as it were, a *secondary function* which strengthens its stability afresh. Instead of an example from pathology, let us take a glaring instance from daily life. A capable working-man, who earns his living, is crippled by an accident in the course of his occupation. The injured man can no longer work, but eventually he obtains a small disablement pension, and he learns how to exploit his mutilation by begging. His new, though worsened, means of livelihood is based precisely on the very thing that deprived him of his former means of livelihood. If you could put an end to his injury you would make him, to begin with, without means of subsistence; the question would arise of whether he was still capable of taking up his earlier work again. What corresponds in the case of neuroses to a secondary exploitation like this of an illness may be described as the *secondary* gain from illness in contrast to the primary one.[1]

[1] [The distinction between the two different kinds of gain from illness had been indicated by Freud in a letter to Fliess of November 18, 1897 (Freud, 1950a, Letter 76), though it was first made explicit in the paper (1909a) quoted in the last footnote. The question had already been discussed at some length in the 'Dora'

In general, however, I should like to recommend that, while not under-estimating the *practical* importance of the gain from illness, you should not let yourselves be impressed by it theoretically. After all, apart from the exceptions I recognized earlier [p. 382], it always calls to mind the examples of 'animal intelligence' illustrated by Oberländer in *Fliegende Blätter*.[1] An Arab was riding his camel along a narrow path cut in the steep face of a mountain. At a turn in the path he suddenly found himself face to face with a lion, which prepared to make a spring. He saw no way out: on one side a perpendicular cliff and on the other a precipice; retreat and flight were impossible. He gave himself up for lost. But the animal thought otherwise. He took one leap with his rider into the abyss—and the lion was left in the lurch. The help provided by a neurosis has as a rule no better success with the patient. This may be because dealing with a conflict by forming symptoms is after all an automatic process which cannot prove adequate to meeting the demands of life, and in which the subject has abandoned the use of his best and highest powers. If there were a choice, it would be preferable to go down in an honourable struggle with fate.

But I still owe you further enlightenment, Gentlemen, on my reasons for not starting my account of the theory of the neuroses with the common neurotic state. You may perhaps suppose that it was because in that case I should have had greater difficulty in proving the sexual causation of the neuroses. But you would be wrong there. In the case of the transference neuroses one must work one's way through the interpretation of symptoms before one can arrive at that discovery. In the common forms of what are known as the 'actual neuroses' [2] the aetiological significance of sexual life is a crude fact that springs to the

case history (1905*e*), where the instances of the crippled beggar and of the ill-treated wife appear again. But the analysis there was later considered incorrect by Freud, who added a long footnote in 1923, which gives perhaps the clearest account of the matter.]

[1] [See footnote 2, p. 28.]

[2] ['*Aktualneurosen*'. '*Aktual*', like the French '*actuel*', has the sense of 'contemporary', 'of the present moment'. The epithet is applied to this group of neuroses because their causes are purely contemporary and do not, as in the case of the psychoneuroses, have their origin in the patient's past life. 'Actual neuroses' is the accepted translation.]

observer's eyes. I came upon it more than twenty years ago when one day I asked myself the question of why in the examination of neurotics their sexual activities were so regularly excluded from consideration. At that time I sacrificed my popularity with my patients for the sake of these enquiries; but after only a brief effort I was able to declare that 'if the *vita sexualis* is normal, there can be no neurosis'—and by this I meant no 'actual neurosis'.[1] No doubt this statement passes too lightly over people's individual differences; it suffers, too, from the indefiniteness inseparable from the judgement of what is 'normal'. But as a rough guide it retains its value to this day. I had by then reached the point of establishing specific relations between particular forms of neurosis and particular sexual noxae; and I have no doubt that I could repeat the same observations to-day if similar pathological material were still at my disposal. I found often enough that a man who indulged in a certain kind of incomplete sexual satisfaction (for instance, manual masturbation) had fallen ill of a particular form of 'actual neurosis', and that this neurosis promptly gave place to another if he replaced this sexual *régime* by another equally far from being irreproachable. I was then in a position to infer the change in a patient's sexual mode of life from an alteration in his condition.[2] I also learnt then to stand obstinately by my suspicions till I had overcome the patients' disingenuousness and compelled them to confirm my views. It is true that thereafter they preferred to go to other doctors who did not make such keen enquiries about their sexual life.

Even at that time I could not fail to notice that the causation of the illness did not always point to sexual life. One person, it was true, fell ill directly from a sexual noxa; but another did so because he had lost his fortune or had been through an exhausting organic illness. The explanation of these varieties came later, when we gained an insight into the suspected interrela-

[1] [This is quoted from a paper on sexuality in the aetiology of the neuroses contributed by Freud to a volume of Löwenfeld's (Freud, 1906a). But he had reached the conclusion more than ten years earlier, and expressed it in almost the same words, in his two papers on anxiety neurosis (1895b and f), where a large part of what follows is already to be found.]

[2] [Cf. an example of this in 'Sexuality in the Aetiology of the Neuroses' (1898a).]

tions between the ego and the libido, and the explanation became the more satisfactory the deeper that insight extended. A
person only falls ill of a neurosis if his ego has lost the capacity to
allocate his libido in some way. The stronger is his ego, the
easier will it be for it to carry out that task. Any weakening
of his ego from whatever cause must have the same effect as an
excessive increase in the claims of the libido and will thus make
it possible for him to fall ill of a neurosis. There are other and
more intimate relations between the ego and the libido;[1] but
these have not yet come within our scope, so I will not bring
them up as part of my present explanation. What remains essential and makes things clear to us is that, in every case and no
matter how the illness is set going, the symptoms of the neurosis
are sustained by the libido and are consequently evidence that
it is being employed abnormally.

Now, however, I must draw your attention to the decisive
difference between the symptoms of the 'actual' neuroses and
those of the psychoneuroses, the first group of which, the transference neuroses, have occupied us so much hitherto. In both
cases the symptoms originate from the libido, and are thus
abnormal employments of it, substitutive satisfactions. But the
symptoms of the 'actual' neuroses—intracranial pressure, sensations of pain, a state of irritation in an organ, weakening or
inhibition of a function—have no 'sense', no psychical meaning.
They are not only manifested predominantly in the body (as
are hysterical symptoms, for instance, as well), but they are also
themselves entirely somatic processes, in the generating of
which all the complicated mental mechanisms we have come
to know are absent. Thus they really are what psychoneurotic
symptoms were so long believed to be. But if so, how can they
correspond to employments of the libido, which we have recognized as a force operating in the *mind*? Well, Gentlemen, that
is a very simple matter. Let me remind you of one of the very
first objections that were brought up against psycho-analysis.
It was said then that it was occupied in finding a purely psychological theory of neurotic phenomena and this was quite hopeless, since psychological theories could never explain an illness.
People had chosen to forget that the sexual function is not a

---

[1] [No doubt an allusion to the subject of narcissism, which is discussed
in Lecture XXVI.]

purely psychical thing any more than it is a purely somatic one. It influences bodily and mental life alike. If in the symptoms of the psychoneuroses we have become acquainted with manifestations of disturbances in the *psychical* operation of the sexual function, we shall not be surprised to find in the 'actual' neuroses the direct *somatic* consequences of sexual disturbances.

Clinical medicine has given us a valuable pointer towards an interpretation of these disturbances, and one that has been taken into account by various enquirers. The 'actual' neuroses, in the details of their symptoms and also in their characteristic of influencing every organic system and every function, exhibit an unmistakable resemblance to the pathological states which arise from the chronic influence of external toxic substances and from a sudden withdrawal of them—to intoxications and conditions of abstinence. The two groups of disorders are brought together still more closely by intermediate conditions such as Grave's disease which we have learnt to recognize as equally due to the operation of toxic substances, but of toxins which are not introduced into the body from outside but originate in the subject's own metabolism. In view of these analogies, we cannot, I think, avoid regarding the neuroses as results of disturbances in the sexual metabolism, whether because more of these sexual toxins is produced than the subject can deal with, or whether because internal and even psychical conditions restrict the proper employment of these substances. The popular mind has from time immemorial paid homage to hypotheses of this kind on the nature of sexual desire, speaking of love as an 'intoxication' and believing that falling in love is brought about by love-philtres—though here the operative agent is to some extent externalized. And for us this would be an occasion for recalling the erotogenic zones and our assertion that sexual excitation can be generated in the most various organs [p. 324]. But for the rest the phrase 'sexual metabolism' or 'chemistry of sexuality' is a term without content; we know nothing about it and cannot even decide whether we are to assume two sexual substances, which would then be named 'male' and 'female',[1] or whether we could be satisfied with *one* sexual toxin which we should have to recognize as the vehicle of all the stimulant

[1] [Elsewhere, e.g. in the *New Introductory Lectures*, p. 595, Freud strongly rejects such a notion.]

effects of the libido. The theoretical structure of psycho-analysis that we have created is in truth a superstructure, which will one day have to be set upon its organic foundation. But we are still ignorant of this.

What characterizes psycho-analysis as a science is not the material which it handles but the technique with which it works. It can be applied to the history of civilization, to the science of religion and to mythology, no less than to the theory of the neuroses, without doing violence to its essential nature. What it aims at and achieves is nothing other than the uncovering of what is unconscious in mental life. The problems of the 'actual' neuroses, whose symptoms are probably generated by direct toxic damage, offer psycho-analysis no points of attack. It can do little towards throwing light on them and must leave the task to biologico-medical research.

And now perhaps you understand better why I did not choose to arrange my material differently. If I had promised you an 'Introduction to the Theory of the Neuroses' the correct path would certainly have led from the simple forms of the 'actual' neuroses to the more complicated psychical illnesses due to disturbance of the libido. As regards the former I should have had to collect from various sources what we have learnt or believe we know, and in connection with the psychoneuroses psycho-analysis would have come up for discussion as the most important technical aid in throwing light on those conditions. But what I intended to give and what I announced was an 'Introduction to Psycho-Analysis'. It was more important for me that you should gain an idea of psycho-analysis than that you should obtain some pieces of knowledge about the neuroses; and for that reason the 'actual' neuroses, unproductive so far as psycho-analysis is concerned, could no longer have a place in the foreground. I believe, too, that I have made the better choice for you. For, on account of the profundity of its hypotheses and the comprehensiveness of its connections, psycho-analysis deserves a place in the interest of every educated person, while the theory of the neuroses is a chapter in medicine like any other.

Nevertheless you will rightly expect that we should devote some interest to the 'actual' neuroses as well. Their intimate clinical connection with the psychoneuroses would alone compel us to do so. I may inform you, then, that we distinguish three pure forms of 'actual' neuroses: neurasthenia, anxiety neurosis and hypochondria.[1] Even this assertion is not uncontradicted. All the names are in use, it is true, but their content is indefinite and fluctuating. There are even doctors who oppose any dividing lines in the chaotic world of neurotic phenomena, any segregation of clinical entities or individual diseases, and who do not even recognize the distinction between the 'actual' neuroses and the psychoneuroses. I think they are going too far and have not chosen the path which leads to progress. The forms of neurosis which I have mentioned occur occasionally in their pure form; more often, however, they are intermixed with each other and with a psychoneurotic disorder. This need not lead us to abandon the distinction between them. Consider the difference between the study of minerals and of rocks in mineralogy. The minerals are described as individuals, no doubt on the basis of the fact that they often occur as crystals, sharply separated from their environment. Rocks consist of aggregations of minerals, which, we may be sure, have not come together by chance but as a result of what determined their origin. In the theory of the neuroses we still know too little of the course of their development to produce anything resembling petrology. But we are certainly doing the right thing if we start by isolating from the mass the individual clinical entities which we recognize and which are comparable to the minerals.

A noteworthy relation between the symptoms of the 'actual' neuroses and of the psychoneuroses makes a further important contribution to our knowledge of the formation of symptoms in the latter. For a symptom of an 'actual' neurosis is often the nucleus and first stage of a psychoneurotic symptom. A relation of this kind can be most clearly observed between neurasthenia and the transference neurosis known as 'conversion hysteria', between anxiety neurosis and anxiety hysteria, but also between hypochondria and the forms of disorder which will be mentioned later [p. 423 ff.] under the name of paraphrenia (dementia praecox and paranoia). Let us take as an example a

[1] [A discussion of hypochondria as a third 'actual' neurosis appears in Section II of Freud's paper on 'Narcissism' (1914c).]

case of hysterical headache or lumbar pain. Analysis shows us that, by condensation and displacement, it has become a substitutive satisfaction for a whole number of libidinal phantasies or memories. But this pain was also at one time a real one and it was then a direct sexual-toxic symptom, the somatic expression of a libidinal excitation. We are far from asserting that *all* hysterical symptoms contain a nucleus of this kind. But it remains a fact that this is especially often the case and that whatever somatic influences (whether normal or pathological) are brought about by libidinal excitation are preferred for the construction of hysterical symptoms. In such cases they play the part of the grain of sand which a mollusc coats with layers of mother-of-pearl. In the same way, the passing indications of sexual excitement which accompany the sexual act are employed by the psychoneurosis as the most convenient and appropriate material for the construction of symptoms.

A similar course of events affords peculiar diagnostic and therapeutic interest. It not at all infrequently happens in the case of a person who is disposed to a neurosis without actually suffering from a manifest one, that a pathological somatic change (through inflammation or injury perhaps) sets the activity of symptom-formation going; so that this activity hastily turns the symptom which has been presented to it by reality into the representative of all the unconscious phantasies which have only been lying in wait to seize hold of some means of expression. In such a case the physician will adopt sometimes one and sometimes another line of treatment. He will either endeavour to remove the organic basis, without bothering about its noisy neurotic elaboration; or he will attack the neurosis which has taken this favourable opportunity for arising and will pay little attention to its organic precipitating cause. The outcome will prove the one or the other line of approach right or wrong; it is impossible to make general recommendations to meet such mixed cases.[1]

[1] [It will be clear from what Freud says in this lecture that the aetiology of the 'actual' neuroses and the distinction between them and the psychoneuroses were established by him at a very early date. The term appears first in a paper on 'Sexuality in the Aetiology of the Neuroses' (1898a), though the notion goes back at least to 1895. A full list of references is given in an Editor's footnote to the paper on ' "Wild" Psycho-Analysis' (1910k).]

LECTURE XXV

ANXIETY[1]

LADIES AND GENTLEMEN,—What I said to you in my last lecture about the general[2] neurotic state will no doubt have struck you as the most incomplete and inadequate of all my pronouncements. I know that is true, and nothing will have surprised you more, I expect, than that there was nothing in it about anxiety,[3] of which most neurotics complain, which they themselves describe as their worst suffering and which does in fact attain enormous intensity in them and may result in their adopting the craziest measures. But there at least I had no intention of giving you short measure. On the contrary, it was my intention to attack the problem of anxiety in neurotics particularly keenly and to discuss it at length with you.

I have no need to introduce anxiety itself to you. Every one of us has experienced that sensation, or, to speak more correctly,

[1] [The problem of anxiety occupied Freud's mind throughout his life, and his views on it went through a number of changes. His first major discussion of it was in his two early papers on anxiety neurosis (1895b and f); his last major discussion of it was in *Inhibitions, Symptoms and Anxiety* (1926d). In an Editor's Introduction to the latter, some account will be found of the development of his views. It should be borne in mind that what he says in the present lecture was subjected later to some important—in one case, fundamental—revisions; these changes were summarized by him in Addendum A to *Inhibitions, Symptoms and Anxiety*. At a still later date, in Lecture XXXII of his *New Introductory Lectures*, p. 545 ff., he restated his final position in a particularly clear form. It must be remembered, however, that, as Freud himself indicates in his Preface (pp. 9–10), the present lecture was his most complete treatment of the subject at the time of its delivery.]

[2] ['*Allgemeine*' in the original. Throughout the last lecture Freud had used the word '*gemeine*' (common).]

[3] ['*Angst*'. Some remarks on the English rendering of this word will be found in an Editor's Appendix to Freud's first paper on anxiety neurosis. Though 'anxiety', in a sense quite different from the colloquial one, is the technical translation, we often find it necessary to render it by such words as 'fear', being 'frightened' or 'afraid', and so on.]

392

that affective state, at one time or other on our own account. But I think the question has never been seriously enough raised of why neurotics in particular suffer from anxiety so much more and so much more strongly than other people. Perhaps it has been regarded as something self-evident: the words '*nervös*' and '*ängstlich*'[1] are commonly used interchangeably, as though they meant the same thing. But we have no right to do so: there are '*ängstlich*' people who are otherwise not at all '*nervös*' and, moreover, '*nervös*' people who suffer from many symptoms, among which a tendency to '*Angst*' is not included.

However that may be, there is no question that the problem of anxiety is a nodal point at which the most various and important questions converge, a riddle whose solution would be bound to throw a flood of light on our whole mental existence. I will not assert that I can give you this complete solution; but you will certainly expect psycho-analysis to approach this subject too in quite a different way from academic medicine. Interest there seems mainly to be centred on tracing the anatomical paths along which the state of anxiety is brought about. We are told that the medulla oblongata is stimulated, and the patient learns that he is suffering from a neurosis of the vagus nerve. The medulla oblongata is a very serious and lovely object. I remember quite clearly how much time and trouble I devoted to its study many years ago. To-day, however, I must remark that I know nothing that could be of less interest to me for the psychological understanding of anxiety than a knowledge of the path of the nerves along which its excitations pass.[2]

It is possible at the start to work upon the subject of anxiety for quite a time without thinking at all of neurotic states. You will understand me at once when I describe this kind of anxiety as 'realistic' anxiety in contrast to 'neurotic' anxiety. Realistic anxiety strikes us as something very rational and intelligible.

---

[1] [These words are by no means equivalent to the colloquial English 'nervous' and 'anxious'. '*Nervös*' might be rendered by 'nervy' or 'jumpy' and '*ängstlich*' by 'nervous' in its colloquial sense. 'Anxious' in its ordinary usage is more like the German '*bekümmert*' or '*besorgt*'.]

[2] [At the age of about thirty Freud had worked for two years at the histology of the medulla oblongata and published three papers on the subject: 1885*d*, 1886*b* and 1886*c*. His own abstracts of these (1897*b*) are included in Vol. III of the *Standard Edition*.]

We may say of it that it is a reaction to the perception of an external danger—that is, of an injury which is expected and foreseen. It is connected with the flight reflex and it may be regarded as a manifestation of the self-preservative instinct. On what occasions anxiety appears—that is to say, in the face of what objects and in what situations—will of course depend to a large extent on the state of a person's knowledge and on his sense of power *vis-à-vis* the external world. We can quite understand how a savage is afraid of a cannon and frightened by an eclipse of the sun, while a white man, who knows how to handle the instrument and can foretell the eclipse, remains without anxiety in these circumstances. On other occasions it is actually superior knowledge that promotes anxiety, because it makes an early recognition of the danger possible. Thus the savage will be terrified at a trail in the jungle that tells an uninformed person nothing, because it warns him of the proximity of a wild animal; and an experienced sailor will look with terror at a small cloud in the sky that seems trivial to a passenger, because it tells him of an approaching hurricane.

On further consideration we must tell ourselves that our judgement that realistic anxiety is rational and expedient calls for drastic revision. For the only expedient behaviour when a danger threatens would be a cool estimate of one's own strength in comparison with the magnitude of the threat and, on the basis of that, a decision as to whether flight or defence, or possibly even attack, offers the best prospect of a successful issue. But in this situation there is no place at all for anxiety; everything that happens would be achieved just as well and probably better if no anxiety were generated. And you can see, indeed, that if the anxiety is excessively great it proves in the highest degree inexpedient; it paralyses all action, including even flight. Usually the reaction to danger consists in a mixture of the affect of anxiety and defensive action. A terrified animal is afraid and flees; but the expedient part of this is the 'flight' and not the 'being afraid'.

Thus one feels tempted to assert that the generation of anxiety is never an expedient thing. It may perhaps help us to see more clearly if we dissect the situation of anxiety more carefully. The first thing about it is *preparedness* for the danger, which manifests itself in increased sensory attention and motor tension. This expectant preparedness can be unhesitatingly recognized as an advantage; indeed, its absence may be made responsible for serious consequences. From it there then proceeds on the one hand motor action—flight in the first instance and at a higher level active defence—and on the other hand what we feel as a state of anxiety. The more the generation of anxiety is limited to a mere abortive beginning—to a signal[1]—the more will the preparedness for anxiety transform itself without disturbance into action and the more expedient will be the shape taken by the whole course of events. Accordingly, the *preparedness* for anxiety seems to me to be the expedient element in what we call anxiety, and the *generation* of anxiety the inexpedient one.

I shall avoid going more closely into the question of whether our linguistic usage means the same thing or something clearly different by '*Angst* [anxiety]', '*Furcht* [fear]' and '*Schreck* [fright]'. I will only say that I think '*Angst*' relates to the state and disregards the object, while '*Furcht*' draws attention precisely to the object. It seems that '*Schreck*', on the other hand, does have a special sense; it lays emphasis, that is, on the effect produced by a danger which is not met by any preparedness for anxiety. We might say, therefore, that a person protects himself from fright by anxiety.[2]

A certain ambiguity and indefiniteness in the use of the word '*Angst*' will not have escaped you. By 'anxiety' we usually understand the subjective state into which we are put by perceiving the 'generation of anxiety' and we call this an affect. And what is an affect in the dynamic sense? It is in any case something highly composite. An affect includes in the first place particular motor innervations or discharges and secondly certain feelings; the latter are of two kinds—perceptions of the motor actions that have occurred and the direct feelings of pleasure and unpleasure which, as we say, give the affect its keynote. But I do not think that with this enumeration we have arrived at the essence of an affect. We seem to see deeper in the

---

[1] [This notion of anxiety serving as a 'signal' was to play a central part in Freud's later accounts of anxiety, in *Inhibitions, Symptoms and Anxiety* (1926d) and below p. 549 in the *New Introductory Lectures*. It appears again below on p. 405.]

[2] [Cf. similar later discussions in Chapter II of *Beyond the Pleasure Principle* (1920g), and in Addendum B to *Inhibitions, Symptoms and Anxiety* (1926d).]

case of some affects and to recognize that the core which holds the combination we have described together is the repetition of some particular significant experience. This experience could only be a very early impression of a very general nature, placed in the prehistory not of the individual but of the species. To make myself more intelligible—an affective state would be constructed in the same way as a hysterical attack and, like it, would be the precipitate of a reminiscence. A hysterical attack may thus be likened to a freshly constructed individual affect, and a normal affect to the expression of a general hysteria which has become a heritage.[1]

Do not suppose that the things I have said to you here about affects are the recognized stock-in-trade of normal psychology. They are on the contrary views that have grown up on the soil of psycho-analysis and are native only to it. What you may gather about affects from psychology—the James-Lange theory, for example—is quite beyond understanding or discussion to us psycho-analysts. But we do not regard our knowledge about affects as very assured either; it is a first attempt at finding our bearings in this obscure region. I will proceed, however. We believe that in the case of the affect of anxiety we know what the early impression is which it repeats. We believe that it is in the *act of birth* that there comes about the combination of un-pleasurable feelings, impulses of discharge and bodily sensations which has become the prototype of the effects of a mortal danger and has ever since been repeated by us as the state of anxiety. The immense increase of stimulation owing to the interruption of the renovation of the blood (internal respira-tion) was at the time the cause of the experience of anxiety; the first anxiety was thus a toxic one. The name '*Angst*'— '*angustiae*', '*Enge*'[2]—emphasizes the characteristic of restriction

[1] [This account of hysterical attacks had been suggested by Freud in a paper on that subject many years earlier (1909a). The view of affects in general which is expressed here may possibly be based on Darwin's explanation of them as relics of actions which originally had a meaning (Darwin, 1872)—an explanation quoted from him by Freud near the end of the Case of Elisabeth von R. (1895d). Freud repeats the present argument in *Inhibitions, Symp-toms and Anxiety* (1926d).]

[2] [These Latin and German words, meaning 'narrow place', 'straits', are from the same root as '*Angst*' (and 'anxiety').]

in breathing which was then present as a consequence of the real situation and is now almost invariably reinstated in the affect. We shall also recognize it as highly relevant that this first state of anxiety arose out of separation from the mother.[1] It is, of course, our conviction that the disposition to repeat the first state of anxiety has been so thoroughly incorporated into the organism through a countless series of generations that a single individual cannot escape the affect of anxiety even if, like the legendary Macduff, he 'was from his mother's womb untimely ripped' and has therefore not himself experienced the act of birth. We cannot say what has become the prototype of the state of anxiety in the case of creatures other than mammals. And in the same way we do not know either what complex of feelings is in such creatures the equivalent to our anxiety.

It may perhaps interest you to learn how anyone could have formed such an idea as that the act of birth is the source and prototype of the affect of anxiety. Speculation had a very small share in it; what I did, rather was to borrow from the *naïve* popular mind. Long years ago, while I was sitting with a number of other young hospital doctors at our mid-day meal in an inn, a house physician from the midwifery department told us of a comic thing that had happened at the last examination for midwives. A candidate was asked what it meant if meconium (excreta) made its appearance at birth in the water coming away, and she promptly replied: 'it means the child's frightened.' She was laughed at and failed in the examination. But silently I took her side and began to suspect that this poor woman from the humbler classes had laid an unerring finger on an important correlation.[2]

If we now pass over to consider neurotic anxiety, what fresh forms and situations are manifested by anxiety in neurotics?

[1] [See below, p. 407.]

[2] [The episode must have occurred in the early eighties, and this is the only record of it. A full history of Freud's belief in a connection between anxiety and birth was given in the Editor's Introduction to *Inhibitions, Symptoms and Anxiety*. From this it seemed that the first known reference to it was in a footnote appearing in the 1909 edition of *The Interpretation of Dreams*, and probably written in the summer of 1908. Since the publication of this Introduction, however, an earlier reference has come to light in the *Minutes of the Vienna Psychoanalytic Society* (1962). At a meeting on April 24, 1907, at which Stekel read a

There is much to be described here. In the first place we find a general apprehensiveness, a kind of freely floating anxiety which is ready to attach itself to any idea that is in any way suitable, which influences judgement, selects what is to be expected, and lies in wait for any opportunity that will allow it to justify itself. We call this state 'expectant anxiety' or 'anxious expectation'. People who are tormented by this kind of anxiety always foresee the most frightful of all possibilities, interpret every chance event as a premonition of evil and exploit every uncertainty in a bad sense. A tendency to an expectation of evil of this sort is to be found as a character trait in many people whom one cannot otherwise regard as sick; one calls them over-anxious or pessimistic. A striking amount of expectant anxiety, however, forms a regular feature of a nervous disorder to which I have given the name of 'anxiety neurosis' and which I include among the 'actual' neuroses.[1]

A second form of anxiety, in contrast to the one I have just described, is bound psychically[2] and attached to particular objects or situations. This is the anxiety of the extremely multifarious and often very strange 'phobias'. Stanley Hall [1914], the respected American psychologist, has recently taken the trouble to present us with a whole series of these phobias in all the magnificence of Greek names. This sounds like a list of the ten Plagues of Egypt, though their number goes far beyond ten.[3] Listen to all the things that can become the object or content of a phobia: darkness, open air, open spaces, cats,

paper on 'The Psychology and Pathology of the Anxiety Neurosis', Adler is reported to have made the following remark: 'One need not venture so far as Freud, who sees anxiety in the process of birth; but anxiety can be traced back into childhood.' Neither in Freud's contribution to the discussion, which was subsequent to Adler's, nor in any other, is the matter referred to again. It would appear from this, however, that Freud's hypothesis was familiarly known in the Vienna Society at least a couple of years before its first publication.]

[1] [Cf. Freud's original account of the anxiety neurosis (1895*b*).]
[2] [Instead of being freely floating.]
[3] [Actually, Stanley Hall enumerates 132 of them. See a review of his paper by Ernest Jones (1916). Stanley Hall (1846–1924) was originally a supporter of Freud's and it was he who invited Freud to lecture in America in 1909, though he later became a follower of Adler.]

spiders, caterpillars, snakes, mice, thunderstorms, sharp points, blood, enclosed spaces, crowds, solitude, crossing bridges, sea voyages and railway journeys, etc., etc. A first attempt at finding one's way about in this confusion suggests a division into three groups. Some of the dreaded objects and situations have something uncanny about them for normal people as well, some relation to danger; and such phobias, therefore, do not strike us as unintelligible, though their strength is greatly exaggerated. Thus most of us have a sense of repulsion if we meet with a snake. Snake phobia, we might say, is a universal human characteristic; and Darwin [1889, 40] has described most impressively how he could not avoid feeling fear of a snake that struck at him, even though he knew that he was protected from it by a thick sheet of glass. We may refer to a second group the cases in which a relation to a danger is still present, though we are accustomed to minimize the danger and not to anticipate it. The majority of situation phobias belong to this group. We know that there is more chance of an accident when we are on a railway-journey than when we stay at home—the chance of a collision; we know, too, that a ship may go down, in which case there is a probability of being drowned; but we do not think about these dangers, and travel by rail and ship without anxiety. It cannot be disputed that we should fall into the river if the bridge collapsed at the moment we were crossing it; but that happens so exceedingly seldom that it does not arise as a danger. Solitude, too, has its dangers and in certain circumstances we avoid it; but there is no question of our not being able to tolerate it under any condition even for a moment. Much the same is true of crowds, of enclosed spaces, of thunderstorms and so on. What in general appears to us strange in these phobias of neurotics is not so much their content as their intensity. The anxiety of phobias is positively overwhelming. And sometimes we get an impression that what neurotics are afraid of are not at all the same things and situations which may in certain circumstances cause anxiety in us too and which they describe by the same names.

We are left with a third group of phobias, which is quite beyond our comprehension. When a strong, grown-up man is unable owing to anxiety to walk along a street or cross a square in his own familiar home-town, when a healthy, well-developed woman is thrown into insensate anxiety because a cat has brushed against the edge of her dress or because a mouse has run across the room, how are we to relate these things to the danger which they obviously constitute for the phobic subject? In the case of such animal phobias there can be no question of an exaggeration of universal human antipathies, since, as though to demonstrate the contrary, there are numerous people who cannot pass by a cat without coaxing it and stroking it. The mouse that these women are so much afraid of is also [in German] one of the chief terms of affection; a girl who is delighted when her lover calls her one will often scream with terror when she sees the pretty creature which bears that name. In the case of the man with agoraphobia the only explanation that we can reach is that he is behaving like a small child. A child is actually taught as part of his education to avoid such situations as dangerous; and our agoraphobic will in fact be saved from his anxiety if we accompany him across the square.

The two forms of anxiety that I have just described—the freely floating expectant anxiety and the sort which is bound to phobias—are independent of each other. One is not a higher stage, as it were, of the other; and they only appear simultaneously in exceptional cases and, so to speak, accidentally. The most powerful general apprehensiveness need not be expressed in phobias; people whose whole existence is restricted by agoraphobia may be entirely free from pessimistic expectant anxiety. Some phobias—for instance, agoraphobia and railway phobia—are demonstrably acquired at a fairly mature age, while others—such as fear of darkness, thunderstorms and animals—seem to have been present from the first. Those of the former kind have the significance of severe illnesses; the latter make their appearance rather as eccentricities or whims. If a person exhibits one of these latter, one may suspect as a rule that he will have other similar ones. I must add that we class all these phobias as *anxiety hysteria*; that is to say, we regard them as a disorder closely related to the familiar conversion hysteria[1] [p. 390].

[1] [Freud's first long discussion of anxiety hysteria was in the case history of 'little Hans' (1909b). Some account of his changing views on phobias is given in an Editor's Appendix to his early paper on 'Obsessions and Phobias' (1895c).]

The third of the forms of neurotic anxiety faces us with the puzzling fact that here the connection between anxiety and a threatening danger is completely lost to view. For instance, anxiety may appear in hysteria as an accompaniment to hysterical symptoms, or in some chance condition of excitement in which, it is true, we should expect some manifestation of affect but least of all one of anxiety; or it may make its appearance, divorced from any determinants and equally incomprehensible to us and to the patient, as an unrelated attack of anxiety. Here there is no sign whatever of any danger or of any cause that could be exaggerated into one. We next learn from these spontaneous attacks that the complex which we describe as a state of anxiety is capable of fragmentation. The total attack can be represented by a single, intensely developed symptom, by a tremor, a vertigo, by palpitation of the heart, or by dyspnoea; and the general feeling by which we recognize anxiety may be absent or have become indistinct. Yet these conditions, which we describe as 'anxiety-equivalents', have to be equated with anxiety in all clinical and aetiological respects.

Two questions now arise. Can we relate neurotic anxiety, in which danger plays little or no part, to realistic anxiety, which is invariably a reaction to danger? And how are we to understand neurotic anxiety? We shall certainly be inclined in the first instance to hold fast to our expectation that where there is anxiety there must be something that one is afraid of.

Clinical observation affords us a number of hints towards understanding neurotic anxiety, and I will give you their tenor:—

(a) It is not difficult to establish the fact that expectant anxiety or general apprehensiveness is closely dependent on certain happenings in sexual life, or, let us say, certain employments of the libido. The simplest and most instructive case of this sort occurs in people who expose themselves to what is known as unconsummated excitation—that is, people in whom violent sexual excitations meet with no sufficient discharge, cannot be brought to a satisfying conclusion—men, for instance, while they are engaged to be married, and women whose husbands are insufficiently potent or, as a precaution, perform the sexual act in an incomplete or curtailed fashion. In such circumstances the libidinal excitation vanishes and anxiety appears in its place whether in the form of expectant anxiety or in attacks and anxiety-equivalents. Interruption of the sexual act as a precaution, if it is practised as a sexual *régime*, is such a regular cause of anxiety neurosis in men, but more particularly in women, that in medical practice it is advisable in such cases to begin by investigating this aetiology. It will then be found on countless occasions that the anxiety neurosis disappears when the sexual abuse is discontinued.

The fact of there being a connection between sexual restraint and anxiety states is, so far as I know, no longer disputed even by physicians who have no contact with psycho-analysis. But I can well believe that an attempt is made to reverse the relation and to put forward the view that the people concerned are such as are already inclined to apprehensiveness and for that reason practise restraint in sexual matters as well. This, however, is decisively contradicted by the behaviour of women, whose sexual activity is essentially of a passive nature—is determined, that is to say, by their treatment by the man. The more passionate a woman is—the more inclined, therefore, to sexual intercourse and the more capable of being satisfied—the more certain she is to react with manifestations of anxiety to a man's impotence or to coitus interruptus, whereas in the case of anaesthetic women or those without much libido such ill-treatment plays a far smaller part.

Of course, the sexual abstinence now so warmly recommended by doctors only has the same importance in generating anxiety states when the libido which is prevented from finding a satisfying discharge is correspondingly strong and has not been dealt with for the greater part by sublimation. Indeed, the decision on whether the outcome is to be illness or not always lies with quantitative factors. Even where what is in question is not illness but the form assumed by a person's character, it is easy to recognize that sexual restriction goes hand in hand with some kind of anxiousness and hesitancy, while intrepidity and impudent daring bring along with them a free indulgence of sexual needs. However much these relations are altered and complicated by a variety of cultural influences, it nevertheless remains true of the average of mankind that anxiety has a close connection with sexual limitation.

I am far from having told you of all the observations that

speak in favour of the genetic relation I have asserted to exist between libido and anxiety. Among them, for instance, is the influence on anxiety disorders of certain phases of life to which, as in the case of puberty and the time of the menopause, a considerable increase in the production of libido may be attributed. In some states of excitement, too, it is possible to observe directly a mixture of libido and anxiety and the final replacement of libido by anxiety. The impression one gains from all these facts is twofold: first, that what is in question is an accumulation of libido which is kept away from its normal employment, and secondly, that here we are entirely in the sphere of somatic processes. How anxiety arises from libido is not at first discernible; we can only recognize that libido is absent and that anxiety is observed in its place.[1]

(*b*) A second pointer is to be found in the analysis of the psychoneuroses, and especially of hysteria. We have seen that in this illness anxiety often appears in company with the symptoms, but that unbound anxiety appears, too, manifested as an attack or as a chronic condition. The patients cannot say what it is they are afraid of, and, by the help of an unmistakable secondary revision [p. 182], link it to the first phobias that come to hand—such as dying, going mad, or having a stroke. If the situation out of which the anxiety (or the symptoms accompanied by anxiety) arose is subjected to analysis, we can as a rule discover what normal course of psychical events has failed to occur and has been replaced by phenomena of anxiety. To express it in another way: we construct the unconscious process as it would have been if it had not experienced any repression and had proceeded unhindered into consciousness. [Pp. 293–4.] This process would have been accompanied by a particular affect, and we now learn to our surprise that this affect accompanying the normal course of events is invariably replaced by anxiety after repression has occurred, no matter what its own quality may be. Thus, when we have a hysterical anxiety-state before us, its unconscious correlate may be an impulse of a similar character—anxiety, shame, embarrassment—or, just as easily, a positive libidinal excitation or a hostile aggressive one, such as rage or anger. Anxiety is therefore the universally

[1] [The last four paragraphs are to a large extent a summary of Freud's first paper on anxiety neurosis (1895*b*).]

current coinage for which *any* affective impulse is or can be exchanged if the ideational content attached to it is subjected to repression.[1]

(*c*) We make a third discovery when we come to patients suffering from obsessional actions, who seem in a remarkable way exempt from anxiety. If we try to hinder their carrying out of their obsessional action—their washing or their ceremonial—or if they themselves venture upon an attempt to give up one of their compulsions, they are forced by the most terrible anxiety to yield to the compulsion. We can see that the anxiety was screened by the obsessional action, and that the latter was only performed in order to avoid the anxiety. In an obsessional neurosis, therefore, anxiety which would otherwise inevitably set in is replaced by the formation of a symptom, and if we turn to hysteria we find a similar relation: the result of the process of repression is either a generating of anxiety pure and simple, or anxiety accompanied by the formation of a symptom, or a more complete formation of a symptom without anxiety. It would thus seem not to be wrong in an abstract sense to assert that in general symptoms are only formed to escape an otherwise unavoidable generating of anxiety. If we adopt this view, anxiety is placed, as it were, in the very centre of our interest in the problems of neurosis.

Our observations on anxiety neurosis led us to conclude that the deflection of the libido from its normal employment, which causes the development of anxiety, takes place in the region of somatic processes [p. 403]. Analyses of hysteria and obsessional neurosis yield the additional conclusion that a similar deflection with the same outcome may also be the result of a refusal on the part of the *psychical* agencies. This much, therefore, we know about the origin of neurotic anxiety. It still sounds fairly indefinite; but for the moment I see no path that would lead us further. The second problem we set ourselves—of establishing a connection between neurotic anxiety, which is libido put to an abnormal employment, and realistic anxiety, which corresponds to a reaction to danger—seems even harder to solve. One might suppose that these were two quite disparate

[1] [See the metapsychological paper on 'Repression' (1915*d*).]

things; and yet we have no means of distinguishing in our feelings between realistic anxiety and neurotic anxiety.

We finally arrive at the connection we are in search of, if we take as our starting-point the opposition we have so often asserted between the ego and the libido. As we know, the generation of anxiety is the ego's reaction to danger and the signal for taking flight. [Cf. p. 395.] If so, it seems plausible to suppose that in neurotic anxiety the ego is making a similar attempt at flight from the demand by its libido, that it is treating this internal danger as though it were an external one. This would therefore fulfil our expectation [p. 401] that where anxiety is shown there is something one is afraid of. But the analogy could be carried further. Just as the attempt at flight from an external danger is replaced by standing firm and the adoption of expedient measures of defence, so too the generation of neurotic anxiety gives place to the formation of symptoms, which results in the anxiety being bound.

The difficulty in understanding now lies elsewhere. The anxiety which signifies a flight of the ego from its libido is after all supposed to be derived from that libido itself. This is obscure and it reminds us not to forget that after all a person's libido is fundamentally something of his and cannot be contrasted with him as something external. It is the topographical dynamics of the generation of anxiety which are still obscure to us—the question of what mental energies are produced in that process and from what mental systems they derive. This is once more a question which I cannot promise to answer: but there are two other tracks which we must not fail to follow and in doing so we shall once more be making use of direct observation and analytic enquiry as a help to our speculations. We will turn to the genesis of anxiety in children and to the source of the neurotic anxiety which is attached to phobias.

Apprehensiveness in children is something very usual, and it seems most difficult to distinguish whether it is neurotic or realistic anxiety. Indeed the value of making the distinction is put in question by the behaviour of children. For on the one hand we are not surprised if a child is frightened of all strangers, or of new situations and things; and we account for this reaction very easily as being due to his weakness and ignorance. Thus we attribute to children a strong inclination to realistic anxiety and we should regard it as quite an expedient arrangement if this apprehensiveness were an innate heritage in them. Children would merely be repeating in this the behaviour of prehistoric men and of modern primitive peoples who as a result of their ignorance and helplessness are afraid of every novelty and of many familiar things which no longer cause us any anxiety to-day. And it would fit in perfectly with our expectation if children's phobias, in part at least, were the same as those which we may attribute to the primaeval periods of human development.

On the other hand we cannot overlook the fact that not all children are anxious to the same degree, and that precisely children who exhibit a special timidity towards objects and in situations of every kind turn out later to be neurotic. Thus the neurotic disposition betrays itself also by an outspoken tendency to realistic anxiety; apprehensiveness appears to be the primary thing and we reach the conclusion that the reason why children and, later, growing youths and girls are afraid of the height of their libido is because in fact they are afraid of everything. The genesis of anxiety from libido would in this way be denied; and if one examined into the determinants of realistic anxiety, consistency would lead one to the view that consciousness of one's own weakness and helplessness—inferiority, according to Adler's terminology,—if it can be prolonged from childhood into adult life, is the final basis of neuroses.

This sounds so simple and seductive that it has a claim on our attention. It is true that it would involve a displacement of the riddle of the neurotic state. The continued existence of the sense of inferiority—and thus, of what determines anxiety and the formation of symptoms—seems so well assured that what calls for an explanation is rather how, as an exception, what we know as health can come about. But what is revealed by a careful examination of apprehensiveness in children? At the very beginning, what children are afraid of is strange *people*; situations only become important because they include people, and impersonal things do not come into account at all until later. But a child is not afraid of these strangers because he attributes evil intentions to them and compares his weakness with their strength, and accordingly assesses them as dangers to his existence, safety and freedom from pain. A child who is mistrustful in this way and terrified of the aggressive instinct which dominates the world is a theoretical construction that has quite miscarried. A child is frightened of a strange face because he is adjusted to the sight of a familiar and beloved figure— ultimately of his mother. It is his disappointment and longing that are transformed into anxiety—his libido, in fact, which has become unemployable, which cannot at that time be held in suspense and is discharged as anxiety. And it can scarcely be a matter of chance, either, that in this situation which is the prototype of the anxiety of children there is a repetition of the determinant of the first state of anxiety during the act of birth—namely, separation from the mother.[1]

In children the first phobias relating to situations are those of darkness and solitude. The former of these often persists throughout life; both are involved when a child feels the absence of some loved person who looks after it—its mother, that is to say. While I was in the next room, I heard a child who was afraid of the dark call out: 'Do speak to me, Auntie! I'm frightened!' 'Why, what good would that do? You can't see me.' To this the child replied: 'If someone speaks, it gets lighter.'[2] Thus a *longing* felt in the dark is transformed into a *fear* of the dark. Far from its being the case that neurotic anxiety is only secondary and a special case of realistic anxiety, we see on the contrary that in a small child something that behaves like realistic anxiety shares its essential feature—origin from unemployed libido—with neurotic anxiety. Innately, children seem to have little true realistic anxiety. In all the situations which can later become determinants of phobias (on heights, on narrow bridges over water, on railway journeys, on ships) children exhibit no anxiety; and, to be sure, the greater

[1] [This was Freud's first explicit insistence on the primary importance of separation from the mother as a factor in the origin of anxiety, though it had been suggested above (p. 397) and implied in earlier writings. References to these will be found in the Editor's Introduction to *Inhibitions, Symptoms and Anxiety* (1926d). In the latter work the matter was discussed at greater length in Chapter VIII. It had also been briefly mentioned at the end of Chapter V in *The Ego and the Id* (1923b), (Norton, 1960).]

[2] [This anecdote had appeared (in a slightly different form) in a footnote to Section 5 of the third of Freud's *Three Essays* (1905d).]

their ignorance the less their anxiety. It would have been a very good thing if they had inherited more of such life-preserving instincts,[1] for that would have greatly facilitated the task of watching over them to prevent their running into one danger after another. The fact is that children, to begin with, over-estimate their strength and behave fearlessly because they are ignorant of dangers. They will run along the brink of the water, climb on to the window-sill, play with sharp objects and with fire—in short, do everything that is bound to damage them and to worry those in charge of them. When in the end realistic anxiety is awakened in them, that is wholly the result of education; for they cannot be allowed to make the instructive experiences themselves.

If, then, there are children who come some way to meet this education in anxiety, and who go on to find dangers themselves that they have not been warned against, this is sufficiently explained by the fact that they have a greater amount of innate libidinal need in their constitution or have been prematurely spoiled by libidinal satisfaction. It is not to be wondered at if such children include, too, the later neurotics: as we know, what most facilitates the development of a neurosis is an incapacity to tolerate a considerable damming-up of libido over any great length of time. You will observe that here once more the constitutional factor comes into its rights—and these, indeed, we have never sought to dispute. We are only on our guard against those who in its favour neglect all other claims, and who introduce the constitutional factor at points at which the combined results of observation and analysis show that it does not belong or must take the last place.

Let me sum up what we have learnt from our observations of the apprehensiveness of children. Infantile anxiety has very little to do with realistic anxiety, but, on the other hand, is closely related to the neurotic anxiety of adults. Like the latter, it is derived from unemployed libido and it replaces the missing love-object by an external object or by a situation.

You will be glad to hear that the analysis of phobias has not much more that is new to teach us. For the same thing happens

---

[1] [This is one of the extremely few occasions on which Freud uses the word '*Instinkt*' instead of his usual '*Trieb*'.]

with them as with children's anxiety: unemployable libido is being constantly transformed into an apparently realistic anxiety and thus a tiny external danger is introduced to represent the claims of the libido. There is nothing to be wondered at in this agreement [between phobias and children's anxiety], for the infantile phobias are not only the prototype of the later ones which we class as 'anxiety hysteria' but are actually their precondition and the prelude to them. Every hysterical phobia goes back to an infantile anxiety and is a continuation of it, even if it has a different content and must thus be given another name. The difference between the two disorders lies in their mechanism. In order that libido shall be changed into anxiety, it no longer suffices in the case of adults for the libido to have become momentarily unemployable in the form of a longing. Adults have long since learnt how to hold such libido in suspense or to employ it in some other way. If, however, the libido belongs to a psychical impulse which has been subjected to repression, then circumstances are re-established similar to those in the case of a child in whom there is still no distinction between conscious and unconscious; and by means of regression to the infantile phobia a passage is opened, as it were, through which the transformation of libido into anxiety can be comfortably accomplished.

As you will recall, we have dealt with repression at great length,[1] but in doing so we have always followed the vicissitudes only of the idea that is to be repressed—naturally, since this was easier to recognize and describe. We have always left on one side the question of what happens to the affect that was attached to the repressed idea; and it is only now that we learn [p. 403] that the immediate vicissitude of that affect is to be transformed into anxiety, whatever quality it may have exhibited apart from this in the normal course of events. This transformation of affect is, however, by far the more important part of the process of repression. It is not so easy to speak of this, since we cannot assert the existence of unconscious affects in the same sense as that of unconscious ideas.[2] An idea remains

---

[1] [In Lecture XIX.]

[2] [For more information on what follows, see the third section of the metapsychological paper on 'The Unconscious' (1915e), and the second chapter of *The Ego and the Id* (1923b), (Norton, 1960).]

the same, except for the one difference, whether it is conscious or unconscious; we can state what it is that corresponds to an unconscious idea. But an affect is a process of discharge and must be judged quite differently from an idea; what corresponds to it in the unconscious cannot be declared without deeper reflection and a clarification of our hypotheses about psychical processes. And that we cannot undertake here. We will, however, emphasize the impression we have now gained that the generation of anxiety is intimately linked to the system of the unconscious.

I have said that transformation into anxiety—it would be better to say discharge in the form of anxiety—is the immediate vicissitude of libido which is subjected to repression. I must add that that vicissitude is not the only or the definitive one. In the neuroses processes are in action which endeavour to bind this generating of anxiety and which even succeed in doing so in various ways. In phobias, for instance, two phases of the neurotic process can be clearly distinguished. The first is concerned with repression and the changing of libido into anxiety, which is then bound to an external danger. The second consists in the erection of all the precautions and guarantees by means of which any contact can be avoided with this danger, treated as it is like an external thing. Repression corresponds to an attempt at flight by the ego from libido which is felt as a danger. A phobia may be compared to an entrenchment against an external danger which now represents the dreaded libido. The weakness of the defensive system in phobias lies, of course, in the fact that the fortress which has been so greatly strengthened towards the outside remains assailable from within. A projection outwards of the danger of libido can never succeed thoroughly.[1] For that reason, in other neuroses other systems of defence are in use against the possible generation of anxiety. That is a most interesting part of the psychology of the neuroses; but unluckily it would lead us too far and it presupposes a deeper specialized knowledge. I will only add one thing more. I have already spoken to you [p. 360] of the 'anticathexis' which is employed by the ego in the process of repression and

---

[1] [More technical accounts of the structure of phobias will be found in 'Repression' (1915d), and 'The Unconscious' (1915e).]

which must be permanently maintained in order that the repression may have stability. This anticathexis has the task of carrying through the various forms of defence against the generating of anxiety after repression.

Let us return to the phobias. I can safely say that you now see how inadequate it is merely to seek to explain their content, to take no interest in anything but how it comes about that this or that object or some particular situation or other has been made into the object of the phobia. The content of a phobia has just about as much importance in relation to it as the manifest façade of a dream has in relation to the dream. It must be admitted, subject to the necessary qualifications, that among the contents of phobias there are a number which, as Stanley Hall [1914, see p. 398] insists, are adapted to serve as objects of anxiety owing to phylogenetic inheritance. It tallies with this, indeed, that many of these anxiety-objects can only establish their connection with danger by a symbolic tie.

We thus find ourselves convinced that the problem of anxiety occupies a place in the question of the psychology of the neuroses which may rightly be described as central. We have received a strong impression of the way in which the generation of anxiety is linked to the vicissitudes of the libido and the system of the unconscious. There is only a single point that we have found disconnected—a gap in our views: the single, yet scarcely disputable, fact that realistic anxiety must be regarded as a manifestation of the ego's self-preservative instincts.[1]

[1] [This difficulty is met at the end of the next lecture, p. 430.]

THE LIBIDO THEORY AND NARCISSISM

LADIES AND GENTLEMEN,—We have repeatedly (and only recently once again [p. 350]) had to deal with the distinction between the ego-instincts and the sexual instincts. In the first place, repression showed us that the two can come into opposition to each other, that the sexual instincts are then ostensibly subdued and are obliged to find satisfaction for themselves along regressive and roundabout paths, and that in doing so they are able to find compensation for their defeat in their indomitability. We next learnt that the two kinds of instincts are from the first differently related to Necessity the educator [p. 355], so that their course of development is not the same and they do not enter into the same connection with the reality principle. Lastly, we seem to have found that the sexual instincts are linked by much closer bonds than the ego-instincts to the affective state of anxiety—a conclusion which seems incomplete in only one important respect. In order to establish it more firmly, therefore, I will bring forward the further noteworthy fact that if hunger and thirst (the two most elementary self-preservative instincts) are unsatisfied, the result is never their transformation into anxiety, whereas the changing of unsatisfied libido into anxiety is, as we have seen, among the best known and most frequently observed of phenomena.

Our right to separate the ego-instincts from the sexual ones cannot, no doubt, be shaken: it is implied in the existence of sexual life as a distinct activity of the individual. The only question is what importance we attribute to this separation, how deep-going we wish to consider it. The answer to this question, however, will be guided by how far we are able to establish the extent to which the sexual instincts behave differently in their somatic and mental manifestations from the others which we are contrasting with them, and how important the consequences are which arise from those differences. Moreover,

412

we have, of course, no motive for asserting an essential difference between the two groups of instincts which is not plainly appreciable. Both of them come before us merely as designations of sources of energy in the individual, and the discussion as to whether they are fundamentally one or essentially different and as to when, if they are one, they became separate from each other—this discussion cannot be conducted on the basis of the connotation of the terms but must keep to the biological facts lying behind them. At the moment we know too little about these, and even if we knew more it would have no relevance for our analytic task.

It is obvious, too, that we shall profit very little if, following Jung's example, we insist upon the original unity of all the instincts and give the name of 'libido' to the energy manifested in all of them. Since no device whatever will make it possible to eliminate the sexual function from mental life, we shall in that case find ourselves obliged to speak of sexual and asexual libido. But the name of libido is properly reserved for the instinctual forces of sexual life, as has hitherto been our practice.

In my opinion, therefore, the question of how far we are to carry the undoubtedly justifiable separation between the sexual and self-preservative instincts is not of much importance for psycho-analysis. Nor is psycho-analysis competent to answer the question. Biology, however, offers a number of suggestive possibilities which speak in favour of the distinction having some importance. Sexuality is, indeed, the single function of the living organism which extends beyond the individual and is concerned with his relation to the species. It is an unmistakable fact that it does not always, like the individual organism's other functions, bring it advantages, but, in return for an unusually high degree of pleasure, brings dangers which threaten the individual's life and often enough destroy it. It is probable, too, that quite special metabolic processes are necessary, differing from all others, in order to maintain a portion of the individual life as a disposition for its descendants. And finally, the individual organism, which regards itself as the main thing and its sexuality as a means, like any other, for its own satisfaction, is from the point of view of biology only an episode in a succession of generations, a short-lived appendage to a germ-plasm endowed with virtual immortality—like the temporary holder of an entail which will outlast him.[1]

The psycho-analytic explanation of the neuroses does not, however, call for such far-ranging considerations. The separate following-up of the sexual and ego-instincts has helped us to find the key to an understanding of the group of transference neuroses. We have been able to trace them back to the basic situation in which the sexual instincts have come into a dispute with the self-preservative instincts, or, to put it in biological (though less precise) terms, a situation in which one aspect of the ego, as an independent individual organism, comes into conflict with its other aspect, as a member of a succession of generations. A dissension of this kind may perhaps only occur in human beings, and on that account neurosis may, generally speaking, constitute their prerogative over the animals. The excessive development of their libido and—what is perhaps made possible precisely by that—their development of a richly articulated mental life seem to have created the determinants for the occurrence of such a conflict. It is at once obvious that these are also the determinants for the great advances that human beings have made beyond what they have in common with the animals; so that their susceptibility to neurosis would only be the reverse side of their other endowments. But these too are only speculations, which are diverting us from our immediate task.

Hitherto it has been a premiss of our work that we can distinguish the ego-instincts from the sexual ones by their manifestations. With the transference neuroses this could be done without difficulty. We termed the cathexes of energy which the ego directs towards the objects of its sexual desires 'libido'; all the others, which are sent out by the self-preservative instincts, we termed 'interest'.[2] By tracing the course of the

[1] [Freud developed this biological argument further in *Beyond the Pleasure Principle* (1920g), particularly in Chapter VI.]

[2] [The term 'ego-interest', sometimes in the alternative forms of 'egoistic interest' or simply 'interest', occurs frequently in this lecture. Freud had first used the term in his paper on narcissism (1914c), and it also appears several times in the metapsychological papers of 1915. The term is used regularly in those passages (as it is in the present one) to distinguish self-preservative forces from the libido. The introduction of the concept of narcissism made this distinction less clear-cut; but it is evident that all through

libidinal cathexes, their transformations and final vicissitudes, we were able to obtain a first insight into the machinery of the mental forces. For this purpose the transference neuroses offered us the most favourable material. But the ego, its composition out of various organizations and their construction and mode of functioning, remained hidden from us; and we were driven to suspect that only the analysis of other neurotic disorders would be able to bring us the necessary insight.

We began at an early date to extend psycho-analytic observations to these other illnesses. Already in 1908 Karl Abraham, after an exchange of thoughts with me, pronounced the main characteristic of dementia praecox (which was reckoned among the psychoses) to be that *in it the libidinal cathexis of objects was lacking*. But the question then arose of what happened to the libido of dementia praecox patients which was turned away from objects. Abraham did not hesitate to give the answer: it is turned back on to the ego and *this reflexive turning-back is the source of the megalomania* in dementia praecox. Megalomania is in every way comparable to the familiar sexual overvaluation of the object in [normal] erotic life.[1] In this way for the first time we learnt to understand a trait in a psychotic illness by relating it to normal erotic life.

I may tell you at once that these first explanations of Abraham's have been accepted in psycho-analysis and have become the basis of our attitude to the psychoses. We thus slowly became familiar with the notion that the libido, which we find attached to objects and which is the expression of an effort to obtain satisfaction in connection with those objects,

this lecture (see, in particular, its last paragraph) Freud was at pains to keep ego-libido (or narcissistic libido) separate from ego-interest (or the self-preservative instinct). Not long afterwards, however, he abandoned this attempt and declared in *Beyond the Pleasure Principle* (1920g), that narcissistic libido 'had necessarily to be identified with the "self-preservative instinct" '. He continued to believe, nevertheless, that there were object-instincts other than libidinal ones—namely those which he described as destructive or death instincts. But after the present work the term 'interest' ceased to appear. A fuller account of this is given in the Editor's Note to 'Instincts and their Vicissitudes' (1915c).]

[1] [This is discussed in the first of Freud's *Three Essays* (1905d).]

can also leave the objects and set the subject's own ego in their place; and this notion was gradually built up more and more consistently. The name for this way of allocating the libido— 'narcissism'—was borrowed by us from a perversion described by Paul Näcke [1899] in which an adult treats his own body with all the caresses that are usually devoted to an outside sexual object.[1]

Reflection will quickly suggest that if any such fixation of the libido to the subject's own body and personality instead of to an object does occur, it cannot be an exceptional or a trivial event. On the contrary it is probable that this narcissism is the universal and original state of things, from which object-love is only later developed, without the narcissism necessarily disappearing on that account. Indeed we had to recall from the history of the development of object-libido that many sexual instincts begin by finding satisfaction in the subject's own body —*auto-erotically*, as we say [p. 314]—and that this capacity for auto-erotism is the basis of the lagging-behind of sexuality in the process of education in the reality principle [p. 355]. Autoerotism would thus be the sexual activity of the narcissistic stage of allocation of the libido.

To put the matter shortly, we pictured the relation of ego-libido to object-libido in a way which I can make plain to you by an analogy from zoology. Think of those simplest of living organisms [the amoebas] which consist of a little-differentiated globule of protoplasmic substance. They put out protrusions, known as pseudopodia, into which they cause the substance of their body to flow over. They are able, however, to withdraw the protrusions once more and form themselves again into a globule. We compare the putting-out of these protrusions, then, to the emission of libido on to objects while the main mass of libido can remain in the ego; and we suppose that in normal circumstances ego-libido can be transformed unhindered into object-libido and that this can once more be taken back into the ego.[2]

[1] [The term is in part due to Havelock Ellis. See a full discussion in an Editor's first footnote to Freud's paper on narcissism (1914c), which is Freud's main exposition of the whole subject.]

[2] [Some discussion of this analogy will be found in the Editor's Appendix B to *The Ego and the Id* (1923b), (Norton, 1960).]

With the help of these ideas we are now able to explain a whole number of mental states or, to express it more modestly, to describe them in terms of the libido theory—states which we must reckon as belonging to normal life, such as the psychical behaviour of a person in love, during an organic illness or when asleep. As regards the state of sleep, we assumed that it was based on turning-away from the external world and adopting a wish to sleep [p. 88]. The mental activity during the night which is manifested in dreams takes place, we found, in obedience to a wish to sleep and is moreover dominated by purely egoistic motives [p. 142].We may now add, on the lines of the libido theory, that sleep is a state in which all object-cathexes, libidinal as well as egoistic, are given up and with-drawn into the ego. May not this throw a fresh light on the recuperating effect of sleep and on the nature of fatigue in general? The picture of the blissful isolation of intra-uterine life which a sleeper conjures up once more before us every night is in this way completed on its psychical side as well. In a sleeper the primal state of distribution of the libido is restored —total narcissism, in which libido and ego-interest, still united and indistinguishable, dwell in the self-sufficing ego.

This is the place for two remarks. First, how do we differenti-ate between the concepts of narcissism and egoism? Well, narcissism, I believe, is the libidinal complement to egoism. When we speak of egoism, we have in view only the individual's *advantage*; when we talk of narcissism we are also taking his libidinal satisfaction into account. As practical motives the two can be traced separately for quite a distance. It is possible to be absolutely egoistic and yet maintain powerful object-cathexes, in so far as libidinal satisfaction in relation to the object forms part of the ego's needs. In that case, egoism will see to it that striving for the object involves no damage to the ego. It is possible to be egoistic and at the same time to be excessively narcissistic—that is to say, to have very little need for an object, whether, once more, for the purpose of direct sexual satisfaction, or in connection with the higher aspirations, derived from sexual need, which we are occasionally in the habit of contrasting with 'sensuality' under the name of 'love'. In all these connections egoism is what is self-evident and constant, while narcissism is the variable element. The opposite to egoism, *altruism*, does not, as a concept, coincide with libidinal object-cathexis, but is distinguished from it by the absence of longings for sexual satisfaction. When someone is completely in love, however, altruism converges with libidinal object-cathexis. As a rule the sexual object attracts a portion of the ego's narcissism to itself, and this becomes noticeable as what is known as the 'sexual overvaluation' of the object. [See above, p. 415.] If in addition there is an altruistic transposition of egoism on to the sexual object, the object becomes supremely powerful; it has, as it were, absorbed the ego.

You will find it refreshing, I believe, if, after what is the essentially dry imagery of science, I present you with a poetic representation of the economic[1] contrast between narcissism and being in love. Here is a quotation from Goethe's *West-östlicher Diwan*:[2]

ZULEIKA

The slave, the lord of victories,
    The crowd, when'er you ask, confess
In sense of personal being lies
    A child of earth's chief happiness.

There's not a life we need refuse
    If our true self we do not miss,
There's not a thing we may not lose
    If one remain the man one is.

HATEM

So it is held, so well may be;
    But down a different track I come;
Of all the bliss earth holds for me
    I in Zuleika find the sum.

Does she expend her being on me,
    Myself grows to myself of cost;
Turns she away, then instantly
    I to my very self am lost.

[1] [I.e. the quantitative factor in the energies concerned. See p. 374 above.]

[2] [The translation is from Ernest Dowden, *West Eastern Divan*, 1914. The word 'divan' in its original Persian sense, which was adopted by Goethe, meant 'a collection of poems'.]

That day with Hatem all were over;
  And yet I should but change my state;
Swift, should she grace some happy lover,
  In him I were incorporate.

My second remark is a supplement to the theory of dreams. We cannot explain the origin of dreams unless we adopt the hypothesis that the repressed unconscious has achieved some degree of independence of the ego, so that it does not acquiesce in the wish to sleep and retains its cathexes even when all the object-cathexes depending on the ego have been withdrawn in order to encourage sleep. Only if that is so can we understand how the unconscious can make use of the lifting or reduction of the censorship which occurs at night, and can succeed in obtaining control over the day's residues so as to construct a forbidden dream-wish out of their material. On the other hand, it may be that these day's residues have to thank an already existing connection with the repressed unconscious for some of their resistance to the withdrawal of libido commanded by the wish to sleep. We will, then, insert this dynamically important feature into our view of the formation of dreams by way of supplement.[1]

Organic illness, painful stimulation or inflammation of an organ, creates a condition which clearly results in a detachment of the libido from its objects. The libido which is withdrawn is found in the ego once more, as an increased cathexis of the diseased part of the body. One may venture to assert, indeed, that the withdrawal of the libido from its objects in these circumstances is more striking than the diversion of egoistic interest from the external world. This seems to offer us a path to an understanding of hypochondria, in which an organ excites the ego's attention in the same way, without being ill so far as we can perceive.

But I shall resist the temptation of going further here or of discussing other situations which can be understood or pictured if we adopt the hypothesis that the object-libido may withdraw into the ego—for I am obliged to meet two objections which, as I know, are now attracting your attention. In the first place

[1] [This had been discussed by Freud at greater length in his 'Metapsychological Supplement to the Theory of Dreams' (1917d [1915]).]

you want to call me to account because in talking of sleep, illness and similar situations I invariably try to separate libido from interest, sexual from ego-instincts, where observations can be fully satisfied by the hypothesis of a single and uniform energy which, being freely mobile, cathects now the object and now the ego, in obedience to one or the other instinct. And in the second place you want to know how I can venture to treat the detaching of the libido from the object as the source of a pathological state, when a transposition of this kind of object-libido into ego-libido (or, more generally, into ego-energy) is among the normal processes of mental dynamics which are repeated daily and every night.

Here is my reply. Your first objection sounds well enough. Consideration of the states of sleep, of illness and of being in love in themselves would probably never have led us to distinguish an ego-libido from an object-libido or libido from interest. But there you are neglecting the investigations from which we started and in the light of which we now look at the mental situations under discussion. The differentiation between libido and interest—that is to say, between the sexual and the self-preservative instincts—was forced upon us by our discovery of the conflict out of which the transference neuroses arise. Since then we cannot give it up. The hypothesis that object-libido can be transformed into ego-libido, that we must therefore take an ego-libido into account, seems to us the only one which is able to resolve the enigma of what are termed the narcissistic neuroses—dementia praecox, for instance—and to account for the resemblances and dissimilarities between them and hysteria or obsessions. We are now applying to illness, sleep and being in love what we have elsewhere found inescapably established. We should proceed further with applications of this kind and see where they will take us to. The only thesis which is not an immediate precipitate of our analytic experience is to the effect that libido remains libido, whether it is directed to objects or to one's own ego, and never turns into egoistic interest, and the converse is also true. This thesis, however, is equivalent to the separation between the sexual and ego-instincts which we have already considered critically and to which we shall continue to hold for heuristic reasons until its possible collapse.

Your second observation, too, raises a justifiable question,

but it is aimed in the wrong direction. It is true that a withdrawal of the object-libido into the ego is not directly pathogenic; it takes place, indeed, as we know, every time before
we go to sleep, only to be reversed when we wake up. The
amoeba withdraws its protrusions only to send them out again
at the first opportunity. But it is quite a different thing when
a particular, very energetic process forces a withdrawal of
libido from objects. Here the libido that has become narcissistic
cannot find its way back to objects, and this interference with
the libido's mobility certainly becomes pathogenic. It seems
that an accumulation of narcissistic libido beyond a certain
amount is not tolerated. We may even imagine that it was for
that very reason that object-cathexes originally came about,
that the ego was obliged to send out its libido so as not to fall
ill as a result of its being dammed up. If it lay within our plan
to go more deeply into dementia praecox, I would show you
that the process which detaches the libido from objects and
cuts off its return to them is closely related to the process of
repression and is to be looked at as its counterpart. But you
would, first and foremost, find yourselves on familiar ground
when you learnt that the determinants of this process are almost
identical—so far as we know at present—with those of repression. The conflict seems to be the same and to be carried on
between the same forces. If the outcome is so different from, for
instance, that in hysteria, the reason can only depend on a
difference in innate disposition. The weak spot in the libidinal
development of these patients lies in a different phase; the
determining fixation, which, as you will recollect [p. 346],
permits the irruption that leads to the formation of symptoms,
lies elsewhere, probably in the stage of primitive narcissism to
which dementia praecox returns in its final outcome. It is very
remarkable that in the case of all the narcissistic neuroses we
have to assume fixation points for the libido going back to far
earlier phases of development than in hysteria or obsessional
neurosis. As you heard, however, the concepts which we arrived
at during our study of the transference neuroses are adequate
in helping us to find our way about in the narcissistic neuroses
which are so much more severe in practice. The conformities go
very far; at bottom the field of phenomena is the same. And
you can imagine how small a prospect anyone has of explaining

these disorders (which belong within the sphere of psychiatry) who is not forearmed for his task with an analytic knowledge of the transference neuroses.

The clinical picture of dementia praecox (which, incidentally, is very changeable) is not determined exclusively by the symptoms arising from the forcing away of the libido from objects and its accumulation in the ego as narcissistic libido. A large part, rather, is played by other phenomena, which are derived from efforts of the libido to attain objects once more and which thus correspond to an attempt at restitution or recovery. These latter symptoms are indeed the more striking and noisy; they exhibit an undeniable resemblance to those of hysteria or, less frequently, of obsessional neurosis, but nevertheless differ from them in every respect. It seems as though in dementia praecox the libido, in its efforts once more to reach objects (that is, the presentations of objects), does in fact snatch hold of something of them, but, as it were, only their shadows—I mean the word-presentations belonging to them. I cannot say more about this now, but I believe that this behaviour of the libido as it strives to find its way back has enabled us to obtain an insight into what really constitutes the difference between a conscious and an unconscious idea.[1]

I have now led you into the region in which the next advances in the work of analysis are to be expected [p. 379]. Since we have ventured to operate with the concept of ego-libido the narcissistic neuroses have become accessible to us; the task before us is to arrive at a dynamic elucidation of these disorders and at the same time to complete our knowledge of mental life by coming to understand the ego. The ego-psychology after which we are seeking must not be based on the data of our self-perceptions but (as in the case of the libido) on the analysis of disturbances and disruptions of the ego. It is likely that we shall have a low opinion of our present knowledge of the vicissitudes

[1] [The view that some of the symptoms in the psychoses represent attempts at recovery was first expressed by Freud in his Schreber analysis (1911c), where an Editor's footnote gives a number of further references. The point, only hinted at here, as to the basic distinction between conscious and unconscious ideas, had been discussed at length in Section VII of the metapsychological paper on the unconscious (1915e).]

of the libido, which we have gained from a study of the transference neuroses, when we have achieved this greater task. But hitherto we have not made much progress with it. The narcissistic neuroses can scarcely be attacked with the technique that has served us with the transference neuroses. You will soon learn why. [Cf. p. 447 below.] What always happens with them is that, after proceeding for a short distance, we come up against a wall which brings us to a stop. Even with the transference neuroses, as you know, we met with barriers of resistance, but we were able to demolish them bit by bit. In the narcissistic neuroses the resistance is unconquerable; at the most, we are able to cast an inquisitive glance over the top of the wall and spy out what is going on on the other side of it. Our technical methods must accordingly be replaced by others; and we do not know yet whether we shall succeed in finding a substitute. Nevertheless, we have no lack of material with these patients either. They make a large number of remarks, even if they do not answer our questions, and for the time being it is our business to interpret these remarks with the help of the understanding we have gained from the symptoms of the transference neuroses. The agreement is great enough to guarantee us some initial advantage. It remains to be seen how far this technique will take us.

There are difficulties in addition which hold up our advance. The narcissistic disorders and the psychoses related to them can only be deciphered by observers who have been trained through the analytic study of the transference neuroses. But our psychiatrists are not students of psycho-analysis and we psycho-analysts see too few psychiatric cases. A race of psychiatrists must first grow up who have passed through the school of psycho-analysis as a preparatory science. A start in that direction is now being made in America, where very many leading psychiatrists lecture to students on the theories of psycho-analysis and where the proprietors of institutions and the directors of insane asylums endeavour to observe their patients in conformity with those theories. Nevertheless we too, over here, have succeeded sometimes in casting a glance over the narcissistic wall, and in what follows I shall tell you a little of what we think we have detected.

The form of disease known as paranoia, chronic systematic insanity, occupies an unsettled position in the attempts at

classification made by present-day psychiatry. There is, however, no doubt of its close affinity to dementia praecox. I once
ventured to suggest that paranoia and dementia praecox should
be brought together under the common designation of 'paraphrenia'.[1] The forms of paranoia are described according to
their content as megalomania, persecution mania, erotomania,
delusions of jealousy, and so on. We shall not expect anything
much in the way of an attempt at an explanation from
psychiatry. Here is an example of one, though, it is true, one
that is out of date and does not carry much weight—an attempt
to derive one symptom from another by means of an intellectual
rationalization: it is suggested that the patient, who, owing to
a primary disposition, believes that he is being persecuted,
infers from his persecution that he must be someone of quite
particular importance and so develops megalomania. According
to our analytic view the megalomania is the direct result of a
magnification of the ego due to the drawing in of the libidinal
object-cathexes—a secondary narcissism which is a return of the
original early infantile one. We have, however, made a few
observations of persecution mania which have induced us to
follow a particular track. The first thing that struck us was that
in the large majority of cases the persecutor was of the same sex
as the persecuted patient. This was still open to an innocent
explanation; but in a few cases that were thoroughly studied
it was clear that the person of the same sex whom the patient
loved most had, since his illness, been turned into his persecutor.
This made a further development possible: namely, the replacement of the beloved person, along the line of familiar resemblances, by someone else—for instance, a father by a schoolmaster
or by some superior. Experiences of this kind in ever increasing
numbers led us to conclude that *paranoia persecutoria* is the
form of the disease in which a person is defending himself
against a homosexual impulse which has become too powerful.[2]
The change over from affection to hatred, which, it is well
known, may become a serious threat to the life of the loved and

[1] [Some comments on Freud's use of this term will be found in
a footnote to his first introduction of it in the last section of the
Schreber analysis (1911*c*).]

[2] [Cf. the third section of Freud's Schreber analysis (1911*c*).]

hated object, corresponds in such cases to the transformation of libidinal impulses into anxiety which is a regular outcome of the process of repression. Listen, for instance, to what is, once again, the most recent instance of my observations in this connection.

A young doctor had to be expelled from the town in which he lived because he had threatened the life of the son of a university professor residing there, who had up till then been his greatest friend. He attributed really fiendish intentions and demonic power to this former friend, whom he regarded as responsible for all the misfortunes that had befallen his family in recent years, for every piece of ill-luck whether in his home or in his social life. But that was not all. He believed that this bad friend and the friend's father, the Professor, had caused the war, too, and brought the Russians into the country. His friend had forfeited his life a thousand times, and our patient was convinced that the criminal's death would put an end to every evil. Yet his affection for him was still so strong that it had paralysed his hand when, on one occasion, he had an opportunity of shooting down his enemy at close range. In the course of the short conversations I had with the patient, it came to light that their friendship went back far into their schooldays. Once at least it had overstepped the bounds of friendship: a night which they had spent together had been an occasion for complete sexual intercourse. Our patient had never acquired the emotional relation to women which would have corresponded to his age and his attractive personality. He had once been engaged to a beautiful young girl of good social position; but she had broken off the engagement because she found that her *fiancé* was without any affection. Years later, his illness broke out just at the moment when he had succeeded for the first time in satisfying a woman completely. When this woman embraced him in gratitude and devotion, he suddenly had a mysterious pain that went round the top of his head like a sharp cut. Later on he interpreted this sensation as though an incision were being made at an autopsy for exposing the brain. And as his friend had become a pathological anatomist, it slowly dawned on him that he alone could have sent this last woman to him to seduce him. From that point onwards his eyes were opened to the other persecutions to which he believed he had been made a victim by the machinations of his one-time friend.

But what about the cases in which the persecutor is not of the same sex as the patient and which appear, therefore, to contradict our explanation of their being a defence against homosexual libido? A little time ago I had an opportunity of examining such a case and was able to derive a confirmation from the apparent contradiction. A girl, who believed she was being persecuted by a man with whom she had had affectionate assignations on two occasions, had in fact first had a delusion that was directed against a woman who could be looked on as a substitute for her mother. It was only after her second assignation that she took the step of detaching the delusion from the woman and transferring it to the man. To begin with, therefore, the precondition of the persecutor being of the same sex as the patient was fulfilled in this case too. In making a complaint to a lawyer and to a doctor, the patient made no mention of this preliminary stage of her delusion and thus gave rise to an appearance of there being a contradiction of our explanation of paranoia.[1]

Homosexual object-choice originally lies closer to narcissism than does the heterosexual kind. When it is a question, therefore, of repelling an undesirably strong homosexual impulse, the path back to narcissism is made particularly easy. Hitherto I have had very little opportunity of talking to you about the foundations of erotic life so far as we have discovered them, and it is too late now to catch up on the omission. This much, however, I can emphasize to you. Object-choice, the step forward in the development of the libido which is made after the narcissistic stage, can take place according to two different types: either according to the *narcissistic type*, where the subject's own ego is replaced by another one that is as similar as possible, or according to the *attachment type*,[2] where people who have become precious through satisfying the other vital needs are chosen as objects by the libido as well. A strong libidinal

---

[1] [The case had been reported in full by Freud not long before (1915*f*).]

[2] ['*Anlehnungstypus.*' This has sometimes been translated '*anaclitic type*'. This is fully discussed in the second section of Freud's paper on narcissism (1914*c*), Cf. above, p. 329.]

fixation to the narcissistic type of object-choice is to be included in the predisposition to manifest homosexuality.

You will recall that at our first meeting of the present academic year I described a case to you of a woman suffering from delusions of jealousy [p. 248]. Now that we are so near its end you would no doubt like to hear how delusions are explained by psycho-analysis. But I have less to tell you about that than you expect. The fact that a delusion cannot be shaken by logical arguments or real experiences is explained in the same way as in the case of an obsession—by its relation to the unconscious, which is represented and held down by the delusion or by the obsession. The difference between the two is based on the difference between the topography and dynamics of the two illnesses.

As with paranoia, so also with melancholia (of which, incidentally, many different clinical forms have been described) we have found a point at which it has become possible to obtain some insight into the internal structure of the disease. We have discovered that the self-reproaches, with which these melancholic patients torment themselves in the most merciless fashion, in fact apply to another person, the sexual object which they have lost or which has become valueless to them through its own fault. From this we can conclude that the melancholic has, it is true, withdrawn his libido from the object, but that, by a process which we must call 'narcissistic identification', the object has been set up in the ego itself, has been, as it were, projected on to the ego. (Here I can only give you a pictorial description and not an ordered account on topographical and dynamic lines.)[1] The subject's own ego is then treated like the object that has been abandoned, and it is subjected to all the acts of aggression and expressions of vengefulness which have been aimed at the object. A melancholic's propensity to suicide is also made more intelligible if we consider that the patient's embitterment strikes with a single blow at his own ego and at the loved and hated object. In melancholia, as well as in other narcissistic disorders, a particular trait in the patient's emotional life emerges with peculiar emphasis—what, since Bleuler, we have been accustomed to describe as 'ambivalence'. By this

[1] [A full account is given in 'Mourning and Melancholia' (1917e [1915]).]

we mean the direction towards the same person of contrary—affectionate and hostile—feelings.[1] Unluckily I have been unable in the course of these lectures to tell you more about this emotional ambivalence. [Cf. p. 443.]

In addition to narcissistic identification, there is a hysterical kind, which has been familiar to us very much longer.[2] I wish it were possible to illustrate for you the differences between the two forms by a few clear specifications. There is something I can tell you about the periodic and cyclical forms of melancholia which I am sure you will be glad to hear. For in favourable circumstances—I have experienced this twice—it is possible by analytic treatment in the lucid intervals to prevent the return of the condition in the same or the opposite emotional mood. We learn from such cases that in melancholia and mania we are concerned once more with a special method of dealing with a conflict whose underlying determinants agree precisely with those of the other neuroses. You can imagine how much more there is for psycho-analysis to learn in this field of knowledge.

I told you too [p. 415] that we hoped that the analysis of the narcissistic disorders would give us an insight into the way in which our ego is put together and built up out of different agencies. We have already made a start with this at one point.[3] From the analysis of delusions of observation we have drawn the conclusion that there actually exists in the ego an agency which unceasingly observes, criticizes and compares, and in that way sets itself over against the other part of the ego. We believe, therefore, that the patient is betraying a truth to us which is not yet sufficiently appreciated when he complains that he is spied upon and observed at every step he takes and that every one of his thoughts is reported and criticized. His

[1] [Some discussion of Freud's use of the term will be found in an Editor's footnote to 'Instincts and their Vicissitudes' (1915c).]

[2] [An early account of hysterical identification occurs in the course of the fourth chapter of The Interpretation of Dreams (1900a). The distinction between the two kinds of identification is explained in the early part of 'Mourning and Melancholia'.]

[3] [For what follows see the third section of 'On Narcissism' (1914c). The later development of these ideas is discussed in the Editor's Introduction to The Ego and the Id (1923b), (Norton, 1960).]

only mistake is in regarding this uncomfortable power as something alien to him and placing it outside himself. He senses an agency holding sway in his ego which measures his actual ego and each of its activities by an *ideal ego* that he has created for himself in the course of his development. We believe, too, that this creation was made with the intention of re-establishing the self-satisfaction which was attached to primary infantile narcissism but which since then has suffered so many disturbances and mortifications. We know the self-observing agency as the ego-censor,[1] the conscience; it is this that exercises the dream-censorship during the night, from which the repressions of inadmissible wishful impulses proceed. When in delusions of observation it becomes split up, it reveals to us its origin from the influences of parents, educators and social environment—from an identification with some of these model figures.

These are a few of the findings which have hitherto been reached from the application of psycho-analysis to the narcissistic disorders. No doubt there are not yet enough of them and they still lack the precision which can only be attained from established familiarity with a new field. We owe all of them to a use of the concept of ego-libido or narcissistic libido, by whose help we can extend to the narcissistic neuroses the views which have proved their value with the transference neuroses. Now, however, you will ask whether it is possible that we shall succeed in subsuming all the disturbances of the narcissistic illnesses and of the psychoses under the libido theory, whether we look upon the libidinal factor in mental life as universally guilty of the causation of illness, and need never attribute the responsibility for it to changes in the functioning of the self-preservative instinct. Well, Ladies and Gentlemen, this question seems to me to call for no urgent reply, and, above all, not to be ripe for judgement. We can confidently leave it over in expectation of the progress of our scientific work. I should not be surprised if it turned out that the power to produce pathogenic

---

[1] [The German form used here is the personal *'Zensor'* in contrast to the impersonal *'Zensur'* in the next part of the sentence, which is the form almost invariably adopted by Freud. Other instances of this very exceptional form occur in the 'Secondary Revision' of Chapter VI of *The Interpretation of Dreams* (1900a), in the paper on narcissism (1914c), and in the *New Introductory Lectures*, p. 479.]

effects was in fact a prerogative of the libidinal instincts, so that the libido theory could celebrate its triumph all along the line from the simplest 'actual' neurosis to the most severe alienation of the personality. We after all know that it is a characteristic feature of the libido that it struggles against submitting to the reality of the universe—to Ananke [p. 355]. But I regard it as extremely probable that the ego-instincts are carried along secondarily by the pathogenic instigation of the libido and forced into functional disturbances. Nor can I think that it would be a disaster to the trend of our researches, if what lies before us is the discovery that in severe psychoses the ego-instincts themselves have gone astray as a primary fact. The future will give the answer—to you, at any rate.

Let me once more, however, return for a moment to anxiety, to throw light on a last obscurity that we left there. I have said [p. 411] that there is something that does not tally with the relation (so thoroughly recognized apart from this) between anxiety and libido: the fact, namely, that realistic anxiety in face of a danger seems to be a manifestation of the self-preserva-tive instinct—which, after all, can scarcely be disputed. How would it be, though, if what was responsible for the affect of anxiety was not the egoistic ego-instincts but the ego-libido? After all, the state of anxiety is in every instance inexpedient, and its inexpedience becomes obvious if it reaches a fairly high pitch. In such cases it interferes with action, whether flight or defence, which alone is expedient and alone serves the cause of self-preservation. If, therefore, we attribute the affective portion of realistic anxiety to ego-libido and the accompanying action to the self-preservative instinct, we shall have got rid of the theoretical difficulty. After all, you do not seriously believe that one runs away because one feels anxiety? No. One feels anxiety and one runs away for a common motive, which is roused by the perception of danger. People who have been through a great mortal danger tell us that they were not at all afraid but merely acted—for instance, that they aimed their rifle at the wild beast—and that is unquestionably what was most expedient.

LECTURE XXVII

TRANSFERENCE[1]

LADIES AND GENTLEMEN,—Since we are now drawing towards the end of our discussions, there is a particular expectation which will be in your minds and which should not be disappointed. You no doubt suppose that I would not have led you through thick and thin of the subject-matter of psycho-analysis only to dismiss you at the end without saying a word about therapy, on which, after all, the possibility of practising psychoanalysis at all is based. The subject, moreover, is one that I cannot withhold from you, since what you learn in connection with it will enable you to make the acquaintance of a new fact in whose absence your understanding of the illnesses investigated by us will remain most markedly incomplete.

You do not, I know, expect me to initiate you into the technique by which analysis for therapeutic ends should be carried out. You only want to know in the most general way the method by which psycho-analytic therapy operates and what, roughly, it accomplishes. And you have an indisputable right to learn this. I shall not, however, tell it you but shall insist on your discovering it for yourselves.

Think it over! You have learnt all that is essential about the determinants of falling ill as well as all the factors that come into effect *after* the patient has fallen ill. Where do these leave room for any therapeutic influence? In the first place there is hereditary disposition. We have not talked about it very often because it is emphatically stressed from other directions and we have

[1] [Freud first broached the idea of transference in his technical contribution to the Breuer and Freud *Studies on Hysteria* (1895d). He returned to it in his 'Dora' analysis (1905e). But his main discussions of the subject before the present one will be found in his papers on technique: in particular 'The Dynamics of Transference' (1912b) deals with the theoretical side of the phenomenon, while 'Observations on Transference-Love' (1915a) is concerned with the technical difficulties raised by the positive transference. Towards the end of his life Freud approached the subject once more in 'Analysis Terminable and Interminable' (1937c).]

nothing new to say about it. But do not suppose that we under-
estimate it; precisely as therapists we come to realize its power
clearly enough. In any case we can do nothing to alter it; we
too must take it as something given, which sets a limit to our
efforts. Next there is the influence of early experiences in childhood, to which we are in the habit of giving prominence in
analysis: they belong to the past and we cannot undo them.
Then comes everything that we have summarized as 'real
frustration'—the misfortunes of life from which arise deprivation of love, poverty, family quarrels, ill-judged choice of a
partner in marriage, unfavourable social circumstances, and
the strictness of the ethical standards to whose pressure the
individual is subject. Here, to be sure, there would be handles
enough for a very effective therapy, but it would have to be of
the kind which Viennese folklore attributes to the Emperor
Joseph[1]—the benevolent interference of a powerful personage
before whose will people bow and difficulties vanish. But who
are we, that we should be able to adopt benevolence of this
kind as an instrument of our therapy? Poor ourselves and
socially powerless, and compelled to earn our livelihood from
our medical activity, we are not even in a position to extend our
efforts to people without means, as other doctors with other
methods of treatment are after all able to do. Our therapy is
too time-consuming and too laborious for that to be possible.
Perhaps, however, you are clutching at one of the factors I
have mentioned and believe that there you have found the
point at which our influence can make its attack. If the ethical
restrictions demanded by society play a part in the deprivation
imposed on the patient, treatment can, after all, give him the
courage, or perhaps a direct injunction, to disregard those
barriers and achieve satisfaction and recovery while forgoing
the fulfilment of an ideal that is exalted, but so often not
adhered to, by society. The patient will thus become healthy
by 'living a full life' sexually. This, it is true, casts a shadow on
analytic treatment for not serving general morality. What it has
given to the individual it will have taken from the community.

But, Ladies and Gentlemen, who has so seriously misinformed you? A recommendation to the patient to 'live a full life'

[1] [Joseph II, whose unconventional methods of distributing charity
were notorious.]

sexually could not possibly play a part in analytic therapy—if only because we ourselves have declared that an obstinate conflict is taking place in him between a libidinal impulse and sexual repression, between a sensual and an ascetic trend. This conflict would not be solved by our helping one of these trends to victory over its opponent. We see, indeed, that in neurotics asceticism has the upper hand; and the consequence of this is precisely that the suppressed sexual tendency finds a way out in symptoms. If, on the contrary, we were to secure victory for sensuality, then the sexual repression that had been put on one side would necessarily be replaced by symptoms. Neither of these two alternative decisions could end the internal conflict; in either case one party to it would remain unsatisfied. There are only a few cases in which the conflict is so unstable that a factor such as the doctor's taking sides could decide it; and such cases do not in fact stand in need of analytic treatment. Anyone on whom the doctor could have so much influence would have found the same way out without the doctor. You must be aware that if an abstinent young man decides in favour of illicit sexual intercourse or if an unsatisfied wife seeks relief with another man, they have not as a rule waited for permission from a doctor or even from their analyst.

In this connection people usually overlook the one essential point—that the pathogenic conflict in neurotics is not to be confused with a normal struggle between mental impulses both of which are on the same psychological footing. In the former case the dissension is between two powers, one of which has made its way to the stage of what is preconscious or conscious while the other has been held back at the stage of the unconscious. For that reason the conflict cannot be brought to an issue; the disputants can no more come to grips than, in the familiar simile, a polar bear and a whale. A true decision can only be reached when they both meet on the same ground. To make this possible is, I think, the sole task of our therapy.

Moreover, I can assure you that you are misinformed if you suppose that advice and guidance in the affairs of life play an integral part in analytic influence. On the contrary, so far as possible we avoid the role of a mentor such as this, and there is nothing we would rather bring about than that the patient should make his decisions for himself. With this purpose, too, we require him to postpone for the term of his treatment any vital decisions on choice of a profession, business undertakings, marriage or divorce, and only to put them in practice when the treatment is finished. You must admit that all this is different from what you pictured. Only in the case of some very youthful or quite helpless or unstable individuals are we unable to put the desired limitation of our role into effect. With them we have to combine the functions of a doctor and an educator; but when this is so we are quite conscious of our responsibility and behave with the necessary caution.[1]

But you must not conclude from my eagerness in defending myself against the charge that neurotics are encouraged in analytic treatment to live a full life—you must not conclude from this that we influence them in favour of conventional virtue. That is at least as far from being the case. It is true that we are not reformers but merely observers; nevertheless, we cannot help observing with a critical eye and we have found it impossible to side with conventional sexual morality or to form a very high opinion of the manner in which society attempts the practical regulation of the problems of sexual life. We can present society with a blunt calculation that what is described as its morality calls for a bigger sacrifice than it is worth and that its proceedings are not based on honesty and do not display wisdom. We do not keep such criticisms from our patients' ears, we accustom them to giving unprejudiced consideration to sexual matters no less than to any others; and if, having grown independent after the completion of their treatment, they decide on their own judgement in favour of some midway position between living a full life and absolute asceticism, we feel our conscience clear whatever their choice. We tell ourselves that anyone who has succeeded in educating himself to truth about himself is permanently defended against the danger of immorality, even though his standard of morality may differ in some respect from that which is customary in society. Moreover, we must guard against over-estimating the importance of the part played by the question of abstinence in influencing neuroses. Only in a minority of cases can the pathogenic situation of frustration and the subsequent damming-up of libido be

1 [Freud discusses this further in the *New Introductory Lectures*, p. 612.]

brought to an end by the sort of sexual intercourse that can be procured without much trouble.

Thus you cannot explain the therapeutic effect of psycho-analysis by its permitting a full sexual life. Look around, then, for something else. I fancy that, while I was rejecting this suggestion of yours, one remark of mine put you on the right track. What we make use of must no doubt be the replacing of what is unconscious by what is conscious, the translation of what is unconscious into what is conscious. Yes, that is it. By carrying what is unconscious on into what is conscious, we lift the repressions, we remove the preconditions for the formation of symptoms, we transform the pathogenic conflict into a normal one for which it must be possible somehow to find a solution. All that we bring about in a patient is this single psychical change: the length to which it is carried is the measure of the help we provide. Where no repressions (or analogous psychical processes) can be undone, our therapy has nothing to expect.

We can express the aim of our efforts in a variety of formulas: making conscious what is unconscious, lifting repressions, filling gaps in the memory—all these amount to the same thing. But perhaps you will be dissatisfied by this admission. You had formed a different picture of the return to health of a neurotic patient—that, after submitting to the tedious labours of a psycho-analysis, he would become another man; but the total result, so it seems, is that he has rather less that is unconscious and rather more that is conscious in him than he had before. The fact is that you are probably under-estimating the importance of an internal change of this kind. The neurotic who is cured has really become another man, though at bottom, of course, he has remained the same; that is to say, he has become what he might have become at best under the most favourable conditions. But that is a very great deal. If you now hear all that has to be done and what efforts it needs to bring about this apparently trivial change in a man's mental life, you will no doubt begin to realize the importance of this difference in psychical levels.

I will digress for a moment to ask if you know what is meant by a causal therapy. That is how we describe a procedure which does not take the symptoms of an illness as its point of attack but sets about removing its *causes*. Well, then, is our psycho-analytic method a causal therapy or not? The reply is not a simple one, but it may perhaps give us an opportunity of realizing the worthlessness of a question framed in this way. In so far as analytic therapy does not make it its first task to remove the symptoms, it is behaving like a causal therapy. In another respect, you may say, it is not. For we long ago traced the causal chain back through the repressions to the instinctual dispositions, their relative intensities in the constitution and the deviations in the course of their development. Supposing, now, that it was possible, by some chemical means, perhaps, to interfere in this mechanism, to increase or diminish the quantity of libido present at a given time or to strengthen one instinct at the cost of another—this then would be a causal therapy in the true sense of the word, for which our analysis would have carried out the indispensable preliminary work of reconnaissance. At present, as you know, there is no question of any such method of influencing libidinal processes; with our psychical therapy we attack at a different point in the combination—not exactly at what we know are the roots of the phenomena, but nevertheless far enough away from the symptoms, at a point which has been made accessible to us by some very remarkable circumstances.

What, then, must we do in order to replace what is unconscious in our patients by what is conscious? There was a time when we thought this was a very simple matter: all that was necessary was for us to discover this unconscious material and communicate it to the patient. But we know already that this was a short-sighted error [p. 281]. *Our* knowledge about the unconscious material is not equivalent to *his* knowledge; if we communicate our knowledge to him, he does not receive it *instead of* his unconscious material but *beside* it; and that makes very little change in it. We must rather picture this unconscious material topographically, we must look for it in his memory at the place where it became unconscious owing to a repression. The repression must be got rid of—after which the substitution of the conscious material for the unconscious can proceed smoothly. How, then, do we lift a repression of this kind? Here our task enters a second phase. First, the search for the repression and then the removal of the resistance which maintains the repression.

How do we remove the resistance? In the same way: by discovering it and showing it to the patient. Indeed, the resistance too is derived from a repression—from the same one that we are endeavouring to resolve, or from one that took place earlier. It was set up by the anticathexis which arose in order to repress the objectionable impulse. Thus we now do the same thing that we tried to do to begin with: interpret, discover and communicate; but now we are doing it at the right place. The anticathexis or the resistance does not form part of the unconscious but of the ego, which is our collaborator, and is so even if it is not conscious. As we know, the word 'unconscious' is being used here in two senses: on the one hand as a phenomenon and on the other as a system. This sounds very difficult and obscure; but is it not only repeating what we have already said in earlier passages?[1] We have long been prepared for it. We expect that this resistance will be given up and the anticathexis withdrawn when our interpretation has made it possible for the ego to recognize it. What are the motive forces that we work with in such a case? First with the patient's desire for recovery, which has induced him to take part with us in our joint work, and secondly with the help of his intelligence, to which we give support by our interpretation. There is no doubt that it is easier for the patient's intelligence to recognize the resistance and to find the translation corresponding to what is repressed if we have previously given him the appropriate anticipatory ideas. If I say to you: 'Look up at the sky! There's a balloon there!' you will discover it much more easily than if I simply tell you to look up and see if you can see anything. In the same way, a student who is looking through a microscope for the first time is instructed by his teacher as to what he will see; otherwise he does not see it at all, though it is there and visible.

And now for the fact![2] In a whole number of nervous diseases—in hysteria, anxiety states, obsessional neurosis—our

---

[1] [See the Editor's footnote 1 on p. 227 above, where these earlier passages are enumerated and references are given to Freud's later, revised views on the subject.]

[2] [See the opening paragraph of the lecture, p. 431.]

expectation is fulfilled. By searching for the repression in this way, by uncovering the resistances, by pointing out what is repressed, we really succeed in accomplishing our task—that is, in overcoming the resistances, lifting the repression and transforming the unconscious material into conscious. In doing so we gain the clearest impression of the way in which a violent struggle takes place in the patient's mind about the overcoming of each resistance—a *normal* mental struggle, on the same psychological ground, between the motives which seek to maintain the anticathexis and those which are prepared to give it up. The former are the old motives which in the past put the repression into effect; among the latter are the newly arrived ones which, we may hope, will decide the conflict in our favour. We have succeeded in reviving the old conflict which led to repression and in bringing up for revision the process that was then decided. The new material that we produce includes, first, the reminder that the earlier decision led to illness and the promise that a different path will lead to recovery, and, secondly, the enormous change in all the circumstances that has taken place since the time of the original rejection. Then the ego was feeble, infantile, and may perhaps have had grounds for banning the demands of the libido as a danger. To-day it has grown strong and experienced, and moreover has a helper at hand in the shape of the doctor. Thus we may expect to lead the revived conflict to a better outcome than that which ended in repression, and, as I have said, in hysteria and in the anxiety and obsessional neuroses success proves us in general to be correct.

There are, however, other forms of illness in which, in spite of the conditions being the same, our therapeutic procedure is never successful. In them, too, it had been a question of an original conflict between the ego and the libido which led to repression—though this may call for a different topographical description; in them, too, it is possible to trace the points in the patient's life at which the repressions occurred; we make use of the same procedure, are ready to make the same promises and give the same help by the offer of anticipatory ideas; and once again the lapse of time between the repressions and the present day favours a different outcome to the conflict. And yet we do not succeed in lifting a single resistance or getting rid of a single repression. These patients, paranoics, melancholics,

sufferers from dementia praecox, remain on the whole un-
affected and proof against psycho-analytic therapy. What can
be the reason for this? Not any lack of intelligence. A certain
amount of intellectual capacity is naturally required in our
patients; but there is certainly no lack of it in, for instance, the
extremely shrewd combinatory paranoics [cf. p. 66 f.]. Nor do
any of the other motives seem to be absent. Thus the melancholics have a very high degree of consciousness, absent in
paranoics, that they are ill and that that is why they suffer so
much; but this does not make them more accessible. We are
faced here by a fact which we do not understand and which
therefore leads us to doubt whether we have really understood
all the determinants of our possible success with the other
neuroses.

If we continue to concern ourselves only with our hysterics
and obsessional neurotics, we are soon met by a second fact for
which we were not in the least prepared. For after a while we
cannot help noticing that these patients behave in a quite
peculiar manner to us. We believed, to be sure, that we had
reckoned with all the motives concerned in the treatment, that
we had completely rationalized the situation between us and
the patients so that it could be looked over at a glance like a
sum in arithmetic; yet, in spite of all this, something seems to
creep in which has not been taken into account in our sum.
This unexpected novelty itself takes many shapes, and I will
begin by describing to you the commoner and more easily
understandable of the forms in which it appears.

We notice, then, that the patient, who ought to want nothing
else but to find a way out of his distressing conflicts, develops a
special interest in the person of the doctor. Everything connected with the doctor seems to be more important to him than
his own affairs and to be diverting him from his illness. For a
time, accordingly, relations with him become very agreeable;
he is particularly obliging, tries wherever possible to show his
gratitude, reveals refinements and merits in his nature which we
should not, perhaps, have expected to find in him. The doctor,
too, thereupon forms a favourable opinion of the patient and
appreciates the good fortune which has enabled him to give his
assistance to such a particularly valuable personality. If the
doctor has an opportunity of talking to the patient's relatives,

he learns to his satisfaction that the liking is a mutual one. The patient never tires in his home of praising the doctor and of extolling ever new qualities in him. 'He's enthusiastic about you,' say his relatives, 'he trusts you blindly; everything you say is like a revelation to him.' Here and there someone in this chorus has sharper eyes and says: 'It's becoming a bore, the way he talks of nothing else but you and has your name on his lips all the time.'

Let us hope that the doctor is modest enough to attribute his patient's high opinion of him to the hopes he can rouse in him and to the widening of his intellectual horizon by the surprising and liberating enlightenment that the treatment brings with it. Under these conditions the analysis makes fine progress too. The patient understands what is interpreted to him and becomes engrossed in the tasks set him by the treatment; the material of memories and associations floods in upon him in plenty, the certainty and appositeness of his interpretations are a surprise to the doctor, and the latter can only take note with satisfaction that here is a patient who readily accepts all the psychological novelties which are apt to provoke the most bitter contradiction among healthy people in the outside world. Moreover the cordial relations that prevail during the work of analysis are accompanied by an objective improvement, which is recognized on all sides, in the patient's illness.

But such fine weather cannot last for ever. One day it clouds over. Difficulties arise in the treatment; the patient declares that nothing more occurs to him. He gives the clearest impression of his interest being no longer in the work and of his cheerfully disregarding the instructions given him to say everything that comes into his head and not to give way to any critical obstacle to doing so. He behaves as though he were outside the treatment and as though he had not made this agreement with the doctor. He is evidently occupied with something, but intends to keep it to himself. This is a situation that is dangerous for the treatment. We are unmistakably confronted by a formidable resistance. But what has happened to account for it?

If we are able once more to clarify the position, we find that the cause of the disturbance is that the patient has transferred on to the doctor intense feelings of affection which are justified neither by the doctor's behaviour nor by the situation that has developed during the treatment. The form in which this affection is expressed and what its aims are depend of course on the personal relation between the two people involved. If those concerned are a young girl and a youngish man, we shall get the impression of a normal case of falling in love; we shall find it understandable that a girl should fall in love with a man with whom she can be much alone and talk of intimate things and who has the advantage of having met her as a helpful superior; and we shall probably overlook the fact that what we should expect from a neurotic girl would rather be an impediment in her capacity for love. The further the personal relations between doctor and patient diverge from this supposed case, the more we shall be surprised to find nevertheless the same emotional relationship constantly recurring. It may still pass muster if a woman who is unhappy in her marriage appears to be seized with a serious passion for a doctor who is still unattached, if she is ready to seek a divorce in order to be his, or if, where there are social obstacles, she even expresses no hesitation about entering into a secret *liaison* with him. Such things come about even outside psycho-analysis. But in these circumstances we are astonished to hear declarations by married women and girls which bear witness to a quite particular attitude to the therapeutic problem: they had always known, they say, that they could only be cured by love, and before the treatment began they had expected that through this relation they would at last be granted what life had hitherto withheld from them; it had only been in this hope that they had taken so much trouble over the treatment and overcome all the difficulties in communicating their thoughts—and we on our part can add: and had so easily understood what is otherwise so hard to believe. But an admission of this sort surprises us: it throws all our calculations to the winds. Can it be that we have left the most important item out of our account?

And indeed, the greater our experience the less we are able to resist making this correction, though having to do so puts our scientific pretensions to shame. On the first few occasions one might perhaps think that the analytic treatment had come up against a disturbance due to a chance event—an event, that is, not intended and not provoked by it. But when a similar affectionate attachment by the patient to the doctor is repeated regularly in every new case, when it comes to light again and again, under the most unfavourable conditions and where there are positively grotesque incongruities, even in elderly women and in relation to grey-bearded men, even where, in our judgement, there is nothing of any kind to entice—then we must abandon the idea of a chance disturbance and recognize that we are dealing with a phenomenon which is intimately bound up with the nature of the illness itself.

This new fact, which we thus recognize so unwillingly, is known by us as *transference*. We mean a transference of feelings on to the person of the doctor, since we do not believe that the situation in the treatment could justify the development of such feelings. We suspect, on the contrary, that the whole readiness for these feelings is derived from elsewhere, that they were already prepared in the patient and, upon the opportunity offered by the analytic treatment, are transferred on to the person of the doctor. Transference can appear as a passionate demand for love or in more moderate forms; in place of a wish to be loved, a wish can emerge between a girl and an old man to be received as a favourite daughter; the libidinal desire can be toned down into a proposal for an inseparable, but ideally non-sensual, friendship. Some women succeed in sublimating the transference and in moulding it till it achieves a kind of viability; others must express it in its crude, original, and for the most part, impossible form. But at bottom it is always the same, and never allows its origin from the same source to be mistaken.

Before we enquire where we are to find a place for this new fact, I will complete my description of it. What happens with male patients? There at least one might hope to escape the troublesome interference caused by difference of sex and by sexual attraction. Our answer, however, must be much the same as in the case of women. There is the same attachment to the doctor, the same overvaluation of his qualities, the same absorption in his interests, the same jealousy of everyone close to him in real life. The sublimated forms of transference are more frequent between one man and another and straightforward sexual demands are rarer, in proportion as manifest homosexuality is unusual as compared with the other ways in which these instinctual components are employed. With his male patients, again, more often than with women, the doctor comes across a form of expression of the transference which seems at first sight to contradict all our previous descriptions— a hostile or *negative* transference.

I must begin by making it clear that a transference is present in the patient from the beginning of the treatment and for a while is the most powerful motive in its advance. We see no trace of it and need not bother about it so long as it operates in favour of the joint work of analysis. If it then changes into a resistance, we must turn our attention to it and we recognize that it alters its relation to the treatment under two different and contrary conditions: firstly, if as an affectionate trend it has become so powerful, and betrays signs of its origin in a sexual need so clearly, that it inevitably provokes an internal opposition to itself, and, secondly, if it consists of hostile instead of affectionate impulses. The hostile feelings make their appearance as a rule later than the affectionate ones and behind them; their simultaneous presence gives a good picture of the emotional ambivalence [p. 427 f.] which is dominant in the majority of our intimate relations with other people. The hostile feelings are as much an indication of an emotional tie as the affectionate ones, in the same way as defiance signifies dependence as much as obedience does, though with a 'minus' instead of a 'plus' sign before it. We can be in no doubt that the hostile feelings towards the doctor deserve to be called a 'transference', since the situation in the treatment quite certainly offers no adequate grounds for their origin; this necessary view of the negative transference assures us, therefore, that we have not gone wrong in our judgement of the positive or affectionate one.

Where the transference arises, what difficulties it raises for us, how we overcome them and what advantages we eventually derive from it—these are questions to be dealt with in detail in a technical guide to analysis, and I shall only touch on them lightly to-day. It is out of the question for us to yield to the patient's demands deriving from the transference; it would be absurd for us to reject them in an unfriendly, still more in an indignant, manner. We overcome the transference by pointing out to the patient that his feelings do not arise from the present situation and do not apply to the person of the doctor, but that they are repeating something that happened to him earlier.[1] In this way we oblige him to transform his repetition into a memory. By that means the transference, which, whether affectionate or hostile, seemed in every case to constitute the greatest threat to the treatment, becomes its best tool, by whose help the most secret compartments of mental life can be opened.

But I should like to say a few words to you to relieve you of your surprise at the emergence of this unexpected phenomenon. We must not forget that the patient's illness, which we have undertaken to analyse, is not something which has been rounded off and become rigid but that it is still growing and developing like a living organism. The beginning of the treatment does not put an end to this development; when, however, the treatment has obtained mastery over the patient, what happens is that the whole of his illness's new production is concentrated upon a single point—his relation to the doctor. Thus the transference may be compared to the cambium layer in a tree between the wood and the bark, from which the new formation of tissue and the increase in the girth of the trunk derive. When the transference has risen to this significance, work upon the patient's memories retreats far into the background. Thereafter it is not incorrect to say that we are no longer concerned with the patient's earlier illness but with a newly created and transformed neurosis which has taken the former's place. We have followed this new edition of the old disorder from its start, we have observed its origin and growth, and we are especially well able to find our way about in it since, as its object, we are situated at its very centre. All the patient's symptoms have abandoned their original meaning and have taken on a new sense which lies in a relation to the transference; or only such symptoms have persisted as are capable of undergoing such a transformation. But the mastering of this new, artificial neurosis coincides with getting rid of the illness which was originally brought to the treatment—with the accomplishment of our therapeutic task. A person who has become normal and free from the operation of repressed instinctual impulses in his rela-

[1] [Cf. for what follows here 'Remembering, Repeating and Working-Through' (1914g).]

tion to the doctor will remain so in his own life after the doctor has once more withdrawn from it.[1]

The transference possesses this extraordinary, and for the treatment, positively central, importance in hysteria, anxiety hysteria and obsessional neurosis, which are for that reason rightly classed together as 'transference neuroses'. No one who has taken in a full impression of the fact of transference from his analytic work will any longer doubt the nature of the suppressed impulses that obtain expression in the symptoms of these neuroses, and will call for no more powerful evidence of their libidinal character. It may be said that our conviction of the significance of symptoms as substitutive satisfactions of the libido only received its final confirmation after the enlistment of the transference.

There is every reason now for us to improve our earlier dynamic account of the therapeutic process and to bring it into harmony with our new realization. If the patient is to fight his way through the normal conflict with the resistances which we have uncovered for him in the analysis [p. 438], he is in need of a powerful stimulus which will influence the decision in the sense which we desire, leading to recovery. Otherwise it might happen that he would choose in favour of repeating the earlier outcome and would allow what had been brought up into consciousness to slip back again into repression. At this point what turns the scale in his struggle is not his intellectual insight—which is neither strong enough nor free enough for such an achievement—but simply and solely his relation to the doctor. In so far as his transference bears a 'plus' sign, it clothes the doctor with authority and is transformed into belief in his communications and explanations. In the absence of such a transference, or if it is a negative one, the patient would never even give a hearing to the doctor and his arguments. In this his belief is repeating the story of its own development; it is a derivative of love and, to start with, needed no arguments. Only later did he allow them enough room to submit them to examination, provided they were brought forward by someone he loved. Without such supports arguments carried no weight, and in

[1] [It may be remarked that Freud very much qualified this assertion in his late technical paper on 'Analysis Terminable and Interminable' (1937c). Cf. the Editor's Note to this.]

most people's lives they never do. Thus in general a man is only accessible from the intellectual side too, in so far as he is capable of a libidinal cathexis of objects; and we have good reason to recognize and to dread in the amount of his narcissism a barrier against the possibility of being influenced by even the best analytic technique.

A capacity for directing libidinal object-cathexes on to people must of course be attributed to every normal person. The tendency to transference of the neurotics I have spoken of is only an extraordinary increase of this universal characteristic. It would indeed be very strange if a human trait so widespread and so important had never been noticed or appreciated. And in fact it *has* been. Bernheim, with an unerring eye, based his theory of hypnotic phenomena on the thesis that everyone is in some way 'suggestible'. His suggestibility was nothing other than the tendency to transference, somewhat too narrowly conceived, so that it did not include negative transference. But Bernheim was never able to say what suggestion actually was and how it came about. For him it was a fundamental fact on whose origin he could throw no light. He did not know that his '*suggestibilité*' depended on sexuality, on the activity of the libido. And it must dawn on us that in our technique we have abandoned hypnosis only to rediscover suggestion in the shape of transference.

But here I will pause, and let you have a word; for I see an objection boiling up in you so fiercely that it would make you incapable of listening if it were not put into words: 'Ah! so you've admitted it at last! You work with the help of suggestion, just like the hypnotists! That is what we've thought for a long time. But, if so, why the roundabout road by way of memories of the past, discovering the unconscious, interpreting and translating back distortions—this immense expenditure of labour, time and money—when the one effective thing is after all only suggestion? Why do you not make direct suggestions against the symptoms, as the others do—the honest hypnotists? Moreover, if you try to excuse yourself for your long détour on the ground that you have made a number of important psychological discoveries which are hidden by direct suggestion—what about the certainty of these discoveries now? Are not they a result of suggestion too, of unintentional suggestion? Is it not possible that you are forcing on the patient what you want and what seems to you correct, in this field as well?'

What you are throwing up at me in this is uncommonly interesting and must be answered. But I cannot do so to-day: we have not the time. Till our next meeting, then. I will answer you, you will see. But to-day I must finish what I have begun. I promised to make you understand by the help of the fact of transference why our therapeutic efforts have no success with the narcissistic neuroses.

I can do so in a few words, and you will see how simply the riddle can be solved and how well everything fits together. Observation shows that sufferers from narcissistic neuroses have no capacity for transference or only insufficient residues of it. They reject the doctor, not with hostility but with indifference. For that reason they cannot be influenced by him either; what he says leaves them cold, makes no impression on them; consequently the mechanism of cure which we carry through with other people—the revival of the pathogenic conflict and the overcoming of the resistance due to repression—cannot be operated with them. They remain as they are. Often they have already undertaken attempts at recovery on their own account which have led to pathological results [p. 422]. We cannot alter this in any way.

On the basis of our clinical impressions we maintained that these patients' object-cathexes must have been given up and that their object-libido must have been transformed into ego-libido [p. 420]. Through this characteristic we distinguished them from the first group of neurotics (sufferers from hysteria, anxiety-hysteria and obsessional neurosis). This suspicion is now confirmed by their behaviour in our attempts at therapy. They manifest no transference and for that reason are inaccessible to our efforts and cannot be cured by us.

LECTURE XXVIII

ANALYTIC THERAPY[1]

LADIES AND GENTLEMEN,—You know what we are going to talk about to-day. You asked me why we do not make use of direct suggestion in psycho-analytic therapy, when we admit that our influence rests essentially on transference—that is, on suggestion; and you added a doubt whether, in view of this predominance of suggestion, we are still able to claim that our psychological discoveries are objective. I promised I would give you a detailed reply.

Direct suggestion is suggestion aimed against the manifestation of the symptoms; it is a struggle between your authority and the motives for the illness. In this you do not concern yourself with these motives; you merely request the patient to suppress their manifestation in symptoms. It makes no difference of principle whether you put the patient under hypnosis or not. Once again Bernheim, with his characteristic perspicacity, maintained that suggestion was the essential element in the phenomena of hypnotism, that hypnosis itself was already a result of suggestion, a suggested state;[2] and he preferred to practise suggestion in a waking state, which can achieve the same effects as suggestion under hypnosis.

Which would you rather hear first on this question—what experience tells us or theoretical considerations?

Let us begin with the former. I was a pupil of Bernheim's, whom I visited at Nancy in 1889 and whose book on suggestion

[1] [This lecture contains Freud's fullest account of the theory of the therapeutic effects of psycho-analysis. His later discussion of the question in his paper on 'Analysis Terminable and Interminable' (1937c) seems in some respects to be at variance with it. Cf. the Editor's Note to that paper. Freud published very little on the details of psychoanalytic technique. See, however, the technical papers in Volume XII of the *Standard Edition*, where a list of his other writings on the subject will be found.]

[2] [Freud subsequently expressed his disagreement with this view of Bernheim's. See footnote at the end of Chapter X of *Group Psychology* (1921c).]

I translated into German.[1] I practised hypnotic treatment for many years, at first by prohibitory suggestion and later in combination with Breuer's method of questioning the patient.[2] I can therefore speak of the results of hypnotic or suggestive therapy on the basis of a wide experience. If, in the words of the old medical aphorism, an ideal therapy should be rapid, reliable and not disagreeable for the patient ['*cito, tuto, jucunde*'], Bernheim's method fulfilled at least two of these requirements. It could be carried through much quicker—or, rather, infinitely quicker—than analytic treatment and it caused the patient neither trouble nor unpleasantness. For the doctor it became, in the long run, *monotonous*: in each case, in the same way, with the same ceremonial, forbidding the most variegated symptoms to exist, without being able to learn anything of their sense and meaning. It was hackwork and not a scientific activity, and it recalled magic, incantations and hocus-pocus. That could not weigh, however, against the patient's interest. But the third quality was lacking: the procedure was not reliable in any respect. It could be used with one patient, but not with another; it achieved a great deal with one and very little with another, and one never knew why. Worse than the capriciousness of the procedure was the lack of permanence in its successes. If, after a short time, one had news of the patient once more, the old ailment was back again or its place had been taken by a new one. One might hypnotize him again. But in the background there was the warning given by experienced workers against robbing the patient of his self-reliance by frequently repeated hypnosis and so making him an addict to this kind of therapy as though it were a narcotic. Admittedly sometimes things went entirely as one would wish: after a few efforts, success was complete and permanent.[3] But the conditions determining such a favourable outcome remained unknown. On one occasion a severe condition in a woman, which I had entirely got rid of by

---

[1] [In fact Freud translated two of Bernheim's books: *De la suggestion et de ses applications à la thérapeutique* (1886, translated 1888–9) and *Hypnotisme, suggestion et psychothérapie* (1891, translated 1892).]

[2] [See p. 292 above.]

[3] [An instance of this kind was reported by Freud in an early paper, 'A Case of Successful Treatment by Hypnotism' (1892–3).]

a short hypnotic treatment, returned unchanged after the patient had, through no action on my part, got annoyed with me; after a reconciliation, I removed the trouble again and far more thoroughly; yet it returned once more after she had fallen foul of me a second time. On another occasion a woman patient, whom I had repeatedly helped out of neurotic states by hypnosis, suddenly, during the treatment of a specially obstinate situation, threw her arms round my neck.[1] After this one could scarcely avoid, whether one wanted to or not, investigating the question of the nature and origin of one's authority in suggestive treatment.

So much for experiences. They show us that in renouncing direct suggestion we are not giving up anything of irreplaceable value. Now let us add a few reflections to this. The practice of hypnotic therapy makes very small demands on either the patient or the doctor. It agrees most beautifully with the estimate in which neuroses are still held by the majority of doctors. The doctor says to the neurotic patient: 'There's nothing wrong with you, it's only a question of nerves; so I can blow away your trouble in two or three minutes with just a few words.' But our views on the laws of energy are offended by the notion of its being possible to move a great weight by a tiny application of force, attacking it directly, without the outside help of any appropriate appliances. In so far as the conditions are comparable, experience shows that this feat is not successfully accomplished in the case of the neuroses either. But I am aware that this argument is not unimpeachable. There is such a thing as a 'trigger-action'.

In the light of the knowledge we have gained from psychoanalysis we can describe the difference between hypnotic and psycho-analytic suggestion as follows. Hypnotic treatment seeks to cover up and gloss over something in mental life; analytic treatment seeks to expose and get rid of something.[2] The former acts like a cosmetic, the latter like surgery. The former makes use of suggestion in order to forbid the symptoms; it strengthens

[1] [Freud described this episode again at the end of Chapter II of his *Autobiographical Study* (1925d), (Norton, 1963).]
[2] [This distinction is developed at some length in an early paper of Freud's 'On Psychotherapy' (1905a).]

the repressions, but, apart from that, leaves all the processes that have led to the formation of the symptoms unaltered. Analytic treatment makes its impact further back towards the roots, where the conflicts are which gave rise to the symptoms, and uses suggestion in order to alter the outcome of those conflicts. Hypnotic treatment leaves the patient inert and unchanged, and for that reason, too, equally unable to resist any fresh occasion for falling ill. An analytic treatment demands from both doctor and patient the accomplishment of serious work, which is employed in lifting internal resistances. Through the overcoming of these resistances the patient's mental life is permanently changed, is raised to a high level of development and remains protected against fresh possibilities of falling ill.[1] This work of overcoming resistances is the essential function of analytic treatment; the patient has to accomplish it and the doctor makes this possible for him with the help of suggestion operating in an *educative* sense. For that reason psychoanalytic treatment has justly been described as a kind of *after-education*.[2]

I hope I have now made it clear to you in what way our method of employing suggestion therapeutically differs from the only method possible in hypnotic treatment. You will understand too, from the fact that suggestion can be traced back to transference, the capriciousness which struck us in hypnotic therapy, while analytic treatment remains calculable within its limits. In using hypnosis we are dependent on the state of the patient's capacity for transference without being able to influence it itself. The transference of a person who is to be hypnotized may be negative or, as most frequently, ambivalent, or he may have protected himself against his transference by adopting special attitudes; of that we learn nothing. In psychoanalysis we act upon the transference itself, resolve what opposes it, adjust the instrument with which we wish to make our impact. Thus it becomes possible for us to derive an entirely fresh advantage from the power of suggestion; we get it into our hands. The patient does not suggest to himself whatever he

[1] [Cf. footnote, p. 445 above.]
[2] [See the paper 'On Psychotherapy' (1905c), where, incidentally, the German word '*Nacherziehung*' ('after-education') is wrongly translated 're-education'.]

pleases: we guide his suggestion so far as he is in any way accessible to its influence.

But you will now tell me that, no matter whether we call the motive force of our analysis transference or suggestion, there is a risk that the influencing of our patient may make the objective certainty of our findings doubtful. What is advantageous to our therapy is damaging to our researches. This is the objection that is most often raised against psycho-analysis, and it must be admitted that, though it is groundless, it cannot be rejected as unreasonable. If it were justified, psycho-analysis would be nothing more than a particularly well-disguised and particularly effective form of suggestive treatment and we should have to attach little weight to all that it tells us about what influences our lives, the dynamics of the mind or the unconscious. That is what our opponents believe; and in especial they think that we have 'talked' the patients into everything relating to the importance of sexual experiences—or even into those experiences themselves—after such notions have grown up in our own depraved imagination. These accusations are contradicted more easily by an appeal to experience than by the help of theory. Anyone who has himself carried out psycho-analyses will have been able to convince himself on countless occasions that it is impossible to make suggestions to a patient in that way. The doctor has no difficulty, of course, in making him a supporter of some particular theory and in thus making him share some possible error of his own. In this respect the patient is behaving like anyone else—like a pupil—but this only affects his intelligence, not his illness. After all, his conflicts will only be successfully solved and his resistances overcome if the anticipatory ideas he is given tally with what is real in him. Whatever in the doctor's conjectures is inaccurate drops out in the course of the analysis;[1] it has to be withdrawn and replaced by something more correct. We endeavour by a careful technique to avoid the occurrence of premature successes due to suggestion; but no harm is done even if they do occur, for we are not satisfied by a first success. We do not regard an analysis as at an end until all the obscurities of the case are cleared up, the gaps in the

[1] [Freud gives a small example of this in the 'Wolf Man' case history (1918b).]

patient's memory filled in, the precipitating causes of the repressions discovered. We look upon successes that set in too soon as obstacles rather than as a help to the work of analysis; and we put an end to such successes by constantly resolving the transference on which they are based. It is this last characteristic which is the fundamental distinction between analytic and purely suggestive therapy, and which frees the results of analysis from the suspicion of being successes due to suggestion. In every other kind of suggestive treatment the transference is carefully preserved and left untouched; in analysis it is itself subjected to treatment and is dissected in all the shapes in which it appears. At the end of an analytic treatment the transference must itself be cleared away; and if success is then obtained or continues, it rests, not on suggestion, but on the achievement by its means of an overcoming of internal resistances, on the internal change that has been brought about in the patient.

The acceptance of suggestions on individual points is no doubt discouraged by the fact that during the treatment we are struggling unceasingly against resistances which are able to transform themselves into negative (hostile) transferences. Nor must we fail to point out that a large number of the individual findings of analysis, which might otherwise be suspected of being products of suggestion, are confirmed from another and irreproachable source. Our guarantors in this case are the sufferers from dementia praecox and paranoia, who are of course far above any suspicion of being influenced by suggestion. The translations of symbols and the phantasies, which these patients produce for us and which in them have forced their way through into consciousness, coincide faithfully with the results of our investigations into the unconscious of transference neurotics and thus confirm the objective correctness of our interpretations, on which doubt is so often thrown. You will not, I think, be going astray if you trust analysis on these points.

I will now complete my picture of the mechanism of cure by clothing it in the formulas of the libido theory. A neurotic is incapable of enjoyment and of efficiency—the former because his libido is not directed on to any real object and the latter because he is obliged to employ a great deal of his available energy on keeping his libido under repression and on warding off its assaults. He would become healthy if the conflict between his ego and his libido came to an end and if his ego had his libido again at its disposal. The therapeutic task consists, therefore, in freeing the libido from its present attachments, which are withdrawn from the ego, and in making it once more serviceable to the ego. Where, then, is the neurotic's libido situated? It is easily found: it is attached to the symptoms, which yield it the only substitutive satisfaction possible at the time. We must therefore make ourselves masters of the symptoms and resolve them—which is precisely the same thing that the patient requires of us. In order to resolve the symptoms, we must go back as far as their origin, we must renew the conflict from which they arose, and, with the help of motive forces which were not at the patient's disposal in the past, we must guide it to a different outcome. This revision of the process of repression can be accomplished only in part in connection with the memory traces of the processes which led to repression. The decisive part of the work is achieved by creating in the patient's relation to the doctor—in the 'transference'—new editions of the old conflicts; in these the patient would like to behave in the same way as he did in the past, while we, by summoning up every available mental force [in the patient], compel him to come to a fresh decision. Thus the transference becomes the battlefield on which all the mutually struggling forces should meet one another.

All the libido, as well as everything opposing it, is made to converge solely on the relation with the doctor. In this process the symptoms are inevitably divested of libido. In place of the patient's true illness there appears the artificially constructed transference illness, in place of the various unreal objects of his libido there appears a single, and once more imaginary, object in the person of the doctor. But, by the help of the doctor's suggestion, the new struggle around this object is lifted to the highest psychical level: it takes place as a normal mental conflict. Since a fresh repression is avoided, the alienation between ego and libido is brought to an end and the subject's mental unity is restored. When the libido is released once more from its temporary object in the person of the doctor, it cannot return to its earlier objects, but is at the disposal of the ego. The forces against which we have been struggling during our work of therapy are, on the one hand, the ego's antipathy to certain trends of the libido—an antipathy expressed in a tendency to repression—and, on the other hand, the tenacity or adhesiveness of the libido [p. 348], which dislikes leaving objects that it has once cathected.

Thus our therapeutic work falls into two phases. In the first, all the libido is forced from the symptoms into the transference and concentrated there; in the second, the struggle is waged around this new object and the libido is liberated from it. The change which is decisive for a favourable outcome is the elimination of repression in this renewed conflict, so that the libido cannot withdraw once more from the ego by flight into the unconscious. This is made possible by the alteration of the ego which is accomplished under the influence of the doctor's suggestion. By means of the work of interpretation, which transforms what is unconscious into what is conscious, the ego is enlarged at the cost of this unconscious; by means of instruction, it is made conciliatory towards the libido and inclined to grant it some satisfaction, and its repugnance to the claims of the libido is diminished by the possibility of disposing of a portion of it by sublimation. The more closely events in the treatment coincide with this ideal description, the greater will be the success of the psycho-analytic therapy. It finds its limits in the lack of mobility of the libido, which may refuse to leave its objects, and the rigidity of narcissism, which will not allow transference on to objects to increase beyond certain bounds. Further light may perhaps be thrown on the dynamics of the process of cure if I say that we get hold of the whole of the libido which has been withdrawn from the dominance of the ego by attracting a portion of it on to ourselves by means of the transference.

It will not be out of place to give a warning that we can draw no direct conclusion from the distribution of the libido during and resulting from the treatment as to how it was distributed during the illness. Suppose we succeeded in bringing a case to a favourable conclusion by setting up and then resolving a strong father-transference to the doctor. It would not be correct to conclude that the patient had suffered previously from a

similar unconscious attachment of his libido to his father. His
father-transference was merely the battlefield on which we
gained control of his libido; the patient's libido was directed
to it from other positions. A battlefield need not necessarily coincide with one of the enemy's key fortresses. The defence of a
hostile capital need not take place just in front of its gates. Not
until after the transference has once more been resolved can
we reconstruct in our thoughts the distribution of libido which
had prevailed during the illness.

From the standpoint of the libido theory, too, we may say
a last word on dreams. A neurotic's dreams help us, like his
parapraxes and his free associations to them, to discover the
sense of his symptoms and to reveal the way in which his libido
is allocated. They show us, in the form of a wish-fulfilment,
what wishful impulses have been subjected to repression and to
what objects the libido withdrawn from the ego has become
attached. For this reason the interpretation of dreams plays a
large part in a psycho-analytic treatment, and in some cases it
is over long periods the most important instrument of our work.
We already know [p. 218] that the state of sleep in itself leads
to a certain relaxation of the repressions. A repressed impulse,
owing to this reduction in the pressure weighing down upon it,
becomes able to express itself far more clearly in a dream than
it can be allowed to be expressed by a symptom during the day.
The study of dreams therefore becomes the most convenient
means of access to a knowledge of the repressed unconscious,
of which the libido withdrawn from the ego forms a part.

But the dreams of neurotics do not differ in any important
respect from those of normal people; it is possible, indeed, that
they cannot be distinguished from them at all. It would be
absurd to give an account of the dreams of neurotics which
could not also apply to the dreams of normal people. We must
therefore say that the difference between neurosis and health
holds only during the day; it is not prolonged into dream-life.
We are obliged to carry over to healthy people a number of
hypotheses which arise in connection with neurotics as a result
of the link between the latter's dreams and their symptoms. We
cannot deny that healthy people as well possess in their mental
life what alone makes possible the formation both of dreams and

of symptoms, and we must conclude that they too have carried out repressions, that they expend a certain amount of energy in order to maintain them, that their unconscious system conceals repressed impulses which are still cathected with energy, and that *a portion of their libido is withdrawn from their ego's disposal.* Thus a healthy person, too, is virtually a neurotic; but dreams appear to be the only symptoms which he is capable of forming. It is true that if one subjects his waking life to a closer examination one discovers something that contradicts this appearance— namely that this ostensibly healthy life is interspersed with a great number of trivial and in practice unimportant symptoms.

The distinction between nervous health and neurosis is thus reduced to a practical question and is decided by the outcome —by whether the subject is left with a sufficient amount of capacity for enjoyment and of efficiency. It probably goes back to the relative sizes of the quota of energy that remains free and of that which is bound by repression, and is of a quantitative not of a qualitative nature. I need not tell you that this discovery is the theoretical justification for our conviction that neuroses are in principle curable in spite of their being based on constitutional disposition.

The identity of the dreams of healthy and neurotic people enables us to infer thus much in regard to defining the characteristics of health. But in regard to dreams themselves we can make a further inference: we must not detach them from their connection with neurotic symptoms, we must not suppose that their essential nature is exhausted by the formula that describes them as a translation of thoughts into an archaic form of expression [p. 199], but we must suppose that they exhibit to us allocations of the libido and object-cathexes that are really present.[1]

We shall soon have reached the end. You are perhaps disappointed that on the topic of the psycho-analytic method of therapy I have only spoken to you about theory and not about the conditions which determine whether a treatment is to be undertaken or about the results it produces. I shall discuss

[1] [Some interesting remarks on the dreams of *psychotic* patients will be found in Section B of 'Some Neurotic Mechanisms' (1922*b*).]

neither: the former because it is not my intention to give you practical instructions on how to carry out a psycho-analysis, and the latter because several reasons deter me from it. At the beginning of our talks [this year, p. 256], I emphasized the fact that under favourable conditions we achieve successes which are second to none of the finest in the field of internal medicine; and I can now add something further—namely that they could not have been achieved by any other procedure. If I were to say more than this I should be suspected of trying to drown the loudly raised voices of depreciation by self-advertisement. The threat has repeatedly been made against psycho-analysts by our medical 'colleagues'—even at public congresses—that a collection of the failures and damaging results of analysis would be published which would open the suffering public's eyes to the worthlessness of this method of treatment. But, apart from the malicious, denunciatory character of such a measure, it would not even be calculated to make it possible to form a correct judgement of the therapeutic effectiveness of analysis. Analytic therapy, as you know, is in its youth; it has taken a long time to establish its technique, and that could only be done in the course of working and under the influence of increasing experience. In consequence of the difficulties in giving instruction, the doctor who is a beginner in psycho-analysis is thrown back to a greater extent than other specialists on his own capacity for further development, and the results of his first years will never make it possible to judge the efficacy of analytic therapy.

Many attempts at treatment miscarried during the early period of analysis because they were undertaken in cases which were altogether unsuited to the procedure and which we should exclude to-day on the basis of our present view of the indications for treatment. But these indications, too, could only be arrived at by experiment. In those days we did not know *a priori* that paranoia and dementia praecox in strongly marked forms are inaccessible, and we had a right to make trial of the method on all kinds of disorders. But most of the failures of those early years were due not to the doctor's fault or an unsuitable choice of patients but to unfavourable external conditions. Here we have only dealt with internal resistances, those of the patient, which are inevitable and can be overcome. The external resistances which arise from the patient's circumstances, from his environment, are of small theoretical interest but of the greatest practical importance. Psycho-analytic treatment may be compared with a surgical operation and may similarly claim to be carried out under arrangements that will be the most favourable for its success. You know the precautionary measures adopted by a surgeon: a suitable room, good lighting, assistants, exclusion of the patient's relatives, and so on. Ask yourselves now how many of these operations would turn out successfully if they had to take place in the presence of all the members of the patient's family, who would stick their noses into the field of the operation and exclaim aloud at every incision. In psycho-analytic treatments the intervention of relatives is a positive danger and a danger one does not know how to meet. One is armed against the patient's internal resistances, which one knows are inevitable, but how can one ward off these external resistances? No kind of explanations make any impression on the patient's relatives; they cannot be induced to keep at a distance from the whole business, and one cannot make common cause with them because of the risk of losing the confidence of the patient, who—quite rightly, moreover—expects the person in whom he has put his trust to take his side. No one who has any experience of the rifts which so often divide a family will, if he is an analyst, be surprised to find that the patient's closest relatives sometimes betray less interest in his recovering than in his remaining as he is. When, as so often, the neurosis is related to conflicts between members of a family, the healthy party will not hesitate long in choosing between his own interest and the sick party's recovery. It is not to be wondered at, indeed, if a husband looks with disfavour on a treatment in which, as he may rightly suspect, the whole cata-logue of his sins will be brought to light. Nor do we wonder at it; but we cannot in that case blame ourselves if our efforts remain unsuccessful and the treatment is broken off pre-maturely because the husband's resistance is added to that of his sick wife. We had in fact undertaken something which in the prevailing circumstances was unrealizable.

Instead of reporting a number of cases, I will tell you the story of a single one, in which, from considerations of medical discretion, I was condemned to play a long-suffering part. I undertook the analytic treatment—it was many years ago—of a girl who had for some time been unable, owing to anxiety, to go out in the street or to stay at home by herself. The patient slowly brought out an admission that her imagination had been seized by chance observations of the affectionate relations between her mother and a well-to-do friend of the family. But she was so clumsy—or so subtle—that she gave her mother a hint of what was being talked about in the analytic sessions. She brought this about by changing her behaviour towards her mother, by insisting on being protected by no one but her mother from her anxiety at being alone and by barring the door to her in her anxiety if she tried to leave the house. Her mother had herself been very neurotic in the past, but had been cured years before in a hydropathic establishment. Or rather, she had there made the acquaintance of the man with whom she was able to enter into a relation that was in every way satisfying to her. The girl's passionate demands took her aback, and she suddenly understood the meaning of her daughter's anxiety: the girl had made herself ill in order to keep her mother prisoner and to rob her of the freedom of movement that her relations with her lover required. The mother quickly made up her mind and brought the obnoxious treatment to an end. The girl was taken to a sanatorium for nervous diseases and was demonstrated for many years as 'a poor victim of psycho-analysis'. All this time, too, I was pursued by the calumny of responsibility for the unhappy end of the treatment. I kept silence, for I thought I was bound by the duty of medical discretion. Long afterwards I learnt from one of my colleagues, who visited the sanatorium and had seen the agoraphobic girl there, that the *liaison* between her mother and the well-to-do friend of the family was common knowledge in the city and that it was probably connived at by the husband and father. Thus it was to this 'secret' that the treatment had been sacrificed.

In the years before the war, when arrivals from many foreign countries made me independent of the favour or disfavour of my own city, I followed a rule of not taking on a patient for treatment unless he was *sui juris*, not dependent on anyone else in the essential relations of his life. This is not possible, however, for every psycho-analyst. Perhaps you may conclude from my warning against relatives that patients designed for psycho-analysis should be removed from their families and that this kind of treatment should accordingly be restricted to inmates of hospitals for nervous diseases. I could not, however, follow you in that. It is much more advantageous for patients (in so far as they are not in a phase of severe exhaustion) to remain during the treatment in the conditions in which they have to struggle with the tasks that face them. But the patients' relatives ought not to cancel out this advantage by their conduct and should not offer any hostile opposition to the doctor's efforts. But how do you propose to influence in that direction factors like these which are inaccessible to us? And you will guess, of course, how much the prospects of a treatment are determined by the patient's social *milieu* and the cultural level of his family.

This presents a gloomy prospect for the effectiveness of psycho-analysis as a therapy—does it not?—even though we are able to explain the great majority of our failures by attributing them to interfering external factors. Friends of analysis have advised us to meet the threatened publication of our failures with statistics of our successes drawn up by ourselves. I did not agree to this. I pointed out that statistics are worthless if the items assembled in them are too heterogeneous; and the cases of neurotic illness which we had taken into treatment were in fact incomparable in a great variety of respects. Moreover, the period of time that could be covered was too short to make it possible to judge the durability of the cures.[1] And it was altogether impossible to report on many of the cases: they concerned people who had kept both their illness and its treatment secret, and their recovery had equally to be kept secret. But the strongest reason for holding back lay in the realization that in matters of therapy people behave highly irrationally, so that one has no prospect of accomplishing anything with them by rational means. A therapeutic novelty is either received with delirious enthusiasm—as, for instance, when Koch introduced his first tuberculin against tuberculosis to the public[2]— or it is treated with abysmal distrust—like Jenner's vaccination, which was in fact a blessing and which even to-day has its irreconcilable opponents. There was obviously a prejudice

[1] [Freud recurs to this question in the *New Introductory Lectures*, p. 616, where the therapeutic value of psychoanalysis is again discussed.]

[2] [In 1890. Its promise was not fulfilled.]

against psycho-analysis. If one had cured a severe case, one might hear people say: 'That proves nothing. He would have recovered on his own account by this time.' And when a woman patient, who had already passed through four cycles of depression and mania, came to be treated by me during an interval after an attack of melancholia and three weeks later started on a phase of mania, all the members of her family—and a high medical authority, too, who was called in for consultation— were convinced that the fresh attack could only be the result of my attempted analysis. Nothing can be done against prejudices. You can see it again to-day in the prejudices which each group of nations at war has developed against the other. The most sensible thing to do is to wait, and to leave such prejudices to the eroding effects of time. One day the same people begin to think about the same things in quite a different way from before; why they did not think so earlier remains a dark mystery.

It is possible that the prejudice against analytic treatment is already diminishing. The constant spread of analytic teachings, the increasing number of doctors practising analysis in a number of countries seems to vouch for this. When I was a young doctor, I found myself in a similar storm of indignation on the doctors' part against treatment by hypnotic suggestion, which is now held up in contrast to analysis by people of 'moderate' views.[1] Hypnotism, however, has not fulfilled its original promise as a therapeutic agent. We psycho-analysts may claim to be its legitimate heirs and we do not forget how much encouragement and theoretical clarification we owe to it. The damaging results attributed to psycho-analysis are restricted essentially to passing manifestations of increased conflict if an analysis is clumsily carried out or if it is broken off in the middle. You have heard an account of what we do with our patients and can form your own judgement as to whether our efforts are calculated to lead to any lasting damage. Abuse of analysis is possible in various directions; in particular, the transference is a dangerous instrument in the hands of an unconscientious doctor. But no medical

---

[1] [Some striking evidence of the medical opposition to hypnotism will be found in an early review by Freud of a book on the subject by the well-known Swiss psychiatrist, August Forel (Freud, 1889a).]

instrument or procedure is guaranteed against abuse; if a knife does not cut, it cannot be used for healing either.

I have finished, Ladies and Gentlemen. It is more than a conventional form of words if I admit that I myself am profoundly aware of the many defects in the lectures I have given you. I regret above all that I have so often promised to return later to a topic I have lightly touched on and have then found no opportunity of redeeming my promise. I undertook to give you an account of a subject which is still incomplete and in process of development, and my condensed summary has itself turned out to be an incomplete one. At some points I have set out the material on which to draw a conclusion and have then myself not drawn it. But I could not pretend to make you into experts; I have only tried to stimulate and enlighten you.

Two

NEW INTRODUCTORY LECTURES
ON PSYCHOANALYSIS

EDITOR'S NOTE

THIS WORK—*Neue Folge der Vorlesungen zur Einführung in die Psychoanalyse,* ("New Series of the Lectures to Serve as an Introduction to Psychoanalysis")—was first published at the beginning of 1933, some fifteen years after the original series of lectures to which it was to be a supplement. The first English translation, by W. J. H. Sprott, appeared in the same year.

In the early part of 1932 the financial affairs of the psychoanalytic publishing business in Vienna had been in a parlous state, and the idea occurred to Freud of coming to its help with a new series of the *Introductory Lectures.* The first and last lectures were ready by the end of May, and the whole book was finished by the end of August. It was actually issued on December 6, a month before the official date of publication.

These lectures differ from the original set in various ways and not merely in that they were never meant to be delivered. As Freud pointed out in his own preface (and as he insisted by his numeration of the lectures), they do not stand on their own legs but are essentially supplementary. What is especially noticeable about them, however, is the way in which they differ in character among themselves. The first lecture, on dreams, is scarcely more than a recapitulation of the dream section of the original series. On the other hand, the third, fourth, and fifth lectures (on the structure of the mind, on anxiety and the theory of the instincts, and on the psychology of women) introduce entirely new material and theories and, in the case of the third and fourth lectures, plunge into theoretical and metapsychological discussions of a difficulty which had been studiously avoided fifteen years earlier. The remaining lectures (the second and the last two) are of a very different order. They deal with a number of miscellaneous topics only indirectly related to psychoanalysis and, moreover, deal with them in what might almost be described as a popular manner. This is not to suggest that they are trivial or uninteresting—far from it. But they call for a very different kind and degree of at-

467

tention than do their fellows. Nevertheless, whatever the reader's choice may be—whether he wishes to know what Freud thought about telepathy, education, religion, or Communism, or whether he wishes to learn Freud's final views on the super-ego, on anxiety, on the death instinct, or on the pre-Oedipus phase in girls—he will certainly find plenty to occupy him in these lectures.

JAMES STRACHEY

PREFACE

MY *Introductory Lectures on Psycho-Analysis* were delivered during the two Winter Terms of 1915–16 and 1916–17 in a lecture room of the Vienna Psychiatric Clinic before an audience gathered from all the Faculties of the University. The first half of the lectures were improvised, and written out immediately afterwards; drafts of the second half were made during the intervening summer vacation at Salzburg, and delivered word for word in the following winter. At that time I still possessed the gift of a phonographic memory.

These new lectures, unlike the former ones, have never been delivered. My age had in the meantime absolved me from the obligation of giving expression to my membership of the University (which was in any case a peripheral one) by delivering lectures; and a surgical operation had made speaking in public impossible for me. If, therefore, I once more take my place in the lecture room during the remarks that follow, it is only by an artifice of the imagination; it may help me not to forget to bear the reader in mind as I enter more deeply into my subject.

The new lectures are by no means intended to take the place of the earlier ones. They do not in any sense form an independent entity with an expectation of finding a circle of readers of its own; they are continuations and supplements, which, in relation to the former series, fall into three groups. A first group contains fresh treatments of subjects which were already dealt with fifteen years ago but which, as a result of a deepening of our knowledge and an alteration in our views, call for a different exposition to-day—that is to say, critical revisions. The two other groups contain what are true extensions, for they deal .with things which either did not exist in psycho-analysis at the time of the first lectures or which were too little in evidence to justify a special chapter-heading. It is inevitable, but not to be regretted, if some of the new lectures unite the characteristics of more than one of these groups.

I have also given expression to the dependence of these new lectures on the *Introductory Lectures* by giving them a numbering continuous with theirs. The first lecture in this volume is accordingly called No. XXIX. Like their predecessors, they offer the professional analyst little that is new; they are addressed to the multitude of educated people to whom we may perhaps attribute a benevolent, even though cautious, interest in the characteristics and discoveries of the young science. This time once again it has been my chief aim to make no sacrifice to an appearance of being simple, complete or rounded-off, not to disguise problems and not to deny the existence of gaps and un-certainties. In no other field of scientific work would it be neces-sary to boast of such modest intentions. They are universally regarded as self-evident; the public expects nothing else. No reader of an account of astronomy will feel disappointed and contemptuous of the science if he is shown the frontiers at which our knowledge of the universe melts into haziness. Only in psychology is it otherwise. There mankind's constitutional unfitness for scientific research comes fully into the open. What people seem to demand of psychology is not progress in know-ledge, but satisfactions of some other sort; every unsolved prob-lem, every admitted uncertainty is made into a reproach against it.

Whoever cares for the science of mental life must accept these injustices along with it.

FREUD

VIENNA, *Summer* 1932

REVISION OF THE THEORY OF DREAMS

LADIES AND GENTLEMEN,—If, after an interval of more than fifteen years, I have brought you together again to discuss with you what novelties, and what improvements it may be, the intervening time has introduced into psycho-analysis, it is right and fitting from more than one point of view that we should turn our attention first to the position of the theory of dreams. It occupies a special place in the history of psycho-analysis and marks a turning-point; it was with it that analysis took the step from being a psychotherapeutic procedure to being a depth-psychology. Since then, too, the theory of dreams has remained what is most characteristic and peculiar about the young science, something to which there is no counterpart in the rest of our knowledge, a stretch of new country, which has been reclaimed from popular beliefs and mysticism. The strangeness of the assertions it was obliged to put forward has made it play the part of a shibboleth, the use of which decided who could become a follower of psycho-analysis and to whom it remained for ever incomprehensible. I myself found it a sheet-anchor during those difficult times when the unrecognized facts of the neuroses used to confuse my inexperienced judgement. Whenever I began to have doubts of the correctness of my wavering conclusions, the successful transformation of a senseless and muddled dream into a logical and intelligible mental process in the dreamer would renew my confidence of being on the right track.

It is therefore of special interest to us, in the particular instance of the theory of dreams, on the one hand to follow the vicissitudes through which psycho-analysis has passed during this interval, and on the other hand to learn what advances it has made in being understood and appreciated by the contemporary world. I may tell you at once that you will be disappointed in both these directions.

Let us look through the volumes of the *Internationale Zeitschrift für (ärztliche) Psychoanalyse* [*International Journal of (Medical) Psycho-Analysis*], in which, since 1913, the authoritative writings

[1] [Cf. Freud's Preface, pp. 469–70 above.]

471

in our field of work have been brought together. In the earlier volumes you will find a recurrent sectional heading 'On Dream-Interpretation', containing numerous contributions on various points in the theory of dreams. But the further you go the rarer do these contributions become, and finally the sectional heading disappears completely. The analysts behave as though they had no more to say about dreams, as though there was nothing more to be added to the theory of dreams. But if you ask how much of dream-interpretation has been accepted by outsiders—by the many psychiatrists and psychotherapists who warm their pot of soup at our fire (incidentally without being very grateful for our hospitality), by what are described as educated people, who are in the habit of assimilating the more striking findings of science, by the literary men and by the public at large—the reply gives little cause for satisfaction. A few formulas have become generally familiar, among them some that we have never put forward—such as the thesis that all dreams are of a sexual nature—but really important things like the fundamental distinction between the manifest content of dreams and the latent dream-thoughts, the realization that the wish-fulfilling function of dreams is not contradicted by anxiety-dreams, the impossibility of interpreting a dream unless one has the dreamer's associations to it at one's disposal, and, above all, the discovery that what is essential in dreams is the process of the dream-work—all this still seems about as foreign to general awareness as it was thirty years ago. I am in a position to say this, since in the course of that period I have received innumerable letters whose writers present their dreams for interpretation or ask for information about the nature of dreams and who declare that they have read my *Interpretation of Dreams*, though in every sentence they betray their lack of understanding of our theory of dreams. But all this shall not deter us from once more giving a connected account of what we know about dreams. You will recall that last time we devoted a whole number of lectures to showing how we came to understand this hitherto unexplained mental phenomenon.[1]

Let us suppose, then, that someone—a patient in analysis,

[1] [Cf. the whole of Part II of *Introductory Lectures on Psycho-Analysis* (1916–17).]

for instance—tells us one of his dreams. We shall assume that in this way he is making us one of the communications to which he has pledged himself by the fact of having started an analytic treatment. It is, to be sure, a communication made by inappropriate means, for dreams are not in themselves social utterances, not a means of giving information. Nor, indeed, do we understand what the dreamer was trying to say to us, and he himself is equally in the dark. And now we have to make a quick decision. On the one hand, the dream may be, as non-analytic doctors assure us, a sign that the dreamer has slept badly, that not every part of his brain has come to rest equally, that some areas of it, under the influence of unknown stimuli, endeavoured to go on working but were only able to do so in a very incomplete fashion. If that is the case, we shall be right to concern ourselves no further with the product of a nocturnal disturbance which has no psychical value: for what could we expect to derive from investigating it that would be of use for our purposes? Or on the other hand—but it is plain that we have from the first decided otherwise. We have—quite arbitrarily, it must be admitted—made the assumption, adopted as a postulate, that even this unintelligible dream must be a fully valid psychical act, with sense and worth, which we can use in analysis like any other communication. Only the outcome of our experiment can show whether we are right. If we succeed in turning the dream into an utterance of value of that kind, we shall evidently have a prospect of learning something new and of receiving communications of a sort which would otherwise be inaccessible to us.

Now, however, the difficulties of our task and the enigmas of our subject rise before our eyes. How do we propose to transform the dream into a normal communication and how do we explain the fact that some of the patient's utterances have assumed a form that is unintelligible both to him and to us?

As you see, Ladies and Gentlemen, this time I am taking the path not of a genetic but of a dogmatic exposition. Our first step is to establish our new attitude to the problem of dreams by introducing two new concepts and names. What has been called the dream we shall describe as the text of the dream or the *manifest* dream, and what we are looking for, what we suspect, so to say, of lying behind the dream, we shall describe as the *latent* dream-thoughts. Having done this, we can express our two tasks as follows. We have to transform the manifest dream into the latent one, and to explain how, in the dreamer's mind, the latter has become the former. The first portion is a *practical* task, for which dream-interpretation is responsible; it calls for a technique. The second portion is a *theoretical* task, whose business it is to explain the hypothetical dream-work; and it can only be a theory. Both of them, the technique of dream-interpretation and the theory of the dream-work, have to be newly created.

With which of the two, then, shall we start? With the technique of dream-interpretation, I think; it will present a more concrete appearance and make a more vivid impression on you.

Well then, the patient has told us a dream, which we are to interpret. We have listened passively, without putting our powers of reflection into action.[1] What do we do next? We decide to concern ourselves as little as possible with what we have heard, with the *manifest* dream. Of course this manifest dream exhibits all sorts of characteristics which are not entirely a matter of indifference to us. It may be coherent, smoothly constructed like a literary composition, or it may be confused to the point of unintelligibility, almost like a delirium; it may contain absurd elements or jokes and apparently witty conclusions; it may seem to the dreamer clear and sharp or obscure and hazy; its pictures may exhibit the complete sensory strength of perceptions or may be shadowy like an indistinct mist; the most diverse characteristics may be present in the same dream, distributed over various portions of it; the dream, finally, may show an indifferent emotional tone or be accompanied by feelings of the strongest joy or distress. You must not suppose that we think nothing of this endless diversity in manifest dreams. We shall come back to it later and we shall find a great deal in it that we can make use of in our interpretations. But for the moment we will disregard it and follow the main road that leads to the interpretation of dreams. That is to say, we ask the dreamer, too, to free himself from the impression of the

[1] [Some illuminating remarks on reflection will be found, in a similar connection, in Chapter II of *The Interpretation of Dreams* (1900a).]

manifest dream, to divert his attention from the dream as a whole on to the separate portions of its content and to report to us in succession everything that occurs to him in relation to each of these portions—what associations present themselves to him if he focuses on each of them separately.

That is a curious technique, is it not?—not the usual way of dealing with a communication or utterance. And no doubt you guess that behind this procedure there are assumptions which have not yet been expressly stated. But let us proceed. In what order are we to get the patient to take up the portions of his dream? There are various possibilities open to us. We can simply follow the chronological order in which they appeared in the account of the dream. That is what may be called the strictest, classical method. Or we can direct the dreamer to begin by looking out for the 'day's residues' in the dream; for experience has taught us that almost every dream includes the remains of a memory or an allusion to some event (or often to several events) of the day before the dream, and, if we follow these connections, we often arrive with one blow at the transition from the apparently far remote dream-world to the real life of the patient. Or, again, we may tell him to start with those elements of the dream's content which strike him by their special clarity and sensory strength; for we know that he will find it particularly easy to get associations to these. It makes no difference by which of these methods we approach the associations we are in search of.[1]

And next, we obtain these associations. What they bring us is of the most various kinds: memories from the day before, the 'dream-day', and from times long past, reflections, discussions, with arguments for and against, confessions and enquiries. Some of them the patient pours out; when he comes to others he is held up for a time. Most of them show a clear connection to some element of the dream; no wonder, since those elements were their starting-point. But it also sometimes happens that the patient introduces them with these words: 'This seems to me to have nothing at all to do with the dream, but I tell it you because it occurs to me.'

[1] [A slightly different list of these alternative methods is given in 'Remarks on the Theory and Practice of Dream-Interpretation' (1923c).]

If one listens to these copious associations, one soon notices that they have more in common with the content of the dream than their starting-points alone. They throw a surprising light on all the different parts of the dream, fill in gaps between them, and make their strange juxtapositions intelligible. In the end one is bound to become clear about the relation between them and the dream's content. The dream is seen to be an abbreviated selection from the associations, a selection made, it is true, according to rules that we have not yet understood: the elements of the dream are like representatives chosen by election from a mass of people. There can be no doubt that by our technique we have got hold of something for which the dream is a substitute and in which lies the dream's psychical value, but which no longer exhibits its puzzling peculiarities, its strangeness and its confusion.

Let there be no misunderstanding, however. The associations to the dream are not yet the latent dream-thoughts. The latter are contained in the associations like an alkali in the mother-liquor, but yet not quite completely contained in them. On the one hand, the associations give us far more than we need for formulating the latent dream-thoughts—namely all the explanations, transitions, and connections which the patient's intellect is bound to produce in the course of his approach to the dream-thoughts. On the other hand, an association often comes to a stop precisely before the genuine dream-thought: it has only come near to it and has only had contact with it through allusions. At that point we intervene on our own; we fill in the hints, draw undeniable conclusions, and give explicit utterance to what the patient has only touched on in his associations. This sounds as though we allowed our ingenuity and caprice to play with the material put at our disposal by the dreamer and as though we misused it in order to interpret *into* his utterances what cannot be interpreted *from* them. Nor is it easy to show the legitimacy of our procedure in an abstract description of it. But you have only to carry out a dream-analysis yourselves or study a good account of one in our literature and you will be convinced of the cogent manner in which interpretative work like this proceeds.

If in general and primarily we are dependent, in interpreting dreams, on the dreamer's associations, yet in relation to certain elements of the dream's content we adopt a quite independent attitude, chiefly because we have to, because as a rule associations fail to materialize in their case. We noticed at an early stage that it is always in connection with the same elements that this happens; they are not very numerous, and repeated experience has taught us that they are to be regarded and interpreted as *symbols* of something else. As contrasted with the other dream-elements, a fixed meaning may be attributed to them, which, however, need not be unambiguous and whose range is determined by special rules with which we are unfamiliar. Since *we* know how to translate these symbols and the dreamer does not, in spite of having used them himself, it may happen that the sense of a dream may at once become clear to us as soon as we have heard the text of the dream, even before we have made any efforts at interpreting it, while it still remains an enigma to the dreamer himself. But I have said so much to you in my earlier lectures about symbolism, our knowledge of it and the problems it poses us, that I need not repeat it to-day.[1]

That, then, is our method of interpreting dreams. The first and justifiable question is: 'Can we interpret *all* dreams by its help?'[2] And the answer is: 'No, not all; but so many that we feel confident in the serviceability and correctness of the procedure.' 'But why not all?' The answer to this has something important to teach us, which at once introduces us into the psychical determinants of the formation of dreams: 'Because the work of interpreting dreams is carried out against a resistance, which varies between trivial dimensions and invincibility (at least so far as the strength of our present methods reaches).' It is impossible during our work to overlook the manifestations of this resistance. At some points the associations are given without hesitation and the first or second idea that occurs to the patient brings an explanation. At other points there is a stoppage and the patient hesitates before bringing out an association, and, if so, we often have to listen to a long chain of ideas before receiving anything that helps us to understand the dream. We are certainly right in thinking that the longer and more roundabout the chain of associations the stronger the

---

[1] [See *Introductory Lectures* (1916–17), Lecture X.]

[2] [Freud had recently written a special note on 'The Limits to the Possibility of Interpretation' (1925*i*).]

resistance. We can detect the same influence at work in the forgetting of dreams. It happens often enough that a patient, despite all his efforts, cannot remember one of his dreams. But after we have been able in the course of a piece of analytic work to get rid of a difficulty which had been disturbing his relation to the analysis, the forgotten dream suddenly re-emerges. Two other observations are also in place here. It very frequently comes about that, to begin with, a portion of a dream is omitted and added afterwards as an addendum. This is to be regarded as an attempt to forget that portion. Experience shows that it is that particular piece which is the most important; there was a greater resistance, we suppose, in the path of communicating it than the other parts of the dream.[1] Furthermore, we often find that a dreamer endeavours to prevent himself from forgetting his dreams by fixing them in writing immediately after waking up. We can tell him that that is no use. For the resistance from which he has extorted the preservation of the text of the dream will then be displaced on to its associations and will make the manifest dream inaccessible to interpretation.[2] In view of these facts we need not feel surprised if a further increase in the resistance suppresses the associations altogether and thus brings the interpretation of the dream to nothing.

From all this we infer that the resistance which we come across in the work of interpreting dreams must also have had a share in their origin. We can actually distinguish between dreams that arose under a slight and under a high pressure of resistance.[3] But this pressure varies as well from place to place within one and the same dream; it is responsible for the gaps, obscurities and confusions which may interrupt the continuity of even the finest of dreams.

But what is creating the resistance and against what is it aimed? Well, the resistance is the surest sign to us of a conflict. There must be a force here which is seeking to express something and another which is striving to prevent its expression.

[1] [Cf. *The Interpretation of Dreams* (1900a), Chapter VII (A).]
[2] [Cf. 'The Handling of Dream-Interpretation in Psycho-Analysis' (1911e).]
[3] [Cf. Section II of 'Remarks on the Theory and Practice of Dream-Interpretation' (1923c).]

What comes about in consequence as a manifest dream may combine all the decisions into which this struggle between two trends has been condensed. At one point one of these forces may have succeeded in putting through what it wanted to say, while at another point it is the opposing agency which has managed to blot out the intended communication completely or to replace it by something that reveals not a trace of it. The commonest and most characteristic cases of dream-construction are those in which the conflict has ended in a compromise, so that the communicating agency has, it is true, been able to say what it wanted but not in the way it wanted—only in a softened down, distorted and unrecognized form. If, then, dreams do not give a faithful picture of the dream-thoughts and if the work of interpretation is required in order to bridge the gap between them, that is the outcome of the opposing, inhibiting and restricting agency which we have inferred from our perception of the resistance while we interpret dreams. So long as we studied dreams as isolated phenomena independent of the psychical structures akin to them, we named this agency the *censor*[1] *of dreams.*

You have long been aware that this censorship is not an institution peculiar to dream-life. You know that the conflict between the two psychical agencies, which we—inaccurately—describe as the 'unconscious repressed' and the 'conscious', dominates our whole mental life and that the resistance against the interpretation of dreams, the sign of the dream-censorship, is nothing other than the resistance due to repression by which the two agencies are separated. You know too that the conflict between these two agencies may under certain conditions produce other psychical structures which, like dreams, are the outcome of compromises; and you will not expect me to repeat to you here everything that was contained in my introduction to the theory of the neuroses in order to demonstrate to you what we know of the determinants of the formation of such compromises. You have realized that the dream is a pathological product, the first member of the class which includes hysterical

---

[1] [This is one of the very rare occasions on which Freud uses the personified form 'Zensor' instead of the impersonal 'Zensur' (censorship).]

symptoms, obsessions and delusions,[1] but that it is distinguished from the others by its transitoriness and by its occurrence under conditions which are part of normal life. For let us bear firmly in mind that, as was already pointed out by Aristotle, dream-life is the way in which our mind works during the state of sleep.[2] The state of sleep involves a turning-away from the real external world, and there we have the necessary condition for the development of a psychosis. The most careful study of the severe psychoses will not reveal to us a single feature that is more characteristic of those pathological conditions. In psychoses, however, the turning-away from reality is brought about in two kinds of way: either by the unconscious repressed becoming excessively strong so that it overwhelms the conscious, which is attached to reality,[3] or because reality has become so intolerably distressing that the threatened ego throws itself into the arms of the unconscious instinctual forces in a desperate revolt. The harmless dream-psychosis is the result of a withdrawal from the external world which is consciously willed and only temporary, and it disappears when relations to the external world are resumed. During the isolation of the sleeping individual an alteration in the distribution of his psychical energy also sets in; a part of the expenditure on repression, which is normally required in order to hold the unconscious down, can be saved, for if the unconscious makes use of its relative liberation for active purposes, it finds its path to motility closed and the only path open to it is the harmless one leading to hallucinatory satisfaction. Now, therefore, a dream can be formed; but the fact of the dream-censorship shows that even during sleep enough of the resistance due to repression is retained.

Here we are presented with a means of answering the question of whether dreams have a function too, whether they are entrusted with any useful achievement. The condition of rest free from stimulus, which the state of sleep wishes to establish,

[1] [This part of the sentence is repeated almost word for word from the second sentence in Freud's preface to the first edition of *The Interpretation of Dreams* (1900a).]

[2] [*The Interpretation of Dreams*, Chapter I.]

[3] [The notion occurs already in one of Freud's very earliest psychological papers, his first one on 'The Neuro-Psychoses of Defence' (1894a).]

is threatened from three directions: in a relatively accidental manner by external stimuli during sleep, and by interests of the previous day which cannot be broken off, and in an unavoidable manner by unsated repressed instinctual impulses which are on the watch for an opportunity of finding expression. In consequence of the diminishing of repressions at night there would be a risk that the rest afforded by sleep would be interrupted whenever an instigation from outside or from inside succeeded in linking up with an unconscious instinctual source. The process of dreaming allows the product of a collaboration of this kind to find an outlet in a harmless hallucinatory experience and in that way assures a continuation of sleep. The fact that a dream occasionally awakens the sleeper, to the accompaniment of a generation of anxiety, is no contradiction of this function but rather, perhaps, a signal that the watchman regards the situation as too dangerous and no longer feels able to control it. And very often then, while we are still asleep, a consolation occurs to us which seeks to prevent our waking up: 'But after all it's only a dream!'

This was what I wanted to say to you, Ladies and Gentlemen, about dream-interpretation, whose task it is to lead the way from the manifest dream to the latent dream-thoughts. When this has been achieved, interest in a dream, so far as practical analysis is concerned, is for the most part at an end. We add the communication we have received in the form of a dream to the rest of the patient's communications and proceed with the analysis. We, however, have an interest in dwelling a little longer on the dream. We are tempted to study the process by which the latent dream-thoughts were transformed into the manifest dream. We call this the 'dream-work'. As you will recall, I described it in such detail in my earlier lectures[1] that I can restrict my present survey to the most concise summary.

The process of the dream-work, then, is something entirely new and strange, nothing resembling which was known before. It has given us our first glimpse of the processes which take place in the unconscious system and has shown us that they are quite other than what we know from our conscious thinking and are bound to appear to the latter preposterous and incorrect.

[1] [*Introductory Lectures*, XI.]

The importance of this finding was then increased by the discovery that in the construction of neurotic symptoms the same mechanisms (we do not venture to say 'processes of thought') are operative as those which have transformed the latent dream-thoughts into the manifest dream.

In what follows I shall not be able to avoid a schematic method of exposition. Let us assume that in a particular case we have before us all the latent thoughts, charged with a greater or less amount of affect, by which the manifest dream has been replaced after its interpretation has been completed. We shall then be struck by one difference among these latent thoughts, and that difference will take us a long way. Almost all these dream-thoughts are recognized by the dreamer or acknowledged by him; he admits that he has thought this, now or at some other time, or that he might have thought it. There is only one single thought that he refuses to accept; it is strange to him or even perhaps repellent; he may possibly reject it with passionate feeling. It now becomes evident to us that the other thoughts are portions of a conscious, or, more accurately, a preconscious train of thinking. They might have been thought in waking life too, and indeed they were probably formed during the previous day. This one repudiated thought, however, or, properly speaking, this one impulse, is a child of night; it belongs to the dreamer's unconscious and on that account it is repudiated and rejected by him. It had to wait for the nightly relaxation of repression in order to arrive at any kind of expression. And in any case this expression is a weakened, distorted and disguised one; without our work of dream-interpretation we should not have found it. This unconscious impulse has to thank its link with the other, unobjectionable, dream-thoughts for the opportunity of slipping past the barrier of the censorship in an inconspicuous disguise. On the other hand, the preconscious dream-thoughts have to thank this same link for the power to occupy mental life during sleep as well. For there is no doubt about it: this unconscious impulse is the true creator of the dream; it is what produces the psychical energy for the dream's construction. Like any other instinctual impulse, it cannot strive for anything other than its own satisfaction; and our experience in interpreting dreams shows us too that that is the sense of all dreaming. In every dream an instinctual wish has to be represented as fulfilled. The shutting-off of mental life from reality at night and the regression to primitive mechanisms which this makes possible enable this wished-for instinctual satisfaction to be experienced in a hallucinatory manner as occurring in the present. As a result of this same regression, ideas are transformed in the dream into visual pictures: the latent dream-thoughts, that is to say, are dramatized and illustrated.

This piece of the dream-work gives us information about some of the most striking and peculiar features of dreams. I will repeat the course of events in dream-formation. As an introduction: the wish to sleep and intentional turning away from the external world. Next, two consequences of this for the mental apparatus: first, the possibility for older and more primitive methods of working to emerge in it—regression; secondly, the lowering of the resistance due to repression which weighs down upon the unconscious. As a result of this last factor the possibility arises for the formation of a dream and this is taken advantage of by the precipitating causes, the internal and external stimuli which have become active. The dream which originates in this way is already a compromise-structure. It has a double function; on the one hand it is ego-syntonic,[1] since, by getting rid of the stimuli which are interfering with sleep, it serves the wish to sleep; on the other hand it allows a repressed instinctual impulse to obtain the satisfaction that is possible in these circumstances, in the form of the hallucinated fulfilment of a wish. The whole process of forming a dream which is permitted by the sleeping ego is, however, subject to the condition of the censorship, which is exercised by the residue of the repression still in operation. I cannot present the process more simply: it is not more simple. But I can proceed now with my description of the dream-work.

Let us go back once more to the latent dream-thoughts. Their most powerful element is the repressed instinctual impulse which has created in them an expression for itself on the basis of the presence of chance stimuli and by transference on to the day's residues—though an expression that is toned down and disguised. Like every instinctual impulse, it too presses for satisfaction by action; but its path to motility is blocked by the physiological regulations implied in the state of sleep; it is

[1] [In conformity with the ego.]

compelled to take the backwards course in the direction of perception and to be content with a hallucinated satisfaction. The
latent dream-thoughts are thus transformed into a collection of
sensory images and visual scenes. It is as they travel on this
course that what seems to us so novel and so strange occurs to
them. All the linguistic instruments by which we express the
subtler relations of thought—the conjunctions and prepositions,
the changes in declension and conjugation—are dropped, because there are no means of representing them; just as in a
primitive language without any grammar, only the raw material
of thought is expressed and abstract terms are taken back to the
concrete ones that are at their basis. What is left over after this
may well appear disconnected. The copious employment of
symbols, which have become alien to conscious thinking, for
representing certain objects and processes is in harmony alike
with the archaic regression in the mental apparatus and with
the demands of the censorship.

But other changes made in the elements of the dream-
thoughts go far beyond this. Such of those elements as allow
any point of contact to be found between them are *condensed* into
new unities. In the process of transforming the thoughts into
pictures, preference is unmistakably given to such as permit of
this putting-together, this condensation; it is as though a force
were at work which was subjecting the material to compression
and concentration. As a result of condensation, one element
in the manifest dream may correspond to numerous elements in
the latent dream-thoughts; but, conversely too, one element
in the dream-thoughts may be represented by several images
in the dream.

Still more remarkable is the other process—*displacement* or
shifting of accent—which in conscious thinking we come across
only as faulty reasoning or as means for a joke. The different
ideas in the dream-thoughts are, indeed, not all of equal value;
they are cathected with quotas of affect of varying magnitude
and are correspondingly judged to be important and deserving
of interest to a greater or less degree. In the dream-work these
ideas are separated from the affects attaching to them. The
affects are dealt with independently; they may be displaced on
to something else, they may be retained, they may undergo
alterations, or they may not appear in the dream at all. The

importance of the ideas that have been stripped of their affect returns in the dream as sensory strength in the dream-pictures; but we observe that this accent has passed over from important elements to indifferent ones. Thus something that played only a minor part in the dream-thoughts seems to be pushed into the foreground in the dream as the main thing, while, on the contrary, what was the essence of the dream-thoughts finds only passing and indistinct representation in the dream. No other part of the dream-work is so much responsible for making the dream strange and incomprehensible to the dreamer. Displacement is the principal means used in the *dream-distortion* to which the dream-thoughts must submit under the influence of the censorship.

After these influences have been brought to bear upon the dream-thoughts the dream is almost complete. A further, somewhat variable, factor also comes into play—known as 'secondary revision'—after the dream has been presented before consciousness as an object of perception. At that point we treat it as we are in general accustomed to treat the contents of our perception: we fill in gaps and introduce connections, and in doing so are often guilty of gross misunderstandings. But this activity, which might be described as a rationalizing one and which at best provides the dream with a smooth façade that cannot fit its true content, may also be omitted or only be expressed to a very modest degree—in which case the dream will display all its rents and cracks openly. It must not be forgotten, on the other hand, that the dream-work does not always operate with equal energy either; it often restricts itself to certain portions of the dream-thoughts only and others of them are allowed to appear in the dream unaltered. In such cases an impression is given of the dream having carried out the most delicate and complex intellectual operations, of its having speculated, made jokes, arrived at decisions and solved problems, whereas all this is a product of our normal mental activity, may have been performed equally well during the day before the dream as during the night, has nothing to do with the dream-work and brings nothing to light that is characteristic of dreams. Nor is it superfluous to insist once more on the contrast within the dream-thoughts themselves between the unconscious instinctual impulse and the day's residues. While the latter exhibit all the multiplicity of our mental acts, the former, which becomes the motive force proper of the forming of the dream, finds its outlet invariably in the fulfilment of a wish.

I could have told you all this fifteen years ago, and indeed I believe I did in fact tell it you then. And now let me bring together such changes and new discoveries as may have been made during the interval. I have said already that I am afraid you will find that it amounts to very little, and you will fail to understand why I obliged you to listen to the same thing twice over, and obliged myself to say it. But fifteen years have passed meanwhile and I hope that this will be my easiest way of re-establishing contact with you. Moreover, these are such fundamental things, of such decisive importance for understanding psycho-analysis, that one may be glad to hear them a second time, and it is in itself worth knowing that they have remained so much the same for fifteen years.

In the literature of this period you will of course find a large quantity of confirmatory material and of presentation of details, of which I intend only to give you samples. I shall also, incidentally, be able to tell you a few things that were in fact already known earlier. What is in question is principally the symbolism in dreams and the other methods of representation in them. Now listen to this. Only quite a short while ago the medical faculty in an American University refused to allow psycho-analysis the status of a science, on the ground that it did not admit of any experimental proof. They might have raised the same objection to astronomy; indeed, experimentation with the heavenly bodies is particularly difficult. There one has to fall back on observation. Nevertheless, some Viennese investigators have actually made a beginning with experimental confirmation of our dream symbolism. As long ago as in 1912 a Dr. Schrötter found that if instructions to dream of sexual matters are given to deeply hypnotized subjects, then in the dream that is thus provoked the sexual material emerges with its place taken by the symbols that are familiar to us. For instance, a woman was told to dream of sexual intercourse with a female friend. In her dream this friend appeared with a travelling-bag on which was pasted the label 'Ladies Only'. Still more impressive experiments were carried out by Betlheim and

Hartmann in 1924. They worked with patients suffering from what is known as the Korsakoff confusional psychosis. They told these patients stories of a grossly sexual kind and observed the distortions which appeared when the patients were instructed to reproduce what they had been told. Once more there emerged the symbols for sexual organs and sexual intercourse that are familiar to us—among them the symbol of the staircase which, as the writers justly remark, could never have been reached by a conscious wish to distort.[1]

In a very interesting series of experiments, Herbert Silberer [1909 and 1912] has shown that one can catch the dream-work red-handed, as it were, in the act of turning abstract thoughts into visual pictures. If he tried to force himself to do intellectual work while he was in a state of fatigue and drowsiness, the thought would often vanish and be replaced by a vision, which was obviously a substitute for it.

Here is a simple example. 'I thought', says Silberer, 'of having to revise an uneven passage in an essay.' The vision: 'I saw myself planing a piece of wood.' It often happened during these experiments that the content of the vision was not the thought that was being dealt with but his own subjective state while he was making the effort—the state instead of the object. This is described by Silberer as a 'functional phenomenon'. An example will show you at once what is meant. The author was endeavouring to compare the opinions of two philosophers on a particular question. But in his sleepy condition one of these opinions kept on escaping him and finally he had a vision that he was asking for information from a disobliging secretary who was bent over his writing-table and who began by disregarding him and then gave him a disagreeable and uncomplying look. The conditions under which the experiments were made probably themselves explain why the vision that was induced represented so often an event of self-observation.[2]

We have not yet finished with symbols. There are some which we believed we recognized but which nevertheless worried

[1] [Longer descriptions of these experiments will be found in Chapter VI (E) of *The Interpretation of Dreams* (1900a).]

[2] [Freud gave a very much fuller account of Silberer's experiments, with a great many quotations, in some passages added in 1914 to *The Interpretation of Dreams* (1900a), Chapter VI (D) and (I).]

us because we could not explain how *this* particular symbol had come to have *that* particular meaning. In such cases confirmations from elsewhere—from philology, folklore, mythology or ritual—were bound to be especially welcome. An instance of this sort is the symbol of an overcoat or cloak [German '*Mantel*']. We have said that in a woman's dreams this stands for a man.[1] I hope it will impress you when you hear that Theodor Reik (1920) gives us this information: 'During the extremely ancient bridal ceremonial of the Bedouins, the bridegroom covers the bride with a special cloak known as "Aba" and speaks the following ritual words: "Henceforth none save I shall cover thee!" ' (Quoted from Robert Eisler [1910, 2, 599 f.]). We have also found several fresh symbols, at least two of which I will tell you of. According to Abraham (1922) a spider in dreams is a symbol of the mother, but of the *phallic* mother, of whom we are afraid; so that the fear of spiders expresses dread of mother-incest and horror of the female genitals. You know, perhaps, that the mythological creation, Medusa's head, can be traced back to the same *motif* of fright at castration.[2] The other symbol I want to talk to you about is that of the *bridge*, which has been explained by Ferenczi (1921 and 1922). First it means the male organ, which unites the two parents in sexual intercourse; but afterwards it develops further meanings which are derived from this first one. In so far as it is thanks to the male organ that we are able to come into the world at all, out of the amniotic fluid, a bridge becomes the crossing from the other world (the unborn state, the womb) to this world (life); and, since men also picture death as a return to the womb (to the water), a bridge also acquires the meaning of something that leads to death, and finally, at a further remove from its original sense, it stands for transitions or changes in condition generally. It tallies with this, accordingly, if a woman who has not overcome her wish to be a man has frequent dreams of bridges that are too short to reach the further shore.

[1] [The symbol is referred to in the *Introductory Lectures*, Lecture X, but the fact that this applies to *women's* dreams is only mentioned among some 'Observations and Examples' published earlier (Freud, 1913*h*).]

[2] [Cf. a posthumously published note by Freud on the subject (1940*c* [1922]).]

In the manifest content of dreams we very often find pictures and situations recalling familiar themes in fairy tales, legends and myths. The interpretation of such dreams thus throws a light on the original interests which created these themes, though we must at the same time not forget, of course, the change in meaning by which this material has been affected in the course of time. Our work of interpretation uncovers, so to say, the raw material, which must often enough be described as sexual in the widest sense, but has found the most varied application in later adaptations. Derivations of this kind are apt to bring down on us the wrath of all non-analytically schooled workers, as though we were seeking to deny or undervalue everything that was later erected on the original basis. Nevertheless, such discoveries are instructive and interesting. The same is true of tracing back the origin of particular themes in plastic art, as, for instance, when M. J. Eisler (1919), following indications in his patients' dreams, gave an analytic interpretation of the youth playing with a little boy represented in the Hermes of Praxiteles. And lastly I cannot resist pointing out how often light is thrown by the interpretation of dreams on mythological themes in particular. Thus, for instance, the legend of the Labyrinth can be recognized as a representation of anal birth: the twisting paths are the bowels and Ariadne's thread is the umbilical cord.

The methods of representation employed by the dream-work —fascinating material, scarcely capable of exhaustion—have been made more and more familiar to us by closer study. I will give you a few examples of them. Thus, for instance, dreams represent the relation of frequency by a multiplication of similar things. Here is a young girl's remarkable dream. She dreamt she came into a great hall and found some one in it sitting on a chair; this was repeated six or eight times or more, but each time it was her father. This is easy to understand when we discover, from accessory details in the interpretation, that this room stood for the womb. The dream then becomes equivalent to the phantasy, familiarly found in girls, of having met their father already during their intra-uterine life when he visited the womb while their mother was pregnant. You should not be confused by the fact that something is reversed in the dream— that her father's 'coming-in' is displaced on to herself; incidentally, this has a special meaning of its own as well. The multiplication of the figure of the father can only express the fact that the event in question occurred repeatedly. After all, it must be allowed that the dream is not taking very much on itself in expressing frequency by multiplicity.[1] It has only needed to go back to the original significance of the former word; to-day it means to us a repetition in time, but it is derived from an accumulation in space. In general, indeed, where it is possible, the dream-work changes temporal relations into spatial ones and represents them as such. In a dream, for instance, one may see a scene between two people who look very small and a long way off, as though one were seeing them through the wrong end of a pair of opera-glasses. Here, both the smallness and the remoteness in space have the same significance: what is meant is remoteness in *time* and we are to understand that the scene is from the remote past.

Again, you may remember that in my earlier lectures I already told you (and illustrated the fact by examples) that we had learnt to make use for our interpretations even of the purely *formal* features of the manifest dream—that is, to transform them into material coming from the latent dream-thoughts.[2] As you already know, all dreams that are dreamt in a single night belong in a single context. But it is not a matter of indifference whether these dreams appear to the dreamer as a continuum or whether he divides them into several parts and into how many. The number of such parts often corresponds to an equal number of separate focal points in the structural formation of the latent dream-thoughts or to contending trends in the dreamer's mental life, each of which finds a dominant, even though never an exclusive, expression in one particular part of the dream. A short introductory dream and a longer main dream following it often stand in the relation of protasis and apodosis [conditional and consequential clauses], of which a very clear instance will be found in the old lectures.[3] A dream

[1] ['*Häufigkeit*' and '*Häufung*' in German. Both words are derived from '*Haufen*'—a 'heap'.]

[2] [Cf. *Introductory Lectures*, XI.]

[3] [*Introductory Lectures*, XII.]

which is described by the dreamer as 'somehow interpolated' will actually correspond to a dependent clause in the dream-thoughts. Franz Alexander (1925) has shown in a study on pairs of dreams that it not infrequently happens that two dreams in one night share the carrying-out of the dream's task by producing a wish-fulfilment in two stages if they are taken together, though each dream separately would not effect that result. Suppose, for instance, that the dream-wish had as its content some illicit action in regard to a particular person. Then in the first dream the person will appear undisguised, but the action will be only timidly hinted at. The second dream will behave differently. The action will be named without disguise, but the person will either be made unrecognizable or replaced by someone indifferent. This, you will admit, gives one an impression of actual cunning. Another and similar relation between the two members of a pair of dreams is found where one represents a punishment and the other the sinful wish-fulfilment. It amounts to this: 'if one accepts the punishment for it, one can go on to allow oneself the forbidden thing.'

I cannot detain you any longer over such minor discoveries or over the discussions relating to the employment of dream-interpretation in the work of analysis. I feel sure you are impatient to hear what changes have been made in our fundamental views on the nature and significance of dreams. I have already warned you that precisely on this there is little to report to you. The most disputed point in the whole theory was no doubt the assertion that all dreams are the fulfilments of wishes. The inevitable and ever recurring objection raised by the layman that there are nevertheless so many anxiety-dreams was, I think I may say, completely disposed of in my earlier lectures.[1] With the division into wishful dreams, anxiety-dreams and punishment dreams, we have kept our theory intact.

Punishment-dreams, too, are fulfilments of wishes, though not of wishes of the instinctual impulses but of those of the critical, censoring and punishing agency in the mind. If we have a pure punishment-dream before us, an easy mental operation will enable us to restore the wishful dream to which the punishment-dream was the correct rejoinder and which, owing

[1] [See *Introductory Lectures*, XIV.]

to this repudiation, was replaced as the manifest dream. As you know, Ladies and Gentlemen, the study of dreams was what first helped us to understand the neuroses, and you will find it natural that our knowledge of the neuroses was later able to influence our view of dreams. As you will hear,[1] we have been obliged to postulate the existence in the mind of a special critical and prohibiting agency which we have named the 'super-ego'. Since recognizing that the censorship of dreams is also a function of this agency, we have been led to examine the part played by the super-ego in the construction of dreams more carefully.

Only two serious difficulties have arisen against the wish-fulfilment theory of dreams. A discussion of them leads far afield and has not yet, indeed, brought us to any wholly satisfying conclusion.

The first of these difficulties is presented in the fact that people who have experienced a shock, a severe psychical trauma —such as happened so often during the war and such as affords the basis for traumatic hysteria—are regularly taken back in their dreams into the traumatic situation. According to our hypotheses about the function of dreams this should not occur. What wishful impulse could be satisfied by harking back in this way to this exceedingly distressing traumatic experience? It is hard to guess.

We meet with the second of these facts almost every day in the course of our analytic work; and it does not imply such an important objection as the other does. One of the tasks of psycho-analysis, as you know, is to lift the veil of amnesia which hides the earliest years of childhood and to bring to conscious memory the manifestations of early infantile sexual life which are contained in them. Now these first sexual experiences of a child are linked to painful impressions of anxiety, prohibition, disappointment and punishment. We can understand their having been repressed; but, that being so, we cannot understand how it is that they have such free access to dream-life, that they provide the pattern for so many dream-phantasies and that dreams are filled with reproductions of these scenes from childhood and with allusions to them. It must be admitted that their unpleasurable character and the dream-work's wish-

[1] [In Lecture XXXI below.]

fulfilling purpose seem far from mutually compatible. But it may be that in this case we are magnifying the difficulty. After all, these same infantile experiences have attached to them all the imperishable, unfulfilled instinctual wishes which throughout life provide the energy for the construction of dreams, and to which we may no doubt credit the possibility, in their mighty uprush, of forcing to the surface, along with the rest, the material of distressing events. And on the other hand the manner and form in which this material is reproduced shows unmistakably the efforts of the dream-work directed to denying the unpleasure by means of distortion and to transforming disappointment into attainment.

With the traumatic neuroses things are different. In their case the dreams regularly end in the generation of anxiety. We should not, I think, be afraid to admit that here the function of the dream has failed. I will not invoke the saying that the exception proves the rule: its wisdom seems to me most questionable. But no doubt the exception does not overturn the rule. If, for the sake of studying it, we isolate one particular psychical function, such as dreaming, from the psychical machinery as a whole, we make it possible to discover the laws that are peculiar to it; but when we insert it once more into the general context we must be prepared to discover that these findings are obscured or impaired by collision with other forces. We say that a dream is the fulfilment of a wish; but if you want to take these latter objections into account, you can say nevertheless that a dream is an *attempt* at the fulfilment of a wish. No one who can properly appreciate the dynamics of the mind will suppose that you have said anything different by this. In certain circumstances a dream is only able to put its intention into effect very incompletely, or must abandon it entirely. Unconscious fixation to a trauma seems to be foremost among these obstacles to the function of dreaming. While the sleeper is obliged to dream, because the relaxation of repression at night allows the upward pressure of the traumatic fixation to become active, there is a failure in the functioning of his dream-work, which would like to transform the memory-traces of the traumatic event into the fulfilment of a wish. In these circumstances it will happen that one cannot sleep, that one gives up sleep from dread of the failure of the function of dreaming. Traumatic neuroses are

here offering us an extreme case; but we must admit that childhood experiences, too, are of a traumatic nature, and we need
not be surprised if comparatively trivial interferences with the
function of dreams may arise under other conditions as well.[1]

[1] [The topic of the last three paragraphs was first raised by Freud in
Chapters II and III of *Beyond the Pleasure Principle* (1920g). Further
allusions to it will be found in Lecture XXXII, p. 570 below.]

LECTURE XXX

DREAMS AND OCCULTISM [1]

LADIES AND GENTLEMEN,—To-day we will proceed along a narrow path, but one which may lead us to a wide prospect.

You will scarcely be surprised by the news that I am going to speak to you on the relation of dreams to occultism. Dreams have, indeed, often been regarded as the gateway into the world of mysticism, and even to-day are themselves looked on by many people as an occult phenomenon. Even we, who have made them into a subject for scientific study, do not dispute that one or more threads link them to those obscure matters. Mysticism, occultism—what is meant by these words? You must not expect me to make any attempt at embracing this ill-circumscribed region with definitions. We all know in a general and indefinite manner what the words imply to us. They refer to some sort of 'other world', lying beyond the bright world governed by relentless laws which has been constructed for us by science.

Occultism asserts that there are in fact 'more things in heaven and earth than are dreamt of in our philosophy'. Well, we need not feel bound by the narrow-mindedness of academic philosophy; we are ready to believe what is shown to us to deserve belief.

We propose to proceed with these things as we do with any other scientific material: first of all to establish whether such events can really be shown to occur, and then and only then, when their factual nature cannot be doubted, to concern ourselves with their explanation. It cannot be denied, however, that even the putting of this decision into action is made hard for us by intellectual, psychological and historical factors. The case is not the same as when we approach other investigations.

[1] [Ernest Jones has given a comprehensive survey of Freud's attitude to occultism in Chapter XIV of the third volume of his biography (1957).]

First, the intellectual difficulty. Let me give you a crude and obvious explanation of what I have in mind. Let us suppose that the question at issue is the constitution of the interior of the earth. We have, as you are aware, no certain knowledge about it. We suspect that it consists of heavy metals in an incandescent state. Then let us imagine that someone puts forward an assertion that the interior of the earth consists of water saturated with carbonic acid—that is to say, with a kind of soda-water. We shall no doubt say that this is most improbable, that it contradicts all our expectations and pays no attention to the known facts which have led us to adopt the metal hypothesis. Nevertheless it is not inconceivable; if someone were to show us a way of testing the soda-water hypothesis we should follow it without objecting. But suppose now that someone else comes along and seriously asserts that the core of the earth consists of jam. Our reaction to this will be quite different. We shall tell ourselves that jam does not occur in nature, that it is a product of human cooking, that, morover, the existence of this material presupposes the presence of fruit-trees and their fruit, and that we cannot see how we can locate vegetation and human cookery in the interior of the earth. The result of these intellectual objections will be a switching of our interest: instead of starting upon an investigation of whether the core of the earth really consists of jam, we shall ask ourselves what sort of person this must be who can arrive at such a notion, or at most we shall ask him where he got it from. The unlucky inventor of the jam theory will be very much insulted and will complain that we are refusing to make an objective investigation of his assertion on the ground of a pretendedly scientific prejudice. But this will be of no help to him. We perceive that prejudices are not always to be reprobated, but that they are sometimes justified and expedient because they save us useless labour. In fact they are only conclusions based on an analogy with other well-founded judgements.

A whole number of occultist assertions have the same sort of effect on us as the jam hypothesis; so that we consider ourselves justified in rejecting them at sight, without further investigation. But all the same, the position is not so simple. A comparison like the one I have chosen proves nothing, or proves as little as comparisons in general. It remains doubtful whether

it fits the case, and it is clear that its choice was already determined by our attitude of contemptuous rejection. Prejudices are
sometimes expedient and justified; but sometimes they are
erroneous and detrimental, and one can never tell when they
are the one and when the other. The history of science itself
abounds in instances which are a warning against premature
condemnation. For a long time it was regarded as a senseless
hypothesis to suppose that the stones, which we now call meteo-
rites, could have reached the earth from outer space or that the
rocks forming mountains, in which the remains of shells are
imbedded, could have once formed the bed of the sea. Incidentally, much the same thing happened to our psycho-
analysis when it brought forward its inference of there being
an unconscious. Thus we analysts have special reason to be
careful in using intellectual considerations for rejecting new
hypotheses and must admit that they do not relieve us from
feelings of antipathy, doubt and uncertainty.

I have spoken of the second factor [that complicates our
approach to the subject] as the psychological one. By that I
mean the general tendency of mankind to credulity and a belief
in the miraculous. From the very beginning, when life takes
us under its strict discipline, a resistance stirs within us against
the relentlessness and monotony of the laws of thought and
against the demands of reality-testing.[1] Reason becomes the
enemy which withholds from us so many possibilities of pleasure.
We discover how much pleasure it gives us to withdraw from
it, temporarily at least, and to surrender to the allurements of
nonsense. Schoolboys delight in the twisting of words; when a
scientific congress is over, the specialists make fun of their own
activities; even earnest-minded men enjoy a joke.[2] More serious
hostility to 'Reason and Science, the highest strength possessed
by man',[3] awaits its opportunity; it hastens to prefer the
miracle-doctor or the practitioner of nature-cures to the 'qualified' physician; it is favourable to the assertions of occultism so

---

[1] [I.e. the process of testing things to see if they are real. This is discussed in 'A Metapsychological Supplement to the Theory of Dreams',
(1917d). See also Introductory Lectures, XXIII.]

[2] [This 'pleasure in nonsense' had been fully discussed by Freud in
Chapter IV of his book on jokes (1905c), (Norton, 1961) pp. 125–7.]

[3] [Goethe, Faust, Part I, Scene 4.]

long as those alleged facts can be taken as breaches of laws and rules; it lulls criticism to sleep, falsifies perceptions and enforces confirmations and agreements which cannot be justified. If this human tendency is taken into account, there is every reason to discount much of the information put forward in occultist literature.

I have called the third doubt the historical one; and by it I mean to point out that there is in fact nothing new in the world of occultism. There emerge in it once more all the signs, miracles, prophecies and apparitions which have been reported to us from ancient times and in ancient books and which we thought had long since been disposed of as the offspring of unbridled imagination or of tendentious fraud, as the product of an age in which man's ignorance was very great and the scientific spirit was still in its cradle. If we accept the truth of what, according to the occultists' information, still occurs to-day, we must also believe in the authenticity of the reports which have come down to us from ancient times. And we must then reflect that the tradition and sacred books of all peoples are brimful of similar marvellous tales and that the religions base their claim to credibility on precisely such miraculous events and find proof in them of the operation of superhuman powers. That being so, it will be hard for us to avoid a suspicion that the interest in occultism is in fact a religious one and that one of the secret motives of the occultist movement is to come to the help of religion, threatened as it is by the advance of scientific thought. And with the discovery of this motive our distrust must increase and our disinclination to embark on the examination of these supposedly occult phenomena.

Sooner or later, however, this disinclination must be overcome. We are faced by a question of fact: is what the occultists tell us true or not? It must, after all, be possible to decide this by observation. At bottom we have cause for gratitude to the occultists. The miraculous stories from ancient times are beyond the reach of our testing. If in our opinion they cannot be substantiated, we must admit that they cannot, strictly speaking, be disproved. But about contemporary happenings, at which we are able to be present, it must be possible for us to reach a definite judgement. If we arrive at a conviction that such miracles do not occur to-day, we need not fear the counter-argument that they may nevertheless have taken place in ancient times: in that case other explanations will be much more plausible. Thus we have settled our doubts and are ready to take part in an investigation of occult phenomena.

But here unluckily we are met by circumstances which are exceedingly unfavourable to our honest intentions. The observations on which our judgement is supposed to depend take place under conditions which make our sensory perceptions uncertain and which blunt our power of attention; they occur in darkness or in dim red light after long periods of blank expectation. We are told that in fact our unbelieving—that is to say, critical—attitude may prevent the expected phenomena from happening. The situation thus brought about is nothing less than a caricature of the circumstances in which we are usually accustomed to carry out scientific enquiries. The observations are made upon what are called 'mediums'—individuals to whom peculiarly 'sensitive' faculties are ascribed, but who are by no means distinguished by outstanding qualities of intellect or character, and who are not, like the miracle-workers of the past, inspired by any great idea or serious purpose. On the contrary, they are looked upon, even by those who believe in their secret powers, as particularly untrustworthy; most of them have already been detected as cheats and we may reasonably expect that the same fate awaits the remainder. Their performances give one the impression of children's mischievous pranks or of conjuring tricks.[1] Never has anything of importance yet emerged from *séances* with these mediums—the revelation of a new source of power, for instance. We do not, it is true, expect to receive hints on pigeon-breeding from the conjurer who produces pigeons by magic from his empty top-hat. I can easily put myself in the place of a person who tries to fulfil the demands of an objective attitude and so takes part in occult *séances*, but who grows tired after a while and turns away in disgust from what is expected of him and goes back unenlightened to his former prejudices. The reproach may be made against such a person that this is not the right way of behaving: that one ought not to lay down in advance what the phenomena one is seeking to study shall be like and in what

[1] [Cf. the similar remarks in Chapter V of *The Future of an Illusion* (1927c).]

circumstances they shall appear. One should, on the contrary, persevere, and give weight to the precautionary and supervisory measures by which efforts have recently been made to provide against the untrustworthiness of mediums. Unfortunately this modern protective technique makes an end of the easy accessibility of occult observations. The study of occultism becomes a specialized and difficult profession—an activity one cannot pursue alongside of one's other interests. And until those concerned in these investigations have reached their conclusions, we are left to our doubts and our own conjectures.

Of these conjectures no doubt the most probable is that there is a real core of yet unrecognized facts in occultism round which cheating and phantasy have spun a veil which it is hard to pierce. But how can we even approach this core? at what point can we attack the problem? It is here, I think, that dreams come to our help, by giving us a hint that from out of this chaos we should pick the subject of *telepathy*.

What we call 'telepathy' is, as you know, the alleged fact that an event which occurs at a particular time comes at about the same moment to the consciousness of someone distant in space, without the paths of communication that are familiar to us coming into question. It is implicitly presupposed that this event concerns a person in whom the other one (the receiver of the intelligence) has a strong emotional interest. For instance, Person A may be the victim of an accident or may die, and Person B, someone nearly attached to him—his mother or daughter or fiancée—learns the fact at about the same time through a visual or auditory perception. In this latter case, then, it is as if she had been informed by telephone, though such was not the case; it is a kind of psychical counterpart to wireless telegraphy. I need not insist to you on the improbability of such events, and there is good reason for dismissing the majority of such reports. A few are left over which cannot be so easily disposed of in this way. Permit me now, for the purpose of what I have to tell you, to omit the cautious little word 'alleged' and to proceed as though I believed in the objective reality of the phenomenon of telepathy. But bear firmly in mind that that is not the case and that I have committed myself to no conviction.

Actually I have little to tell you—only a modest fact. I will also at once reduce your expectations still further by saying that at bottom dreams have little to do with telepathy. Telepathy does not throw any fresh light on the nature of dreams nor do dreams give any direct evidence of the reality of telepathy. Moreover the phenomenon of telepathy is by no means bound up with dreams; it can occur as well during the waking state. The only reason for discussing the relation between dreams and telepathy is that the state of sleep seems particularly suited for receiving telepathic messages. In such cases one has what is called a telepathic dream and, when it is analysed, one forms a conviction that the telepathic news has played the same part as any other portion of the day's residues and that it has been changed in the same way by the dream-work and made to serve its purpose.

During the analysis of one such telepathic dream, something occurred which seems to me of sufficient interest in spite of its triviality to serve as the starting-point of this lecture. When in 1922 I gave my first account of this matter I had only a single observation at my disposal. Since then I have made a number of similar ones, but I will keep to the first example, because it is easiest to describe, and I will take you straight away in medias res.[1]

An obviously intelligent man, who from his own account was not in the least 'inclined towards occultism', wrote to me about a dream he had had which seemed to him remarkable. He began by informing me that his married daughter, who lived at a distance from him, was expecting her first confinement in the middle of December. This daughter meant a great deal to him and he knew too that she was very much attached to him. During the night of November 16–17, then, he dreamt that his wife had given birth to twins. A number of details followed, which I may here pass over, and all of which were never in fact explained. The wife who in the dream had become the mother of twins was his *second* wife, his daughter's stepmother. He did not wish to have a child by his present wife who, he said, had no aptitude for bringing up children sensibly; moreover,

---

[1] [This was first published in very much greater detail, in 'Dreams and Telepathy' (1922*a*).]

at the time of the dream he had long ceased to have sexual relations with her. What led him to write to me was not doubt about the theory of dreams, though the manifest content of his dream would have justified it, for why did the dream, in complete contradiction to his wishes, make his wife give birth to children? Nor, according to him, was there any reason to fear that this unwished-for event might occur. What induced him to report this dream to me was the circumstance that on the morning of November 18 he received a telegram announcing that his daughter had given birth to twins. The telegram had been handed in the day before and the birth had taken place during the night of November 16–17, at about the same time at which he had had the dream of his wife's twin birth. The dreamer asked me whether I thought the coincidence between dream and event was accidental. He did not venture to call the dream a telepathic one, since the difference between its content and the event affected precisely what seemed to him essential in it—the identity of the person who gave birth to the children. But one of his comments shows that he would not have been astonished at an actual telepathic dream: he believed his daughter would have thought particularly of him during her labour.

I feel sure, Ladies and Gentlemen, that you have been able to explain this dream already and understand too why I have told it you. Here was a man who was dissatisfied with his second wife and who would prefer his wife to be like the daughter of his first marriage. This 'like' dropped out, of course, so far as the unconscious was concerned. And now the telepathic message arrived during the night to say that his daughter had given birth to twins. The dream-work took control of the news, allowed the unconscious wish to operate on it—the wish that he could put his daughter in the place of his second wife—and thus arose the puzzling manifest dream, which disguised the wish and distorted the message. We must admit that it is only the *interpretation* of the dream that has shown us that it was a telepathic one: psycho-analysis has revealed a telepathic event which we should not otherwise have discovered.

But pray do not let yourselves be misled! In spite of all this, dream-interpretation has told us nothing about the objective reality of the telepathic event. It may equally be an illusion which can be explained in another way. The man's latent dream-thoughts may have run: 'To-day is the day the confinement should take place if my daughter is really out in her reckoning by a month, as I suspect. And when I saw her last she looked just as though she was going to have twins. How my dead wife who was so fond of children would have rejoiced over twins!' (I base this last factor on some associations of the dreamer's which I have not mentioned.) In that case the instigation to the dream would have been well-grounded suspicions on the dreamer's part and not a telepathic message; but the outcome would remain the same. You see then that even the interpretation of this dream has told us nothing on the question of whether we are to allow objective reality to telepathy. That could only be decided by a thorough-going investigation of all the circumstances of the case—which was unfortunately no more possible in this instance than in any of the others in my experience. Granted that the telepathy hypothesis offers by far the simplest explanation, yet that does not help us much. The simplest explanation is not always the correct one; the truth is often no simple matter, and before deciding in favour of such a far-reaching hypothesis we should like to have taken every precaution.

We may now leave the subject of dreams and telepathy: I have nothing more to say to you on it. But kindly observe that what seemed to us to teach us something about telepathy was not the dream but the interpretation of the dream, its psycho-analytic working-over. Accordingly, in what follows we may leave dreams entirely on one side and may follow an expectation that the employment of psycho-analysis may throw a little light on other events described as occult. There is, for instance, the phenomenon of thought-transference, which is so close to telepathy and can indeed without much violence be regarded as the same thing. It claims that mental processes in one person—ideas, emotional states, conative impulses—can be transferred to another person through empty space without employing the familiar methods of communication by means of words and signs. You will realize how remarkable, and perhaps even of what great practical importance, it would be if something of the kind really happened. It may be noted, incidentally, that strangely enough precisely this phenomenon is referred to least frequently in the miraculous stories of the past.

I have formed an impression in the course of the psycho-analytic treatment of patients that the activities of professional fortune-tellers conceal an opportunity for making particularly unobjectionable observations on thought-transference. These are insignificant and even inferior people, who immerse themselves in some sort of performance[1]—lay out cards, study writing or lines upon the palm of the hand, or make astrological calculations—and at the same time, after having shown themselves familiar with portions of their visitor's past or present circumstances, go on to prophesy their future. As a rule their clients exhibit great satisfaction over these achievements and feel no resentment if later on these prophecies are not fulfilled. I have come across several such cases and have been able to study them analytically, and in a moment I will tell you the most remarkable of these instances. Their convincingness is unfortunately impaired by the numerous reticences to which I am compelled by the obligation of medical discretion. I have, however, of set purpose avoided distortions. So listen now to the story of one of my women patients, who had an experience of this kind with a fortune-teller.[2]

She had been the eldest of a numerous family and had grown

---

[1] [In Section I of his earlier, posthumously published, paper, 'Psycho-Analysis and Telepathy' (1941d [1921]), Freud had elaborated on the significance of the fortune-teller's distracting his attention by some meaningless activity as a means of releasing an unconscious mental process. He there compared the use of a similar 'distracting contrivance' in the making of some kinds of jokes; see for this Chapter V of his book on jokes (1905c), pp. 151–3. Much earlier, in his technical contribution to *Studies on Hysteria* (1895d), he had brought forward the same explanation for certain techniques for producing hypnosis, and in particular for his own early method of eliciting forgotten facts by pressure on the patient's forehead; and this he afterwards developed in a discussion of hypnotism in Chapter X of his *Group Psychology* (1921c). Compare also some remarks near the end of Chapter VI of *The Psychopathology of Everyday Life* (1901b) on the fact that attention directed to an automatic action *interferes* with its performance, p. 132.]

[2] [This case is reported at greater length, with some slight variations, in 'Psycho-Analysis and Telepathy', and much more briefly in Section C of 1925i.]

up with an extremely strong attachment to her father. She had married young and had found entire satisfaction in her marriage. Only one thing was wanting to her happiness: she had remained childless, so she could not bring her beloved husband completely into the place of her father. When, after long years of disappointment, she decided to undergo a gynaecological operation, her husband revealed to her that the blame was his: an illness before their marriage had made him incapable of procreating children. She took the disappointment badly, became neurotic and clearly suffered from fears of being tempted [into unfaithfulness to her husband]. To cheer her up, he took her with him on a business trip to Paris. They were sitting there one day in the hall of their hotel when she noticed a stir among the hotel servants. She asked what was going on and was told that Monsieur le Professeur had arrived and was giving consultations in a little room over there. She expressed a wish to have a try. Her husband rejected the idea, but while he was not watching she slipped into the consulting-room and faced the fortune-teller. She was 27 years old, but looked much younger and had taken off her wedding-ring. Monsieur le Professeur made her lay her hand on a tray filled with ashes and carefully studied the imprint; he then told her all kinds of things about hard struggles that lay before her, and ended with the comforting assurance that all the same she would still get married and would have two children by the time she was 32. When she told me this story she was 43 years old, seriously ill and without any prospect of ever having a child. Thus the prophecy had not come true; yet she spoke of it without any sort of bitterness but with an unmistakable expression of satisfaction, as though she were recalling a cheerful event. It was easy to establish that she had not the slightest notion of what the two numbers in the prophecy [2 and 32] might mean or whether they meant anything at all.

You will say that this is a stupid and incomprehensible story and ask why I have told it you. I should be entirely of your opinion if—and this is the salient point—analysis had not made it possible to arrive at an interpretation of the prophecy which is convincing precisely from the explanation it affords of the details. For the two numbers find their place in the life of my patient's *mother*. She had married late—not till she was over thirty, and in the family they had often dwelt on the fact of the success with which she had hastened to make up for lost time. Her two first children (with our patient the elder) had been born with the shortest possible interval between them, in a single calendar year; and she had in fact two children by the time she was 32. What Monsieur le Professeur had said to my patient meant therefore: 'Take comfort from the fact of being so young. You'll have the same destiny as your mother, who also had to wait a long time for children, and you'll have two children by the time you're 32.' But to have the same destiny as her mother, to put herself in her mother's place, to take her place with her father—that had been the strongest wish of her youth, the wish on account of whose non-fulfilment she was just beginning to fall ill. The prophecy promised her that the wish would still be fulfilled in spite of everything; how could she fail to feel friendly to the prophet? Do you regard it as possible, however, that Monsieur le Professeur was familiar with the facts of the intimate family history of his chance client? Out of the question! How, then, did he arrive at the knowledge which enabled him to give expression to my patient's strongest and most secret wish by including the two numbers in his pro- phecy? I can see only two possible explanations. Either the story as it was told me is untrue and the events occurred other- wise, or thought-transference exists as a real phenomenon. One can suppose, no doubt, that after an interval of 16 years the patient had introduced the two numbers concerned into her recollection from her unconscious. I have no basis for this suspicion, but I cannot exclude it, and I imagine that you will be readier to believe in a way out of that kind than in the reality of thought-transference. If you do decide on the latter course, do not forget that it was only analysis that created the occult fact—uncovered it when it lay distorted to the point of being unrecognizable.

If it were a question of *one* case only like that of my patient, one would shrug it aside. No one would dream of erecting upon a single observation a belief which implies taking such a decisive line. But you must believe me when I assure you that this is not the only case in my experience. I have collected a whole number of such prophecies and from all of them I gained the

impression that the fortune-teller had merely brought to expression the thoughts, and more especially the secret wishes, of
those were were questioning him, and that we were therefore
justified in analysing these prophecies as though they were subjective products, phantasies or dreams of the people concerned.
Not every case, of course, is equally convincing and in not
every case is it equally possible to exclude more rational explanations; but, taking them as a whole, there remains a strong
balance of probability in favour of thought-transference as a
fact. The importance of the subject would justify me in producing all my cases to you; but that I cannot do, owing to the
prolixity of description that would be involved and to the
inevitable breach of the obligations of discretion. I will try so
far as possible to appease my conscience in giving you a few
more examples.

One day I was visited by a highly intelligent young man, a
student preparing for his final examinations for a doctorate, but
unable to take them since, as he complained, he had lost all
interest and power of concentration and even any faculty for
orderly memory.[1] The previous history of this condition of
quasi-paralysis was soon revealed: he had fallen ill after carrying
out a great act of self-discipline. He had a sister, to whom he
was attached by an intense but always restrained devotion, just
as she was to him. 'What a pity we can't get married!' they
would often say to each other. A respectable man fell in love
with the sister; she responded to his affection, but her parents
did not assent to the union. In their difficulty the young couple
turned to her brother, nor did he refuse his help. He made it
possible for them to correspond with each other, and his influence eventually persuaded the parents to consent. In the
course of the engagement, however, an occurrence took place
whose meaning it was easy to guess. He went with his future
brother-in-law on a difficult mountain-climb without a guide;
they lost their way and were in danger of not returning safe and
sound. Shortly after his sister's marriage he fell into this condition of mental exhaustion.
  The influence of psycho-analysis restored his ability to work

[1] [This case too appears in rather greater detail in 'Psycho-Analysis
and Telepathy'.]

and he left me in order to go in for his examinations; but after he had passed them successfully he came back to me for a short time in the autumn of the same year. It was then that he related a remarkable experience to me which he had had before the summer. In his University town there lived a fortune-teller who enjoyed great popularity. Even the Princes of the Royal House used to consult her before important undertakings. Her mode of operation was very simple. She asked to be given the date of the relevant person's birth; she required to know nothing else about him, not even his name. She then proceeded to consult her astrological books, made long calculations and finally uttered a prophecy relating to the person in question. My patient decided to call upon her mystical arts in connection with his brother-in-law. He visited her and told her the relevant date. After carrying out her calculations she made her prophecy: 'The person in question will die in July or August of this year of crayfish- or oyster-poisoning.' My patient finished his story with the words: 'It was quite marvellous!'

From the first I had listened with irritation. After this exclamation of his I went so far as to ask: 'What do you see that's so marvellous in this prophecy? Here we are in late autumn and your brother-in-law isn't dead or you'd have told me long ago. So the prophecy hasn't come true.' 'No doubt that's so,' he replied, 'but here is what's marvellous. My brother-in-law is passionately devoted to crayfish and oysters and in the previous summer—that's to say, *before* my visit to the fortune-teller—he had an attack of oyster-poisoning[1] of which he nearly died.' What was I to say to this? I could only feel annoyed that this highly-educated man (who had moreover been through a successful analysis) should not have a clearer view of the position. I for my part, rather than believe that it is possible to calculate the onset of an attack of crayfish- or oyster-poisoning from astrological tables, prefer to suppose that my patient had not yet overcome his hatred for his rival, the repression of which had earlier led to his falling ill, and that the fortune-teller was simply giving expression to his own expectation: 'a taste of that kind isn't to be given up, and one day, all the same, it will be the end of him.' I must admit that I cannot think of any other

[1] ['Crayfish-poisoning' in the 'Psycho-Analysis and Telepathy' version.]

explanation for this case, unless, perhaps, that my patient was having a joke with me. But neither then nor at a later time did he give me grounds for such a suspicion, and he seemed to be meaning what he said seriously.

Here is another case.[1] A young man in a position of consequence was involved in a *liaison* with a *demi-mondaine* which was characterized by a curious compulsion. He was obliged from time to time to provoke her with derisive and insulting remarks till she was driven to complete desperation. When he had brought her to that point, he was relieved, became reconciled with her and made her a present. But now he wanted to be free of her: the compulsion seemed to him uncanny. He noticed that this *liaison* was damaging his reputation; he wanted to have a wife of his own and to raise a family. But since he could not get free from this *demi-mondaine* by his own strength, he called analysis to his help. After one of these abusive scenes, when the analysis had already started, he got her to write something on a piece of paper, so as to show it to a graphologist. The report that he received from him was that the writing was that of someone in extreme despair, who would certainly commit suicide in the next few days. This did not, it is true, occur and the lady remained alive; but the analysis succeeded in loosening his bonds. He left the lady and turned to a young girl who he expected would be able to make him a good wife. Soon afterwards a dream appeared which could only hint at a dawning doubt as to the girl's worthiness. He obtained a specimen of her writing too, took it to the same authority, and was given a verdict on her writing which confirmed his apprehensions. He therefore abandoned the idea of making her his wife.

In order to form an opinion of the graphologist's reports, especially the first one, we must know something of our subject's secret history. In his early youth he had (in accordance with his passionate nature) fallen in love to the pitch of frenzy with a married woman who was still young but nevertheless older than he was. When she rejected him, he made an attempt at suicide which, there can be no doubt, was seriously intended.

[1] [Also reported with some further details in 'Psycho-Analysis and Telepathy', though the present account is in some respects fuller.]

It was only by a hair's breadth that he escaped death and he was only restored after a long period of nursing. But this wild action made a deep impression on the woman he loved; she granted him her favours, he became her lover and thenceforward remained secretly attached to her and served her with a truly chivalrous devotion. More than twenty years later, when they had both grown older—but the woman, naturally, more than he—the need was awakened in him to detach himself from her, to make himself free, to lead a life of his own, to set up a house and raise a family. And along with this feeling of satiety there arose in him his long-suppressed craving for vengeance on his mistress. As he had once tried to kill himself because she had spurned him, so he wished now to have the satisfaction of her seeking death because he left her. But his love was still too strong for it to be possible for this wish to become conscious in him; nor was he in a position to do her enough harm to drive her into death. In this frame of mind he took on the *demi-mondaine* as a sort of whipping-boy, to satisfy his thirst for revenge *in corpore vili*; and he allowed himself to practise upon her all the torments which he might expect would bring about with her the result he wished to produce on his mistress. The fact that the vengeance applied to the latter was betrayed by his making her into a confidante and adviser in his *liaison* instead of concealing his defection from her. The wretched woman, who had long fallen from giving to receiving favours, probably suffered more from his confidences than the *demi-mondaine* did from his brutalities. The compulsion of which he complained in regard to this substitutive figure, and which drove him to analysis, had of course been transferred on to her from his old mistress; it was from her that he wanted to free himself but could not. I am not an authority on handwriting and have no high opinion of the art of divining character from it; still less do I believe in the possibility of foretelling the writer's future in this way. You can see, however, whatever one may think of the value of graphology, that there is no mistaking the fact that the expert, when he promised that the writer of the specimen presented to him would commit suicide in the next few days, had once again only brought to light a powerful secret wish of the person who was questioning him. Something of the same kind happened afterwards in the case of the second report. What was

there concerned, however, was not an unconscious wish; it was
the questioner's dawning doubt and apprehension that found a
clear expression from the graphologist's mouth. Incidentally,
my patient succeeded, with the help of analysis, in finding an
object for his love outside the magic circle in which he had been
spellbound.

Ladies and Gentlemen,—You have now heard how dream-
interpretation and psycho-analysis in general assist occultism.
I have shown you from examples that by their application
occult facts have been brought to light which would otherwise
have remained unknown. Psycho-analysis cannot give a direct
answer to the question that no doubt interests you the most—
whether we are to believe in the objective reality of these findings. But the material revealed by its help makes an impression
which is at all events favourable to an affirmative reply. Your
interest will not come to a stop at this point, however. You will
want to know what conclusions are justified by the incomparably richer material in which psycho-analysis has no part.
But I cannot follow you there: it lies outside my province. The
only further thing I could do would be to report observations to
you which have at least so much relation to analysis that they
were made during psycho-analytic treatment and were even
perhaps made possible by its influence. I will tell you one such
example—the one which has left the strongest impression behind on me. I shall tell it at great length and shall ask for your
attention to a large number of details, though even so I shall
have to suppress much that would have greatly increased the
convincing force of the observation. It is an example in which
the fact came clearly to light and did not need to be developed
by analysis. In discussing it, however, we shall not be able to do
without the help of analysis. But I will tell you in advance that
this example too of apparent thought-transference in the analytic situation is not exempt from all doubts and that it does not
allow us to take up an unqualified position in support of the
reality of occult phenomena.[1]

Listen then:—One autumn day in the year 1919, at about

[1] [This case is the one which should have been the 'third case' to be
included in 'Psycho-Analysis and Telepathy'. The circumstances of its

10.45 a.m., Dr. David Forsyth,[1] who had just arrived from London, sent in his card to me while I was working with a patient. (My respected colleague from London University will not, I feel sure, regard it as an indiscretion if in this way I betray the fact that he spent some months being initiated by me into the arts of psycho-analytic technique.) I only had time to greet him and to make an appointment to see him later. Dr. Forsyth had a claim to my particular interest; he was the first foreigner to come to me after I had been cut off by the war-years and to bring a promise of better times. Soon afterwards, at eleven o'clock, Herr P., one of my patients, arrived—an intelligent and agreeable man, between forty and fifty years of age, who had originally come to me on account of difficulties with women. His case did not promise any therapeutic success; I had long before proposed our stopping the treatment, but he had wished to continue it, evidently because he felt comfortable in a well-tempered father-transference to me. At that period money played no part: there was too little of it about. The sessions which I spent with him were stimulating and refreshing for me as well, and consequently, in disregard of the strict rules of medical practice, analytic work was being carried on up to a foreseen time-limit.

That day P. returned to his attempts at having erotic relations with women and once again mentioned a pretty, piquante, penniless girl, with whom he felt he might succeed, if the fact of her being a virgin did not scare him off any serious attempt. He had often talked of her before but that day he told me for the first time that, though of course she had no notion of the true grounds of his impediment, she used to call him 'Herr von Vorsicht' [Mr. Foresight]. I was struck by this information; Dr. Forsyth's visiting card lay beside me, and I showed it to him.

---

omission were explained by Freud in that paper. As was indicated there, the original draft survived. It resembled the version given here so closely that it was doubtful whether it was necessary to print it separately. It should be added, however, that the manuscript has once again unaccountably disappeared.]

[1] [Dr. David Forsyth (1877–1941), Consulting Physician to Charing Cross Hospital, London, was an original member of the London Society for Psycho-Analysis, founded in 1913.]

These are the facts of the case. I expect they will seem to you paltry; but listen a little longer, there is more behind them.

When he was young, P. had spent some years in England and since then had retained a permanent interest in English literature. He possessed a rich English library and used to bring me books from it. I owe to him an acquaintance with such authors as Bennett and Galsworthy, of whom till then I had read little. One day he lent me a novel of Galsworthy's with the title *The Man of Property*, whose scene is laid in the bosom of a family invented by the author, bearing the name of 'Forsyte'. Galsworthy himself was evidently captivated by this creation of his, for in later volumes he repeatedly came back to the members of this family and finally collected all the tales relating to them under the title of *The Forsyte Saga*. Only a few days before the occurrence I am speaking of, he had brought me a fresh volume from this series. The name 'Forsyte', and everything typical that the author had sought to embody in it, had played a part, too, in my conversations with P. and it had become part of the secret language which so easily grows up between two people who see a lot of each other. Now the name 'Forsyte' in these novels differs little from that of my visitor 'Forsyth' and, as pronounced by a German, the two can scarcely be distinguished; and there is an English word with a meaning—'foresight'—which we should also pronounce in the same way and which would be translated '*Voraussicht*' or '*Vorsicht*'. Thus P. had in fact selected from his personal concerns the very name with which I was occupied at the same time as a result of an occurrence of which he was unaware.

That begins to look better, you will agree. But we shall, I think, receive a stronger impression of the striking phenomenon and even obtain an insight into its determinants, if we throw some analytic light upon two other associations brought up by P. during the same session.

Firstly: One day of the previous week I had waited in vain for Herr P. at eleven o'clock, and had then gone out to visit Dr. Anton von Freund[1] in his *pension*. I was surprised to find that Herr P. lived on another floor of the same building in which the *pension* was located. In connection with this I had later told P. that I had in a sense paid him a visit in his house; but I know

[1] [A prominent Hungarian psycho-analyst.]

definitely that I did not tell him the name of the person I visited in the *pension*. And now, shortly after mentioning 'Herr von Vorsicht' he asked me whether perhaps the Freud-Ottorego who was giving a course of lectures on English at the Volks-universität[1] was my daughter. And for the first time during our long period of intercourse he gave my name the distorted form to which I have indeed become habituated by functionaries, officials and compositors: instead of 'Freud' he said 'Freund'.

Secondly: At the end of the same session he told me a dream, from which he had woken in a fright—a regular *'Alptraum'*, he said. He added that not long ago he had forgotten the English word for that, and when someone had asked him said that the English for *'Alptraum'* was 'a mare's nest'. This was nonsense, of course, he went on; 'a mare's nest' meant something incredible, a cock-and-bull story: the translation of *'Alptraum'* was 'nightmare'. The only element in common between this association and the previous one seemed to be the element 'English'. I was however reminded of a small incident which had occurred about a month earlier. P. was sitting with me in the room when another visitor, a dear friend from London, Dr. Ernest Jones, unexpectedly came in after a long separation. I signed to him to go into the next room while I finished with P. The latter, however, had at once recognized him from his photograph hanging in the waiting-room, and even expressed a wish to be introduced to him. Now Jones is the author of a monograph on the *Alptraum*—the nightmare. I did not know whether P. was acquainted with it; he avoided reading ana-lytic literature.

I should like to begin by putting before you an investigation of what analytic understanding can be arrived at of the back-ground of P.'s associations and of the motives for them. P. was placed similarly to me in relation to the name 'Forsyte' or 'Forsyth'; it meant the same to him, and it was entirely to him that I owed my acquaintance with the name. The remarkable fact was that he brought the name into the analysis unheralded, only the briefest time after it had become significant to me in another sense owing to a new event—the London doctor's arrival. But the manner in which the name emerged in his ana-

[1] ['People's University', providing what is known in England as 'Adult Education'.]

lytic session is perhaps not less interesting than the fact itself. He did not say, for instance: 'The name "Forsyte", out of the novels you are familiar with, has just occurred to me.' He was able, without any conscious relation to that source, to weave the name into his own experiences and to produce it thence—a thing that might have happened long before but had not happened till then. What he *did* say now was: 'I'm a Forsyth too: that's what the girl calls me.' It is hard to mistake the mixture of jealous demand and melancholy self-depreciation which finds its expression in this remark. We shall not be going astray if we complete it in some such way as this: 'It's mortifying to me that your thoughts should be so intensely occupied with this new arrival. Do come back to me; after all I'm a Forsyth too— though it's true I'm only a Herr von Vorsicht [gentleman of foresight], as the girl says.' And thereupon his train of thought, passing along the associative threads of the element 'English' went back to two earlier events, which were able to stir up the same feelings of jealousy. 'A few days ago you paid a visit to my house—not, alas, to me but to a Herr von Freund.' This thought caused him to distort the name 'Freud' into 'Freund'. The 'Freud-Ottorego' from the lecture-syllabus must come in here because as a teacher of English she provided the manifest association. And now came the recollection of another visitor a few weeks before, of whom he was no doubt equally jealous, but for whom he also felt he was no match, for Dr. Jones was able to write a monograph on the nightmare whereas he was at best only able to produce such dreams himself. His mention of his mistake about the meaning of 'a mare's nest' comes into this connection, for it can only mean to say: 'After all I'm not a genuine Englishman any more than I'm a genuine Forsyth.'

Now I cannot describe his feelings of jealousy as either out of place or unintelligible. He had been warned that his analysis, and at the same time our contact, would come to an end as soon as foreign pupils and patients returned to Vienna; and that was in fact what happened shortly afterwards. What we have so far achieved, however, has been a piece of analytic work—the explanation of three associations brought up by him in the same session and nourished by the same motive: and this has not much to do with the other question of whether these associations could or could not have been made without thought-transference.

This question arises in the case of each of the three associations and thus falls into three separate questions: Could P. have known that Dr. Forsyth had just paid me his first visit? Could he know the name of the person I had visited in his house? Did he know that Dr. Jones had written a monograph on the nightmare? Or was it only *my* knowledge about these things that was revealed in his associations? It will depend on the reply to these separate questions whether my observation allows of a conclusion favourable to thought-transference.

Let us leave the first question aside for a while; the other two can be dealt with more easily. The case of my visit to his *pension* makes a particularly convincing impression at first sight. I am certain that in my short, joking reference to my visit to his house I mentioned no name. I think it is most unlikely that P. made enquiries at the *pension* as to the name of the person concerned; I believe rather that the existence of that person remained entirely unknown to him. But the evidential value of this case is totally destroyed by a chance circumstance. The man whom I had visited at the *pension* was not only called 'Freund'; he was a true friend to us all.[1] He was Dr. Anton von Freund whose donation had made the foundation of our publishing house possible. His early death, together with that of our colleague Karl Abraham a few years later, are the gravest misfortunes which have befallen the growth of psycho-analysis. It is possible, therefore, that I had said to Herr P.: 'I visited a friend [*Freund*] in your house' and with this possibility the occult interest of his second association vanishes.

The impression made by the third association evaporates equally quickly. Could P. know that Jones had published a monograph on the nightmare if he never read any analytic literature? Yes, he could. He possessed books from our publishing house and could in any case have seen the titles of the new publications advertised on the wrappers. This cannot be proved, but neither can it be disproved. We can reach no decision, therefore, along this path. To my regret, this observation of mine suffers from the same weakness as so many similar ones: it was written down too late and was discussed at a time when I was no longer seeing Herr P. and could not question him further.

[1] ['*Freund*' is, of course, the German word for 'friend'. Freud had written a moving obituary of him (1920c).]

Let us go back to the first event, which even taken by itself supports the apparent fact of thought-transference. Could P. know that Dr. Forsyth had been with me a quarter of an hour before him? Could he have any knowledge at all of his existence or of his presence in Vienna? We must not give way to an inclination to deny both questions flatly. I can see a way that leads to a partly affirmative answer. I may after all have told Herr P. that I was expecting a doctor from England for instruction in analysis, as a first dove after the Deluge. This might have happened in the summer of 1919, for Dr. Forsyth had made arrangements with me by letter some months before his arrival. I may even have mentioned his name, though that seems to me most improbable. In view of the other connection which the name carried for both of us, a discussion of it must inevitably have followed, of which something would have remained in my memory. Nevertheless such a discussion may have taken place and I may have totally forgotten it afterwards, so that it became possible for the emergence of 'Herr von Vorsicht' in the analytic session to strike me as a miracle. If one regards oneself as a sceptic, it is a good plan to have occasional doubts about one's scepticism too. It may be that I too have a secret inclination towards the miraculous which thus goes half way to meet the creation of occult facts.

If we have thus got one miraculous possibility out of the way, there is another waiting for us, and the most difficult of all. Assuming that Herr P. knew that there was a Dr. Forsyth and that he was expected in Vienna in the autumn, how is it to be explained that he became receptive to his presence on the very day of his arrival and immediately after his first visit? One might say it was chance—that is, leave it unexplained. But it was precisely in order to exclude chance that I discussed P.'s other two associations, in order to show you that he was really occupied with jealous thoughts about people who visited me. Or one might, not to neglect the most extreme possibility, experiment with the hypothesis that P. had observed a special excitement about me (which, to be sure, I myself knew nothing of) and drew his conclusion from it. Or Herr P. (though he arrived a quarter of an hour after the Englishman left) met him on the short stretch of street which they both had to pass along, recognized him by his characteristically English appearance and, being in a permanent state of jealous expectation, thought: 'Ah, so that's Dr. Forsyth with whose arrival my analysis is to come to an end! And he's probably just come straight from the Professor.' I cannot carry these rationalistic speculations any further. We are once again left with a *non liquet* [not proven]; but I must confess that I have a feeling that here too the scales weigh in favour of thought-transference. Moreover, I am certainly not alone in having been in the position of experiencing 'occult' events like this in the analytic situation. Helene Deutsch published some similar observations in 1926 and studied the question of their being determined by the transference relations between patient and analyst.

I am sure you will not feel very well satisfied with my attitude to this problem—with my not being entirely convinced but prepared to be convinced. You may perhaps say to yourselves: 'Here's another case of a man who has done honest work as a scientist all through his life and has grown feeble-minded, pious and credulous in his old age.' I am aware that a few great names must be included in this class, but you should not reckon me among them. At least I have not become pious, and I hope not credulous. It is only that, if one has gone about all one's life bending in order to avoid a painful collision with the facts, so too in one's old age one still keeps one's back ready to bow before new realities. No doubt you would like me to hold fast to a moderate theism and show myself relentless in my rejection of everything occult. But I am incapable of currying favour and I must urge you to have kindlier thoughts on the objective possibility of thought-transference and at the same time of telepathy as well.

You will not forget that here I am only treating these problems in so far as it is possible to approach them from the direction of psycho-analysis. When they first came into my range of vision more than ten years ago, I too felt a dread of a threat against our scientific *Weltanschauung*, which, I feared, was bound to give place to spiritualism or mysticism if portions of occultism were proved true.[1] To-day I, think otherwise. In my opinion it

---

[1] [These thoughts were expressed by Freud at considerable length in the introductory portion of his posthumously published paper on 'Psycho-Analysis and Telepathy' (1941*d*).]

shows no great confidence in science if one does not think it capable of assimilating and working over whatever may perhaps turn out to be true in the assertions of occultists. And particularly so far as thought-transference is concerned, it seems actually to favour the extension of the scientific—or, as our opponents say, the mechanistic—mode of thought to the mental phenomena which are so hard to lay hold of. The telepathic process is supposed to consist in a mental act in one person instigating the same mental act in another person. What lies between these two mental acts may easily be a physical process into which the mental one is transformed at one end and which is transformed back once more into the same mental one at the other end. The analogy with other transformations, such as occur in speaking and hearing by telephone, would then be unmistakable. And only think if one could get hold of this physical equivalent of the psychical act! It would seem to me that psycho-analysis, by inserting the unconscious between what is physical and what was previously called 'psychical', has paved the way for the assumption of such processes as telepathy. If only one accustoms oneself to the idea of telepathy, one can accomplish a great deal with it—for the time being, it is true, only in imagination. It is a familiar fact that we do not know how the common purpose comes about in the great insect communities: possibly it is done by means of a direct psychical transference of this kind. One is led to a suspicion that this is the original, archaic method of communication between individuals and that in the course of phylogenetic evolution it has been replaced by the better method of giving information with the help of signals which are picked up by the sense organs. But the older method might have persisted in the background and still be able to put itself into effect under certain conditions—for instance, in passionately excited mobs. All this is still uncertain and full of unsolved riddles; but there is no reason to be frightened by it.

If there is such a thing as telepathy as a real process, we may suspect that, in spite of its being so hard to demonstrate, it is quite a common phenomenon. It would tally with our expectations if we were able to point to it particularly in the mental life of children. Here we are reminded of the frequent anxiety felt by children over the idea that their parents know all their thoughts without having to be told them—an exact counterpart and per-haps the source of the belief of adults in the omniscience of God. A short time ago Dorothy Burlingham, a trustworthy witness, in a paper on child analysis and the mother [1932] published some observations which, if they can be confirmed, would be bound to put an end to the remaining doubts on the reality of thought-transference. She made use of the situation, no longer a rare one, in which a mother and child are simultaneously in analysis, and reported some remarkable events such as the following. One day the mother spoke during her analytic session of a gold coin that had played a particular part in one of the scenes of her childhood. Immediately afterwards, after she had returned home, her little boy, about ten years old, came to her room and brought her a gold coin which he asked her to keep for him. She asked him in astonishment where he had got it from. He had been given it on his birthday; but his birthday had been several months earlier and there was no reason why the child should have remembered the gold coin precisely then. The mother reported the occurrence to the child's analyst and asked her to find out from the child the reason for his action. But the child's analysis threw no light on the matter; the action had forced its way that day into the child's life like a foreign body. A few weeks later the mother was sitting at her writing-desk to write down, as she had been told to do, an account of the experience, when in came the boy and asked for the gold coin back, as he wanted to take it with him to show in his analytic session. Once again the child's analysis could discover no explanation of his wish.

And this brings us back to psycho-analysis, which was what we started out from.

THE DISSECTION OF THE PSYCHICAL
PERSONALITY[1]

LADIES AND GENTLEMEN,—I know you are aware in regard to
your own relations, whether with people or things, of the importance of your starting-point. This was also the case with
psycho-analysis. It has not been a matter of indifference for the
course of its development or for the reception it met with that it
began its work on what is, of all the contents of the mind, most
foreign to the ego—on symptoms. Symptoms are derived from
the repressed, they are, as it were, its representatives before the
ego; but the repressed *is* foreign territory to the ego—internal
foreign territory—just as reality (if you will forgive the unusual
expression) is external foreign territory. The path led from
symptoms to the unconscious, to the life of the instincts, to sexuality; and it was then that psycho-analysis was met by the brilliant objection that human beings are not merely sexual creatures but have nobler and higher impulses as well. It might have
been added that, exalted by their consciousness of these higher
impulses, they often assume the right to think nonsense and to
neglect facts.

You know better. From the very first we have said that
human beings fall ill of a conflict between the claims of instinctual life and the resistance which arises within them against it;
and not for a moment have we forgotten this resisting, repelling,
repressing agency, which we thought of as equipped with its
special forces, the ego-instincts, and which coincides with the
ego of popular psychology. The truth was merely that, in view of
the laborious nature of the progress made by scientific work,
even psycho-analysis was not able to study every field simultaneously and to express its views on every problem in a single
breath. But at last the point was reached when it was possible

[1] [The greater part of the material in this lecture is derived (with some
amplifications) from Chapters I, II, III and V of *The Ego and the Id*
(1923*b*).]

for us to divert our attention from the repressed to the repressing forces, and we faced this ego, which had seemed so self-evident, with the secure expectation that here once again we should find things for which we could not have been prepared. It was not easy, however, to find a first approach; and that is what I intend to talk to you about to-day.

I must, however, let you know of my suspicion that this account of mine of ego-psychology will affect you differently from the introduction into the psychical underworld which preceded it. I cannot say with certainty why this should be so. I thought first that you would discover that whereas what I reported to you previously were, in the main, facts, however strange and peculiar, now you will be listening principally to opinions—that is, to speculations. But that does not meet the position. After further consideration I must maintain that the amount of intellectual working-over of the factual material in our ego-psychology is not much greater than it was in the psychology of the neuroses. I have been obliged to reject other explanations as well of the result I anticipate: I now believe that it is somehow a question of the nature of the material itself and of our being unaccustomed to dealing with it. In any case, I shall not be surprised if you show yourselves even more reserved and cautious in your judgement than hitherto.

The situation in which we find ourselves at the beginning of our enquiry may be expected itself to point the way for us. We wish to make the ego the matter of our enquiry, our very own ego. But is that possible? After all, the ego is in its very essence a subject; how can it be made into an object? Well, there is no doubt that it can be. The ego can take itself as an object, can treat itself like other objects, can observe itself, criticize itself, and do Heaven knows what with itself. In this, one part of the ego is setting itself over against the rest. So the ego can be split; it splits itself during a number of its functions—temporarily at least. Its parts can come together again afterwards. That is not exactly a novelty, though it may perhaps be putting an unusual emphasis on what is generally known. On the other hand, we are familiar with the notion that pathology, by making things larger and coarser, can draw our attention to normal conditions which would otherwise have escaped us. Where it points to a breach or a rent, there may normally be an articulation present. If we throw a crystal to the floor, it breaks; but not into haphazard pieces. It comes apart along its lines of cleavage into fragments whose boundaries, though they were invisible, were predetermined by the crystal's structure. Mental patients are split and broken structures of this same kind. Even we cannot withhold from them something of the reverential awe which peoples of the past felt for the insane. They have turned away from external reality, but for that very reason they know more about internal, psychical reality and can reveal a number of things to us that would otherwise be inaccessible to us.

We describe one group of these patients as suffering from delusions of being observed. They complain to us that perpetually, and down to their most intimate actions, they are being molested by the observation of unknown powers—presumably persons—and that in hallucinations they hear these persons reporting the outcome of their observation: 'now he's going to say this, now he's dressing to go out' and so on. Observation of this sort is not yet the same thing as persecution, but it is not far from it; it presupposes that people distrust them, and expect to catch them carrying out forbidden actions for which they would be punished. How would it be if these insane people were right, if in each of us there is present in his ego an agency like this which observes and threatens to punish, and which in them has merely become sharply divided from their ego and mistakenly displaced into external reality?

I cannot tell whether the same thing will happen to you as to me. Ever since, under the powerful impression of this clinical picture, I formed the idea that the separation of the observing agency from the rest of the ego might be a regular feature of the ego's structure, that idea has never left me, and I was driven to investigate the further characteristics and connections of the agency which was thus separated off. The next step is quickly taken. The content of the delusions of being observed already suggests that the observing is only a preparation for judging and punishing, and we accordingly guess that another function of this agency must be what we call our conscience. There is scarcely anything else in us that we so regularly separate from our ego and so easily set over against it as precisely our conscience. I feel an inclination to do something that I think will give me pleasure, but I abandon it on the ground that my conscience does not allow it. Or I have let myself be persuaded by too great an expectation of pleasure into doing something to which the voice of conscience has objected and after the deed my conscience punishes me with distressing reproaches and causes me to feel remorse for the deed. I might simply say that the special agency which I am beginning to distinguish in the ego is conscience. But it is more prudent to keep the agency as something independent and to suppose that conscience is one of its functions and that self-observation, which is an essential preliminary to the judging activity of conscience, is another of them. And since when we recognize that something has a separate existence we give it a name of its own, from this time forward I will describe this agency in the ego as the '*super-ego*'.

I am now prepared to hear you ask me scornfully whether our ego-psychology comes down to nothing more than taking commonly used abstractions literally and in a crude sense, and transforming them from concepts into things—by which not much would be gained. To this I would reply that in ego-psychology it will be difficult to escape what is universally known; it will rather be a question of new ways of looking at things and new ways of arranging them than of new discoveries. So hold to your contemptuous criticism for the time being and await further explanations. The facts of pathology give our efforts a background that you would look for in vain in popular psychology. So I will proceed.

Hardly have we familiarized ourselves with the idea of a super-ego like this which enjoys a certain degree of autonomy, follows its own intentions and is independent of the ego for its supply of energy, than a clinical picture forces itself on our notice which throws a striking light on the severity of this agency and indeed its cruelty, and on its changing relations to the ego. I am thinking of the condition of melancholia,[1] or, more precisely, of melancholic attacks, which you too will have heard plenty about, even if you are not psychiatrists. The most striking feature of this illness, of whose causation and mechanism we know much too little, is the way in which the super-ego —'conscience', you may call it, quietly—treats the ego. While a melancholic can, like other people, show a greater or lesser

[1] [Modern terminology would probably speak of 'depression'.]

degree of severity to himself in his healthy periods, during a melancholic attack his super-ego becomes over-severe, abuses the poor ego, humiliates it and ill-treats it, threatens it with the direst punishments, reproaches it for actions in the remotest past which had been taken lightly at the time—as though it had spent the whole interval in collecting accusations and had only been waiting for its present access of strength in order to bring them up and make a condemnatory judgement on their basis. The super-ego applies the strictest moral standard to the help-less ego which is at its mercy; in general it represents the claims of morality, and we realize all at once that our moral sense of guilt is the expression of the tension between the ego and the super-ego. It is a most remarkable experience to see morality, which is supposed to have been given us by God and thus deeply implanted in us, functioning [in these patients] as a periodic phenomenon. For after a certain number of months the whole moral fuss is over, the criticism of the super-ego is silent, the ego is rehabilitated and again enjoys all the rights of man till the next attack. In some forms of the disease, indeed, something of a contrary sort occurs in the intervals; the ego finds itself in a blissful state of intoxication, it celebrates a triumph, as though the super-ego had lost all its strength or had melted into the ego; and this 'liberated, manic ego permits itself a truly unin-hibited satisfaction of all its appetites. Here are happenings rich in unsolved riddles!

No doubt you will expect me to give you more than a mere illustration when I inform you that we have found out all kinds of things about the formation of the super-ego—that is to say, about the origin of conscience. Following a well-known pro-nouncement of Kant's which couples the conscience within us with the starry Heavens, a pious man might well be tempted to honour these two things as the masterpieces of creation. The stars are indeed magnificent, but as regards conscience God has done an uneven and careless piece of work, for a large majority of men have brought along with them only a modest amount of it or scarcely enough to be worth mentioning. We are far from overlooking the portion of psychological truth that is contained in the assertion that conscience is of divine origin; but the thesis needs interpretation. Even if conscience is something 'within us', yet it is not so from the first. In this it is a real contrast to sexual life, which is in fact there from the beginning of life and not only a later addition. But, as is well known, young children are amoral and possess no internal inhibitions against their impulses striving for pleasure. The part which is later taken on by the super-ego is played to begin with by an external power, by parental authority. Parental influence governs the child by offering proofs of love and by threatening punishments which are signs to the child of loss of love and are bound to be feared on their own account. This realistic anxiety is the precursor of the later moral anxiety.[1] So long as it is dominant there is no need to talk of a super-ego and of a conscience. It is only subsequently that the secondary situation develops (which we are all too ready to regard as the normal one), where the external restraint is internalized and the super-ego takes the place of the parental agency and observes, directs and threatens the ego in exactly the same way as earlier the parents did with the child.

The super-ego, which thus takes over the power, function and even the methods of the parental agency, is however not merely its successor but actually the legitimate heir of its body. It proceeds directly out of it, we shall learn presently by what process. First, however, we must dwell upon a discrepancy between the two. The super-ego seems to have made a one-sided choice and to have picked out only the parents' strictness and severity, their prohibiting and punitive function, whereas their loving care seems not to have been taken over and maintained. If the parents have really enforced their authority with severity we can easily understand the child's in turn developing a severe super-ego. But, contrary to our expectation, experience shows that the super-ego can acquire the same characteristic of relentless severity even if the upbringing had been mild and kindly and had so far as possible avoided threats and punishments. We shall come back later to this contradiction when we deal with the transformations of instinct during the formation of the super-ego.[2]

I cannot tell you as much as I should like about the metamorphosis of the parental relationship into the super-ego, partly

[1] ['*Gewissensangst*', literally 'conscience anxiety'.]
[2] [See p. 573 below.]

because that process is so complicated that an account of it will not fit into the framework of an introductory course of lectures such as I am trying to give you, but partly also because we ourselves do not feel sure that we understand it completely. So you must be content with the sketch that follows.

The basis of the process is what is called an 'identification'— that is to say, the assimilation of one ego to another one,[1] as a result of which the first ego behaves like the second in certain respects, imitates it and in a sense takes it up into itself. Identification has been not unsuitably compared with the oral, cannibalistic incorporation of the other person. It is a very important form of attachment to someone else, probably the very first, and not the same thing as the choice of an object. The difference between the two can be expressed in some such way as this. If a boy identifies himself with his father, he wants to *be like* his father; if he makes him the object of his choice, he wants to *have* him, to possess him. In the first case his ego is altered on the model of his father; in the second case that is not necessary. Identification and object-choice are to a large extent independent of each other; it is however possible to identify oneself with someone whom, for instance, one has taken as a sexual object, and to alter one's ego on his model. It is said that the influencing of the ego by the sexual object occurs particularly often with women and is characteristic of femininity. I must already have spoken to you in my earlier lectures of what is by far the most instructive relation between identification and object-choice. It can be observed equally easily in children and adults, in normal as in sick people. If one has lost an object or has been obliged to give it up, one often compensates oneself by identifying oneself with it and by setting it up once more in one's ego, so that here object-choice regresses, as it were, to identification.[2]

I myself am far from satisfied with these remarks on identification; but it will be enough if you can grant me that the installation of the super-ego can be described as a successful

---

[1] [I.e. one ego coming to resemble another one.]

[2] [The matter is in fact only very briefly alluded to in the *Introductory Lectures* (see the later part of Lecture XXVI). Identification was the subject of Chapter VII of *Group Psychology* (1921c). The formation of the super-ego was discussed at length in Chapter III of *The Ego and the Id* (1923b), (Norton, 1961).]

instance of identification with the parental agency. The fact that speaks decisively for this view is that this new creation of a superior agency within the ego is most intimately linked with the destiny of the Oedipus complex, so that the super-ego appears as the heir of that emotional attachment which is of such importance for childhood. With his abandonment of the Oedipus complex a child must, as we can see, renounce the intense object-cathexes which he has deposited with his parents, and it is as a compensation for this loss of objects that there is such a strong intensification of the identifications with his parents which have probably long been present in his ego. Identifications of this kind as precipitates of object-cathexes that have been given up will be repeated often enough later in the child's life; but it is entirely in accordance with the emotional importance of this first instance of such a transformation that a special place in the ego should be found for its outcome. Close investigation has shown us, too, that the super-ego is stunted in its strength and growth if the surmounting of the Oedipus complex is only incompletely successful. In the course of development the super-ego also takes on the influences of those who have stepped into the place of parents—educators, teachers, people chosen as ideal models. Normally it departs more and more from the original parental figures; it becomes, so to say, more impersonal. Nor must it be forgotten that a child has a different estimate of its parents at different periods of its life. At the time at which the Oedipus complex gives place to the super-ego they are something quite magnificent; but later they lose much of this. Identifications then come about with these later parents as well, and indeed they regularly make important contributions to the formation of character; but in that case they only affect the ego, they no longer influence the super-ego, which has been determined by the earliest parental imagos.[1]

I hope you have already formed an impression that the hypothesis of the super-ego really describes a structural relation and is not merely a personification of some such abstraction as that of conscience. One more important function remains to be mentioned which we attribute to this super-ego. It is also the

[1] [This point was discussed by Freud in a paper on 'The Economic Problem of Masochism' (1924c).]

vehicle of the ego ideal by which the ego measures itself, which it emulates, and whose demand for ever greater perfection it strives to fulfil. There is no doubt that this ego ideal is the precipitate of the old picture of the parents, the expression of admiration for the perfection which the child then attributed to them.[1]

I am sure you have heard a great deal of the sense of inferiority which is supposed particularly to characterize neurotics. It especially haunts the pages of what are known as *belles lettres*. An author who uses the term 'inferiority complex' thinks that by so doing he has fulfilled all the demands of psycho-analysis and has raised his composition to a higher psychological plane. In fact 'inferiority complex' is a technical term that is scarcely used in psycho-analysis. For us it does not bear the meaning of anything simple, let alone elementary. To trace it back to the self-perception of possible organic defects, as the school of what are known as 'Individual Psychologists'[2] likes to do, seems to us a short-sighted error. The sense of inferiority has strong erotic roots. A child feels inferior if he notices that he is not loved, and so does an adult. The only bodily organ which is really regarded as inferior is the atrophied penis, a girl's clitoris.[3] But the major part of the sense of inferiority derives from the ego's relation to

---

[1] [There is some obscurity in this passage, and in particular over the phrase '*der Träger des Ichideals*', here translated 'the vehicle of the ego ideal'. When Freud first introduced the concept in his paper on narcissism (1914c), he distinguished between the ego ideal itself and 'a special psychical agency which performs the task of seeing that narcissistic satisfaction from the ego ideal is ensured and which, with this end in view, constantly watches the actual ego and measures it by that ideal' Similarly, in Lecture XXVI of the *Introductory Lectures* (1916–17) he speaks of a person sensing 'an agency holding sway in his ego which measures his actual ego and each of its activities by an ideal ego that he has created for himself in the course of his development.' In some of Freud's later writings this distinction between the ideal and the agency enforcing it became blurred. It seems possible that it is revived here and that the super-ego is being identified with the enforcing agency. The use of the term '*Idealfunktion*' three paragraphs lower down (p530) raises the same question.]

[2] [Their views are discussed in Lecture XXXIV, p. 604 ff. below.]

[3] [Cf. a footnote of Freud's to his paper on the anatomical distinction between the sexes (1925j.]

its super-ego; like the sense of guilt it is an expression of the tension between them. Altogether, it is hard to separate the sense of inferiority and the sense of guilt. It would perhaps be right to regard the former as the erotic complement to the moral sense of inferiority. Little attention has been given in psycho-analysis to the question of the delimitation of the two concepts.

If only because the inferiority complex has become so popular, I will venture to entertain you here with a short digression. A historical personality of our own days, who is still alive though at the moment he has retired into the background, suffers from a defect in one of his limbs owing to an injury at the time of his birth. A very well-known contemporary writer who is particularly fond of compiling the biographies of celebrities has dealt, among others, with the life of the man I am speaking of.[1] Now in writing a biography it may well be difficult to suppress a need to plumb the psychological depths. For this reason our author has ventured on an attempt to erect the whole of the development of his hero's character on the sense of inferiority which must have been called up by his physical defect. In doing so, he has overlooked one small but not insignificant fact. It is usual for mothers whom Fate has presented with a child who is sickly or otherwise at a disadvantage to try to compensate him for his unfair handicap by a superabundance of love. In the instance before us, the proud mother behaved otherwise; she withdrew her love from the child on account of his infirmity. When he had grown up into a man of great power, he proved unambiguously by his actions that he had never forgiven his mother. When you consider the importance of a mother's love for the mental life of a child, you will no doubt make a tacit correction of the biographer's inferiority theory.

But let us return to the super-ego. We have allotted it the functions of self-observation, of conscience and of [maintaining] the ideal.[2] It follows from what we have said about its origin that it presupposes an immensely important biological fact and a fateful psychological one: namely, the human child's long dependence on its parents and the Oedipus complex, both of which, again, are intimately interconnected. The super-ego is

[1] [*Wilhelm II*, by Emil Ludwig (1926).]
[2] ['*Idealfunktion.*' Cf. footnote 1, p. 529 above.]

the representative for us of every moral restriction, the advocate of a striving towards perfection—it is, in short, as much as we have been able to grasp psychologically of what is described as the higher side of human life. Since it itself goes back to the influence of parents, educators and so on, we learn still more of its significance if we turn to those who are its sources. As a rule parents and authorities analogous to them follow the precepts of their own super-egos in educating children. Whatever understanding their ego may have come to with their super-ego, they are severe and exacting in educating children. They have forgotten the difficulties of their own childhood and they are glad to be able now to identify themselves fully with their own parents who in the past laid such severe restrictions upon them. Thus a child's super-ego is in fact constructed on the model not of its parents but of its parents' super-ego; the contents which fill it are the same and it becomes the vehicle of tradition and of all the time-resisting judgements of value which have propagated themselves in this manner from generation to generation. You may easily guess what important assistance taking the super-ego into account will give us in our understanding of the social behaviour of mankind—in the problem of delinquency, for instance—and perhaps even what practical hints on education. It seems likely that what are known as materialistic views of history sin in under-estimating this factor. They brush it aside with the remark that human 'ideologies' are nothing other than the product and superstructure of their contemporary economic conditions. That is true, but very probably not the whole truth. Mankind never lives entirely in the present. The past, the tradition of the race and of the people, lives on in the ideologies of the super-ego, and yields only slowly to the influences of the present and to new changes; and so long as it operates through the super-ego it plays a powerful part in human life, independently of economic conditions. [Cf. p. 642 ff.]

In 1921 I endeavoured to make use of the differentiation between the ego and the super-ego in a study of group psychology. I arrived at a formula such as this: a psychological group is a collection of individuals who have introduced the same person into their super-ego and, on the basis of this common element, have identified themselves with one another in their ego.[1] This

[1] [See the end of Chapter VIII of *Group Psychology* (1921c).]

applies, of course, only to groups that have a leader. If we possessed more applications of this kind, the hypothesis of the super-ego would lose its last touch of strangeness for us, and we should become completely free of the embarrassment that still comes over us when, accustomed as we are to the atmosphere of the underworld, we move in the more superficial, higher strata of the mental apparatus. We do not suppose, of course, that with the separation off of the super-ego we have said the last word on the psychology of the ego. It is rather a first step; but in this case it is not only the first step that is hard.

Now, however, another problem awaits us—at the opposite end of the ego, as we might put it. It is presented to us by an observation during the work of analysis, an observation which is actually a very old one. As not infrequently happens, it has taken a long time to come to the point of appreciating its importance. The whole theory of psycho-analysis is, as you know, in fact built up on the perception of the resistance offered to us by the patient when we attempt to make his unconscious conscious to him. The objective sign of this resistance is that his associations fail or depart widely from the topic that is being dealt with. He may also recognize the resistance *subjectively* by the fact that he has distressing feelings when he approaches the topic. But this last sign may also be absent. We then say to the patient that we infer from his behaviour that he is now in a state of resistance; and he replies that he knows nothing of that, and is only aware that his associations have become more difficult. It turns out that we were right; but in that case his resistance was unconscious too, just as unconscious as the repressed, at the lifting of which we were working. We should long ago have asked the question: from what part of his mind does an unconscious resistance like this arise? The beginner in psycho-analysis will be ready at once with the answer: it is, of course, the resistance of the unconscious. An ambiguous and unserviceable answer! If it means that the resistance arises from the repressed, we must rejoin: certainly not! We must rather attribute to the repressed a strong upward drive, an impulsion to break through into consciousness. The resistance can only be a manifestation of the ego, which originally put the repression into force and now wishes to maintain it. That, moreover, is the view we always took. Since we have come to assume a special agency in the ego, the super-ego, which represents demands of a restrictive and rejecting character, we may say that repression is the work of this super-ego and that it is carried out either by itself or by the ego in obedience to its orders. If then we are met by the case of the resistance in analysis not being conscious to the patient, this means either that in quite important situations the super-ego and the ego can operate unconsciously, or—and this would be still more important—that portions of both of them, the ego and the super-ego themselves, are unconscious. In both cases we have to reckon with the disagreeable discovery that on the one hand (super-) ego and conscious and on the other hand repressed and unconscious are far from coinciding.

And here, Ladies and Gentlemen, I feel that I must make a pause to take breath—which you too will welcome as a relief—and, before I go on, to apologize to you. My intention is to give you some addenda to the introductory lectures on psycho-analysis which I began fifteen years ago, and I am obliged to behave as though you as well as I had in the interval done nothing but practise psycho-analysis. I know that that assumption is out of place; but I am helpless, I cannot do otherwise. This is no doubt related to the fact that it is in general so hard to give anyone who is not himself a psycho-analyst an insight into psycho-analysis. You can believe me when I tell you that we do not enjoy giving an impression of being members of a secret society and of practising a mystical science. Yet we have been obliged to recognize and express as our conviction that no one has a right to join in a discussion of psycho-analysis who has not had particular experiences which can only be obtained by being analysed oneself. When I gave you my lectures fifteen years ago I tried to spare you certain speculative portions of our theory; but it is precisely from them that are derived the new acquisitions of which I must speak to you to-day.

I return now to our topic. In face of the doubt whether the ego and super-ego are themselves unconscious or merely produce unconscious effects, we have, for good reasons, decided in favour of the former possibility. And it is indeed the case that large portions of the ego and super-ego can remain unconscious and are normally unconscious. That is to say, the individual knows nothing of their contents and it requires an expenditure of effort to make them conscious. It is a fact that ego and conscious, repressed and unconscious do not coincide. We feel a need to make a fundamental revision of our attitude to the problem of conscious–unconscious. At first we are inclined greatly to reduce the value of the criterion of being conscious since it has shown itself so untrustworthy. But we should be doing it an injustice. As may be said of our life, it is not worth much, but it is all we have. Without the illumination thrown by the quality of consciousness, we should be lost in the obscurity of depth-psychology; but we must attempt to find our bearings afresh.

There is no need to discuss what is to be called conscious: it is removed from all doubt. The oldest and best meaning of the word 'unconscious' is the descriptive one; we call a psychical process unconscious whose existence we are obliged to assume —for some such reason as that we infer it from its effects—, but of which we know nothing. In that case we have the same relation to it as we have to a psychical process in another person, except that it is in fact one of our own. If we want to be still more correct, we shall modify our assertion by saying that we call a process unconscious if we are obliged to assume that it is being activated *at the moment*, though *at the moment* we know nothing about it. This qualification makes us reflect that the majority of conscious processes are conscious only for a short time; very soon they become *latent*, but can easily become conscious again. We might also say that they had become unconscious, if it were at all certain that in the condition of latency they are still something psychical. So far we should have learnt nothing new; nor should we have acquired the right to introduce the concept of an unconscious into psychology. But then comes the new observation that we were already able to make in parapraxes. In order to explain a slip of the tongue, for instance, we find ourselves obliged to assume that the intention to make a particular remark was present in the subject. We infer it with certainty from the interference with his remark which has occurred; but the intention did not put itself through and was thus unconscious. If, when we subsequently put it before the speaker, he recognizes it as one familiar to him, then it was only temporarily unconscious to him; but if he repudiates it as something foreign to him, then it was permanently unconscious.[1] From this experience we retrospectively obtain the right also to pronounce as something unconscious what had been described as latent. A consideration of these dynamic relations permits us now to distinguish two kinds of unconscious—one which is easily, under frequently occurring circumstances, transformed into something conscious, and another with which this transformation is difficult and takes place only subject to a considerable expenditure of effort or possibly never at all. In order to escape the ambiguity as to whether we mean the one or the other unconscious, whether we are using the word in the descriptive or in the dynamic sense, we make use of a permissible and simple way out. We call the unconscious which is only latent, and thus easily becomes conscious, the 'preconscious' and retain the term 'unconscious' for the other. We now have three terms, 'conscious', 'preconscious' and 'unconscious', with which we can get along in our description of mental phenomena. Once again: the preconscious is also unconscious in the purely descriptive sense, but we do not give it that name, except in talking loosely or when we have to make a defence of the existence in mental life of unconscious processes in general.

You will admit, I hope, that so far that is not too bad and allows of convenient handling. Yes, but unluckily the work of psycho-analysis has found itself compelled to use the word 'unconscious' in yet another, third, sense, and this may, to be sure, have led to confusion. Under the new and powerful impression of there being an extensive and important field of mental life which is normally withdrawn from the ego's knowledge so that the processes occurring in it have to be regarded as unconscious in the truly dynamic sense, we have come to understand the term 'unconscious' in a topographical or systematic sense as well; we have come to speak of a 'system' of the preconscious and a 'system' of the unconscious, of a conflict between the ego and the system *Ucs.*, and have used the word more and more to denote a mental province rather than a quality of what is mental. The discovery, actually an inconvenient one, that portions of the ego and super-ego as well are unconscious in the dynamic sense, operates at this point as a relief—it makes possible

[1] [Cf. *Introductory Lectures,* IV.]

the removal of a complication. We perceive that we have no right to name the mental region that is foreign to the ego 'the system *Ucs.*', since the characteristic of being unconscious is not restricted to it. Very well; we will no longer use the term 'unconscious' in the systematic sense and we will give what we have hitherto so described a better name and one no longer open to misunderstanding. Following a verbal usage of Nietzsche's and taking up a suggestion by Georg Groddeck [1923],[1] we will in future call it the 'id'.[2] This impersonal pronoun seems particularly well suited for expressing the main characteristic of this province of the mind—the fact of its being alien to the ego. The super-ego, the ego and the id—these, then, are the three realms, regions, provinces, into which we divide an individual's mental apparatus, and with the mutual relations of which we shall be concerned in what follows.

But first a short interpolation. I suspect that you feel dissatisfied because the three qualities of the characteristic of consciousness and the three provinces of the mental apparatus do not fall together into three peaceable couples, and you may regard this as in some sense obscuring our findings. I do not think, however, that we should regret it, and we should tell ourselves that we had no right to expect any such smooth arrangement. Let me give you an analogy; analogies, it is true, decide nothing, but they can make one feel more at home. I am imagining a country with a landscape of varying configuration —hill-country, plains, and chains of lakes—, and with a mixed population: it is inhabited by Germans, Magyars and Slovaks, who carry on different activities. Now things might be partitioned in such a way that the Germans, who breed cattle, live in the hill-country, the Magyars, who grow cereals and wine, live in the plains, and the Slovaks, who catch fish and plait

[1] [A German physician by whose unconventional ideas Freud was much attracted.]
[2] [In German '*Es*', the ordinary word for 'it'.]

reeds, live by the lakes. If the partitioning could be neat and clear-cut like this, a Woodrow Wilson would be delighted by it;[1] it would also be convenient for a lecture in a geography lesson. The probability is, however, that you will find less orderliness and more mixing, if you travel through the region. Germans, Magyars and Slovaks live interspersed all over it; in the hill-country there is agricultural land as well, cattle are bred in the plains too. A few things are naturally as you expected, for fish cannot be caught in the mountains and wine does not grow in the water. Indeed, the picture of the region that you brought with you may on the whole fit the facts; but you will have to put up with deviations in the details.

You will not expect me to have much to tell you that is new about the id apart from its new name. It is the dark, inaccessible part of our personality; what little we know of it we have learnt from our study of the dream-work and of the construction of neurotic symptoms, and most of that is of a negative character and can be described only as a contrast to the ego. We approach the id with analogies: we call it a chaos, a cauldron full of seething excitations. We picture it as being open at its end to somatic influences, and as there taking up into itself instinctual needs which find their psychical expression in it,[2] but we cannot say in what substratum. It is filled with energy reaching it from the instincts, but it has no organization, produces no collective will, but only a striving to bring about the satisfaction of the instinctual needs subject to the observance of the pleasure principle. The logical laws of thought do not apply in the id, and this is true above all of the law of contradiction. Contrary impulses exist side by side, without cancelling each other out or diminishing each other: at the most they may converge to form compromises under the dominating economic pressure towards

[1] [It may be remarked that only a year or so before writing this Freud had finished his collaboration with W. C. Bullitt (then American Ambassador in Berlin) on a study of President Wilson, of whose political judgement he was highly critical. The work has not hitherto (1965) been published.]

[2] [Freud is here regarding instincts as something physical, of which mental processes are the representatives.]

the discharge of energy. There is nothing in the id that could be compared with negation; and we perceive with surprise an exception to the philosophical theorem that space and time are necessary forms of our mental acts.[1] There is nothing in the id that corresponds to the idea of time; there is no recognition of the passage of time, and—a thing that is most remarkable and awaits consideration in philosophical thought—no alteration in its mental processes is produced by the passage of time. Wishful impulses which have never passed beyond the id, but impressions, too, which have been sunk into the id by repression, are virtually immortal; after the passage of decades they behave as though they had just occurred. They can only be recognized as belonging to the past, can only lose their importance and be deprived of their cathexis of energy, when they have been made conscious by the work of analysis, and it is on this that the therapeutic effect of analytic treatment rests to no small extent.

Again and again I have had the impression that we have made too little theoretical use of this fact, established beyond any doubt, of the unalterability by time of the repressed. This seems to offer an approach to the most profound discoveries. Nor, unfortunately, have I myself made any progress here.

The id of course knows no judgements of value: no good and evil, no morality. The economic or, if you prefer, the quantitative factor, which is intimately linked to the pleasure principle, dominates all its processes. Instinctual cathexes seeking discharge—that, in our view, is all there is in the id. It even seems that the energy of these instinctual impulses is in a state different from that in the other regions of the mind, far more mobile and capable of discharge;[2] otherwise the displacements and condensations would not occur which are characteristic of

---

[1] [The reference is to Kant.]

[2] [This difference was referred to by Freud in many passages. See, in particular, Section V of the metapsychological paper on 'The Unconscious' (1915e), and Chapter IV of *Beyond the Pleasure Principle* (1920g). In both these passages Freud attributes the distinction to Breuer, apparently having in mind a footnote to Section 2 (A) of Breuer's theoretical contribution to *Studies on Hysteria* (1895d).]

the id and which so completely disregard the *quality* of what is cathected—what in the ego we should call an idea. We would give much to understand more about these things! You can see, incidentally, that we are in a position to attribute to the id characteristics other than that of its being unconscious, and you can recognize the possibility of portions of the ego and super-ego being unconscious without possessing the same primitive and irrational characteristics.[1]

We can best arrive at the characteristics of the actual ego, in so far as it can be distinguished from the id and from the super-ego, by examining its relation to the outermost superficial portion of the mental apparatus, which we describe as the system *Pcpt.-Cs.*[2] This system is turned towards the external world, it is the medium for the perceptions arising thence, and during its functioning the phenomenon of consciousness arises in it. It is the sense-organ of the entire apparatus; moreover it is receptive not only to excitations from outside but also to those arising from the interior of the mind. We need scarcely look for a justification of the view that the ego is that portion of the id which was modified by the proximity and influence of the external world, which is adapted for the reception of stimuli and as a protective shield against stimuli, comparable to the cortical layer by which a small piece of living substance is surrounded. The relation to the external world has become the decisive factor for the ego; it has taken on the task of representing the external world to the id—fortunately for the id, which could not escape destruction if, in its blind efforts for the satisfaction of its instincts, it disregarded that supreme external power. In accomplishing this function, the ego must observe the external world, must lay down an accurate picture of it in the memory-traces of its perceptions, and by its exercise of the function of 'reality-testing'[3] must put aside whatever in this picture of the external world is an addition derived from internal sources of excitation. The ego controls the approaches to motility under

'The Unconscious' he remarks that in his opinion this distinction represents the deepest insight we have gained up to the present into the nature of nervous energy. Cf. a further footnote on p. 553 below.]

[1] [This account of the id is in the main based on Section V of the paper on 'The Unconscious'.]

[2] [Perceptual-conscious.]   [3] [See footnote 1, p. 497 above.]

the id's orders; but between a need and an action it has interposed a postponement in the form of the activity of thought,[1] during which it makes use of the mnemic residues of experience. In that way it has dethroned the pleasure principle which dominates the course of events in the id without any restriction and has replaced it by the reality principle, which promises more certainty and greater success.

The relation to time, which is so hard to describe, is also introduced into the ego by the perceptual system; it can scarcely be doubted that the mode of operation of that system is what provides the origin of the idea of time.[2] But what distinguishes the ego from the id quite especially is a tendency to synthesis in its contents, to a combination and unification in its mental processes which are totally lacking in the id. When presently we come to deal with the instincts in mental life we shall, I hope, succeed in tracing this essential characteristic of the ego back to its source.[3] It alone produces the high degree of organization which the ego needs for its best achievements. The ego develops from perceiving the instincts to controlling them; but this last is only achieved by the [psychical] representative of the instinct[4] being allotted its proper place in a considerable assemblage, by its being taken up into a coherent context. To adopt a popular mode of speaking, we might say that the ego stands for reason and good sense while the id stands for the untamed passions.

So far we have allowed ourselves to be impressed by the merits and capabilities of the ego; it is now time to consider the other side as well. The ego is after all only a portion of the id, a

---

[1] [This is further discussed below, p. 553.]

[2] [Freud gave some indication of what he had in mind by this at the end of his paper on the 'Mystic Writing-Pad' (1925a).]

[3] [Freud does not seem, in fact, to have returned to the subject in these lectures.—He had discussed this characteristic of the ego at length in Chapter III of *Inhibitions, Symptoms and Anxiety* (1926d). Though he had stressed the synthetic tendency of the ego particularly in his later writings (e.g. among many others in Chapter II of *The Questions of Lay Analysis* (1926e), (Norton, 1950), the concept was implicit in his picture of the ego from the earliest times. See, for instance, the term he almost invariably used during the Breuer period for ideas that had to be repressed: 'incompatible'—i.e. that could not be synthesized by the ego. So in Section II of the first paper on the neuro-psychoses of defence (1894a).]

[4] [See footnote 2, p. 537 above.]

portion that has been expediently modified by the proximity of the external world with its threat of danger. From a dynamic point of view it is weak, it has borrowed its energies from the id, and we are not entirely without insight into the methods—we might call them dodges—by which it extracts further amounts of energy from the id. One such method, for instance, is by identifying itself with actual or abandoned objects. The object-cathexes spring from the instinctual demands of the id. The ego has in the first instance to take note of them. But by identifying itself with the object it recommends itself to the id in place of the object and seeks to divert the id's libido on to itself. We have already seen [p. 528] that in the course of its life the ego takes into itself a large number of precipitates like this of former object-cathexes. The ego must on the whole carry out the id's intentions, it fulfils its task by finding out the circumstances in which those intentions can best be achieved. The ego's relation to the id might be compared with that of a rider to his horse. The horse supplies the locomotive energy, while the rider has the privilege of deciding on the goal and of guiding the powerful animal's movement. But only too often there arises between the ego and the id the not precisely ideal situation of the rider being obliged to guide the horse along the path by which it itself wants to go.

There is one portion of the id from which the ego has separated itself by resistances due to repression. But the repression is not carried over into the id: the repressed merges into the remainder of the id.

We are warned by a proverb against serving two masters at the same time. The poor ego has things even worse: it serves three severe masters and does what it can to bring their claims and demands into harmony with one another. These claims are always divergent and often seem incompatible. No wonder that the ego so often fails in its task. Its three tyrannical masters are the external world, the super-ego and the id. When we follow the ego's efforts to satisfy them simultaneously—or rather, to obey them simultaneously—we cannot feel any regret at having personified this ego and having set it up as a separate organism. It feels hemmed in on three sides, threatened by three kinds of danger, to which, if it is hard pressed, it reacts by generating anxiety. Owing to its origin from the experiences of the perceptual system, it is earmarked for representing the demands of the external world, but it strives too to be a loyal servant of the id, to remain on good terms with it, to recommend itself to it as an object and to attract its libido to itself. In its attempts to mediate between the id and reality, it is often obliged to cloak the *Ucs.* commands of the id with its own *Pcs.* rationalizations, to conceal the id's conflicts with reality, to profess, with diplomatic disingenuousness, to be taking notice of reality even when the id has remained rigid and unyielding. On the other hand it is observed at every step it takes by the strict super-ego, which lays down definite standards for its conduct, without taking any account of its difficulties from the direction of the id and the external world, and which, if those standards are not obeyed, punishes it with tense feelings of inferiority and of guilt. Thus the ego, driven by the id, confined by the super-ego, repulsed by reality, struggles to master its economic task of bringing about harmony among the forces and influences working in and upon it; and we can understand how it is that so often we cannot suppress a cry: 'Life is not easy!' If the ego is obliged to admit its weakness, it breaks out in anxiety—realistic anxiety regarding the external world, moral anxiety regarding the super-ego and neurotic anxiety regarding the strength of the passions in the id.

I should like to portray the structural relations of the mental personality, as I have described them to you, in the unassuming sketch which I now present you with:

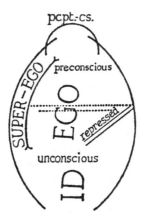

As you see here, the super-ego merges into the id; indeed, as heir to the Oedipus complex it has intimate relations with the id; it is more remote than the ego from the perceptual system.[1] The id has intercourse with the external world only through the ego—at least, according to this diagram. It is certainly hard to say to-day how far the drawing is correct. In one respect it is undoubtedly not. The space occupied by the unconscious id ought to have been incomparably greater than that of the ego or the preconscious. I must ask you to correct it in your thoughts.

And here is another warning, to conclude these remarks, which have certainly been exacting and not, perhaps, very illuminating. In thinking of this division of the personality into an ego, a super-ego and an id, you will not, of course, have pictured sharp frontiers like the artificial ones drawn in political geography. We cannot do justice to the characteristics of the mind by linear outlines like those in a drawing or in primitive painting, but rather by areas of colour melting into one another as they are presented by modern artists. After making the separation we must allow what we have separated to merge together once more. You must not judge too harshly a first attempt at giving a pictorial representation of something so intangible as psychical processes. It is highly probable that the development of these divisions is subject to great variations in different individuals; it is possible that in the course of actual functioning they may change and go through a temporary phase of involution. Particularly in the case of what is phylogenetically the last and most delicate of these divisions—the differentiation between the ego and the super-ego—something of the sort seems to be true. There is no question but that the same thing results from psychical illness. It is easy to imagine, too, that certain mystical practices may succeed in upsetting the normal

[1] [If this diagram is compared with the similar one in Chapter II of *The Ego and the Id* (1923b), it will be seen that the earlier diagram differs principally from the present one in the fact that the super-ego is not indicated in it. Its absence is justified in a later passage in the same work. In the original edition of these lectures this picture was printed upright, like its predecessor in *The Ego and the Id*. For some reason, perhaps to economize space, it was turned over on to its side, though otherwise unchanged, in both *G.S.* and *G.W.*]

relations between the different regions of the mind, so that, for instance, perception may be able to grasp happenings in the depths of the ego and in the id which were otherwise inaccessible to it. It may safely be doubted, however, whether this road will lead us to the ultimate truths from which salvation is to be expected. Nevertheless it may be admitted that the therapeutic efforts of psycho-analysis have chosen a similar line of approach. Its intention is, indeed, to strengthen the ego, to make it more independent of the super-ego, to widen its field of perception and enlarge its organization, so that it can appropriate fresh portions of the id.[1] Where id was, there ego shall be. It is a work of culture—not unlike the draining of the Zuider Zee.

[1] [Freud had said something similar in the last chapter of *The Ego and the Id*.]

LECTURE XXXII

ANXIETY AND INSTINCTUAL LIFE

LADIES AND GENTLEMEN,—You will not be surprised to hear that I have a number of novelties to report to you about our conception [*Auffassung*] of anxiety and of the basic instincts of mental life; nor will you be surprised to learn that none of these novelties can claim to offer a final solution of these still unsettled problems. I have a particular reason for using the word 'conception' here. These are the most difficult problems that are set to us, but their difficulty does not lie in any insufficiency of observations; what present us with these riddles are actually the commonest and most familiar of phenomena. Nor does the difficulty lie in the recondite nature of the speculations to which they give rise; speculative consideration plays little part in this sphere. But it is truly a matter of conceptions—that is to say, of introducing the right abstract ideas, whose application to the raw material of observation will produce order and clarity in it.

I devoted a lecture (the twenty-fifth) to anxiety in my previous series; and I must briefly recapitulate what I said in it. We described anxiety as an affective state—that is to say, a combination of certain feelings in the pleasure-unpleasure series with the corresponding innervations of discharge and a perception of them, but probably also the precipitate of a particular important event, incorporated by inheritance—something that may thus be likened to an individually acquired hysterical attack.[1] The event which we look upon as having left behind it an affective trace of this sort is the process of birth, at the time of which the effects upon the heart's action and upon respiration characteristic of anxiety were expedient ones. The very first anxiety would thus have been a toxic one. We then started off from a distinction between realistic anxiety and neurotic anxiety, of which the former was a reaction, which seemed intelligible to us, to a danger—that is, to an expected injury

[1] [Cf. the clearer account in *Introductory Lectures*, XXV.]

from outside—while the latter was completely enigmatic, and appeared to be pointless.

In an analysis of realistic anxiety we brought it down to the state of increased sensory attention and motor tension which we describe as 'preparedness for anxiety'. It is out of this that the anxiety reaction develops. Here two outcomes are possible. Either the generation of anxiety—the repetition of the old traumatic experience—is limited to a signal, in which case the remainder of the reaction can adapt itself to the new situation of danger and can proceed to flight or defence; or the old situation can retain the upper hand and the total reaction may consist in no more than a generation of anxiety, in which case the affective state becomes paralysing and will be inexpedient for present purposes.

We then turned to neurotic anxiety and pointed out that we observe it under three conditions. We find it first as a freely floating, general apprehensiveness, ready to attach itself temporarily, in the form of what is known as 'expectant anxiety', to any possibility that may freshly arise—as happens, for instance, in a typical anxiety neurosis. Secondly, we find it firmly attached to certain ideas in the so-called 'phobias', in which it is still possible to recognize a relation to external danger but in which we must judge the fear exaggerated out of all proportion. Thirdly and lastly, we find anxiety in hysteria and other forms of severe neurosis, where it either accompanies symptoms or emerges independently as an attack or more persistent state, but always without any visible basis in an external danger. We then asked ourselves two questions: 'What are people afraid of in neurotic anxiety?' and 'How are we to bring it into relation with realistic anxiety felt in the face of external dangers?'

Our investigations were far from remaining unsuccessful: we reached a few important conclusions. In regard to anxious expectation clinical experience revealed that it had a regular connection with the libidinal economics of sexual life. The commonest cause of anxiety neurosis is unconsummated excitation. Libidinal excitation is aroused but not satisfied, not employed; apprehensiveness then appears instead of this libido that has been diverted from its employment. I even thought I was justified in saying that this unsatisfied libido was directly changed into anxiety. This view found support in some quite regularly occurring phobias of small children. Many of these phobias are very puzzling to us, but others, such as the fear of being alone and the fear of strangers, can be explained with certainty. Loneliness as well as a strange face arouse the child's longing for his familiar mother; he is unable to control this libidinal excitation, he cannot hold it in suspense but changes it into anxiety. This infantile anxiety must therefore be regarded not as of the realistic but as of the neurotic kind. Infantile phobias and the expectation of anxiety in anxiety neurosis offer us two examples of one way in which neurotic anxiety originates: by a direct transformation of libido. We shall at once come to know of a second mechanism, but it will turn out not to be very different from the first.

For we consider that what is responsible for the anxiety in hysteria and other neuroses is the process of repression. We believe it is possible to give a more complete account of this than before, if we separate what happens to the idea that has to be repressed from what happens to the quota of libido attaching to it. It is the idea which is subjected to repression and which may be distorted to the point of being unrecognizable; but its quota of affect is regularly transformed into anxiety—and this is so whatever the nature of the affect may be, whether it is aggressiveness or love. It makes no essential difference, then, for what reason a quota of libido has become unemployable: whether it is on account of the infantile weakness of the ego, as in children's phobias, or on account of somatic processes in sexual life, as in anxiety neurosis, or owing to repression, as in hysteria. Thus in reality the two mechanisms that bring about neurotic anxiety coincide.

In the course of these investigations our attention was drawn to a highly significant relation between the generation of anxiety and the formation of symptoms—namely, that these two represent and replace each other. For instance, an agoraphobic patient may start his illness with an attack of anxiety in the street. This would be repeated every time he went into the street again. He will now develop the symptom of agoraphobia; this may also be described as an inhibition, a restriction of the ego's functioning, and by means of it he spares himself anxiety attacks. We can witness the converse of this if we interfere in the formation of symptoms, as is possible, for instance, with obsessions. If we prevent a patient from carrying out a washing ceremonial, he falls into a state of anxiety which he finds hard to tolerate and from which he had evidently been protected by his symptom. And it seems, indeed, that the generation of anxiety is the earlier and the formation of symptoms the later of the two, as though the symptoms are created in order to avoid the outbreak of the anxiety state. This is confirmed too by the fact that the first neuroses of childhood are phobias—states in which we see so clearly how an initial generation of anxiety is replaced by the later formation of a symptom; we get an impression that it is from these interrelations that we shall best obtain access to an understanding of neurotic anxiety. And at the same time we have also succeeded in answering the question of what it is that a person is afraid of in neurotic anxiety and so in establishing the connection between neurotic and realistic anxiety. What he is afraid of is evidently his own libido. The difference between this situation and that of realistic anxiety lies in two points: that the danger is an internal instead of an external one and that it is not consciously recognized.

In phobias it is very easy to observe the way in which this internal danger is transformed into an external one—that is to say, how a neurotic anxiety is changed into an apparently realistic one. In order to simplify what is often a very complicated business, let us suppose that the agoraphobic patient is invariably afraid of feelings of temptation that are aroused in him by meeting people in the street. In his phobia he brings about a displacement and henceforward is afraid of an external situation. What he gains by this is obviously that he thinks he will be able to protect himself better in that way. One can save oneself from an external danger by flight; fleeing from an internal danger is a difficult enterprise.

At the conclusion of my earlier lecture on anxiety I myself expressed the opinion that, although these various findings of our enquiry were not mutually contradictory, somehow they did not fit in with one another. Anxiety, it seems, in so far as it is an affective state, is the reproduction of an old event which brought a threat of danger; anxiety serves the purposes of self-preservation and is a signal of a new danger; it arises from libido that has in some way become unemployable and it also arises during the process of repression; it is replaced by the formation of a symptom, is, as it were, psychically bound—one has a feeling that something is missing here which would bring all these pieces together into a whole.

Ladies and Gentlemen, the dissection of the mental personality into a super-ego, an ego and an id, which I put before you in my last lecture, has obliged us to take our bearings afresh in the problem of anxiety as well. With the thesis that the ego is the sole seat of anxiety[1]—that the ego alone can produce and feel anxiety—we have established a new and stable position from which a number of things take on a new aspect. And indeed it is difficult to see what sense there would be in speaking of an 'anxiety of the id' or in attributing a capacity for apprehensiveness to the super-ego. On the other hand, we have welcomed a desirable element of correspondence in the fact that the three main species of anxiety, realistic, neurotic and moral, can be so easily connected with the ego's three dependent relations—to the external world, to the id and to the super-ego [p.542]. Along with this new view, moreover, the function of anxiety as a signal announcing a situation of danger (a notion, incidentally, not unfamiliar to us) comes into prominence, the question of what the material is out of which anxiety is made loses interest, and the relations between realistic and neurotic anxiety have become surprisingly clarified and simplified. It is also to be remarked that we now understand the apparently complicated cases of the generation of anxiety better than those which were considered simple.

For we have recently been examining the way in which anxiety is generated in certain phobias which we class as anxiety hysteria, and have chosen cases in which we were dealing with the typical repression of wishful impulses arising from the Oedipus complex. We should have expected to find that it was a libidinal cathexis of the boy's mother as object which, as

[1] [This was first stated, in slightly different words, near the end of *The Ego and the Id* (1923b). It was discussed at several points in *Inhibitions, Symptoms and Anxiety* (1926d). The greater part of what follows on the subject of anxiety is derived from the latter work.]

a result of repression, had been changed into anxiety and which now emerged, expressed in symptomatic terms, attached to a substitute for his father. I cannot present you with the detailed steps of an investigation such as this; it will be enough to say that the surprising result was the opposite of what we expected. It was not the repression that created the anxiety; the anxiety was there earlier; it was the anxiety that made the repression.[1] But what sort of anxiety can it have been? Only anxiety in the face of a threatening external danger—that is to say, a realistic anxiety. It is true that the boy felt anxiety in the face of a demand by his libido—in this instance, anxiety at being in love with his mother; so the case was in fact one of neurotic anxiety. But this being in love only appeared to him as an internal danger, which he must avoid by renouncing that object, because it conjured up an external situation of danger. And in every case we examine we obtain the same result. It must be confessed that we were not prepared to find that internal instinctual danger would turn out to be a determinant and preparation for an external, real, situation of danger.

But we have not made any mention at all so far of what the real danger is that the child is afraid of as a result of being in love with his mother. The danger is the punishment of being castrated, of losing his genital organ. You will of course object that after all that is not a real danger. Our boys are not castrated because they are in love with their mothers during the phase of the Oedipus complex. But the matter cannot be dismissed so simply. Above all, it is not a question of whether castration is really carried out; what is decisive is that the danger is one that threatens from outside and that the child believes in it. He has some ground for this, for people threaten him often enough with cutting off his penis during the phallic phase,[2] at the time of his early masturbation, and hints at that punishment must regularly find a phylogenetic reinforcement in him. It is our suspicion that during the human family's primaeval period castration used actually to be carried out by a jealous and cruel father upon growing boys, and that circumcision, which so frequently plays a part in puberty rites among primi-

---

[1] [Cf. Chapter IV of Inhibitions, Symptoms and Anxiety. The cases examined there were those of 'Little Hans' and the 'Wolf Man'.]

[2] [This phase is discussed later in this lecture, p. 562 f.]

tive peoples, is a clearly recognizable relic of it. We are aware that here we are diverging widely from the general opinion; but we must hold fast to the view that fear of castration is one of the commonest and strongest motives for repression and thus for the formation of neuroses. The analysis of cases in which circumcision, though not, it is true, castration, has been carried out on boys as a cure or punishment for masturbation (a far from rare occurrence in Anglo-American society) has given our conviction a last degree of certainty. It is very tempting at this point to go more deeply into the castration complex, but I will stick to our subject.

Fear of castration is not, of course, the only motive for repression: indeed, it finds no place in women, for though they have a castration complex they cannot have a fear of being castrated. Its place is taken in their sex by a fear of loss of love, which is evidently a later prolongation of the infant's anxiety if it finds its mother absent. You will realize how real a situation of danger is indicated by this anxiety. If a mother is absent or has withdrawn her love from her child, it is no longer sure of the satisfaction of its needs and is perhaps exposed to the most distressing feelings of tension. Do not reject the idea that these determinants of anxiety may at bottom repeat the situation of the original anxiety at birth, which, to be sure, also represented a separation from the mother. Indeed, if you follow a train of thought suggested by Ferenczi [1925], you may add the fear of castration to this series, for a loss of the male organ results in an inability to unite once more with the mother (or a substitute for her) in the sexual act. I may mention to you incidentally that the very frequent phantasy of returning into the mother's womb is a substitute for this wish to copulate. There would be many interesting things and surprising connections to tell you at this point, but I cannot go outside the framework of an introduction to psycho-analysis. I will only draw your attention to the fact that here psychological researches trench upon the facts of biology.

Otto Rank, to whom psycho-analysis is indebted for many excellent contributions, also has the merit of having expressly emphasized the significance of the act of birth and of separation from the mother [Rank, 1924]. Nevertheless we have all found it impossible to accept the extreme inferences which he has drawn from this factor as bearing on the theory of the neuroses and even on analytic therapy. The core of his theory—that the experience of anxiety at birth is the model of all later situations of danger—he found already there.[1] If we dwell on these situations of danger for a moment, we can say that in fact a particular determinant of anxiety (that is, situation of danger) is allotted to every age of development as being appropriate to it. The danger of psychical helplessness fits the stage of the ego's early immaturity; the danger of loss of an object (or loss of love) fits the lack of self-sufficiency in the first years of child-hood; the danger of being castrated fits the phallic phase; and finally fear of the super-ego, which assumes a special position, fits the period of latency. In the course of development the old determinants of anxiety should be dropped, since the situations of danger corresponding to them have lost their importance owing to the strengthening of the ego. But this only occurs most incompletely. Many people are unable to surmount the fear of loss of love; they never become sufficiently independent of other people's love and in this respect carry on their behaviour as infants. Fear of the super-ego should normally never cease, since, in the form of moral anxiety, it is indispensable in social relations, and only in the rarest cases can an individual become independent of human society. A few of the old situations of danger, too, succeed in surviving into later periods by making contemporary modifications in their determinants of anxiety. Thus, for instance, the danger of castration persists under the mark of syphilidophobia. It is true that as an adult one knows that castration is no longer customary as a punishment for the indulgence of sexual desires, but on the other hand one has learnt that instinctual liberty of that kind is threatened by serious diseases. There is no doubt that the people we describe as neurotics remain infantile in their attitude to danger and

[1] [Freud had first published it in a footnote added to the second (1909) edition of *The Interpretation of Dreams,* but there is reason to believe that his theory had been known considerably earlier among his adherents in Vienna. His criticism of Rank's birth theory occurs chiefly in Chapters VIII and X of *Inhibitions, Symptoms and Anxiety.*]

have not surmounted obsolete determinants of anxiety. We may take this as a factual contribution to the characterization of neurotics; it is not so easy to say why it should be so.

I hope you have not lost the thread of what I am saying and remember that we are investigating the relations between anxiety and repression. In the course of this we have learnt two new things: first, that anxiety makes repression and not, as we used to think, the other way round, and [secondly] that the instinctual situation which is feared goes back ultimately to an external situation of danger. The next question will be: how do we now picture the process of a repression under the influence of anxiety? The answer will, I think, be as follows. The ego notices that the satisfaction of an emerging instinctual demand would conjure up one of the well-remembered situations of danger. This instinctual cathexis must therefore be somehow suppressed, stopped, made powerless. We know that the ego succeeds in this task if it is strong and has drawn the instinctual impulse concerned into its organization. But what happens in the case of repression is that the instinctual impulse still belongs to the id and that the ego feels weak. The ego thereupon helps itself by a technique which is at bottom identical with normal thinking. Thinking is an experimental action carried out with small amounts of energy, in the same way as a general shifts small figures about on a map before setting his large bodies of troops in motion.[1] Thus the ego anticipates the satisfaction of

[1] [This postponing activity of thought has already been mentioned in the last lecture (p. 540) as one of the main functions of the ego. The conception of thinking as an experimental, small-scale kind of acting— an essential element in 'reality-testing'—is among the earliest and most fundamental of Freud's theories, closely related to his distinction between the primary and secondary psychical processes (cf. p. 538 and footnote 3). It appears first in Sections 16, 17 and 18 of Part I of the 'Project' of 1895 and is discussed again in Section 3 of Part III of the same work (1950a). There the discussion is in ostensibly neurological terms, but it reappears as pure psychology in Chapters VII (E) of The Interpretation of Dreams (1900a). It will be found again in Chapter VII of the book on jokes (1905c), p. 192, in the paper on the 'Two Principles of Mental Functioning' (1911b), in Section V of 'The Unconscious' (1915e), in Chapter V of The Ego and the Id (1923b), and in 'Negation' (1925h). It makes a final appearance in Chapter VIII of the Outline of Psycho-Analysis (1940 [1938]), Freud's last major work. (Norton, 1949).]

the questionable instinctual impulse and permits it to bring about the reproduction of the unpleasurable feelings at the beginning of the feared situation of danger. With this the automatism of the pleasure-unpleasure principle is brought into operation and now carries out the repression of the dangerous instinctual impulse.

'Stop a moment!' you will exclaim; 'we can't follow you any further there!' You are quite right; I must add a little more before it can seem acceptable to you. First, I must admit that I have tried to translate into the language of our normal thinking what must in fact be a process that is neither conscious nor preconscious, taking place between quotas of energy in some unimaginable substratum. But that is not a strong objection, for it cannot be done in any other way. What is more important is that we should distinguish clearly what happens in the ego and what happens in the id when there is a repression. We have just said what the ego does: it makes use of an experimental cathexis and starts up the pleasure-unpleasure automatism by means of a signal of anxiety. After that, several reactions are possible or a combination of them in varying proportions. Either the anxiety attack is fully generated and the ego withdraws entirely from the objectionable excitation; or, in place of the experimental cathexis it opposes the excitation with an anticathexis, and this combines with the energy of the repressed impulse to form a symptom; or the anticathexis is taken up into the ego as a reaction-formation, as an intensification of certain of the ego's dispositions, as a permanent alteration of it.[1] The more the generation of anxiety can be restricted to a mere signal, so much the more does the ego expend on actions of defence which amount to the psychical binding of the repressed [impulse], and so much the closer, too, does the process approximate to a normal working-over of it,[2] though no doubt without attaining to it.

[1] [This idea of an alteration of the ego as a result of an anticathexis is already to be found in some of Freud's very early writings, e.g. at the end of the second paper on 'The Neuro-Psychoses of Defence' (1896*b*). It had occurred more recently in Chapter XI (A) of *Inhibitions, Symptoms and Anxiety* (1926*d*), and was to be discussed further in Sections II and V of the very late technical paper 'Analysis Terminable and Interminable' (1937*c*).]

[2] [The concept of 'working-over' as a normal method of dealing

Incidentally, here is a point on which we may dwell for a moment. You yourselves have no doubt assumed that what is known as 'character', a thing so hard to define, is to be ascribed entirely to the ego. We have already made out a little of what it is that creates character. First and foremost there is the incorporation of the former parental agency as a super-ego, which is no doubt its most important and decisive portion, and, further, identifications with the two parents of the later period and with other influential figures, and similar identifications formed as precipitates of abandoned object-relations [cf. p. 528]. And we may now add as contributions to the construction of character which are never absent the reaction-formations which the ego acquires—to begin with in making its repressions and later, by a more normal method, when it rejects unwished-for instinctual impulses.[1]

Now let us go back and turn to the id. It is not so easy to guess what occurs during repression in connection with the instinctual impulse that is being fought against. The main question which our interest raises is as to what happens to the energy, to the libidinal charge, of that excitation—how is it employed? You recollect that the earlier hypothesis was that it is precisely this that is transformed by repression into anxiety.[2] We no longer feel able to say that. The modest reply will rather be that what happens to it is probably not always the same thing. There is probably an intimate correspondence which we ought to get to know about between what is occurring at the time in the ego and in the id in connection with the repressed impulse. For since we have decided that the pleasure-

with a disagreeable mental event is an old one of Freud's. Thus, in a lecture on hysteria delivered at the date of the Breuer and Freud 'Preliminary Communication', he said: 'Incidentally, a healthy psychical mechanism has other methods of dealing with the effect of a psychical trauma . . .—namely by working it over associatively . . .' (1893h).]

[1] [The earlier part of this paragraph is derived from a discussion at the beginning of Chapter III of *The Ego and the Id* (1923b). The later part is based on Chapter XI (A) of *Inhibitions, Symptoms and Anxiety*.]

[2] [Cf. the metapsychological paper on 'Repression' (1915d), and *Introductory Lectures*, XXV.]

unpleasure principle, which is set in action by the signal of anxiety, plays a part in repression, we must alter our expectations. That principle exercises an entirely unrestricted dominance over what happens in the id. We can rely on its bringing about quite profound changes in the instinctual impulse in question. We are prepared to find that repression will have very various consequences, more or less far-reaching. In some cases the repressed instinctual impulse may retain its libidinal cathexis, and may persist in the id unchanged, although subject to constant pressure from the ego. In other cases what seems to happen is that it is totally destroyed, while its libido is permanently diverted along other paths. I expressed the view that this is what happens when the Oedipus complex is dealt with normally—in this desirable case, therefore, being not simply repressed but destroyed in the id.[1] Clinical experience has further shown us that in many cases, instead of the customary result of repression, a degradation of the libido takes place—a regression of the libidinal organization to an earlier stage. This can, of course, only occur in the id, and if it occurs it will be under the influence of the same conflict which was introduced by the signal of anxiety. The most striking example of this kind is provided by the obsessional neurosis, in which libidinal regression and repression operate together.

I fear, Ladies and Gentlemen, that you will find this exposition hard to follow, and you will guess that I have not stated it exhaustively. I am sorry to have had to rouse your displeasure. But I can set myself no other aim than to give you an impression of the nature of our findings and of the difficulties involved in working them out. The deeper we penetrate into the study of mental processes the more we recognize their abundance and complexity. A number of simple formulas which to begin with seemed to meet our needs have later turned out to be inadequate. We do not tire of altering and improving them. In my lecture on the theory of dreams [the first in the present series] I introduced you to a region in which for fifteen years there has scarcely been a new discovery. Here, where we are dealing with anxiety, you see everything in a state of flux and change. These novelties, moreover, have not yet been thor-

---

[1] [Cf. 'The Dissolution of the Oedipus Complex' (1942d).]

oughly worked through and perhaps this too adds to the difficulties of demonstrating them. But have patience! We shall soon be able to take leave of the subject of anxiety. I cannot promise that it will have been settled to our satisfaction, but it is to be hoped that we shall have made a little bit of progress. And in the meantime we have made all sorts of new discoveries. Now, for instance, our study of anxiety leads us to add a new feature to our description of the ego. We have said that the ego is weak in comparison with the id, that it is its loyal servant, eager to carry out its orders and to fulfil its demands. We have no intention of withdrawing this statement. But on the other hand this same ego is the better organized part of the id, with its face turned towards reality. We must not exaggerate the separation between the two of them too much, and we must not be surprised if the ego on its part can bring its influence to bear on the processes in the id. I believe the ego exercises this influence by putting into action the almost omnipotent pleasure-unpleasure principle by means of the signal of anxiety. On the other hand, it shows its weakness again immediately afterwards, for by the act of repression it renounces a portion of its organization and has to allow the repressed instinctual impulse to remain permanently withdrawn from its influence.

And now, only one more remark on the problem of anxiety. Neurotic anxiety has changed in our hands into realistic anxiety, into fear of particular external situations of danger. But we cannot stop there, we must take another step—though it will be a step backward. We ask ourselves what it is that is actually dangerous and actually feared in a situation of danger of this kind. It is plainly not the injury to the subject as judged objectively, for this need be of no significance psychologically, but something brought about by it in the mind. Birth, for instance, our model for an anxiety state, can after all scarcely be regarded on its own account as an injury, although it may involve a danger of injuries. The essential thing about birth, as about every situation of danger, is that it calls up in mental experience a state of highly tense excitation, which is felt as unpleasure and which one is not able to master by discharging it. Let us call a state of this kind, before which the efforts of the pleasure principle break down, a 'traumatic' moment.[1] Then,

[1] [This phrase, with its echo of Charcot, goes back to Freud's very

if we take in succession neurotic anxiety, realistic anxiety and the situation of danger, we arrive at this simple proposition: what is feared, what is the object of the anxiety, is invariably the emergence of a traumatic moment, which cannot be dealt with by the normal rules of the pleasure principle. We understand at once that our endowment with the pleasure principle does not guarantee us against objective injuries but only against a particular injury to our psychical economics. It is a long step from the pleasure principle to the self-preservative instinct; the intentions of the two of them are very far from coinciding from the start. But we see something else besides; perhaps it is the solution we are in search of. Namely, that in all this it is a question of relative quantities. It is only the magnitude of the sum of excitation that turns an impression into a traumatic moment, paralyses the function of the pleasure principle and gives the situation of danger its significance. And if that is how things are, if these puzzles can be solved so prosaically, why should it not be possible for similar traumatic moments to arise in mental life without reference to hypothetical situations of danger—traumatic moments, then, in which anxiety is not aroused as a signal but is generated anew for a fresh reason. Clinical experience declares decidedly that such is in fact the case. It is only the *later* repressions that exhibit the mechanism we have described, in which anxiety is awakened as a signal of an earlier situation of danger. The first and original repressions arise directly from traumatic moments, when the ego meets with an excessively great libidinal demand; they construct their anxiety afresh, although, it is true, on the model of birth. The same may apply to the generation of anxiety in anxiety neurosis owing to somatic damage to the sexual function. We shall no longer maintain that it is the libido itself that is turned into anxiety in such cases.[1] But I can see no objection to there being a twofold origin of anxiety—one as a direct consequence of the

earliest discussions of hysteria. See, for instance, Section I of his first paper on 'The Neuro-Psychoses of Defence' (1894a).]

[1] [In Chapter VIII of *Inhibitions, Symptoms and Anxiety* Freud still maintained, at least as a possibility, that in anxiety neurosis 'what finds discharge in the generating of anxiety is precisely the surplus of unutilized libido'. With the present sentence the last trace of the old theory is abandoned.]

traumatic moment and the other as a signal threatening a repetition of such a moment.

I feel sure you are rejoicing, Ladies and Gentlemen, at not
having to listen to any more about anxiety. But you have
gained nothing by it: what follows is no better. It is my design
to introduce you to-day as well to the field of the libido theory
or theory of the instincts, where there have equally been a
number of new developments. I will not claim that we have
made great advances in it, so that it would be worth your
taking any amount of trouble to learn about them. No. This is
a region in which we are struggling laboriously to find our bearings and make discoveries; you will only be witnesses of our
efforts. Here too I shall have to go back to some of the things I
told you earlier.

The theory of the instincts is so to say our mythology. Instincts are mythical entities, magnificent in their indefiniteness.
In our work we cannot for a moment disregard them, yet we
are never sure that we are seeing them clearly. You know how
popular thinking deals with the instincts. People assume as
many and as various instincts as they happen to need at the
moment—a self-assertive instinct, an imitative instinct, an instinct of play, a gregarious instinct and many others like them.
People take them up, as it were, make each of them do its particular job, and then drop them again. We have always been
moved by a suspicion that behind all these little *ad hoc* instincts
there lay concealed something serious and powerful which we
should like to approach cautiously. Our first step was modest
enough. We told ourselves we should probably not be going
astray if we began by separating two main instincts or classes of
instincts or groups of instincts in accordance with the two great
needs—hunger and love. However jealously we usually defend
the independence of psychology from every other science, here
we stood in the shadow of the unshakable biological fact that
the living individual organism is at the command of two intentions, self-preservation and the preservation of the species,
which seem to be independent of each other, which, so far as
we know at present, have no common origin and whose interests are often in conflict in animal life. Actually what we
are talking now is biological psychology, we are studying the

psychical accompaniments of biological processes. It was as representing this aspect of the subject that the 'ego-instincts' and the 'sexual instincts' were introduced into psycho-analysis. We included in the former everything that had to do with the preservation, assertion and magnification of the individual. To the latter we had to attribute the copiousness called for by infantile and perverse sexual life. In the course of investigating the neuroses we came to know the ego as the restricting and repressing power and the sexual trends as the restricted and repressed one; we therefore believed that we had clear evidence not only of the difference between the two groups of instincts but also of the conflict between them. The first object of our study was only the sexual instincts, whose energy we named 'libido'. It was in relation to them that we sought to clarify our ideas of what an instinct is and what is to be attributed to it. Here we have the libido theory.

An instinct, then, is distinguished from a stimulus by the fact that it arises from sources of stimulation within the body, that it operates as a constant force and that the subject cannot avoid it by flight, as is possible with an external stimulus. We can distinguish an instinct's source, object and aim. Its source is a state of excitation in the body, its aim is the removal of that excitation; on its path from its source to its aim the instinct becomes operative psychically. We picture it as a certain quota of energy which presses in a particular direction. It is from this pressing that it derives its name of 'Trieb'.[1] People speak of 'active' and 'passive' instincts, but it would be more correct to speak of instincts with active and passive aims: for an expenditure of activity is needed to achieve a passive aim as well. The aim can be achieved in the subject's own body; as a rule an external object is brought in, in regard to which the instinct achieves its external aim; its internal aim invariably remains the bodily change which is felt as satisfaction. It has not become clear to us whether the relation of the instinct to its somatic source gives it a specific quality and if so what. The evidence of analytic experience shows that it is an undoubted fact that instinctual impulses from one source attach themselves to those

[1] [The German word is often translated 'drive' but 'instinct' has been used throughout the *Standard Edition* for reasons stated in the General Preface in Volume I.]

from other sources and share their further vicissitudes and that in general one instinctual satisfaction can be replaced by another. But it must be admitted that we do not understand this very well. The relations of an instinct to its aim and object are also open to alterations; both can be exchanged for other ones, though its relation to its object is nevertheless the more easily loosened. A certain kind of modification of the aim and change of the object, in which our social valuation is taken into account, is described by us as 'sublimation'. Besides this, we have grounds for distinguishing instincts which are 'inhibited in their aim'—instinctual impulses from sources well known to us with an unambiguous aim, but which come to a stop on their way to satisfaction, so that a lasting object-cathexis comes about and a permanent trend [of feeling]. Such, for instance, is the relation of tenderness, which undoubtedly originates from the sources of sexual need and invariably renounces its satisfaction.[1]

You see how many of the characteristics and vicissitudes of the instincts still escape our comprehension. A further distinction should be mentioned here which is exhibited between the sexual and self-preservative instincts and which would be of the greatest theoretical importance if it applied to the groups as a whole. The sexual instincts are noticeable to us for their plasticity, their capacity for altering their aims, their replaceability, which admits of one instinctual satisfaction being replaced by another, and their readiness for being deferred, of which we have just given a good example in the aim-inhibited instincts. We should be glad to deny these characteristics to the self-preservative instincts, and to say of them that they are inflexible, admit of no delay, are imperative in a very different sense and have a quite other relation to repression and to anxiety. But a little reflection tells us that this exceptional position applies, not to all the ego-instincts, but only to hunger and thirst, and is evidently based on a peculiar character of the sources of those instincts. A good part of the confusing impression made by all this is that we have not given separate consideration to the alterations which the influence of the organized ego makes in the instinctual impulses that belonged originally to the id.

We find ourselves on firmer ground when we investigate the

[1] [The contents of this paragraph are largely repeated from the first portion of 'Instincts and their Vicissitudes' (1915c).]

manner in which the life of the instincts serves the sexual function. Here we have acquired quite definite knowledge, with which you too are already familiar. It is not the case, then, that we recognize a sexual instinct which is from the first the vehicle of an urge towards the aim of the sexual function—the union of the two sex-cells. What we see is a great number of component instincts arising from different areas and regions of the body, which strive for satisfaction fairly independently of one another and find that satisfaction in something that we may call 'organ-pleasure'.[1] The genitals are the latest of these 'erotogenic zones' and the name of 'sexual' pleasure cannot be withheld from their organ-pleasure. These impulses which strive for pleasure are not all taken up into the final organization of the sexual function. A number of them are set aside as unserviceable, by repression or some other means; a few of them are diverted from their aim in the remarkable manner I have mentioned [p. 97] and used to strengthen other impulses; yet others persist in minor roles, and serve for the performance of introductory acts, for the production of fore-pleasure.[2] You have heard how in the course of this long-drawn-out development several phases of preliminary organization can be recognized and also how this history of the sexual function explains its aberrations and atrophies. The first of these 'pregenital' phases is known to us as the *oral* one because, in conformity with the way in which an infant in arms is nourished, the erotogenic zone of the mouth dominates what may be called the sexual activity of that period of life. At a second level the *sadistic* and *anal* impulses come to the fore, undoubtedly in connection with the appearance of the teeth, the strengthening of the muscular apparatus and the control of the sphincter functions. We have learnt a number of interesting details about this remarkable stage of development in particular.[3] Thirdly comes the *phallic* phase in which in both sexes

---

[1] [This term had been discussed by Freud at some length in *Introductory Lectures,* XXI. The same lecture covers the contents of much of the first part of the present paragraph.]

[2] [A long discussion of fore-pleasure is given in Section I of the third of Freud's *Three Essays on the Theory of Sexuality* (1905d). In the book on jokes (1905c) p. 137 the subject recurs at several points.]

[3] [These are discussed below, pp. 546–66.]

the male organ (and what corresponds to it in girls) attains an importance which can no longer be overlooked.[1] We have reserved the name of *genital* phase for the definitive sexual organization which is established after puberty and in which the female genital organ for the first time meets with the recognition which the male one acquired long before.

So far all this is trite repetition. And you must not suppose that the many things I have not mentioned this time no longer hold good. This repetition was necessary so that I might use it as the starting-point for a report on the advances in our knowledge. We can boast of having learnt much that is new, particularly about the early organizations of the libido, and of having obtained a clearer grasp of the significance of what is old; and I will give you at least a few examples to demonstrate this. Abraham showed in 1924 that two stages can be distinguished in the sadistic-anal phase. The earlier of these is dominated by the destructive trends of destroying and losing, the later one by trends friendly towards objects—those of keeping and possessing. It is in the middle of this phase, therefore, that consideration for the object makes its first appearance as a precursor of a later erotic cathexis. We are equally justified in making a similar subdivision in the first, oral phase. In the first sub-stage what is in question is only oral incorporation, there is no ambivalence at all in the relation to the object—the mother's breast. The second stage, characterized by the emergence of the biting activity, may be described as the 'oral-sadistic' one; it exhibits for the first time the phenomena of ambivalence, which become so much clearer afterwards, in the following sadistic-anal phase. The value of these new distinctions is to be seen especially if we look for the dispositional points in the development of the libido in the case of particular neuroses, such as obsessional neurosis or melancholia.[2] You must here recall to mind what we have learnt about the connection between fixation of the libido, disposition and regression.[3]

[1] [See 'The Infantile Genital Organization' (1923e).]

[2] [I.e. the points in libidinal development at which a fixation lays down a disposition to some particular neurosis. Cf. 'The Disposition to Obsessional Neurosis' (1913i). The term 'dispositional point' occurs in Section III of the Schreber analysis (1911c).]

[3] [In *Introductory Lectures*, XXII.]

Our attitude to the phases of the organization of the libido has in general shifted a little. Whereas earlier we chiefly emphasized the way in which each of them passed away before the next, our attention now is directed to the facts that show us how much of each earlier phase persists alongside of and behind the later configurations and obtains a permanent representation in the libidinal economy and character of the subject. Still more significant have studies become which have taught us how frequently under pathological conditions regressions to earlier phases occur and that particular regressions are characteristic of particular forms of illness.[1] But I cannot go into that here, it forms part of the specialized psychology of the neuroses.

We have been able to study transformations of instinct and similar processes particularly in anal erotism, the excitations arising from the sources of the erotogenic anal zone, and we were surprised at the multiplicity of uses to which these instinctual impulses are put. It may not be easy, perhaps, to get free from the contempt into which this particular zone has fallen in the course of evolution. Let us therefore allow ourselves to be reminded by Abraham that embryologically the anus corresponds to the primitive mouth, which has migrated down to the end of the bowel.[2] We have learnt, then, that after a person's own faeces, his excrement, has lost its value for him, this instinctual interest derived from the anal source passes over on to objects that can be presented as *gifts*. And this is rightly so, for faeces were the first gift that an infant could make, something he could part with out of love for whoever was looking after him. After this, corresponding exactly to analogous changes of meaning that occur in linguistic development, this ancient interest in faeces is transformed into the high valuation of *gold* and *money* but also makes a contribution to the affective cathexis of *baby* and *penis*. It is a universal conviction among children, who long retain the cloaca theory, that babies are born from the bowel like a piece of faeces:[3] defaecation is the model of the act of birth. But the penis too has its fore-runner in the column

---

[1] [This is probably once again a reference to Abraham's important publication of 1924.]

[2] [Abraham, 1924; English translation, p. 500.]

[3] [Cf. Freud's early paper on 'The Sexual Theories of Children' (1908c).]

of faeces which fills and stimulates the mucous membrane of the bowel. When a child, unwillingly enough, comes to realize that there are human creatures who do not possess a penis, that organ appears to him as something detachable from the body and becomes unmistakably analogous to the excrement, which was the first piece of bodily material that had to be renounced. A great part of anal erotism is thus carried over into a cathexis of the penis. But the interest in that part of the body has, in addition to its anal-erotic root, an oral one which is perhaps more powerful still: for when sucking has come to an end, the penis also becomes heir of the mother's nipple.

If one is not aware of these profound connections, it is impossible to find one's way about in the phantasies of human beings, in their associations, influenced as they are by the unconscious, and in their symptomatic language. Faeces—money —gift—baby—penis are treated there as though they meant the same thing, and they are represented too by the same symbols. Nor must you forget that I have only been able to give you very incomplete information. I may hurriedly add, perhaps, that interest in the vagina, which awakens later, is also essentially of anal-erotic origin. This is not to be wondered at, for the vagina itself, to borrow an apt phrase from Lou Andreas-Salomé [1916], is 'taken on lease' from the rectum:[1] in the life of homosexuals, who have failed to accomplish some part of normal sexual development, the vagina is once more represented by it. In dreams a locality often appears which was earlier a simple room but is now divided into two by a wall, or the other way round. This always means the relation of the vagina to the bowel.[2] It is also easy to follow the way in which in girls what is an entirely unfeminine wish to possess a penis is normally transformed into a wish for a baby, and then for a man as the bearer of the penis and giver of the baby; so that here we can see too how a portion of what was originally anal-erotic interest obtains admission into the later genital organization.[3]

[1] [Her paper was summarized by Freud in a footnote added in 1920 to the second of his *Three Essays* (1905d).]

[2] [This example had been added in 1919 to Chapter VI (E) of *The Interpretation of Dreams* (1900a).]

[3] [The greater part of the last two paragraphs is derived from 'Transformations of Instinct' (1917c), but there are a few additional points

During our studies of the pregenital phases of the libido we have also gained a few fresh insights into the formation of character. We noticed a triad of character-traits which are found together with fair regularity: orderliness, parsimoniousness and obstinacy; and we inferred from the analysis of people exhibiting these traits that they have arisen from their anal erotism becoming absorbed and employed in a different way. We therefore speak of an 'anal character' in which we find this remarkable combination and we draw a contrast to some extent between the anal character and unmodified anal erotism.[1] We also discovered a similar but perhaps still firmer link between ambition and urethral erotism. A striking allusion to this connection is to be seen in the legend that Alexander the Great was born during the same night in which a certain Herostratus set fire to the celebrated temple of Artemis at Ephesus out of a sheer desire for fame. So the ancients would seem not to have been unaware of the connection. You know, of course, how much urination has to do with fire and extinguishing fire.[2] We naturally expect that other character traits as well will turn out similarly to be precipitates or reaction-formations related to particular pregenital libidinal structures; but we have not yet been able to show this.

It is now time, however, for me to go back both in history and in my subject-matter and once more to take up the most general problems of instinctual life. To begin with, the opposition between the ego-instincts and the sexual instincts lay at the base of our libido theory. When later on we began to study the ego itself more closely and arrived at the conception of narcissism, this distinction itself lost its foundation. In rare cases one can observe that the ego has taken itself as an object and is behaving as though it were in love with itself. Hence the term 'narcissism', borrowed from the Greek myth.[3] But that is only

here. The subject had already been alluded to in *Introductory Lectures* XX.]

[1] [These connections had in fact been indicated in quite an early paper of Freud's, 'Character and Anal Erotism' (1908b).]

[2] [Freud had very recently devoted a short paper to this subject (1932a).]

[3] [Of Narcissus, who was in love with himself.]

an extreme exaggeration of a normal state of affairs. We came to understand that the ego is always the main reservoir of libido, from which libidinal cathexes of objects go out and into which they return again, while the major part of this libido remains permanently in the ego.[1] Thus ego libido is being constantly changed into object libido and object libido into ego libido. But in that case they could not be different in their nature and it could have no sense to distinguish the energy of the one from the energy of the other; we could either drop the term 'libido' or use it as synonymous with psychical energy in general.

We did not maintain this position for long. Our feeling of their being a contrariety in instinctual life soon found another and sharper expression. It is not my wish, however, to put before you the origin of this novelty in the theory of the instincts; it too is based essentially on biological considerations. I shall offer it to you as a ready-made product. Our hypothesis is that there are two essentially different classes of instincts: the sexual instincts, understood in the widest sense—Eros, if you prefer that name—and the aggressive instincts, whose aim is destruction. When it is put to you like this, you will scarcely regard it as a novelty. It looks like an attempt at a theoretical transfiguration of the commonplace opposition between loving and hating, which coincides, perhaps, with the other polarity, of attraction and repulsion, which physics assumes in the inorganic world. But it is a remarkable thing that this hypothesis is nevertheless felt by many people as an innovation and, indeed, as a most undesirable one which should be got rid of as quickly as possible. I presume that a strong affective factor is coming into effect in this rejection. Why have we ourselves needed such a long time before we decided to recognize an aggressive instinct? Why did we hesitate to make use, on behalf of our theory, of facts which were obvious and familiar to everyone? We should probably have met with little resistance if we had wanted to ascribe an instinct with such an aim to animals. But to include it in the

---

[1] [But cf. the statement on p. 541 above that 'the object-cathexes spring from the instinctual demands of the id'. See also, however, the reference to a combined ego and id with regard to the destructive instinct on p. 569 below.]

human constitution appears sacrilegious; it contradicts too many religious presumptions and social conventions. No, man must be naturally good or at least good-natured. If he occasionally shows himself brutal, violent or cruel, these are only passing disturbances of his emotional life, for the most part provoked, or perhaps only consequences of the inexpedient social regulations which he has hitherto imposed on himself.

Unfortunately what history tells us and what we ourselves have experienced does not speak in this sense but rather justifies a judgement that belief in the 'goodness' of human nature is one of those evil illusions by which mankind expect their lives to be beautified and made easier while in reality they only cause damage. We need not continue this controversy, since we have argued in favour of a special aggressive and destructive instinct in men not on account of the teachings of history or of our experience in life but on the basis of general considerations to which we were led by examining the phenomena of sadism and masochism. As you know, we call it sadism when sexual satisfaction is linked to the condition of the sexual object's suffering pain, ill-treatment and humiliation, and masochism when the need is felt of being the ill-treated object oneself. As you know too, a certain admixture of these two trends is included in normal sexual relations, and we speak of perversions when they push the other sexual aims into the background and replace them by their own aims.[1] And you will scarcely have failed to notice that sadism has a more intimate relation with masculinity and masochism with femininity, as though there were a secret kinship present; though I must add that we have made no progress along that path. Both phenomena, sadism and masochism alike, but masochism quite especially, present a truly puzzling problem to the libido theory; and it is only proper if what was a stumbling-block for the one theory should become the cornerstone of the theory replacing it.

It is our opinion, then, that in sadism and in masochism we have before us two excellent examples of a mixture of the two classes of instinct, of Eros and aggressiveness; and we proceed to the hypothesis that this relation is a model one—that every instinctual impulse that we can examine consists of similar

[1] [For this see *Introductory Lectures*, XX and XXI.]

fusions or alloys of the two classes of instinct. These fusions, of course, would be in the most varied ratios. Thus the erotic instincts would introduce the multiplicity of their sexual aims into the fusion, while the others would only admit of mitigations or gradations in their monotonous trend. This hypothesis opens a prospect to us of investigations which may some day be of great importance for the understanding of pathological processes. For fusions may also come apart, and we may expect that functioning will be most gravely affected by defusions of such a kind. But these conceptions are still too new; no one has yet tried to apply them in our work.[1]

Let us go back to the special problem presented to us by masochism. If for a moment we leave its erotic components on one side, it affords us a guarantee of the existence of a trend that has self-destruction as its aim. If it is true of the destructive instinct as well [as of the libido] that the ego—but what we have in mind here is rather the id, the whole person[2]—originally includes all the instinctual impulses, we are led to the view that masochism is older than sadism, and that sadism is the destructive instinct directed outwards, thus acquiring the characteristic of aggressiveness. A certain amount of the original destructive instinct may still remain in the interior. It seems that we can only perceive it under two conditions: if it is combined with erotic instincts into masochism or if—with a greater or lesser erotic addition—it is directed against the external world as aggressiveness. And now we are struck by the significance of the possibility that the aggressiveness may not be able to find satisfaction in the external world because it comes up against real obstacles. If this happens, it will perhaps retreat and increase the amount of self-destructiveness holding sway in the interior. We shall hear how this is in fact what occurs and how important a process this is. Impeded aggressiveness seems to involve a grave injury. It really seems as though it is necessary for us to destroy some other thing or person in order not to destroy ourselves, in order to guard against the impulsion to self-destruction. A sad disclosure indeed for the moralist!

But the moralist will console himself for a long time to come with the improbability of our speculations. A queer instinct,

---

[1] [See for this question Chapter IV of *The Ego and the Id* (1923b).]
[2] [Cf. footnote 1, p. 567.]

indeed, directed to the destruction of its own organic home! Poets, it is true, talk of such things; but poets are irresponsible people and enjoy the privilege of poetic licence. Incidentally, such ideas are not foreign even to physiology: consider the notion, for instance, of the mucous membrane of the stomach digesting itself. It must be admitted, however, that our self-destructive instinct calls for support on a wider basis. One cannot, after all, venture on a hypothesis of such a wide range merely because a few poor fools have linked their sexual satisfaction to a peculiar condition. A more profound study of the instincts will, I believe, give us what we need. The instincts rule not only mental but also vegetative life, and these organic instincts exhibit a characteristic which deserves our deepest interest. (We shall not be able to judge until later whether it is a general characteristic of instincts.) For they reveal an effort to restore an earlier state of things. We may suppose that from the moment at which a state of things that has once been attained is upset, an instinct arises to create it afresh and brings about phenomena which we can describe as a 'compulsion to repeat'. Thus the whole of embryology is an example of the compulsion to repeat. A power of regenerating lost organs extends far up into the animal kingdom, and the instinct for recovery to which, alongside of therapeutic assistance, our cures are due must be the residue of this capacity which is so enormously developed in the lower animals. The spawning migrations of fishes, the migratory flights of birds, and possibly all that we describe as manifestations of instinct[1] in animals, take place under the orders of the compulsion to repeat, which expresses the *conservative nature* of the instincts. Nor have we far to look in the mental field for its manifestations. We have been struck by the fact that the forgotten and repressed experiences of childhood are reproduced during the work of analysis in dreams and reactions, particularly in those occurring in the transference, although their revival runs counter to the interest of the pleasure principle; and we have explained this by supposing that in these cases a compulsion to repeat is overcoming even the pleasure principle. Outside analysis, too, something similar can be observed. There are people in whose lives the same reactions are perpetually being repeated uncorrected, to their own detri-

[1] ['*Instinkt*' in the original; '*Triebe*' two lines below.]

ment, or others who seem to be pursued by a relentless fate, though closer investigation teaches us that they are unwittingly bringing this fate on themselves. In such cases we attribute a 'daemonic' character to the compulsion to repeat.

But how can this conservative characteristic of instincts help us to understand our self-destructiveness? What earlier state of things does an instinct such as this want to restore? Well, the answer is not far to seek and opens wide perspectives. If it is true that—at some immeasurably remote time and in a manner we cannot conceive—life once proceeded out of inorganic matter, then, according to our presumption, an instinct must have arisen which sought to do away with life once more and to re-establish the inorganic state. If we recognize in this instinct the self-destructiveness of our hypothesis, we may regard the self-destructiveness as an expression of a 'death instinct' which cannot fail to be present in every vital process. And now the instincts that we believe in divide themselves into two groups—the erotic instincts, which seek to combine more and more living substance into ever greater unities, and the death instincts, which oppose this effort and lead what is living back into an inorganic state. From the concurrent and opposing action of these two proceed the phenomena of life which are brought to an end by death.

You may perhaps shrug your shoulders and say: 'That isn't natural science, it's Schopenhauer's philosophy!' But, Ladies and Gentlemen, why should not a bold thinker have guessed something that is afterwards confirmed by sober and pains-taking detailed research? Moreover, there is nothing that has not been said already, and similar things had been said by many people before Schopenhauer. Furthermore, what we are saying is not even genuine Schopenhauer. We are not asserting that death is the only aim of life; we are not overlooking the fact that there is life as well as death. We recognize two basic instincts and give each of them its own aim. How the two of them are mingled in the process of living, how the death instinct is made to serve the purposes of Eros, especially by being turned outwards as aggressiveness—these are tasks which are left to future investigation. We have not gone beyond the point at which this prospect lies open before us. The question, too, of whether the conservative character may not belong to all instincts without exception, whether the erotic instincts as well may not be seeking to bring back an earlier state of things when they strive to bring about a synthesis of living things into greater unities—this question, too, we must leave unanswered.[1]

We have travelled somewhat far from our basis. I will tell you in retrospect the starting-point of these reflections on the theory of the instincts. It was the same as that which led us to revise the relation between the ego and the unconscious—the impression derived from the work of analysis that the patient who puts up a resistance is so often unaware of that resistance. Not only the fact of the resistance is unconscious to him, however, but its motives as well. We were obliged to search out these motives or motive, and to our surprise we found them in a powerful need for punishment which we could only class with masochistic wishes. The practical significance of this discovery is not less than its theoretical one, for the need for punishment is the worst enemy of our therapeutic efforts. It is satisfied by the suffering which is linked to the neurosis, and for that reason holds fast to being ill. It seems that this factor, an unconscious need for punishment, has a share in every neurotic illness. And here those cases in which the neurotic suffering can be replaced by suffering of another kind are wholly convincing. I will report an experience of this kind.

I once succeeded in freeing an unmarried woman, no longer young, from the complex of symptoms which had condemned her for some fifteen years to an existence of torment and had excluded her from any participation in life. She now felt she was well, and she plunged into eager activity, in order to develop her by no means small talent and to snatch a little recognition, enjoyment, and success, late though the moment was. But every one of her attempts ended either with people letting her know or with herself recognizing that she was too old to accomplish anything in that field. After each outcome of this kind a relapse into illness would have been the obvious thing, but she was no longer able to bring that about. Instead, she met

---

[1] [This discussion of the compulsion to repeat and of the death instinct is almost wholly derived from *Beyond the Pleasure Principle* (1920g). A fuller account of masochism will be found in the rather later paper 'The Economic Problem of Masochism' (1924c).]

each time with an accident which put her out of action for a time and caused her suffering. She fell down and sprained her ankle or hurt her knee, or she injured her hand in something she was doing. When she was made aware of how great her own share might be in these apparent accidents, she, so to say, changed her technique. Instead of accidents, indispositions appeared on the same provocations—catarrhs, sore throats, influenzal conditions, rheumatic swellings—till at last she made up her mind to resign her attempts and the whole agitation came to an end.

There is, as we think, no doubt about the origin of this unconscious need for punishment. It behaves like a piece of conscience, like a prolongation of our conscience into the unconscious; and it must have the same origin as conscience and correspond, therefore, to a piece of aggressiveness that has been internalized and taken over by the super-ego. If only the words went together better, we should be justified for all practical purposes in calling it an 'unconscious sense of guilt'. Theoretically we are in fact in doubt whether we should suppose that all the aggressiveness that has returned from the external world is bound by the super-ego and accordingly turned against the ego, or that a part of it is carrying on its mute and uncanny activity as a free destructive instinct in the ego and the id. A distribution of the latter kind is the more probable; but we know nothing more about it. There is no doubt that, when the super-ego was first instituted, in equipping that agency use was made of the piece of the child's aggressiveness towards his parents for which he was unable to effect a discharge outwards on account of his erotic fixation as well as of external difficulties; and for that reason the severity of the super-ego need not simply correspond to the strictness of the upbringing [see p. 526 above]. It is very possible that, when there are later occasions for suppressing aggressiveness, the instinct may take the same path that was opened to it at that decisive point of time.

People in whom this unconscious sense of guilt is excessively strong betray themselves in analytic treatment by the negative therapeutic reaction which is so disagreeable from the prognostic point of view.[1] When one has given them the solution

[1] [See a long footnote in Chapter V of *The Ego and the Id* (1923*b*).]

of a symptom, which should normally be followed by at least its temporary disappearance, what they produce instead is a momentary exacerbation of the symptom and of the illness. It is often enough to praise them for their behaviour in the treatment or to say a few hopeful words about the progress of the analysis in order to bring about an unmistakable worsening of their condition. A non-analyst would say that the 'will to recovery' was absent. If you follow the analytic way of thinking, you will see in this behaviour a manifestation of the unconscious sense of guilt, for which being ill, with its sufferings and impediments, is just what is wanted. The problems which the unconscious sense of guilt has opened up, its connections with morality, education, crime and delinquency, are at present the preferred field of work for psycho-analysts.[1]

And here, at an unexpected point, we have emerged from the psychical underworld into the open market-place. I cannot lead you any further, but before I take leave of you for to-day I must detain you with one more train of thought. It has become our habit to say that our civilization has been built up at the cost of sexual trends which, being inhibited by society, are partly, it is true, repressed but have partly been made usable for other aims. We have admitted, too, that, in spite of all our pride in our cultural attainments, it is not easy for us to fulfil the requirements of this civilization or to feel comfortable in it, because the instinctual restrictions imposed on us constitute a heavy psychical burden. Well, what we have come to see about the sexual instincts, applies equally and perhaps still more to the other ones, the aggressive instincts. It is they above all that make human communal life difficult and threaten its survival. Restriction of the individual's aggressiveness is the first and perhaps the severest sacrifice which society requires of him. ·We have learnt the ingenious way in which the taming of this unruly thing has been achieved. The institution of the super-ego which takes over the dangerous aggressive impulses, introduces a garrison, as it were, into regions that are inclined to rebellion. But on the other hand, if we look at it purely psychologically, we must

[1] [The main discussions of the sense of guilt will be found in Chapter V of *The Ego and the Id* (1923*b*), 'The Economic Problem of Masochism' (1924*c*) and Chapters VII and VIII of *Civilization and its Discontents* (1930*a*).]

recognize that the ego does not feel happy in being thus sacrificed to the needs of society, in having to submit to the destructive trends of aggressiveness which it would have been glad to employ itself against others. It is like a prolongation in the mental sphere of the dilemma of 'eat or be eaten' which dominates the organic animate world. Luckily the aggressive instincts are never alone but always alloyed with the erotic ones. These latter have much to mitigate and much to avert under the conditions of the civilization which mankind has created.[1]

[1] [The aggressive and destructive instincts had been discussed at length by Freud shortly before in *Civilization and its Discontents* (1930a) (Norton, 1962) particularly in Chapters V and VI.]

LECTURE XXXIII

FEMININITY[1]

LADIES AND GENTLEMEN,—All the while I am preparing to talk to you I am struggling with an internal difficulty. I feel uncertain, so to speak, of the extent of my licence. It is true that in the course of fifteen years of work psycho-analysis has changed and grown richer; but, in spite of that, an introduction to psycho-analysis might have been left without alteration or supplement. It is constantly in my mind that these lectures are without a *raison d'être*. For analysts I am saying too little and nothing at all that is new; but for you I am saying too much and saying things which you are not equipped to understand and which are not in your province. I have looked around for excuses and I have tried to justify each separate lecture on different grounds. The first one, on the theory of dreams, was supposed to put you back again at one blow into the analytic atmosphere and to show you how durable our views have turned out to be. I was led on to the second one, which followed the paths from dreams to what is called occultism, by the opportunity of speaking my mind without constraint on a department of work in which prejudiced expectations are fighting to-day against passionate resistances, and I could hope that your judgement, educated to tolerance on the example of psycho-analysis, would not refuse to accompany me on the excursion. The third lecture, on the dissection of the personality, certainly made the hardest demands upon you with its unfamiliar subject-matter; but it was impossible for me to keep this first beginning of an ego-psychology back from you, and if we had possessed it fifteen years ago I should have had to mention it to you then. My last lecture, finally, which you were probably

[1] [This lecture is mainly based on two earlier papers: 'Some Psychical Consequences of the Anatomical Distinction between the Sexes' (1925*j*) and 'Female Sexuality' (1931*b*). The last section, however, dealing with women in adult life, contains new material. Freud returned to the subject once again in Chapter VII of the posthumous *Outline of Psycho-Analysis* (1940*a* [1938]).]

576

able to follow only by great exertions, brought forward necessary corrections—fresh attempts at solving the most important
conundrums; and my introduction would have been leading
you astray if I had been silent about them. As you see, when one
starts making excuses it turns out in the end that it was all inevitable, all the work of destiny. I submit to it, and I beg you to
do the same.

To-day's lecture, too, should have no place in an introduction; but it may serve to give you an example of a detailed piece
of analytic work, and I can say two things to recommend it. It
brings forward nothing but observed facts, almost without any
speculative additions, and it deals with a subject which has
a claim on your interest second almost to no other. Throughout
history people have knocked their heads against the riddle of
the nature of femininity—

> Häupter in Hieroglyphenmützen,
> Häupter in Turban und schwarzem Barett,
> Perückenhäupter und tausend andre
> Arme, schwitzende Menschenhäupter. . . .[1]

Nor will *you* have escaped worrying over this problem—
those of you who are men; to those of you who are women this
will not apply—you are yourselves the problem. When you
meet a human being, the first distinction you make is 'male or
female?' and you are accustomed to make the distinction with
unhesitating certainty. Anatomical science shares your certainty at one point and not much further. The male sexual product, the spermatozoon, and its vehicle are male; the ovum and
the organism that harbours it are female. In both sexes organs
have been formed which serve exclusively for the sexual functions; they were probably developed from the same [innate]
disposition into two different forms. Besides this, in both sexes
the other organs, the bodily shapes and tissues, show the influence of the individual's sex, but this is inconstant and its
amount variable; these are what are known as the secondary

[1] Heads in hieroglyphic bonnets,
Heads in turbans and black birettas,
Heads in wigs and thousand other
Wretched, sweating heads of humans. . . .
        (Heine, *Nordsee* [Second Cycle, VII, 'Fragen'].)

sexual characters. Science next tells you something that runs counter to your expectations and is probably calculated to confuse your feelings. It draws your attention to the fact that portions of the male sexual apparatus also appear in women's bodies, though in an atrophied state, and vice versa in the alternative case. It regards their occurrence as indications of *bisexuality*,[1] as though an individual is not a man or a woman but always both—merely a certain amount more the one than the other. You will then be asked to make yourselves familiar with the idea that the proportion in which masculine and feminine are mixed in an individual is subject to quite considerable fluctuations. Since, however, apart from the very rarest cases, only one kind of sexual product—ova or semen—is nevertheless present in one person, you are bound to have doubts as to the decisive significance of those elements and must conclude that what constitutes masculinity or femininity is an unknown characteristic which anatomy cannot lay hold of.

Can psychology do so perhaps? We are accustomed to employ 'masculine' and 'feminine' as mental qualities as well, and have in the same way transferred the notion of bisexuality to mental life. Thus we speak of a person, whether male or female, as behaving in a masculine way in one connection and in a feminine way in another. But you will soon perceive that this is only giving way to anatomy or to convention. You cannot give the concepts of 'masculine' and 'feminine' *any* new connotation. The distinction is not a psychological one; when you say 'masculine', you usually mean 'active', and when you say 'feminine', you usually mean 'passive'. Now it is true that a relation of the kind exists. The male sex-cell is actively mobile and searches out the female one, and the latter, the ovum, is immobile and waits passively. This behaviour of the elementary sexual organisms is indeed a model for the conduct of sexual individuals during intercourse. The male pursues the female for the purpose of sexual union, seizes hold of her and penetrates into her. But by this you have precisely reduced the character-

[1] [Bisexuality was discussed by Freud in the first edition of his *Three Essays on the Theory of Sexuality* (1905d). The passage includes a long footnote to which he made additions in later issues of the work.]

istic of masculinity to the factor of aggressiveness so far as psychology is concerned. You may well doubt whether you have gained any real advantage from this when you reflect that in some classes of animals the females are the stronger and more aggressive and the male is active only in the single act of sexual union. This is so, for instance, with the spiders. Even the functions of rearing and caring for the young, which strike us as feminine *par excellence*, are not invariably attached to the female sex in animals. In quite high species we find that the sexes share the task of caring for the young between them or even that the male alone devotes himself to it. Even in the sphere of human sexual life you soon see how inadequate it is to make masculine behaviour coincide with activity and feminine with passivity. A mother is active in every sense towards her child; the act of lactation itself may equally be described as the mother suckling the baby or as her being sucked by it. The further you go from the narrow sexual sphere the more obvious will the 'error of superimposition'[1] become. Women can display great activity in various directions, men are not able to live in company with their own kind unless they develop a large amount of passive adaptability. If you now tell me that these facts go to prove precisely that both men and women are bisexual in the psychological sense, I shall conclude that you have decided in your own minds to make 'active' coincide with 'masculine' and 'passive' with 'feminine'. But I advise you against it. It seems to me to serve no useful purpose and adds nothing to our knowledge.[2]

One might consider characterizing femininity psychologically as giving preference to passive aims. This is not, of course, the same thing as passivity; to achieve a passive aim may call for a large amount of activity. It is perhaps the case that in a woman, on the basis of her share in the sexual function, a preference for passive behaviour and passive aims is carried over into her life to a greater or lesser extent, in proportion to the

[1] [I.e. mistaking two different things for a single one. The term was explained in *Introductory Lectures*, XX.]

[2] [The difficulty of finding a psychological meaning for 'masculine' and 'feminine' was discussed in a long footnote added in 1915 to Section 4 of the third of his *Three Essays* (1905d), and again at the beginning of a still longer footnote at the end of Chapter IV of *Civilization and its Discontents* (1930a).]

limits, restricted or far-reaching, within which her sexual life thus serves as a model. But we must beware in this of under-estimating the influence of social customs, which similarly force women into passive situations. All this is still far from being cleared up. There is one particularly constant relation between femininity and instinctual life which we do not want to over-look. The suppression of women's aggressiveness which is pre-scribed for them constitutionally and imposed on them socially favours the development of powerful masochistic impulses, which succeed, as we know, in binding erotically the destruc-tive trends which have been diverted inwards. Thus masochism, as people say, is truly feminine. But if, as happens so often, you meet with masochism in men, what is left to you but to say that these men exhibit very plain feminine traits?

And now you are already prepared to hear that psychology too is unable to solve the riddle of femininity. The explanation must no doubt come from elsewhere, and cannot come till we have learnt how in general the differentiation of living organ-isms into two sexes came about. We know nothing about it, yet the existence of two sexes is a most striking characteristic of organic life which distinguishes it sharply from inanimate nature. However, we find enough to study in those human in-dividuals who, through the possession of female genitals, are characterized as manifestly or predominantly feminine. In con-formity with its peculiar nature, psycho-analysis does not try to describe what a woman is—that would be a task it could scarcely perform—but sets about enquiring how she comes into being, how a woman develops out of a child with a bisexual dis-position. In recent times we have begun to learn a little about this, thanks to the circumstance that several of our excellent women colleagues in analysis have begun to work at the ques-tion. The discussion of this has gained special attractiveness from the distinction between the sexes. For the ladies, whenever some comparison seemed to turn out unfavourable to their sex, were able to utter a suspicion that we, the male analysts, had been unable to overcome certain deeply-rooted prejudices against what was feminine, and that this was being paid for in the partiality of our researches. We, on the other hand, standing on the ground of bisexuality, had no difficulty in avoiding impoliteness. We had only to say: 'This doesn't apply to *you*.

You're the exception; on this point you're more masculine than feminine.'

We approach the investigation of the sexual development of women with two expectations. The first is that here once more the constitution will not adapt itself to its function without a struggle. The second is that the decisive turning-points will already have been prepared for or completed before puberty. Both expectations are promptly confirmed. Furthermore, a comparison with what happens with boys tells us that the development of a little girl into a normal woman is more difficult and more complicated, since it includes two extra tasks, to which there is nothing corresponding in the development of a man. Let us follow the parallel lines from their beginning. Undoubtedly the material is different to start with in boys and girls: it did not need psycho-analysis to establish that. The difference in the structure of the genitals is accompanied by other bodily differences which are too well known to call for mention. Differences emerge too in the instinctual disposition which give a glimpse of the later nature of women. A little girl is as a rule less aggressive, defiant and self-sufficient; she seems to have a greater need for being shown affection and on that account to be more dependent and pliant. It is probably only as a result of this pliancy that she can be taught more easily and quicker to control her excretions: urine and faeces are the first gifts that children make to those who look after them [see p. 100 above], and controlling them is the first concession to which the instinctual life of children can be induced. One gets an impression, too, that little girls are more intelligent and livelier than boys of the same age; they go out more to meet the external world and at the same time form stronger object-cathexes. I cannot say whether this lead in development has been confirmed by exact observations, but in any case there is no question that girls cannot be described as intellectually backward. These sexual differences are not, however, of great consequence: they can be outweighed by individual variations. For our immediate purposes they can be disregarded.

Both sexes seem to pass through the early phases of libidinal development in the same manner. It might have been expected that in girls there would already have been some lag in aggressiveness in the sadistic-anal phase, but such is not the case. Analysis of children's play has shown our women analysts that the aggressive impulses of little girls leave nothing to be desired in the way of abundance and violence. With their entry into the phallic phase the differences between the sexes are completely eclipsed by their agreements. We are now obliged to recognize that the little girl is a little man. In boys, as we know, this phase is marked by the fact that they have learnt how to derive pleasurable sensations from their small penis and connect its excited state with their ideas of sexual intercourse. Little girls do the same thing with their still smaller clitoris. It seems that with them all their masturbatory acts are carried out on this penis-equivalent, and that the truly feminine vagina is still undiscovered by both sexes. It is true that there are a few isolated reports of early vaginal sensations as well, but it could not be easy to distinguish these from sensations in the anus or vestibulum; in any case they cannot play a great part. We are entitled to keep to our view that in the phallic phase of girls the clitoris is the leading erotogenic zone. But it is not, of course, going to remain so. With the change to femininity the clitoris should wholly or in part hand over its sensitivity, and at the same time its importance, to the vagina. This would be one of the two tasks which a woman has to perform in the course of her development, whereas the more fortunate man has only to continue at the time of his sexual maturity the activity that he has previously carried out at the period of the early efflorescence of his sexuality.

We shall return to the part played by the clitoris; let us now turn to the second task with which a girl's development is burdened. A boy's mother is the first object of his love, and she remains so too during the formation of his Oedipus complex and, in essence, all through his life. For a girl too her first object must be her mother (and the figures of wet-nurses and foster-mothers that merge into her). The first object-cathexes occur in attachment to the satisfaction of the major and simple vital needs,[1] and the circumstances of the care of children are the same for both sexes. But in the Oedipus situation the girl's father has become her love-object, and we expect that in the normal course of development she will find her way from

[1] [Cf. *Introductory Lectures*, XXI.]

this paternal object to her final choice of an object. In the course of time, therefore, a girl has to change her erotogenic zone and her object—both of which a boy retains. The question then arises of how this happens: in particular, how does a girl pass from her mother to an attachment to her father? or, in other words, how does she pass from her masculine phase to the feminine one to which she is biologically destined?

It would be a solution of ideal simplicity if we could suppose that from a particular age onwards the elementary influence of the mutual attraction between the sexes makes itself felt and impels the small woman towards men, while the same law allows the boy to continue with his mother. We might suppose in addition that in this the children are following the pointer given them by the sexual preference of their parents. But we are not going to find things so easy; we scarcely know whether we are to believe seriously in the power of which poets talk so much and with such enthusiasm but which cannot be further dissected analytically. We have found an answer of quite another sort by means of laborious investigations, the material for which at least was easy to arrive at. For you must know that the number of women who remain till a late age tenderly dependent on a paternal object, or indeed on their real father, is very great. We have established some surprising facts about these women with an intense attachment of long duration to their father. We knew, of course, that there had been a preliminary stage of attachment to the mother, but we did not know that it could be so rich in content and so long-lasting, and could leave behind so many opportunities for fixations and dispositions. During this time the girl's father is only a troublesome rival; in some cases the attachment to her mother lasts beyond the fourth year of life. Almost everything that we find later in her relation to her father was already present in this earlier attachment and has been transferred subsequently on to her father. In short, we get an impression that we cannot understand women unless we appreciate this phase of their pre-Oedipus attachment to their mother.

We shall be glad, then, to know the nature of the girl's libidinal relations to her mother. The answer is that they are of very many different kinds. Since they persist through all three phases of infantile sexuality, they also take on the characteristics of the different phases and express themselves by oral, sadistic-anal and phallic wishes. These wishes represent active as well as passive impulses; if we relate them to the differentiation of the sexes which is to appear later—though we should avoid doing so as far as possible—we may call them masculine and feminine. Besides this, they are completely ambivalent, both affectionate and of a hostile and aggressive nature. The latter often only come to light after being changed into anxiety ideas. It is not always easy to point to a formulation of these early sexual wishes; what is most clearly expressed is a wish to get the mother with child and the corresponding wish to bear her a child—both belonging to the phallic period and sufficiently surprising, but established beyond doubt by analytic observation. The attractiveness of these investigations lies in the surprising detailed findings which they bring us. Thus, for instance, we discover the fear of being murdered or poisoned, which may later form the core of a paranoic illness, already present in this pre-Oedipus period, in relation to the mother. Or another case: you will recall an interesting episode in the history of analytic research which caused me many distressing hours. In the period in which the main interest was directed to discovering infantile sexual traumas, almost all my women patients told me that they had been seduced by their father. I was driven to recognize in the end that these reports were untrue and so came to understand that hysterical symptoms are derived from phantasies and not from real occurrences. It was only later that I was able to recognize in this phantasy of being seduced by the father the expression of the typical Oedipus complex in women. And now we find the phantasy of seduction once more in the pre-Oedipus prehistory of girls; but the seducer is regularly the mother. Here, however, the phantasy touches the ground of reality, for it was really the mother who by her activities over the child's bodily hygiene inevitably stimulated, and perhaps even roused for the first time, pleasurable sensations in her genitals.[1]

---

[1] [In his early discussions of the aetiology of hysteria Freud often mentioned seduction by adults as among its commonest causes (see, for instance, Section I of the second paper on the neuro-psychoses of defence (1896c), and Section II (b) of 'The Aetiology of Hysteria' (1896c). But nowhere in these early publications did he specifically inculpate the girl's father. Indeed, in some additional footnotes written

I have no doubt you are ready to suspect that this portrayal of the abundance and strength of a little girl's sexual relations with her mother is very much overdrawn. After all, one has opportunities of seeing little girls and notices nothing of the sort. But the objection is not to the point. Enough can be seen in the children if one knows how to look. And besides, you should consider how little of its sexual wishes a child can bring to pre-conscious expression or communicate at all. Accordingly we are only within our rights if we study the residues and conse-quences of this emotional world in retrospect, in people in whom these processes of development had attained a specially clear and even excessive degree of expansion. Pathology has always done us the service of making discernible by isolation and exaggeration conditions which would remain concealed in a normal state. And since our investigations have been carried out on people who were by no means seriously abnormal, I think we should regard their outcome as deserving belief.

We will now turn our interest on to the single question of what it is that brings this powerful attachment of the girl to her mother to an end. This, as we know, is its usual fate: it is des-tined to make room for an attachment to her father. Here we come upon a fact which is a pointer to our further advance. This step in development does not involve only a simple change of object. The turning away from the mother is accompanied by hostility; the attachment to the mother ends in hate. A hate of that kind may become very striking and last all through life; it may be carefully overcompensated later on; as a rule one part

in 1924 for the *Gesammelte Schriften* reprint of *Studies on Hysteria,* he admitted to having on two occasions suppressed the fact of the father's responsibility. He made this quite clear, however, in the letter to Fliess of September 21, 1897 (Freud, 1950a, Letter 69), in which he first ex-pressed his scepticism about these stories told by his patients. His first published admission of his mistake was given several years later in a hint in the second of the *Three Essays* (1905d), but a much fuller account of the position followed in his contribution on the aetiology of the neuroses to a volume by Löwenfeld (1906a). Later on he gave two accounts of the effects that this discovery of his mistake had on his own mind—in his 'History of the Psycho-Analytic Movement' (1914d), and in his *Autobiographical Study* (1925d), (Norton, 1963). The further discovery which is described in the present paragraph of the text had already been indicated in the paper on 'Female Sexuality' (1931b).]

of it is overcome while another part persists. Events of later years naturally influence this greatly. We will restrict ourselves, however, to studying it at the time at which the girl turns to her father and to enquiring into the motives for it. We are then given a long list of accusations and grievances against the mother which are supposed to justify the child's hostile feelings; they are of varying validity which we shall not fail to examine. A number of them are obvious rationalizations and the true sources of enmity remain to be found. I hope you will be interested if on this occasion I take you through all the details of a psycho-analytic investigation.

The reproach against the mother which goes back furthest is that she gave the child too little milk—which is construed against her as lack of love. Now there is some justification for this reproach in our families. Mothers often have insufficient nourishment to give their children and are content to suckle them for a few months, for half or three-quarters of a year. Among primitive peoples children are fed at their mother's breast for two or three years. The figure of the wet-nurse who suckles the child is as a rule merged into the mother; when this has not happened, the reproach is turned into another one— that the nurse, who fed the child so willingly, was sent away by the mother too early. But whatever the true state of affairs may have been, it is impossible that the child's reproach can be justified as often as it is met with. It seems, rather, that the child's avidity for its earliest nourishment is altogether insatiable, that it never gets over the pain of losing its mother's breast. I should not be surprised if the analysis of a primitive child, who could still suck at its mother's breast when it was already able to run about and talk, were to bring the same reproach to light. The fear of being poisoned is also probably connected with the withdrawal of the breast. Poison is nourishment that makes one ill. Perhaps children trace back their early illnesses too to this frustration. A fair amount of intellectual education is a prerequisite for believing in chance; primitive people and uneducated ones, and no doubt children as well, are able to assign a ground for everything that happens. Perhaps originally it was a reason on animistic lines. Even to-day in some strata of our population no one can die without having been killed by someone else—preferably by the doctor.

And the regular reaction of a neurotic to the death of someone closely connected with him is to put the blame on himself for having caused the death.

The next accusation against the child's mother flares up when the next baby appears in the nursery. If possible the connection with oral frustration is preserved: the mother could not or would not give the child any more milk because she needed the nourishment for the new arrival. In cases in which the two children are so close in age that lactation is prejudiced by the second pregnancy, this reproach acquires a real basis, and it is a remarkable fact that a child, even with an age difference of only 11 months, is not too young to take notice of what is happening. But what the child grudges the unwanted intruder and rival is not only the suckling but all the other signs of maternal care. It feels that it has been dethroned, despoiled, prejudiced in its rights; it casts a jealous hatred upon the new baby and develops a grievance against the faithless mother which often finds expression in a disagreeable change in its behaviour. It becomes 'naughty', perhaps, irritable and disobedient and goes back on the advances it has made towards controlling its excretions. All of this has been very long familiar and is accepted as self-evident; but we rarely form a correct idea of the strength of these jealous impulses, of the tenacity with which they persist and of the magnitude of their influence on later development. Especially as this jealousy is constantly receiving fresh nourishment in the later years of childhood and the whole shock is repeated with the birth of each new brother or sister. Nor does it make much difference if the child happens to remain the mother's preferred favourite. A child's demands for love are immoderate, they make exclusive claims and tolerate no sharing.

An abundant source of a child's hostility to its mother is provided by its multifarious sexual wishes, which alter according to the phase of the libido and which cannot for the most part be satisfied. The strongest of these frustrations occur at the phallic period, if the mother forbids pleasurable activity with the genitals—often with severe threats and every sign of displeasure—activity to which, after all, she herself had introduced the child. One would think these were reasons enough to account for a girl's turning away from her mother. One would judge, if so, that the estrangement follows inevitably from the nature of children's sexuality, from the immoderate character of their demand for love and the impossibility of fulfilling their sexual wishes. It might be thought indeed that this first love-relation of the child's is doomed to dissolution for the very reason that it is the first, for these early object-cathexes are regularly ambivalent to a high degree. A powerful tendency to aggressiveness is always present beside a powerful love, and the more passionately a child loves its object the more sensitive does it become to disappointments and frustrations from that object; and in the end the love must succumb to the accumulated hostility. Or the idea that there is an original ambivalence such as this in erotic cathexes may be rejected, and it may be pointed out that it is the special nature of the mother-child relation that leads, with equal inevitability, to the destruction of the child's love; for even the mildest upbringing cannot avoid using compulsion and introducing restrictions, and any such intervention in the child's liberty must provoke as a reaction an inclination to rebelliousness and aggressiveness. A discussion of these possibilities might, I think, be most interesting; but an objection suddenly emerges which forces our interest in another direction. All these factors—the slights, the disappointments in love, the jealousy, the seduction followed by prohibition—are, after all, also in operation in the relation of a *boy* to his mother and are yet unable to alienate him from the maternal object. Unless we can find something that is specific for girls and is not present or not in the same way present in boys, we shall not have explained the termination of the attachment of girls to their mother.

I believe we have found this specific factor, and indeed where we expected to find it, even though in a surprising form. Where we expected to find it, I say, for it lies in the castration complex. After all, the anatomical distinction [between the sexes] must express itself in psychical consequences. It was, however, a surprise to learn from analyses that girls hold their mother responsible for their lack of a penis and do not forgive her for their being thus put at a disadvantage.

As you hear, then, we ascribe a castration complex to women as well. And for good reasons, though its content cannot be the same as with boys. In the latter the castration complex arises after they have learnt from the sight of the female genitals that the organ which they value so highly need not necessarily accompany the body. At this the boy recalls to mind the threats he brought on himself by his doings with that organ, he begins to give credence to them and falls under the influence of fear of castration, which will be the most powerful motive force in his subsequent development. The castration complex of girls is also started by the sight of the genitals of the other sex. They at once notice the difference and, it must be admitted, its significance too. They feel seriously wronged, often declare that they want to 'have something like it too', and fall a victim to 'envy for the penis', which will leave ineradicable traces on their development and the formation of their character and which will not be surmounted in even the most favourable cases without a severe expenditure of psychical energy. The girl's recognition of the fact of her being without a penis does not by any means imply that she submits to the fact easily. On the contrary, she continues to hold on for a long time to the wish to get something like it herself and she believes in that possibility for improbably long years; and analysis can show that, at a period when knowledge of reality has long since rejected the fulfilment of the wish as unattainable, it persists in the unconscious and retains a considerable cathexis of energy. The wish to get the longed-for penis eventually in spite of everything may contribute to the motives that drive a mature woman to analysis, and what she may reasonably expect from analysis—a capacity, for instance, to carry on an intellectual profession—may often be recognized as a sublimated modification of this repressed wish.

One cannot very well doubt the importance of envy for the penis. You may take it as an instance of male injustice if I assert that envy and jealousy play an even greater part in the mental life of women than of men. It is not that I think these characteristics are absent in men or that I think they have no other roots in women than envy for the penis; but I am inclined to attribute their greater amount in women to this latter influence. Some analysts, however, have shown an inclination to depreciate the importance of this first instalment of penis-envy in the phallic phase. They are of opinion that what we find of this attitude in women is in the main a secondary structure which has come about on the occasion of later conflicts by regression to this early infantile impulse. This, however, is a general problem of depth psychology. In many pathological—or even unusual—instinctual attitudes (for instance, in all sexual perversions) the question arises of how much of their strength is to be attributed to early infantile fixations and how much to the influence of later experiences and developments. In such cases it is almost always a matter of complemental series such as we put forward in our discussion of the aetiology of the neuroses.[1] Both factors play a part in varying amounts in the causation; a less on the one side is balanced by a more on the other. The infantile factor sets the pattern in all cases but does not always determine the issue, though it often does. Precisely in the case of penis-envy I should argue decidedly in favour of the preponderance of the infantile factor.

The discovery that she is castrated is a turning-point in a girl's growth. Three possible lines of development start from it: one leads to sexual inhibition or to neurosis, the second to change of character in the sense of a masculinity complex, the third, finally, to normal femininity. We have learnt a fair amount, though not everything, about all three.

The essential content of the first is as follows: the little girl has hitherto lived in a masculine way, has been able to get pleasure by the excitation of her clitoris and has brought this activity into relation with her sexual wishes directed towards her mother, which are often active ones; now, owing to the influence of her penis-envy, she loses her enjoyment in her phallic sexuality. Her self-love is mortified by the comparison with the boy's far superior equipment and in consequence she renounces her masturbatory satisfaction from her clitoris, repudiates her love for her mother and at the same time not infrequently represses a good part of her sexual trends in general. No doubt her turning away from her mother does not occur all at once, for to begin with the girl regards her castration as an individual misfortune, and only gradually extends it to other females and finally to her mother as well. Her love was directed to her *phallic* mother; with the discovery that her mother is castrated it becomes possible to drop her as an object, so that

[1] [See *Introductory Lectures*, XXII and XXIII.]

the motives for hostility, which have long been accumulating, gain the upper hand. This means, therefore, that as a result of the discovery of women's lack of a penis they are debased in value for girls just as they are for boys and later perhaps for men.

You all know the immense aetiological importance attributed by our neurotic patients to their masturbation. They make it responsible for all their troubles and we have the greatest difficulty in persuading them that they are mistaken. In fact, however, we ought to admit to them that they are right, for masturbation is the executive agent of infantile sexuality, from the faulty development of which they are indeed suffering. But what neurotics mostly blame is the masturbation of the period of puberty; they have mostly forgotten that of early infancy, which is what is really in question. I wish I might have an opportunity some time of explaining to you at length how important all the factual details of early masturbation become for the individual's subsequent neurosis or character: whether or not it was discovered, how the parents struggled against it or permitted it, or whether he succeeded in suppressing it himself. All of this leaves permanent traces on his development. But I am on the whole glad that I need not do this. It would be a hard and tedious task and at the end of it you would put me in an embarrassing situation by quite certainly asking me to give you some practical advice as to how a parent or educator should deal with the masturbation of small children.[1] From the development of girls, which is what my present lecture is concerned with, I can give you the example of a child herself trying to get free from masturbating. She does not always succeed in this. If envy for the penis has provoked a powerful impulse against clitoridal masturbation but this nevertheless refuses to give way, a violent struggle for liberation ensues in which the girl, as it were, herself takes over the role of her deposed mother and gives expression to her entire dissatisfaction with her inferior clitoris in her efforts against obtaining satisfaction from it. Many years later, when her

[1] [Freud's fullest discussion of masturbation was in his contributions to a symposium on the subject in the Vienna Psycho-Analytical Society (1912f).]

masturbatory activity has long since been suppressed, an interest still persists which we must interpret as a defence against a temptation that is still dreaded. It manifests inself in the emergence of sympathy for those to whom similar difficulties are attributed, it plays a part as a motive in contracting a marriage and, indeed, it may determine the choice of a husband or lover. Disposing of early infantile masturbation is truly no easy or indifferent business.

Along with the abandonment of clitoridal masturbation a certain amount of activity is renounced. Passivity now has the upper hand, and the girl's turning to her father is accomplished principally with the help of passive instinctual impulses. You can see that a wave of development like this, which clears the phallic activity out of the way, smooths the ground for femininity. If too much is not lost in the course of it through repression, this femininity may turn out to be normal. The wish with which the girl turns to her father is no doubt originally the wish for the penis which her mother has refused her and which she now expects from her father. The feminine situation is only established, however, if the wish for a penis is replaced by one for a baby, if, that is, a baby takes the place of a penis in accordance with an ancient symbolic equivalence [p. 564 f.]. It has not escaped us that the girl has wished for a baby earlier, in the undisturbed phallic phase: that, of course, was the meaning of her playing with dolls. But that play was not in fact an expression of her femininity; it served as an identification with her mother with the intention of substituting activity for passivity. *She* was playing the part of her mother and the doll was herself: now she could do with the baby everything that her mother used to do with her. Not until the emergence of the wish for a penis does the doll-baby become a baby from the girl's father, and thereafter the aim of the most powerful feminine wish. Her happiness is great if later on this wish for a baby finds fulfilment in reality, and quite especially so if the baby is a little boy who brings the longed-for penis with him.[1] Often enough in her combined picture of 'a baby from her father' the emphasis is laid on the baby and her father left unstressed. In this way the ancient masculine wish for the possession of a penis is still faintly visible through the femininity now achieved. But per-

[1] [See p. 597 below.]

haps we ought rather to recognize this wish for a penis as being *par excellence* a feminine one.

With the transference of the wish for a penis-baby on to her father, the girl has entered the situation of the Oedipus complex. Her hostility to her mother, which did not need to be freshly created, is now greatly intensified, for she becomes the girl's rival, who receives from her father everything that she desires from him. For a long time the girl's Oedipus complex concealed her pre-Oedipus attachment to her mother from our view, though it is nevertheless so important and leaves such lasting fixations behind it. For girls the Oedipus situation is the outcome of a long and difficult development; it is a kind of preliminary solution, a position of rest which is not soon abandoned, especially as the beginning of the latency period is not far distant. And we are now struck by a difference between the two sexes, which is probably momentous, in regard to the relation of the Oedipus complex to the castration complex. In a boy the Oedipus complex, in which he desires his mother and would like to get rid of his father as being a rival, develops naturally from the phase of his phallic sexuality. The threat of castration compels him, however, to give up that attitude. Under the impression of the danger of losing his penis, the Oedipus complex is abandoned, repressed and, in the most normal cases, entirely destroyed [see p. 556], and a severe super-ego is set up as its heir. What happens with a girl is almost the opposite. The castration complex prepares for the Oedipus complex instead of destroying it; the girl is driven out of her attachment to her mother through the influence of her envy for the penis and she enters the Oedipus situation as though into a haven of refuge. In the absence of fear of castration the chief motive is lacking which leads boys to surmount the Oedipus complex. Girls remain in it for an indeterminate length of time; they demolish it late and, even so, incompletely. In these circumstances the formation of the super-ego must suffer; it cannot attain the strength and independence which give it its cultural significance, and feminists are not pleased when we point out to them the effects of this factor upon the average feminine character.

To go back a little. We mentioned [p. 590] as the second possible reaction to the discovery of female castration the development of a powerful masculinity complex. By this we mean that the girl refuses, as it were, to recognize the unwelcome fact and, defiantly rebellious, even exaggerates her previous masculinity, clings to her clitoridal activity and takes refuge in an identification with her phallic mother or her father. What can it be that decides in favour of this outcome? We can only suppose that it is a constitutional factor, a greater amount of activity, such as is ordinarily characteristic of a male. However that may be, the essence of this process is that at this point in development the wave of passivity is avoided which opens the way to the turn towards femininity. The extreme achievement of such a masculinity complex would appear to be the influencing of the choice of an object in the sense of manifest homosexuality. Analytic experience teaches us, to be sure, that female homosexuality is seldom or never a direct continuation of infantile masculinity. Even for a girl of this kind it seems necessary that she should take her father as an object for some time and enter the Oedipus situation. But afterwards, as a result of her inevitable disappointments from her father, she is driven to regress into her early masculinity complex. The significance of these disappointments must not be exaggerated; a girl who is destined to become feminine is not spared them, though they do not have the same effect. The predominance of the constitutional factor seems indisputable; but the two phases in the development of female homosexuality are well mirrored in the practices of homosexuals, who play the parts of mother and baby with each other as often and as clearly as those of husband and wife.

What I have been telling you here may be described as the prehistory of women. It is a product of the very last few years and may have been of interest to you as an example of detailed analytic work. Since its subject is woman, I will venture on this occasion to mention by name a few of the women who have made valuable contributions to this investigation. Dr. Ruth Mack Brunswick [1928] was the first to describe a case of neurosis which went back to a fixation in the pre-Oedipus stage and had never reached the Oedipus situation at all. The case took the form of jealous paranoia and proved accessible to therapy. Dr. Jeanne Lampl-de Groot [1927] has established the incredible phallic activity of girls towards their mother by some assured observations, and Dr. Helene Deutsch [1932] has shown that the erotic actions of homosexual women reproduce the relations between mother and baby.

It is not my intention to pursue the further behaviour of femininity through puberty to the period of maturity. Our knowledge, moreover, would be insufficient for the purpose. But I will bring a few features together in what follows. Taking its prehistory as a starting-point, I will only emphasize here that the development of femininity remains exposed to disturbance by the residual phenomena of the early masculine period. Regressions to the fixations of the pre-Oedipus phases very frequently occur; in the course of some women's lives there is a repeated alternation between periods in which masculinity or femininity gains the upper hand. Some portion of what we men call 'the enigma of women' may perhaps be derived from this expression of bisexuality in women's lives. But another question seems to have become ripe for judgement in the course of these researches. We have called the motive force of sexual life 'the libido'. Sexual life is dominated by the polarity of masculine–feminine; thus the notion suggests itself of considering the relation of the libido to this antithesis. It would not be surprising if it were to turn out that each sexuality had its own special libido appropriated to it, so that one sort of libido would pursue the aims of a masculine sexual life and another sort those of a feminine one. But nothing of the kind is true. There is only one libido, which serves both the masculine and the feminine sexual functions. To it itself we cannot assign any sex; if, following the conventional equation of activity and masculinity, we are inclined to describe it as masculine, we must not forget that it also covers trends with a passive aim. Nevertheless the juxtaposition 'feminine libido' is without any justification. Furthermore, it is our impression that more constraint has been applied to the libido when it is pressed into the service of the feminine function, and that—to speak teleologically—Nature takes less careful account of its [that function's] demands than in the case of masculinity. And the reason for this may lie—thinking once again teleologically—in the fact that the accomplishment of the aim of biology has been entrusted to the aggressiveness of men and has been made to some extent independent of women's consent.

The sexual frigidity of women, the frequency of which appears to confirm this disregard, is a phenomenon that is still insufficiently understood. Sometimes it is psychogenic and in that case accessible to influence; but in other cases it suggests the hypothesis of its being constitutionally determined and even of there being a contributory anatomical factor.

I have promised to tell you of a few more psychical peculiarities of mature femininity, as we come across them in analytic observation. We do not lay claim to more than an average validity for these assertions; nor is it always easy to distinguish what should be ascribed to the influence of the sexual function and what to social breeding. Thus, we attribute a larger amount of narcissism to femininity, which also affects women's choice of object, so that to be loved is a stronger need for them than to love. The effect of penis-envy has a share, further, in the physical vanity of women, since they are bound to value their charms more highly as a late compensation for their original sexual inferiority.[1] Shame, which is considered to be a feminine characteristic *par excellence* but is far more a matter of convention than might be supposed, has as its purpose, we believe, concealment of genital deficiency. We are not forgetting that at a later time shame takes on other functions. It seems that women have made few contributions to the discoveries and inventions in the history of civilization; there is, however, one technique which they may have invented—that of plaiting and weaving. If that is so, we should be tempted to guess the unconscious motive for the achievement. Nature herself would seem to have given the model which this achievement imitates by causing the growth at maturity of the pubic hair that conceals the genitals. The step that remained to be taken lay in making the threads adhere to one another, while on the body they stick into the skin and are only matted together. If you reject this idea as fantastic and regard my belief in the influence of lack of a penis on the configuration of femininity as an *idée fixe*, I am of course defenceless.

The determinants of women's choice of an object are often made unrecognizable by social conditions. Where the choice is able to show itself freely, it is often made in accordance with the narcissistic ideal of the man whom the girl had wished to

[1] [Cf. Section II of 'On Narcissism' (1914c).]

become. If the girl has remained in her attachment to her father —that is, in the Oedipus complex—her choice is made according to the paternal type. Since, when she turned from her mother to her father, the hostility of her ambivalent relation remained with her mother, a choice of this kind should guarantee a happy marriage. But very often the outcome is of a kind that presents a general threat to such a settlement of the conflict due to ambivalence. The hostility that has been left behind follows in the train of the positive attachment and spreads over on to the new object. The woman's husband, who to begin with inherited from her father, becomes after a time her mother's heir as well. So it may easily happen that the second half of a woman's life may be filled by the struggle against her husband, just as the shorter first half was filled by her rebellion against her mother. When this reaction has been lived through, a second marriage may easily turn out very much more satisfying.[1] Another alteration in a woman's nature, for which lovers are unprepared, may occur in a marriage after the first child is born. Under the influence of a woman's becoming a mother herself, an identification with her own mother may be revived, against which she had striven up till the time of her marriage, and this may attract all the available libido to itself, so that the compulsion to repeat reproduces an unhappy marriage between her parents. The difference in a mother's reaction to the birth of a son or a daughter shows that the old factor of lack of a penis has even now not lost its strength. A mother is only brought unlimited satisfaction by her relation to a son; this is altogether the most perfect, the most free from ambivalence of all human relationships.[2] A mother can transfer to her son the ambition which she has been obliged to suppress in herself, and she can expect from him the satisfaction of all that has been left over in her of her masculinity complex. Even a marriage is not made secure until the wife

---

[1] [This had already been remarked upon earlier, in 'The Taboo of Virginity' (1918a).]

[2] [This point seems to have been made by Freud first in a footnote to Chapter VI of Group Psychology (1921c). He repeated it in the Introductory Lectures, XIII, and in Chapter V of Civilization and its Discontents (1930a). That exceptions may occur is shown by the example above, p. 530.]

has succeeded in making her husband her child as well and in acting as a mother to him.

A woman's identification with her mother allows us to distinguish two strata: the pre-Oedipus one which rests on her affectionate attachment to her mother and takes her as a model, and the later one from the Oedipus complex which seeks to get rid of her mother and take her place with her father. We are no doubt justified in saying that much of both of them is left over for the future and that neither of them is adequately surmounted in the course of development. But the phase of the affectionate pre-Oedipus attachment is the decisive one for a woman's future: during it preparations are made for the acquisition of the characteristics with which she will later fulfil her role in the sexual function and perform her invaluable social tasks. It is in this identification too that she acquires her attractiveness to a man, whose Oedipus attachment to his mother it kindles into passion. How often it happens, however, that it is only his son who obtains what he himself aspired to! One gets an impression that a man's love and a woman's are a phase apart psychologically.

The fact that women must be regarded as having little sense of justice is no doubt related to the predominance of envy in their mental life; for the demand for justice is a modification of envy and lays down the condition subject to which one can put envy aside. We also regard women as weaker in their social interests and as having less capacity for sublimating their instincts than men. The former is no doubt derived from the dissocial quality which unquestionably characterizes all sexual relations. Lovers find sufficiency in each other, and families too resist inclusion in more comprehensive associations.[1] The aptitude for sublimation is subject to the greatest individual variations. On the other hand I cannot help mentioning an impression that we are constantly receiving during analytic practice. A man of about thirty strikes us as a youthful, somewhat unformed individual, whom we expect to make powerful use of the possibilities for development opened up to him by analysis. A woman of the same age, however, oftens frightens us by her psychical rigidity and unchange-

[1] [Cf. some remarks on this in Chapter XII (D) of *Group Psychology* (1921c).]

ability. Her libido has taken up final positions and seems incapable of exchanging them for others. There are no paths open to further development; it is as though the whole process had already run its course and remains thenceforward insusceptible to influence—as though, indeed, the difficult development to femininity had exhausted the possibilities of the person concerned. As therapists we lament this state of things, even if we succeed in putting an end to our patient's ailment by doing away with her neurotic conflict.

That is all I had to say to you about femininity. It is certainly incomplete and fragmentary and does not always sound friendly. But do not forget that I have only been describing women in so far as their nature is determined by their sexual function. It is true that that influence extends very far; but we do not overlook the fact that an individual woman may be a human being in other respects as well. If you want to know more about femininity, enquire from your own experiences of life, or turn to the poets, or wait until science can give you deeper and more coherent information.

EXPLANATIONS, APPLICATIONS AND ORIENTATIONS

LADIES AND GENTLEMEN,—Perhaps you will allow me for once, as a relief from the dry tone of these lectures, to talk to you about some things which have very little theoretical significance but which concern you closely in so far as you are friendlily disposed to psycho-analysis. Let us imagine, for instance, that in your leisure hours you take up a German, English or American novel, in which you expect to find an account of contemporary people and society. After a few pages you come upon a first comment on psycho-analysis and soon afterwards upon others, even though the context does not seem to call for them. You must not imagine that it is a question of applying depth-psychology to a better understanding of the characters in the book or of their actions—though, incidentally, there are other and more serious works in which an attempt of that kind is in fact made. No, these are for the most part facetious remarks intended by the author to display his wide reading and intellectual superiority. Nor will you always form an impression that he really knows what he is talking about. Again, you may go as a recreation to a social gathering—and this need not necessarily happen in Vienna. After a short time the conversation turns upon psycho-analysis and you will hear the greatest variety of people passing their judgement on it, mostly in voices of unwavering certainty. It is quite usual for the judgement to be contemptuous or often slanderous or at least, once again, facetious. If you are so imprudent as to betray the fact that you know something about the subject, they fall upon you with one accord, ask for information and explanations and soon convince you that all these severe judgements had been arrived at without any basis of knowledge, that scarcely any of these critics had ever opened an analytic book or, if they had, had gone beyond the first resistance aroused by their contact with this new material.

You may perhaps expect an introduction to psycho-analysis

to give you instructions, too, on what arguments you should use to correct these obvious errors about analysis, what books you should recommend to give more accurate information, or even what examples you should bring up in the discussion from your reading or experience in order to alter the company's attitude. I must beg you to do none of this. It would be useless. The best plan would be for you to conceal your superior knowledge altogether. If that is no longer possible, limit yourself to saying that, so far as you can make out, psycho-analysis is a special branch of knowledge, very hard to understand and to form an opinion on, which is concerned with very serious things, so that a few jokes will not bring one to close quarters with it—and that it would be better to find some other plaything for social entertainment. Nor, of course, will you join in attempts at interpretation, if unwary people repeat their dreams; and you will resist the temptation to curry favour for analysis by retailing reports of its cures.

But you may raise the question of why these people—both the ones who write books and the conversationalists—behave so badly; and you may incline to the view that the responsibility for this lies not only on them but also on psycho-analysis. I think so too. What you come upon as prejudice in literature and society is an after-effect of an earlier judgement—the judgement, namely, that was formed upon the young psycho-analysis by the representatives of official science. I once complained of this in a historical account I wrote,[1] and I shall not do so again—perhaps that once was too often—but it is a fact that there was no violation of logic, and no violation of propriety and good taste, to which the scientific opponents of psycho-analysis did not give way at that time. The situation recalled what was actually put in practice in the Middle Ages when an evil-doer, or even a mere political opponent, was put in the pillory and given over to maltreatment by the mob. You may not realize clearly, perhaps, how far upwards in our society mob-characteristics extend, and what misconduct people will be guilty of when they feel themselves part of a crowd and relieved of personal responsibility. At the beginning of that time I was more or less alone and I soon saw that there was no future

---

[1] ['On the History of the Psycho-Analytic Movement' (1914d).]

in polemics but that it was equally senseless to lament and to invoke the help of kindlier spirits, for there were not courts to which such appeals could be made. So I took another road. I made a first application of psycho-analysis by explaining to myself that this behaviour of the crowd was a manifestation of the same resistance which I had to struggle against in individual patients. I refrained from polemics myself and influenced my adherents, when little by little they appeared, in the same direction. This procedure was the right one. The interdict which lay upon psycho-analysis in those days has been lifted since then. But, just as an abandoned faith survives as a superstition, just as a theory which has been given up by science continues to exist as a popular belief, so the original outlawing of psycho-analysis by scientific circles persists to-day in the facetious contempt of the laymen who write books or make conversation. So this will no longer surprise you.

But you must not expect to hear the glad tidings that the struggle about analysis is over and has ended in its recognition as a science and its admission as a subject for instruction at universities. There is no question of that. The struggle continues, though in more polite forms. What is also new is that a sort of buffer-layer has formed in scientific society between analysis and its opponents. This consists of people who allow the validity of some portions of analysis and admit as much, subject to the most entertaining qualifications, but who on the other hand reject other portions of it, a fact which they cannot proclaim too loudly. It is not easy to divine what determines their choice in this. It seems to depend on personal sympathies. One person will take objection to sexuality, another to the unconscious; what seems particularly unpopular is the fact of symbolism. Though the structure of psycho-analysis is unfinished, it nevertheless presents, even to-day, a unity from which elements cannot be broken off at the caprice of whoever comes along: but these eclectics seem to disregard this. I have never had the impression that these half- or quarter-adherents based their rejection on an examination of the facts. Some distinguished men, too, are included in this category. They, to be sure, are excused by the fact that their time and their interest belong to other things—to those things, namely, in mastering which they have achieved so much. But in that case would they not do better to suspend their judgement instead of taking sides so decisively? With one of these great men I once succeeded in effecting a rapid conversion. He was a world-famous critic, who had followed the spiritual currents of the time with benevolent understanding and prophetic penetration. I only came to know him when he was past his eightieth year; but he was still enchanting in his talk. You will easily guess whom I mean.[1] Nor was it I who introduced the subject of psycho-analysis. It was he who did so, by comparing himself with me in the most modest fashion. 'I am only a literary man,' he said, 'but you are a natural scientist and discoverer. However, there is one thing I must say to you: I have never had sexual feelings towards my mother.' 'But there is no need at all for you to have known them,' was my reply; 'to grown-up people those are unconscious feelings.' 'Oh! so *that's* what you think!' he said with relief, and pressed my hand. We went on talking together on the best of terms for another few hours. I heard later that in the few remaining years of his life he often spoke of analysis in a friendly way and was pleased at being able to use a word that was new to him—'repression'.

There is a common saying that we should learn from our enemies. I confess I have never succeeded in doing so; but I thought all the same that it might be instructive for you if I undertook a review of all the reproaches and objections which the opponents of psycho-analysis have raised against it, and if I went on to point out the injustices and offences against logic which could so easily be revealed in them. But 'on second thoughts' [2] I told myself that it would not be at all interesting but would become tedious and distressing and would be precisely what I have been so carefully avoiding all these years. So

[1] [It was Georg Brandes, the celebrated Danish scholar (1842–1927), for whom Freud had always had an admiration. Freud had heard him lecture in Vienna in March 1900. He was enthusiastic, and, on his wife's suggestion, sent a copy of *The Interpretation of Dreams* to Brandes at his hotel; but it is not known whether there was any reaction. See Letter 131 of the Fliess correspondence (Freud, 1950a). Ernest Jones mentions their meeting (which took place in 1925) in the third volume of his biography (1957, 120). Freud gave another account of it in a letter of April 19, 1927, to one of his nieces (Letter 229 in Freud, 1960a).]

[2] [In English in the original.]

you must forgive me if I pursue this path no further and if I spare you the judgements of our so-called scientific opponents. After all it is nearly always a question of people whose one qualification is the impartiality which they have preserved by keeping at a distance from the experiences of psycho-analysis. But I know there are other cases in which you will not let me off so lightly. 'Nevertheless', you will tell me, 'there are such a number of people to whom your last remark does not apply. They have not evaded analytic experience, they have analysed patients and have perhaps been analysed themselves; for a time they have even been your collaborators. Yet they have arrived at other views and theories on the basis of which they have seceded from you and founded independent schools of psycho-analysis. You ought to throw some light for us on the possibility and significance of these secessionist movements which have been so frequent in the history of analysis.'

Well, I will try to do so; but only in brief, since they contribute less to an understanding of analysis than you might expect. I feel sure you will be thinking in the first place of Adler's 'Individual Psychology', which, in America for instance, is regarded as a line of thought collateral with our psycho-analysis and on a par with it and which is regularly mentioned alongside of it. Actually, Individual Psychology has very little to do with psycho-analysis but, as a result of certain historical circumstances, leads a kind of parasitic existence at its expense. The determinants which we have attributed to this group of opponents apply to the founders of Individual Psychology only to a limited extent. Its very name is inappropriate and seems to have been the product of embarrassment. We cannot allow the legitimate use of the term as an antithesis to 'group psychology' to be interfered with; moreover, our own activity is concerned for the most part and primarily with the psychology of human individuals. I shall not enter to-day upon an objective criticism of Adler's Individual Psychology; there is no place for it in the plan of these introductory lectures. Besides, I have already attempted it once, and feel no temptation to change anything in what I said then.[1] I will, however, illustrate the impression

[1] [Freud's main criticism of Adler's views was made in his 'History of the Psycho-Analytic Movement' (1914*d*). It will perhaps seem surprising that Jung's defection is not alluded to in the present lecture,

his views produce by a small episode dating from the years before analysis.

In the neighbourhood of the little Moravian town in which I was born, and which I left when I was a three-year-old child,[1] there is a modest health-resort, prettily situated in the woods. During my schooldays I went there several times in the holidays. Some twenty years later the illness of a near relative was the occasion for my visiting the place again. In the course of a conversation with the physician attached to the spa, who had attended my relative, I enquired among other things about his relations with the peasants—Slovaks, I believe—who constituted his whole *clientèle* during the winter. He told me that his medical practice proceeded as follows. In his consulting hours the patients came into his room and stood in a row. One after another stepped forward and described his complaint: he had back-ache or pains in his stomach or had tired legs, and so on. The doctor then examined him and, after satisfying himself as to what was the matter, called out the diagnosis, which was the same in every case. He translated the word to me; it meant approximately 'bewitched'. I asked in astonishment whether the peasants made no objection to his verdict being the same with every patient. 'Oh, no!' he replied, 'they are very pleased with it: it is what they expected. Each of them, as he went back to his place in the row, showed the others by looks and gestures that I was a fellow who understood things.' Little did I guess at the time in what circumstances I should come across an analogous situation once again.

For, whether a man is a homosexual or a necrophilic, a hysteric suffering from anxiety, an obsessional neurotic cut off from society, or a raving lunatic, the 'Individual Psychologist' of the Adlerian school will declare that the impelling motive of his condition is that he wishes to assert himself, to overcompensate for his inferiority, to remain 'on top', to pass from the

apart from the short unidentified reference on p. 607 below, and that Freud expected Adler's views to be given first place by his readers. This is in agreement with some remarks in the 'History' in which he says that 'of the two movements under discussion Adler's is indubitably the more important'.]

[1] [Freiberg, afterwards re-named Příbor.]

feminine to the masculine line. In my young student days we used to hear something very much the same in the out-patients' department when a case of hysteria was introduced: hysterical patients, we were told, produce their symptoms to make themselves interesting, to draw attention to themselves. It is a remarkable thing how these ancient pieces of wisdom keep on cropping up. But even at that time this fragment of psychology did not seem to cover the riddle of hysteria. It left unexplained, for instance, why the patients used no other methods for attaining their purpose. There must, of course, be *something* correct in this theory of the 'Individual Psychologists': a small particle is taken for the whole. The self-preservative instinct will try to profit by every situation; the ego will seek to turn even illness to its advantage. In psycho-analysis this is known as the 'secondary gain from illness'.[1] Though, indeed, when we think of the facts of masochism, of the unconscious need for punishment and of neurotic self-injury, which make plausible the hypothesis of there being instinctual impulses that run contrary to self-preservation, we even feel shaken in our belief in the general validity of the commonplace truth on which the theoretical structure of Individual Psychology is erected. But a theory such as this is bound to be very welcome to the great mass of the people, a theory which recognizes no complications, which introduces no new concepts that are hard to grasp, which knows nothing of the unconscious, which gets rid at a single blow of the universally oppressive problem of sexuality and which restricts itself to the discovery of the artifices by which people seek to make life easy. For the mass of the people themselves take things easily: they call for no more than a single reason by way of explanation, they do not thank science for its diffuseness, they want to have simple solutions and to know that problems are solved. When we consider how very far Individual Psychology goes in meeting these demands, we cannot suppress the recollection of a sentence in *Wallenstein*:

> Wär' der Gedank' nicht so verwünscht gescheidt,
> Man wär' versucht, ihn herzlich dumm zu nennen.[2]

---

[1] [Cf. *Introductory Lectures*, XXIV.]

[2] [Were the idea not so confounded clever,
I'd be inclined to call it really stupid.
          Schiller, *Die Piccolomini*, II, 7.]

Criticism from specialist circles, which is so relentless against psycho-analysis, has in general handled Individual Psychology with kid gloves. It is true that in America one of the most highly respected psychiatrists published a paper against Adler under the title 'Enough', in which he gave energetic expression to his boredom at the 'compulsion to repeat' of Individual Psychology. If others have treated it far more amiably, no doubt their antagonism to analysis has had much to do with it.

I need not say much about other schools which have branched off from our psycho-analysis. The fact that they have done so cannot be used either for or against the validity of psycho-analytic theories. You have only to think of the strong emotional factors that make it hard for many people to fit themselves in with others or to subordinate themselves, and of the still greater difficulty justly insisted on by the dictum 'Quot capita tot sensus'.[1] When the differences of opinion had gone beyond a certain point, the most sensible thing was to part and thereafter to proceed along our different ways—especially when the theoretical divergence involved a change in practical procedure. Suppose, for instance, that an analyst[2] attaches little value to the influence of the patient's personal past and looks for the causation of neuroses exclusively in present-day motives and in expectations of the future. In that case he will also neglect the analysis of childhood; he will have to adopt an entirely different technique and will have to make up for the omission of the events from the analysis of childhood by increasing his didactic influence and by directly indicating certain particular aims in life. We for our part will then say: 'This may be a school of wisdom; but it is no longer analysis.' Or someone else[3] may arrive at the view that the experience of anxiety at birth sows the seed of all later neurotic disturbances. It may thereupon seem to him legitimate to restrict analysis to the consequences of this single impression and to promise therapeutic success from a treatment lasting from three to four months. As you will observe, I have chosen two examples which start from diametrically opposite premises. It is an almost universal characteristic of these 'secessionist movements' that each

[1] [More usually given in the form (derived from Terence, *Phormio*, II, 4) 'Quot homines tot sententiae (As many men, so many opinions)'.]

[2] [The allusion is to Jung.]   [3] [Here Rank is referred to.]

of them takes hold of one fragment out of the wealth of themes in psycho-analysis and makes itself independent on the basis of this seizure—selecting the instinct for mastery, for instance, or ethical conflict, or the [importance of the] mother, or genitality, and so on. If it appears to you that secessions of this sort are already more numerous to-day in the history of psycho-analysis than in other intellectual movements, I am not sure that I should agree with you. If it is the case, the responsibility must be laid on the intimate relations which exist in psycho-analysis between theoretical views and therapeutic treatment. Mere differences of opinion would be tolerable for far longer. People like accusing us psycho-analysts of intolerance. The only manifestation of this ugly characteristic has been precisely our parting from those who think differently from us. No other harm has been done to them. On the contrary, they have fallen on their feet, and are better off than they were before. For by their separation they have usually freed themselves of one of the burdens which weigh us down—the odium of infantile sexuality, perhaps, or the absurdity of symbolism—and are regarded by their environment as passably respectable, which is still not true of those of us who are left behind. Moreover, apart from one notable exception, it was they who excluded themselves.[1]

What further claims do you make in the name of tolerance? That when someone has uttered an opinion which we regard as completely false we should say to him: 'Thank you very much for having given voice to this contradiction. You are guarding us against the danger of complacency and are giving us an opportunity of showing the Americans that we are really as "broad-minded" [2] as they always wish. To be sure, we do not believe a word of what you are saying, but that makes no difference. Probably you are just as right as we are. After all, who can possibly know who is right? In spite of our antagonism, pray allow us to represent your point of view in our publications. We hope that you will be kind enough in exchange to find a place for our views which you deny.' In the future, when the misuse of Einstein's relativity has been entirely achieved, this will obviously become the regular custom in scientific affairs. For the moment, it is true, we have not gone quite so far. We restrict ourselves, in the old fashion, to putting forward only our own convictions, we

[1] [This may possibly refer to Stekel.]   [2] [In English in the original.]

expose ourselves to the risk of error because it cannot be guarded against, and we reject what is in contradiction to us. We have made plentiful use in psycho-analysis of the right to change our opinions if we think we have found something better.

One of the first applications of psycho-analysis was to teach us to understand the opposition offered to us by our contemporaries because we practised psycho-analysis. Other applications, of an objective nature, may claim a more general interest. Our first purpose, of course, was to understand the disorders of the human mind, because a remarkable experience had shown that here understanding and cure almost coincide, that a traversable road leads from the one to the other.[1] And for a long time it was our only purpose. Then, however, we perceived the close relations, the internal identity indeed, between pathological processes and what are known as normal ones. Psycho-analysis became a depth-psychology; and, since nothing that men make or do is understandable without the co-operation of psychology, the applications of psycho-analysis to numerous fields of knowledge, in particular to those of the mental sciences, came about of their own accord, pushed their way to the front and called for ventilation. These tasks unluckily came up against obstacles which, rooted as they were in the circumstances, have not yet been overcome even to-day. An application of this kind presupposes specialized knowledge which an analyst does not possess, while those who possess it, the specialists, know nothing of analysis and perhaps want to know nothing. The result has been that analysts, as amateurs with an equipment of greater or less adequacy, often hastily scraped together, have made excursions into such fields of knowledge as mythology, the history of civilization, ethnology, the science of religion and so on. They were no better treated by the experts resident in those fields than are trespassers in general: their methods and their findings, in so far as they attracted attention, were in the first instance rejected. But these conditions are constantly improving, and in every region there is a growing number of people who study psycho-analysis in order to make use of it in their special subject, and in order, as colonists, to

[1] [Breuer's treatment of his first patient. See *Introductory Lectures,* XVIII.]

replace the pioneers. Here we may expect a rich harvest of new discoveries. Applications of analysis are always confirmations of it as well. There, too, where scientific work is further removed from practical activity, the inevitable differences of opinion will no doubt take a less embittered form.

I feel a strong temptation to conduct you through all the applications of psycho-analysis to the mental sciences. They are things worth knowing by anyone with intellectual interests; and not to hear about abnormality and illness for a time would be a well-deserved relaxation. But I must renounce the idea: it would once more carry us outside the framework of these lectures and, I must honestly admit, I should not be equal to the task. It is true that in a few of these regions I myself took the first step; but to-day I no longer embrace the whole field, and I should have to do a great deal of studying in order to master what has been accomplished since my beginnings. Any of you who are disappointed by my refusal may make up for it in the pages of our periodical *Imago*, which is designed to cover the non-medical applications of analysis.[1]

But there is one topic which I cannot pass over so easily—not, however, because I understand particularly much about it or have contributed very much to it. Quite the contrary: I have scarcely concerned myself with it at all.[2] I must mention it because it is so exceedingly important, so rich in hopes for the future, perhaps the most important of all the activities of analysis. What I am thinking of is the application of psycho-analysis to education, to the upbringing of the next generation.

[1] [See *Introductory Lectures*, X, *Standard Ed.*]

[2] [Though this is perhaps the longest of Freud's discussions on the relations between analysis and education, it is in fact far from being the only one. Apart from numerous incidental references, the question was considered by him at some length in Section III of Chapter III of the 'Little Hans' case history (1909*b*); and he dealt with it again in his prefaces to two books, one by Pfister (1913*b*), and the other by Aichhorn (1925*f*). The special problems connected with sex education were the theme of an early paper on 'The Sexual Enlightenment of Children' (1907*c*) and were touched on again thirty years later in the last paragraph of Section IV of 'Analysis Terminable and Interminable' (1937*c*). Lastly it may be mentioned that the question of religious education had come up at several points in Chapters IX and X of *The Future of an Illusion* (1927*c*).]

I am glad that I am at least able to say that my daughter, Anna Freud, has made this study her life-work and has in that way compensated for my neglect.

The road that led to this application is easily traced. When in the treatment of an adult neurotic we followed up the determinants of his symptoms, we were regularly led back to his early childhood. A knowledge of the later aetiological factors was not sufficient either for understanding the case or for producing a therapeutic effect. We were therefore compelled to make ourselves acquainted with the psychical peculiarities of childhood; we learnt a quantity of things which could not have been learnt except through analysis, and we were able to put right many opinions that were generally held about childhood. We recognized that particular importance attached to the first years of childhood—up to the age of five, perhaps—for several reasons. Firstly, because those years include the early efflorescence of sexuality which leaves behind it decisive instigating factors for the sexual life of maturity. Secondly, because the impressions of this period impinge upon an immature and feeble ego, and act upon it like traumas. The ego cannot fend off the emotional storms which they provoke in any way except by repression and in this manner acquires in childhood all its dispositions to later illnesses and functional disturbances. We realized that the difficulty of childhood lies in the fact that in a short span of time a child has to appropriate the results of a cultural evolution which stretches over thousands of years, including the acquisition of control over his instincts and adaptation to society—or at least the first beginnings of these two. He can only achieve a part of this modification through his own development; much must be imposed on him by education.[1] We are not surprised that children often carry out this task very imperfectly. During these early times many of them pass through states that may be put on a par with neuroses—and this is certainly so in the case of all those who produce manifest illnesses later on. In some children the neurotic illness does not wait till maturity but breaks out already in childhood and gives parents and doctors plenty of trouble.

[1] [The German word '*Erziehung*', which is here and elsewhere in this discussion translated 'education', has a much wider meaning than the English word and includes 'upbringing' in a general sense.]

We had no misgivings over applying analytic treatment to children who either exhibited unambiguous neurotic symptoms or who were on the road to an unfavourable development of character. The apprehension expressed by opponents of analysis that the child would be injured by it proved unfounded. What we gained from these undertakings was that we were able to confirm on the living subject what we had inferred (from historical documents, as it were) in the case of adults. But the gain for the children was also very satisfactory. It turned out that a child is a very favourable subject for analytic therapy; the results are thorough and lasting. The technique of treatment worked out for adults must, of course, be largely altered for children. A child is psychologically a different object from an adult. As yet he possesses no super-ego, the method of free association does not carry far with him, transference (since the real parents are still on the spot) plays a different part. The internal resistances against which we struggle in adults are replaced for the most part in children by external difficulties. If the parents make themselves vehicles of the resistance, the aim of the analysis—and even the analysis itself—is often imperilled. Hence it is often necessary to combine with a child's analysis a certain amount of analytic influencing of his parents. On the other hand, the inevitable deviations of analyses of children from those of adults are diminished by the circumstance that some of our patients have retained so many infantile character-traits that the analyst (once again adapting himself to his subject) cannot avoid making use with them of certain of the techniques of child-analysis. It has automatically happened that child-analysis has become the domain of women analysts, and no doubt this will remain true.

The recognition that most of our children pass through a neurotic phase in the course of their development carries with it the germ of a hygienic challenge. The question may be raised whether it would not be expedient to come to a child's help with an analysis even if he shows no signs of a disturbance, as a measure for safeguarding his health, just as to-day we inoculate healthy children against diphtheria without waiting to see if they fall ill of it. The discussion of this question has only an academic interest at present, but I may venture to consider it here. The mere suggestion would seem to the great bulk of our contemporaries to be a monstrous outrage, and in view of the attitude towards analysis of most people in a parental position any hope of putting through such an idea must be abandoned for the time being. Prophylaxis such as this against neurotic illness, which would probably be very effective, also presupposes a quite other constitution of society. The watchword for the application of psycho-analysis to education is to be found to-day elsewhere. Let us make ourselves clear as to what the first task of education is. The child must learn to control his instincts. It is impossible to give him liberty to carry out all his impulses without restriction. To do so would be a very instructive experiment for child-psychologists; but life would be impossible for the parents and the children themselves would suffer grave damage, which would show itself partly at once and partly in later years. Accordingly, education must inhibit, forbid and suppress, and this it has abundantly seen to in all periods of history. But we have learnt from analysis that precisely this suppression of instincts involves the risk of neurotic illness. As you will remember, we have examined in detail how this occurs.[1] Thus education has to find its way between the Scylla of non-interference and the Charybdis of frustration. Unless this problem is entirely insoluble, an optimum must be discovered which will enable education to achieve the most and damage the least. It will therefore be a matter of deciding how much to forbid, at what times and by what means. And in addition we have to take into account the fact that the objects of our educational influence have very different innate constitutional dispositions, so that it is quite impossible that the same educational procedure can be equally good for all children. A moment's reflection tells us that hitherto education has fulfilled its task very badly and has done children great damage. If it discovers the optimum and carries out its task ideally, it can hope to wipe out one of the factors in the aetiology of falling ill—the influence of the accidental traumas of childhood. It cannot in any case get rid of the other factor—the power of an insubordinate instinctual constitution. If now we consider the difficult problems that confront the educator—how he has to recognize the child's constitutional individuality, to infer from

[1] [See *Introductory Lectures,* in particular Lectures **XXII** and **XXIII**.]

small indications what is going on in his immature mind, to give him the right amount of love and yet to maintain an effective degree of authority—we shall tell ourselves that the only appropriate preparation for the profession of educator is a thorough psycho-analytic training. It would be best that he should have been analysed himself, for, when all is said and done, it is impossible to assimilate analysis without experiencing it personally. The analysis of teachers and educators seems to be a more efficacious prophylactic measure than the analysis of children themselves, and there are less difficulties in the way of putting it into practice.

We may mention, though only as an incidental consideration, an indirect way in which the upbringing of children may be helped by analysis and which may with time acquire a greater influence. Parents who have themselves experienced an analysis and owe much to it, including an insight into the faults of their own upbringing, will treat their children with better understanding and will spare them much of what they themselves were not spared.

Parallel with the efforts of analysts to influence education, other investigations are being made into the origin and prevention of delinquency and crime. Here again I am only opening the door for you and showing you the rooms that lie beyond it, without leading you inside.[1] I am certain that if you remain loyal to your interest in psycho-analysis you will be able to learn much that is new and valuable on these subjects. I must not, however, leave the topic of education without referring to one particular aspect of it. It has been said—and no doubt justly—that every education has a partisan aim, that it endeavours to bring the child into line with the established order of society, without considering how valuable or how stable that order may be in itself. If [it is argued] one is convinced of the defects in our present social arrangements, education with a psycho-analytic alignment cannot justifiably be put at their service as well: it must be given another and higher aim, liberated from the prevailing demands of society. In my opinion, however, this argument is out of place here. Such a demand goes beyond the legitimate function of analysis. In the same way, it is not the

[1] [See, in this connection, Freud's preface to Aichhorn's *Wayward Youth* (Freud, 1925*f*).]

business of a doctor who is called in to treat a case of pneumonia to concern himself with whether the patient is an honest man or a suicide or a criminal, whether he deserves to remain alive or whether one ought to wish him to. This other aim which it is desired to give to education will also be a partisan one, and it is not the affair of an analyst to decide between the parties. I am leaving entirely on one side the fact that psycho-analysis would be refused any influence on education if it admitted to intentions inconsistent with the established social order. Psycho-analytic education will be taking an uninvited responsibility on itself if it proposes to mould its pupils into rebels. It will have played its part if it sends them away as healthy and efficient as possible. It itself contains enough revolutionary factors to ensure that no one educated by it will in later life take the side of reaction and suppression. It is even my opinion that revolutionary children are not desirable from any point of view.

I propose further, Ladies and Gentlemen, to say a few words to you about psycho-analysis as a form of therapy. I discussed the theoretical side of this question fifteen years ago[1] and I cannot formulate it in any other manner to-day; I have now to tell you of our experience during this interval. As you know, psycho-analysis originated as a method of treatment; it has far outgrown this, but it has not abandoned its home-ground and it is still linked to its contact with patients for increasing its depth and for its further development. The accumulated impressions from which we derive our theories could be arrived at in no other way. The failures we meet with as therapists are constantly setting us new tasks and the demands of real life are an effective guard against an overgrowth of the speculation which we cannot after all do without in our work. I have already discussed long ago the means used by psycho-analysis in helping patients, when it does help them, and the method by which it does so;[2] to-day I shall enquire how much it achieves.

You are perhaps aware that I have never been a therapeutic enthusiast; there is no danger of my misusing this lecture by

[1] [In *Introductory Lectures*, XXVII and XXVIII.]

[2] [See last footnote and the papers on technique in Volume XII of the *Standard Edition*.]

indulging in eulogies. I would rather say too little than too much. During the period at which I was the only analyst, people who were ostensibly friendly to my ideas used to say to me: 'That's all very nice and clever; but show me a case that you have cured by analysis.' This was one of the many formulas which in the course of time have succeeded one another in performing the function of pushing the uncomfortable novelty aside. To-day it is as out of date as many others: the analyst, too, has a heap of letters in his files from grateful patients who have been cured. The analogy does not stop at that. Psycho-analysis is really a method of treatment like others. It has its triumphs and its defeats, its difficulties, its limitations, its indications. At one time a complaint was made against analysis that it was not to be taken seriously as a treatment since it did not dare to issue any statistics of its successes. Since then, the Psycho-Analytic Institute in Berlin, which was founded by Dr. Max Eitingon, has published a statement of its results during its first ten years.[1] Its therapeutic successes give grounds neither for boasting nor for being ashamed. But statistics of that kind are in general uninstructive; the material worked upon is so heterogeneous that only very large numbers would show anything. It is wiser to examine one's individual experiences. And here I should like to add that I do not think our cures can compete with those of Lourdes. There are so many more people who believe in the miracles of the Blessed Virgin than in the existence of the unconscious. If we turn to mundane competitors, we must compare psycho-analytic treatment with other kinds of psychotherapy. To-day organic physical methods of treating neurotic states need scarcely be mentioned. Analysis as a psycho-therapeutic procedure does not stand in opposition to other methods used in this specialized branch of medicine; it does not diminish their value nor exclude them. There is no theoretical inconsistency in a doctor who likes to call himself a psychotherapist using analysis on his patients alongside of any other method of treatment according to the peculiarities of the case and the favourable or unfavourable external circumstances. It is in fact technique that necessitates the specialization in medical practice. Thus in the same way surgery and orthopaedics were obliged to separate. Psycho-analytic activity is

---

[1] [Freud contributed a preface to this (1930*b*).]

arduous and exacting; it cannot well be handled like a pair of glasses that one puts on for reading and takes off when one goes for a walk. As a rule psycho-analysis possesses a doctor either entirely or not at all. Those psychotherapists who make use of analysis among other methods, occasionally, do not to my knowledge stand on firm analytic ground; they have not accepted the whole of analysis but have watered it down—have drawn its fangs, perhaps; they cannot be counted as analysts. This is, I think, to be regretted. But co-operation in medical practice between an analyst and a psychotherapist who restricts himself to other techniques would serve quite a useful purpose.

Compared with the other psychotherapeutic procedures psycho-analysis is beyond any doubt the most powerful. It is just and fair, too, that this should be so for it is also the most laborious and time-consuming; it would not be used on slight cases. In suitable cases it is possible by its means to get rid of disturbances and bring about changes for which in pre-analytic times one would not have ventured to hope. But it has its very appreciable limits. The therapeutic ambition of some of my adherents has made the greatest efforts to overcome these obstacles so that every sort of neurotic disorder might be curable by psycho-analysis. They have endeavoured to compress the work of analysis into a shorter duration, to intensify transference so that it may be able to overcome any resistance, to unite other forms of influence with it so as to compel a cure. These efforts are certainly praiseworthy, but, in my opinion, they are vain. They bring with them, too, a danger of being oneself forced away from analysis and drawn into a boundless course of experimentation.[1] The expectation that every neurotic phenomenon can be cured may, I suspect, be derived from the layman's belief that the neuroses are something quite unnecessary which have no right whatever to exist. Whereas in fact they are severe, constitutionally fixed illnesses, which rarely restrict themselves to only a few attacks but persist as a rule over long periods or throughout life. Our analytic experience that they can be extensively influenced, if the historical precipitating

[1] [It may well be that in writing these sentences Freud had his friend Ferenczi in mind, whose obituary, which he was to write a few months later, contains an echo of these ideas.]

causes and accidental auxiliary factors of the illness can be
dealt with, has led us to neglect the constitutional factor in our
therapeutic practice, and in any case we can do nothing about
it; but in theory we ought always to bear it in mind. The radical inaccessibility of the psychoses to analytic treatment should,
in view of their close relationship to the neuroses, restrict our
pretensions in regard to these latter. The therapeutic effectiveness of psycho-analysis remains cramped by a number of
weighty and scarcely assailable factors. In the case of children,
where one might count on the greatest successes, the difficulties
are the external ones connected with their relation to their
parents, though these difficulties are after all a necessary part of
being a child. In the case of adults the difficulties arise in the
first instance from two factors: the amount of psychical rigidity
present and the form of the illness with all that that covers in the
way of deeper determinants.

The first of these factors is often unjustly overlooked. However great may be the plasticity of mental life and the possibility
of reviving old conditions, not everything can be brought to life
again. Some changes seem to be definitive and correspond to
scars formed when a process has run its course. On other occasions one has an impression of a general stiffening of mental
life; the psychical processes, to which one could very well indicate other paths, seem incapable of abandoning the old ones.
But perhaps this is the same thing as what I mentioned just now,
only looked at differently. All too often one seems to see that it
is only the treatment's lack of the necessary motive force that
prevents one from bringing the change about. One particular
dependent relation, one special instinctual component, is too
powerful in comparison with the opposing forces that we are
able to mobilize. This is quite generally true with the psychoses.
We understand them well enough to know the point at which
the levers should be applied, but they would not be able to
move the weight. It is here, indeed, that hope for the future
lies: the possibility that our knowledge of the operation of the
hormones (you know what they are) may give us the means of
successfully combating the quantitative factors of the illnesses:
but we are far from that to-day. I realize that the uncertainty in
all these matters is a constant instigation towards perfecting
analysis and in particular the transference. Beginners in analy-

sis especially are left in doubt in case of a failure whether they should blame the peculiarities of the case or their own clumsy handling of the therapeutic procedure. But, as I have said already, I do not think much can be achieved by efforts in this direction.

The second limitation upon analytic successes is given by the form of the illness. You know already that the field of application of analytic therapy lies in the transference neuroses—phobias, hysteria, obsessional neurosis—and further, abnormalities of character which have been developed in place of these illnesses. Everything differing from these, narcissistic and psychotic conditions, is unsuitable to a greater or less extent. It would be entirely legitimate to guard against failures by carefully excluding such cases. This precaution would lead to a great improvement in the statistics of analysis. There is, however, a pitfall here. Our diagnoses are very often made only after the event. They resemble the Scottish King's test for identifying witches that I read about in Victor Hugo.[1] This king declared that he was in possession of an infallible method of recognizing a witch. He had the women stewed in a cauldron of boiling water and then tasted the broth. Afterwards he was able to say: 'That was a witch', or 'No, that was not one.' It is the same with us, except that *we* are the sufferers. We cannot judge the patient who comes for treatment (or, in the same way, the candidate who comes for training) till we have studied him analytically for a few weeks or months. We are in fact buying a pig in a poke. The patient brings along indefinite general ailments which do not admit of a conclusive diagnosis. After this period of testing it may turn out that the case is an unsuitable one. If so we send him away if he is a candidate, or continue the trial a little longer if he is a patient on the chance that we may yet see things in a more favourable light. The patient has his revenge by adding to our list of failures, and the rejected candidate does so perhaps, if he is paranoid, by writing books on psycho-analysis himself. As you see, our precautions have been of no avail.

I am afraid these detailed discussions are exhausting your

---

[1] [The origin of this anecdote has not been found. Freud had already used it in his contribution to a discussion on masturbation (1912*f*).]

interest. But I should be still more sorry if you were to think it is my intention to lower your opinion of psycho-analysis as a therapy. Perhaps I really made a clumsy start. For I wanted to do the opposite: to excuse the therapeutic limitations of analysis by pointing out their inevitability. With the same aim in view I turn to another point: the reproach against analytic treatment that it takes a disproportionately long time. On this it must be said that psychical changes do in fact only take place slowly; if they occur rapidly, suddenly, that is a bad sign. It is true that the treatment of a fairly severe neurosis may easily extend over several years; but consider, in case of success, how long the illness would have lasted. A decade, probably, for every year of treatment: the illness, that is to say (as we see so often in untreated cases), would not have ended at all. In some cases we have reasons for resuming an analysis many years afterwards. Life had developed fresh pathological reactions to fresh precipitating causes; but in the meantime our patient had been well. The first analysis had not in fact brought to light all his pathological dispositions, and it was natural for the analysis to have been stopped when success was achieved. There are also severely handicapped people who are kept under analytic supervision all through their lives and are taken back into analysis from time to time. But these people would otherwise have been altogether incapable of existence and we must feel glad that they can be kept on their feet by this piecemeal and recurrent treatment. The analysis of character disorders also calls for long periods of treatment; but it is often successful; and do you know of any other therapy with which such a task could even be approached? Therapeutic ambition may feel unsatisfied by such results; but we have learnt from the example of tuberculosis and lupus that success can only be obtained when the treatment has been adapted to the characteristics of the illness.[1]

I have told you that psycho-analysis began as a method of treatment; but I did not want to commend it to your interest as a method of treatment but on account of the truths it contains, on account of the information it gives us about what

[1] [One of the very last of Freud's writings, 'Analysis Terminable and Interminable' (1937c), is devoted to a long discussion of the limitations of psycho-analytic therapy.]

concerns human beings most of all—their own nature—and on account of the connections it discloses between the most different of their activities. As a method of treatment it is one among many, though, to be sure, *primus inter pares*. If it was without therapeutic value it would not have been discovered, as it was, in connection with sick people and would not have gone on developing for more than thirty years.

LECTURE XXXV

THE QUESTION
OF A WELTANSCHAUUNG[1]

Ladies and Gentlemen,—At our last meeting we were occupied with little everyday concerns—putting our own modest house in order, as it were. I propose that we should now take a bold leap and venture upon answering a question which is constantly being asked in other quarters: does psycho-analysis lead to a particular *Weltanschauung* and, if so, to which?

'*Weltanschauung*' is, I am afraid, a specifically German concept, the translation of which into foreign languages might well raise difficulties. If I try to give you a definition of it, it is bound to seem clumsy to you. In my opinion, then, a *Weltanschauung* is an intellectual construction which solves all the problems of our existence uniformly on the basis of one overriding hypothesis, which, accordingly, leaves no question unanswered and in which everything that interests us finds its fixed place. It will easily be understood that the possession of a *Weltanschauung* of this kind is among the ideal wishes of human beings. Believing in it one can feel secure in life, one can know what to strive for, and how one can deal most expediently with one's emotions and interests.

If that is the nature of a *Weltanschauung*, the answer as regards psycho-analysis is made easy. As a specialist science, a branch of psychology—a depth-psychology or psychology of the unconscious—it is quite unfit to construct a *Weltanschauung* of its own: it must accept the scientific one. But the *Weltanschauung* of science already departs noticeably from our definition. It is true that it too assumes the *uniformity* of the explanation of the

---

[1] [This word might be translated 'A View of the Universe', but Freud himself explains its meaning in the second paragraph below. As it appears more than thirty times in the course of this lecture, the simplest plan seems to be to leave it in German; and in any case it has almost naturalized itself in our language. Freud had already approached the topic of this lecture in a passage at the end of Chapter II of *Inhibitions, Symptoms and Anxiety* (1926d).]

universe; but it does so only as a programme, the fulfilment of which is relegated to the future. Apart from this it is marked by negative characteristics, by its limitation to what is at the moment knowable and by its sharp rejection of certain elements that are alien to it. It asserts that there are no sources of knowledge of the universe other than the intellectual working-over of carefully scrutinized observations—in other words, what we call research—and alongside of it no knowledge derived from revelation, intuition or divination. It seems as though this view came very near to being generally recognized in the course of the last few centuries that have passed; and it has been left to *our* century to discover the presumptuous objection that a *Weltanschauung* like this is alike paltry and cheerless, that it overlooks the claims of the human intellect and the needs of the human mind.

This objection cannot be too energetically repudiated. It is quite without a basis, since the intellect and the mind are objects for scientific research in exactly the same way as any non-human things. Psycho-analysis has a special right to speak for the scientific *Weltanschauung* at this point, since it cannot be reproached with having neglected what is mental in the picture of the universe. Its contribution to science lies precisely in having extended research to the mental field. And, incidentally, without such a psychology science would be very incomplete. If, however, the investigation of the intellectual and emotional functions of men (and of animals) is included in science, then it will be seen that nothing is altered in the attitude of science as a whole, that no new sources of knowledge or methods of research have come into being. Intuition and divination would be such, if they existed; but they may safely be reckoned as illusions, the fulfilments of wishful impulses. It is easy to see, too, that these demands upon a *Weltanschauung* are only based on emotion. Science takes notice of the fact that the human mind produces these demands and is ready to examine their sources; but it has not the slightest reason to regard them as justified. On the contrary it sees this as a warning carefully to separate from knowledge everything that is illusion and an outcome of emotional demands like these.

This does not in the least mean that these wishes are to be pushed contemptuously on one side or their value for human life under-estimated. We are ready to trace out the fulfilments of them which they have created for themselves in the products of art and in the systems of religion and philosophy; but we cannot nevertheless overlook the fact that it would be illegitimate and highly inexpedient to allow these demands to be transferred to the sphere of knowledge. For this would be to lay open the paths which lead to psychosis, whether to individual or group psychosis, and would withdraw valuable amounts of energy from endeavours which are directed towards reality in order, so far as possible, to find satisfaction in it for wishes and needs.

From the standpoint of science one cannot avoid exercising one's critical faculty here and proceeding with rejections and dismissals. It is not permissible to declare that science is one field of human mental activity and that religion and philosophy are others, at least its equal in value, and that science has no business to interfere with the other two: that they all have an equal claim to be true and that everyone is at liberty to choose from which he will draw his convictions and in which he will place his belief. A view of this kind is regarded as particularly superior, tolerant, broad-minded and free from illiberal prejudices. Unfortunately it is not tenable and shares all the pernicious features of an entirely unscientific *Weltanschauung* and is equivalent to one in practice. It is simply a fact that the truth cannot be tolerant, that it admits of no compromises or limitations, that research regards every sphere of human activity as belonging to it and that it must be relentlessly critical if any other power tries to take over any part of it.

Of the three powers which may dispute the basic position of science, religion alone is to be taken seriously as an enemy. Art is almost always harmless and beneficent; it does not seek to be anything but an illusion. Except for a few people who are spoken of as being 'possessed' by art, it makes no attempt at invading the realm of reality. Philosophy is not opposed to science, it behaves like a science and works in part by the same methods; it departs from it, however, by clinging to the illusion of being able to present a picture of the universe which is without gaps and is coherent, though one which is bound to collapse with every fresh advance in our knowledge. It goes astray in its method by over-estimating the epistemological value of our logical operations and by accepting other sources of knowledge such as intuition. And it often seems that the poet's derisive comment is not unjustified when he says of the philosopher:

> Mit seinen Nachtmützen und Schlafrockfetzen
> Stopft er die Lücken des Weltenbaus.[1]

But philosophy has no direct influence on the great mass of mankind; it is of interest to only a small number even of the top layer of intellectuals and is scarcely intelligible to anyone else. On the other hand, religion is an immense power which has the strongest emotions of human beings at its service. It is well known that at an earlier date it comprised everything that played an intellectual part in men's lives, that it took the place of science when there was scarcely yet such a thing as science, and that it constructed a *Weltanschauung*, consistent and self-contained to an unparalleled degree, which, although it has been profoundly shaken, persists to this day.

If we are to give an account of the grandiose nature of religion, we must bear in mind what it undertakes to do for human beings. It gives them information about the origin and coming into existence of the universe, it assures them of its protection and of ultimate happiness in the ups and downs of life and it directs their thoughts and actions by precepts which it lays down with its whole authority. Thus it fulfils three functions. With the first of them it satisfies the human thirst for knowledge; it does the same thing that science attempts to do with *its* means, and at that point enters into rivalry with it. It is to its second function that it no doubt owes the greatest part of its influence. Science can be no match for it when it soothes the fear that men feel of the dangers and vicissitudes of life, when it assures them of a happy ending and offers them comfort in unhappiness. It is true that science can teach us how to avoid certain dangers and that there are some sufferings which it can

[1] Heine, ['Die Heimkehr', LVIII. Literally: 'With his nightcaps and the tatters of his dressing-gown he patches up the gaps in the structure of the universe.' The lines were favourite ones with Freud. He alluded to them in connection with the secondary revision of dreams in Chapter VI (I) of *The Interpretation of Dreams* (1900*a*), and again in a letter to Jung of February 25, 1908 (Jones, 1955, 488). Many years earlier he had quoted them in full in a letter to his future wife, apparently in 1883 (Jones, 1953, 214).]

successfully combat; it would be most unjust to deny that it is a powerful helper to men; but there are many situations in which it must leave a man to his suffering and can only advise him to submit to it. In its third function, in which it issues precepts and lays down prohibitions and restrictions, religion is furthest away from science. For science is content to investigate and to establish facts, though it is true that from its applications rules and advice are derived on the conduct of life. In some circumstances these are the same as those offered by religion, but, when this is so, the reasons for them are different.

The convergence between these three aspects of religion is not entirely clear. What has an explanation of the origin of the universe to do with the inculcation of certain particular ethical precepts? The assurances of protection and happiness are more intimately linked with the ethical requirements. They are the reward for fulfilling these commands; only those who obey them may count upon these benefits, punishment awaits the disobedient. Incidentally, something similar is true of science. Those who disregard its lessons, so it tells us, expose themselves to injury.

The remarkable combination in religion of instruction, consolation and requirements can only be understood if it is subjected to a genetic analysis. This may be approached from the most striking point of the aggregate, from its instruction on the origin of the universe; for why, we may ask, should a cosmogony be a regular component of religious systems? The doctrine is, then, that the universe was created by a being resembling a man, but magnified in every respect, in power, wisdom, and the strength of his passions—an idealized super-man. Animals as creators of the universe point to the influence of totemism, upon which we shall have a few words at least to say presently. It is an interesting fact that this creator is always only a single being, even when there are believed to be many gods. It is interesting, too, that the creator is usually a man, though there is far from being a lack of indications of female deities; and some mythologies actually make the creation begin with a male god getting rid of a female deity,[1] who is degraded into being a monster. Here the most interesting problems of detail open

[1] [Freud had considerably more to say about female deities in Essay III, Part I, Section D, of *Moses and Monotheism* (1939a).]

out; but we must hurry on. Our further path is made easy to recognize, for this god-creator is undisguisedly called 'father'. Psycho-analysis infers that he really is the father, with all the magnificence in which he once appeared to the small child. A religious man pictures the creation of the universe just as he pictures his own origin.

This being so, it is easy to explain how it is that consoling assurances and strict ethical demands are combined with a cosmogony. For the same person to whom the child owed his existence, the father (or more correctly, no doubt, the parental agency compounded of the father and mother), also protected and watched over him in his feeble and helpless state, exposed as he was to all the dangers lying in wait in the external world; under his father's protection he felt safe. When a human being has himself grown up, he knows, to be sure, that he is in possession of greater strength, but his insight into the perils of life has also grown greater, and he rightly concludes that fundamentally he still remains just as helpless and unprotected as he was in his childhood, that faced by the world he is still a child. Even now, therefore, he cannot do without the protection which he enjoyed as a child. But he has long since recognized, too, that his father is a being of narrowly restricted power, and not equipped with every excellence. He therefore harks back to the mnemic image of the father whom in his childhood he so greatly overvalued. He exalts the image into a deity and makes it into something contemporary and real. The effective strength of this mnemic image and the persistence of his need for protection jointly sustain his belief in God.

The third main item in the religious programme, the ethical demand, also fits into this childhood situation with ease. I may remind you of Kant's famous pronouncement in which he names, in a single breath, the starry heavens and the moral law within us [see p. 525 above].[1] However strange this juxtaposition may sound—for what have the heavenly bodies to do

---

[1] [In the original edition the present sentence read: 'In a famous pronouncement the philosopher Kant named the existence of the starry heavens and that of the moral law within us as the most powerful witnesses to the greatness of God.' It was changed to the form translated above in *G.S.* (1934)—the earlier quotation of the same passage having no doubt been previously overlooked.]

with the question of whether one human creature loves another or kills him?—it nevertheless touches on a great psychological truth. The same father (or parental agency) which gave the child life and guarded him against its perils, taught him as well what he might do and what he must leave undone, instructed him that he must adapt himself to certain restrictions on his instinctual wishes, and made him understand what regard he was expected to have for his parents and brothers and sisters, if he wanted to become a tolerated and welcome member of the family circle and later on of larger associations. The child is brought up to a knowledge of his social duties by a system of loving rewards and punishments, he is taught that his security in life depends on his parents (and afterwards other people) loving him and on their being able to believe that he loves them. All these relations are afterwards introduced by men unaltered into their religion. Their parents' prohibitions and demands persist within them as a moral conscience. With the help of this same system of rewards and punishments, God rules the world of men. The amount of protection and happy satisfaction assigned to an individual depends on his fulfilment of the ethical demands; his love of God and his consciousness of being loved by God are the foundations of the security with which he is armed against the dangers of the external world and of his human environment. Finally, in prayer he has assured himself a direct influence on the divine will and with it a share in the divine omnipotence.

I feel sure that while you have been listening to me you have been bothered by a number of questions which you would be glad to hear answered. I cannot undertake to do so here and now, but I feel confident that none of these detailed enquiries would upset our thesis that the religious *Weltanschauung* is determined by the situation of our childhood. That being so, it is all the more remarkable that, in spite of its infantile nature, it nevertheless had a precursor. There is no doubt that there was a time without religion, without gods. This is known as the stage of animism. At that time, too, the world was peopled with spiritual beings resembling men—we call them demons. All the objects in the external world were their habitation, or perhaps were identical with them; but there was no superior power which had created them all and afterwards ruled them and to which one could turn for protection and help. The demons of animism were for the most part hostile in their attitude to human beings, but it appears that human beings had more self-confidence then than later on. They were certainly in a constant state of the most acute fear of these evil spirits; but they defended themselves against them by certain actions to which they ascribed the power to drive them away. Nor apart from this did they regard themselves as defenceless. If they desired something from Nature—if they wished for rain, for instance—they did not direct a prayer to the weather-god, but they performed a magical act which they expected to influence Nature directly: they themselves did something which resembled rain. In their struggle against the powers of the world around them their first weapon was *magic*, the earliest fore-runner of the technology of to-day. Their reliance on magic was, as we suppose, derived from their overvaluation of their own intellectual operations, from their belief in the 'omnipotence of thoughts', which, incidentally, we come upon again in our obsessional neurotic patients.[1] We may suppose that human beings at that period were particularly proud of their acquisitions in the way of language, which must have been accompanied by a great facilitation of thinking. They attributed magical power to words. This feature was later taken over by religion. 'And God said "Let there be light!" and there was light.' Moreover the fact of their magical actions shows that animistic men did not simply rely on the power of their wishes. They expected results, rather, from the performance of an action which would induce Nature to imitate it. If they wanted rain, they themselves poured out water; if they wanted to encourage the earth to be fruitful, they demonstrated a dramatic performance of sexual intercourse to it in the fields.

You know how hard it is for anything to die away when once it has achieved psychical expression. So you will not be surprised to hear that many of the utterances of animism have persisted to this day, for the most part as what we call superstition, alongside of and behind religion. But more than this, you will scarcely be able to reject a judgement that the philosophy of

[1] [For all of this see the third essay in *Totem and Taboo* (1912–13), (Norton, 1952), particularly Section 3.]

today has retained some essential features of the animistic mode of thought—the overvaluation of the magic of words and the belief that the real events in the world take the course which our thinking seeks to impose on them. It would seem, it is true, to be an animism without magical actions. On the other hand, we may suppose that even in those days there were ethics of some sort, precepts upon the mutual relations of men; but nothing suggests that they had any intimate connection with animistic beliefs. They were probably the direct expression of men's relative powers and of their practical needs.

It would be well worth knowing what brought about the transition from animism to religion, but you may imagine the obscurity which to-day still veils these primaeval ages of the evolution of the human spirit. It appears to be a fact that the first form assumed by religion was the remarkable phenomenon of totemism, the worship of animals, in whose train the first ethical commandments, the taboos, made their appearance. In a volume called *Totem and Taboo* [1912–13], I once elaborated a notion which traced this transformation back to a revolution in the circumstances of the human family. The main achievement of religion as compared with animism lies in the psychical binding of the fear of demons. Nevertheless a vestige of this primaeval age, the Evil Spirit, has kept a place in the religious system.

This being the prehistory of the religious *Weltanschauung*, let us turn now to what has happened since then and to what is still going on before our eyes. The scientific spirit, strengthened by the observation of natural processes, has begun, in the course of time, to treat religion as a human affair and to submit it to a critical examination. Religion was not able to stand up to this. What first gave rise to suspicion and scepticism were its tales of miracles, for they contradicted everything that had been taught by sober observation and betrayed too clearly the influence of the activity of the human imagination. After this its doctrines explaining the origin of the universe met with rejection, for they gave evidence of an ignorance which bore the stamp of ancient times and to which, thanks to their increased familiarity with the laws of nature, people knew they were superior. The idea that the universe came into existence through acts of copulation or creation analogous to the origin of individual people had ceased to be the most obvious and self-evident hypothesis since the distinction between animate creatures with a mind and an inanimate Nature had impressed itself on human thought—a distinction which made it impossible to retain belief in the original animism. Nor must we overlook the influence of the comparative study of different religious systems and the impression of their mutual exclusiveness and intolerance.

Strengthened by these preliminary exercises, the scientific spirit gained enough courage at last to venture on an examination of the most important and emotionally valuable elements of the religious *Weltanschauung*. People may always have seen, though it was long before they dared to say so openly, that the pronouncements of religion promising men protection and happiness if they would only fulfil certain ethical requirements had also shown themselves unworthy of belief. It seems not to be the case that there is a Power in the universe which watches over the well-being of individuals with parental care and brings all their affairs to a happy ending. On the contrary, the destinies of mankind can be brought into harmony neither with the hypothesis of a Universal Benevolence nor with the partly contradictory one of a Universal Justice. Earthquakes, tidal waves, conflagrations, make no distinction between the virtuous and pious and the scoundrel or unbeliever. Even where what is in question is not inanimate Nature but where an individual's fate depends on his relations to other people, it is by no means the rule that virtue is rewarded and that evil finds its punishment. Often enough the violent, cunning or ruthless man seizes the envied good things of the world and the pious man goes away empty. Obscure, unfeeling and unloving powers determine men's fate; the system of rewards and punishments which religion ascribes to the government of the universe seems not to exist. Here once again is a reason for dropping a portion of the animistic theory which had been rescued from animism by religion.

The last contribution to the criticism of the religious *Weltanschauung* was effected by psycho-analysis, by showing how religion originated from the helplessness of children and by tracing its contents to the survival into maturity of the wishes and needs of childhood. This did not precisely mean a contradiction of religion, but it was nevertheless a necessary rounding-off of our knowledge about it, and in one respect at least it was a contradiction, for religion itself lays claim to a divine origin. And, to be sure, it is not wrong in this, provided that our interpretation of God is accepted.

In summary, therefore, the judgement of science on the religious *Weltanschauung* is this. While the different religions wrangle with one another as to which of them is in possession of the truth, our view is that the question of the truth of religious beliefs may be left altogether on one side. Religion is an attempt to master the sensory world in which we are situated by means of the wishful world which we have developed within us as a result of biological and psychological necessities. But religion cannot achieve this. Its doctrines bear the imprint of the times in which they arose, the ignorant times of the childhood of humanity. Its consolations deserve no trust. Experience teaches us that the world is no nursery. The ethical demands on which religion seeks to lay stress need, rather, to be given another basis; for they are indispensable to human society and it is dangerous to link obedience to them with religious faith. If we attempt to assign the place of religion in the evolution of mankind, it appears not as a permanent acquisition but as a counterpart to the neurosis which individual civilized men have to go through in their passage from childhood to maturity.[1]

You are of course free to criticize this description of mine; I will even go half way to meet you on this. What I told you about the gradual crumbling away of the religious *Weltanschauung* was certainly incomplete in its abbreviated form. The order of the different processes was not given quite correctly; the co-operation of various forces in the awakening of the scientific spirit was not followed out. I also left out of account the alterations which took place in the religious *Weltanschauung* itself during the period of its undisputed sway and afterwards under the influence of growing criticism. Finally, I restricted my remarks, strictly

[1] [The possibility of society suffering from neuroses analogous to individual ones was mentioned by Freud in Chapter VIII of *The Future of an Illusion* (1927c), and near the end of *Civilization and its Discontents* (1930a). He discussed it at much greater length in Essay III, Part I, Section C of *Moses and Monotheism* (1939a). The analogy between religious practices and obsessive actions had been pointed out much earlier (Freud, 1907b).]

speaking, to one single form taken by religion, that of the Western peoples. I constructed an anatomical model, so to speak, for the purpose of a hurried demonstration which was to be as impressive as possible. Let us leave on one side the question of whether my knowledge would in any case have been sufficient to do the thing better and more completely. I am aware that you can find everything I said to you said better elsewhere. Nothing in it is new. But let me express a conviction that the most careful working-over of the material of the problems of religion would not shake our conclusions.

The struggle of the scientific spirit against the religious *Weltanschauung* is, as you know, not at an end: it is still going on to-day under our eyes. Though as a rule psycho-analysis makes little use of the weapon of controversy, I will not hold back from looking into this dispute. In doing so I may perhaps throw some further light on our attitude to *Weltanschauungen*. You will see how easily some of the arguments brought forward by the supporters of religion can be answered, though it is true that others may evade refutation.

The first objection we meet with is to the effect that it is an impertinence on the part of science to make religion a subject for its investigations, for religion is something sublime, superior to any operation of the human intellect, something which may not be approached with hair-splitting criticisms. In other words, science is not qualified to judge religion: it is quite serviceable and estimable otherwise, so long as it keeps to its own sphere. But religion is not its sphere, and it has no business there. If we do not let ourselves be put off by this brusque repulse and enquire further what is the basis of this claim to a position exceptional among all human concerns, the reply we receive (if we are thought worthy of any reply) is that religion cannot be measured by human measurements, for it is of divine origin and was given us as a revelation by a Spirit which the human spirit cannot comprehend. One would have thought that there was nothing easier than the refutation of this argument: it is a clear case of *petitio principii*, of 'begging the question' [1]—I know of no good German equivalent expression. The actual question raised is whether there *is* a divine spirit and a revelation by it; and the matter is certainly not decided by saying that this question

[1] [In English in the original.]

cannot be asked, since the deity may not be put in question. The position here is what it occasionally is during the work of analysis. If a usually sensible patient rejects some particular suggestion on specially foolish grounds, this logical weakness is evidence of the existence of a specially strong motive for the denial—a motive which can only be of an affective nature, an emotional tie.

We may also be given another answer, in which a motive of this kind is openly admitted: religion may not be critically examined because it is the highest, most precious, and most sublime thing that the human spirit has produced, because it gives expression to the deepest feelings and alone makes the world tolerable and life worthy of men. We need not reply by disputing this estimate of religion but by drawing attention to another matter. What we do is to emphasize the fact that what is in question is not in the least an invasion of the field of religion by the scientific spirit, but on the contrary an invasion by religion of the sphere of scientific thought. Whatever may be the value and importance of religion, it has no right in any way to restrict thought—no right, therefore, to exclude itself from having thought applied to it.

Scientific thinking does not differ in its nature from the normal activity of thought, which all of us, believers and un- believers, employ in looking after our affairs in ordinary life. It has only developed certain features: it takes an interest in things even if they have no immediate, tangible use; it is concerned carefully to avoid individual factors and affective influences; it examines more strictly the trustworthiness of the sense-percep- tions on which it bases its conclusions; it provides itself with new perceptions which cannot be obtained by everyday means and it isolates the determinants of these new experiences in experi- ments which are deliberately varied. Its endeavour is to arrive at correspondence with reality—that is to say, with what exists outside us and independently of us and, as experience has taught us, is decisive for the fulfilment or disappointment of our wishes. This correspondence with the real external world we call 'truth'. It remains the aim of scientific work even if we leave the practical value of that work out of account. When, there- fore, religion asserts that it can take the place of science, that, because it is beneficent and elevating, it must also be true, that is in fact an invasion which must be repulsed in the most general interest. It is asking a great deal of a person who has learnt to conduct his ordinary affairs in accordance with the rules of experience and with a regard to reality, to suggest that he shall hand over the care of what are precisely his most intimate interests to an agency which claims as its privilege freedom from the precepts of rational thinking. And as regards the protection which religion promises its believers, I think none of us would be so much as prepared to enter a motor-car if its driver announced that he drove, unperturbed by traffic regulations, in accordance with the impulses of his soaring imagination.

The prohibition against thought issued by religion to assist in its self-preservation is also far from being free from danger either for the individual or for human society. Analytic experience has taught us that a prohibition like this, even if it is originally limited to a particular field, tends to widen out and thereafter to become the cause of severe inhibitions in the subject's conduct of life. This result may be observed, too, in the female sex, following from their being forbidden to have anything to do with their sexuality even in thought.[1] Biography is able to point to the damage done by the religious inhibition of thought in the life stories of nearly all eminent individuals in the past. On the other hand intellect—or let us call it by the name that is familiar to us, reason—is among the powers which we may most expect to exercise a unifying influence on men—on men who are held together with such difficulty and whom it is therefore scarcely possible to rule. It may be imagined how impossible human society would be, merely if everyone had his own multiplication table and his own private units of length and weight. Our best hope for the future is that intellect—the scientific spirit, reason—may in process of time establish a dictatorship in the mental life of man. The nature of reason is a guarantee that afterwards it will not fail to give man's emotional impulses and what is determined by them the position they deserve. But the common compulsion exercised by such a dominance of reason will prove to be the strongest uniting bond among men and lead the way to further unions. Whatever, like

[1] [This had been considered in Chapter IX of *The Future of an Illusion* (1927c).]

religion's prohibition against thought, opposes such a development, is a danger for the future of mankind.

It may then be asked why religion does not put an end to this dispute which is so hopeless for it by frankly declaring: 'It is a fact that I cannot give you what is commonly called "truth"; if you want that, you must keep to science. But what I have to offer you is something incomparably more beautiful, more consoling and more uplifting than anything you could get from science. And because of that, I say to you that it is true in another, higher sense.' It is easy to find the answer to this. Religion cannot make this admission because it would involve its forfeiting all its influence on the mass of mankind. The ordinary man only knows one kind of truth, in the ordinary sense of the word. He cannot imagine what a higher or a highest truth may be. Truth seems to him no more capable of comparative degrees than death; and he cannot join in the leap from the beautiful to the true. Perhaps you will think as I do that he is right in this.

So the struggle is not at an end. The supporters of the religious *Weltanschauung* act upon the ancient dictum: the best defence is attack. 'What', they ask, 'is this science which presumes to disparage our religion—our religion which has brought salvation and consolation to millions of people over many thousands of years? What has it accomplished so far? What can we expect from it in the future? On its own admission it is incapable of bringing consolation and exaltation. Let us leave them on one side then, though that is no light renunciation. But what about its theories? Can it tell us how the universe came about and what fate lies before it? Can it even draw us a coherent picture of the universe, or show us where we are to look for the unexplained phenomena of life or how the forces of the mind are able to act upon inert matter? If it could do this we should not refuse it our respect. But none of these, no problem of this kind, has been solved by it hitherto. It gives us fragments of alleged discovery, which it cannot bring into harmony with one another; it collects observations of uniformities in the course of events which it dignifies with the name of laws and submits to its risky interpretations. And consider the small degree of certainty which it attaches to its findings! Everything it teaches is only provisionally true: what is praised to-day as the highest wisdom will be rejected to-morrow and replaced by something else, though once more only tentatively. The latest error is then described as the truth. And for this truth we are to sacrifice our highest good!'

I expect, Ladies and Gentlemen, that, in so far as you your-selves are supporters of the scientific *Weltanschauung* which is attacked in these words, you will not be too profoundly shaken by this criticism. And here I should like to recall to you a re-mark that once went the rounds in Imperial Austria. The old gentleman[1] once shouted at the Committee of a parliamentary party that was troublesome to him: 'This isn't ordinary oppo-sition any more! It's *factious* opposition!' Similarly, as you will recognize, the reproaches against science for not having yet solved the problems of the universe are exaggerated in an un-just and malicious manner; it has truly not had time enough yet for these great achievements. Science is very young—a human activity which developed late. Let us bear in mind, to select only a few dates, that only some three hundred years have passed since Kepler discovered the laws of planetary move-ment, that the life of Newton, who analysed light into the colours of the spectrum and laid down the theory of gravitation, ended in 1727—that is to say, little more than two hundred years ago—and that Lavoisier discovered oxygen shortly before the French Revolution. The life of an individual is very short in comparison with the duration of human evolution; I may be a very old man to-day,[2] but nevertheless I was already alive when Darwin published his book on the origin of species. In the same year as that, 1859, Pierre Curie, the discoverer of rad-ium, was born. And if you go further back, to the beginnings of exact science among the Greeks, to Archimedes, to Aristarchus of Samos (about 250 B.C.) who was the fore-runner of Coper-nicus, or even to the first beginnings of astronomy among the Babylonians, you will only have covered a small fraction of the length of time which anthropologists require for the evolution of man from an ape-like ancestral form, and which certainly comprises more than a hundred thousand years. And we must not forget that the last century has brought such a wealth of new discoveries, such a great acceleration of scientific advance

[1] [The Emperor Francis Joseph was popularly so named.]
[2] [Freud was 76 when he wrote this.]

that we have every reason to view the future of science with confidence.

We must admit to some extent the correctness of the other criticisms. The path of science is indeed slow, hesitating, laborious. This fact cannot be denied or altered. No wonder the gentlemen in the other camp are dissatisfied. They are spoilt: revelation gave them an easier time. Progress in scientific work is just as it is in an analysis. We bring expectations with us into the work, but they must be forcibly held back. By observation, now at one point and now at another, we come upon something new; but to begin with the pieces do not fit together. We put forward conjectures, we construct hypotheses, which we withdraw if they are not confirmed, we need much patience and readiness for any eventuality, we renounce early convictions so as not to be led by them into overlooking unexpected factors, and in the end our whole expenditure of effort is rewarded, the scattered findings fit themselves together, we get an insight into a whole section of mental events, we have completed our task and now we are free for the next one. In analysis, however, we have to do without the assistance afforded to research by experiment.

Moreover, there is a good deal of exaggeration in this criticism of science. It is not true that it staggers blindly from one experiment to another, that it replaces one error by another. It works as a rule like a sculptor at his clay model, who tirelessly alters his rough sketch, adds to it and takes away from it, till he has arrived at what he feels is a satisfactory degree of resemblance to the object he sees or imagines. Besides, at least in the older and more mature sciences, there is even to-day a solid ground-work which is only modified and improved but no longer demolished. Things are not looking so bad in the business of science.

And what, finally, is the aim of these passionate disparagements of science? In spite of its present incompleteness and of the difficulties attaching to it, it remains indispensable to us and nothing can take its place. It is capable of undreamt-of improvements, whereas the religious *Weltanschauung* is not. This is complete in all essential respects; if it was a mistake, it must remain one for ever. No belittlement of science can in any way alter the fact that it is attempting to take account of our dependence on the real external world, while religion is an illusion and it derives its strength from its readiness to fit in with our instinctual wishful impulses.[1]

I am under an obligation to go on to consider other *Weltanschauungen* which are in opposition to the scientific one; but I do so unwillingly, for I know that I am not properly competent to judge them. So you must bear this proviso in mind in listening to the following remarks, and if your interest has been aroused you should seek better instruction elsewhere.

And here I must first mention the various systems of philosophy which have ventured to draw a picture of the universe as it is reflected in the mind of thinkers who were for the most part turned away from the world. But I have already attempted to give a general account of the characteristics of philosophy [p. 624 f. above] and I am probably as unqualified as few people have ever been to form an estimate of the different systems. So I will invite you to join me in turning to a consideration of two other phenomena which, particularly in our days, it is impossible to disregard.

The first of these *Weltanschauungen* is as it were a counterpart to political anarchism, and is perhaps a derivative of it. There have certainly been intellectual nihilists of this kind in the past, but just now the relativity theory of modern physics seems to have gone to their head. They start out from science, indeed, but they contrive to force it into self-abrogation, into suicide; they set it the task of getting itself out of the way by refuting its own claims. One often has an impression in this connection that this nihilism is only a temporary attitude which is to be retained until this task has been performed. Once science has been disposed of, the space vacated may be filled by some kind of mysticism or, indeed, by the old religious *Weltanschauung*. According to the anarchist theory there is no such thing as truth, no assured knowledge of the external world. What we give out as being scientific truth is only the product of our own needs as they are bound to find utterance under changing external conditions: once again, they are illusion. Fundamentally, we

[1] [Freud's most elaborate evaluation of religion had been made in *The Future of an Illusion* (1927c).]

find only what we need and see only what we want to see. We have no other possibility. Since the criterion of truth—correspondence with the external world—is absent, it is entirely a matter of indifference what opinions we adopt. All of them are equally true and equally false. And no one has a right to accuse anyone else of error.

A person of an epistemological bent might find it tempting to follow the paths—the sophistries—by which the anarchists succeed in enticing such conclusions from science. No doubt we should come upon situations similar to those derived from the familiar paradox of the Cretan who says that all Cretans are liars.[1] But I have neither the desire nor the capacity for going into this more deeply. All I can say is that the anarchist theory sounds wonderfully superior so long as it relates to opinions about abstract things: it breaks down with its first step into practical life. Now the actions of men are governed by their opinions, their knowledge; and it is the same scientific spirit that speculates about the structure of atoms or the origin of man and that plans the construction of a bridge capable of bearing a load. If what we believe were really a matter of indifference, if there were no such thing as knowledge distinguished among our opinions by corresponding to reality, we might build bridges just as well out of cardboard as out of stone, we might inject our patients with a decagram of morphine instead of a centigram, and might use tear-gas as a narcotic instead of ether. But even the intellectual anarchists would violently repudiate such practical applications of their theory.

The other opposition has to be taken far more seriously, and in this instance I feel the liveliest regret at the inadequacy of my information. I suspect that you know more about this business than I do and that you took up your position long ago in favour of Marxism or against it. Karl Marx's investigations into the economic structure of society and into the influence of different economic systems upon every department of human life have in our days acquired an undeniable authority. How far his views in detail are correct or go astray, I cannot of course tell. I un-

[1] [The simplest form of this paradox (known as the 'Epimenides') is provided by a man who says 'I am lying'. If he is lying, he is speaking the truth; and if he is speaking the truth, he is lying.]

derstand that this is not an easy matter even for others better instructed than I am. There are assertions contained in Marx's theory which have struck me as strange: such as that the development of forms of society is a process of natural history, or that the changes in social stratification arise from one another in the manner of a dialectical process. I am far from sure that I understand these assertions aright; nor do they sound to me 'materialistic' but, rather, like a precipitate of the obscure Hegelian philosophy in whose school Marx graduated. I do not know how I can shake off my lay opinion that the class structure of society goes back to the struggles which, from the beginning of history, took place between human hordes[1] only slightly differing from each other. Social distinctions, so I thought, were originally distinctions between clans or races. Victory was decided by psychological factors, such as the amount of constitutional aggressiveness, but also by the firmness of the organization within the horde, and by material factors, such as the possession of superior weapons. Living together in the same area, the victors became the masters and the vanquished the slaves. There is no sign to be seen in this of a natural law or of a conceptual [dialectical] evolution. On the other hand the influence exercised upon the social relations of mankind by progressive control over the forces of Nature is unmistakable. For men always put their newly acquired instruments of power at the service of their aggressiveness and use them against one another. The introduction of metals—bronze and iron—made an end to whole epochs of civilization and their social institutions. I really believe that it was gunpowder and fire-arms that abolished chivalry and aristocratic rule, and that the Russian despotism was already doomed before it lost the War, because no amount of inbreeding among the ruling families of Europe could have produced a race of Tsars capable of withstanding the explosive force of dynamite.

It is possible, indeed, that with our present economic crisis, following after the Great War, we are only paying the price of our latest tremendous victory over nature, the conquest of the air. That does not sound very illuminating, but the first links at least in the chain are clearly recognizable. English politics

---

[1] [Freud always uses the term 'horde' to mean comparatively *small* groups.]

were based on the security which was guaranteed by the seas that washed her coasts. In the moment at which Blériot flew across the Channel in his aeroplane this protective isolation was breached; and in the night during which (in peace-time and on an exercise) a German Zeppelin cruised over London the war against Germany was no doubt a foregone conclusion.[1] Nor must the U-boat threat be forgotten in this connection.

I am almost ashamed to comment to you on a subject of such importance and complexity with these few inadequate remarks, and I know too that I have told you nothing that is new to you. I merely want to draw your attention to the fact that the relation of mankind to their control over Nature, from which they derive their weapons for fighting their fellow-men, must necessarily also affect their economic arrangements. We seem to have come a long way from the problem of a *Weltanschauung*, but we shall very soon be back to it. The strength of Marxism clearly lies, not in its view of history or the prophecies of the future that are based on it, but in its sagacious indication of the decisive influence which the economic circumstances of men have upon their intellectual, ethical and artistic attitudes. A number of connections and implications were thus uncovered, which had previously been almost totally overlooked. But it cannot be assumed that economic motives are the only ones that determine the behaviour of human beings in society. The undoubted fact that different individuals, races and nations behave differently under the same economic conditions is alone enough to show that economic motives are not the sole dominating factors. It is altogether incomprehensible how psychological factors can be overlooked where what is in question are the reactions of living human beings; for not only were these reactions concerned in establishing the economic conditions, but even under the domination of those conditions men can only bring their original instinctual impulses into play—their self-preservative instinct, their aggressiveness, their need to be loved, their drive towards obtaining pleasure and avoiding unpleasure. In an earlier enquiry I also pointed out the important claims made by the super-ego, which represents tradition and the ideals of the past and will for a time resist the incentives of a new economic

[1] I was told of this from trustworthy sources during the first year of the war.

situation.[1] And finally we must not forget that the mass of human beings who are subjected to economic necessities also undergo the process of cultural development—of civilization as other people may say[2]—which, though no doubt influenced by all the other factors, is certainly independent of them in its origin, being comparable to an organic process and very well able on its part to exercise an influence on the other factors.[3] It displaces instinctual aims and brings it about that people become antagonistic to what they had previously tolerated. Moreover, the progressive strengthening of the scientific spirit seems to form an essential part of it. If anyone were in a position to show in detail the way in which these different factors—the general inherited human disposition, its racial variations and its cultural transformations—inhibit and promote one another under the conditions of social rank, profession and earning capacity—if anyone were able to do this, he would have supplemented Marxism so that it was made into a genuine social science. For sociology too, dealing as it does with the behaviour of people in society, cannot be anything but applied psychology. Strictly speaking there are only two sciences: psychology, pure and applied, and natural science.

The newly achieved discovery of the far-reaching importance of economic relations brought with it a temptation not to leave alterations in them to the course of historical development but to put them into effect oneself by revolutionary action. Theoretical Marxism, as realized in Russian Bolshevism, has acquired

---

[1] [See above, p. 531.]

[2] [Cf. a parallel passage in *Why War?* (1933*b*), and Freud's sweeping comment on this verbal point in *The Future of an Illusion* (1927*c*): 'I scorn to distinguish between culture and civilization.']

[3] [The notion of a 'process of civilization' was very much in Freud's mind at this time. He had discussed it at several points in *Civilization and its Discontents* (1930*a*); and he mentioned it again in *Why War?* (1933*b*). But the idea was closely linked with one of much longer standing—the hypothesis, namely, of *repression* as an organic process. He himself brought out the connection fully in the two long footnotes at the beginning and end of Chapter IV of *Civilization and its Discontents.*]

the energy and the self-contained and exclusive character of a *Weltanschauung*, but at the same time an uncanny likeness to what it is fighting against. Though originally a portion of science and built up, in its implementation, upon science and technology, it has created a prohibition of thought which is just as ruthless as was that of religion in the past. Any critical examination of Marxist theory is forbidden, doubts of its correctness are punished in the same way as heresy was once punished by the Catholic Church. The writings of Marx have taken the place of the Bible and the Koran as a source of revelation, though they would seem to be no more free from contradictions and obscurities than those older sacred books.

And although practical Marxism has mercilessly cleared away all idealistic systems and illusions, it has itself developed illusions which are no less questionable and unprovable than the earlier ones. It hopes in the course of a few generations so to alter human nature that people will live together almost without friction in the new order of society, and that they will undertake the duties of work without any compulsion. Meanwhile it shifts elsewhere the instinctual restrictions which are essential in society; it diverts the aggressive tendencies which threaten all human communities to the outside and finds support in the hostility of the poor against the rich and of the hitherto powerless against the former rulers. But a transformation of human nature such as this is highly improbable. The enthusiasm with which the mass of the people follow the Bolshevist instigation at present, so long as the new order is incomplete and is threatened from outside, gives no certainty for a future in which it would be fully built up and in no danger. In just the same way as religion, Bolshevism too must compensate its believers for the sufferings and deprivations of their present life by promises of a better future in which there will no longer be any unsatisfied need. This Paradise, however, is to be in this life, instituted on earth and thrown open within a foreseeable time. But we must remember that the Jews as well, whose religion knows nothing of an after-life, expected the arrival of a Messiah on earth, and that the Christian Middle Ages at many times believed that the Kingdom of God was at hand.

There is no doubt of how Bolshevism will reply to these objections. It will say that so long as men's nature has not yet been transformed it is necessary to make use of the means which affect them to-day. It is impossible to do without compulsion in their education, without the prohibition of thought and without the employment of force to the point of bloodshed; and if the illusions were not awakened in them, they could not be brought to acquiesce in this compulsion. And we should be politely asked to say how things could be managed differently. This would defeat us. I could think of no advice to give. I should admit that the conditions of this experiment would have deterred me and those like me from undertaking it; but we are not the only people concerned. There are men of action, unshakable in their convictions, inaccessible to doubt, without feeling for the sufferings of others if they stand in the way of their intentions. We have to thank men of this kind for the fact that the tremendous experiment of producing a new order of this kind is now actually being carried out in Russia. At a time when the great nations announce that they expect salvation only from the maintenance of Christian piety, the revolution in Russia—in spite of all its disagreeable details—seems none the less like the message of a better future. Unluckily neither our scepticism nor the fanatical faith of the other side gives a hint as to how the experiment will turn out. The future will tell us; perhaps it will show that the experiment was undertaken prematurely, that a sweeping alteration of the social order has little prospect of success until new discoveries have increased our control over the forces of Nature and so made easier the satisfaction of our needs. Only then perhaps may it become possible for a new social order not only to put an end to the material need of the masses but also to give a hearing to the cultural demands of the individual. Even then, to be sure, we shall still have to struggle for an incalculable time with the difficulties which the untameable character of human nature presents to every kind of social community.

Ladies and Gentlemen,—Allow me in conclusion to sum up what I had to say of the relation of psycho-analysis to the question of a *Weltanschauung*. Psycho-analysis, in my opinion, is incapable of creating a *Weltanschauung* of its own. It does not need one; it is a part of science and can adhere to the scientific *Weltanschauung*. This, however, scarcely deserves such a grandiloquent title, for it is not all-comprehensive, it is too incomplete and makes no claim to being self-contained and to the construction of systems. Scientific thought is still very young among human beings; there are too many of the great problems which it has not yet been able to solve. A *Weltanschauung* erected upon science has, apart from its emphasis on the real external world, mainly negative traits, such as submission to the truth and rejection of illusions. Any of our fellow-men who is dissatisfied with this state of things, who calls for more than this for his momentary consolation, may look for it where he can find it. We shall not grudge it him, we cannot help him, but nor can we on his account think differently.

Appendixes

BIBLIOGRAPHY
AND AUTHOR INDEX

[Titles of books and periodicals are in italics; titles of papers are in inverted commas. Abbreviations are in accordance with the *World List of Scientific Periodicals* (London, 1952). Further abbreviations used in this volume will be found in the List at the end of this bibliography. Numerals in thick type refer to volumes; ordinary numerals refer to pages. The figures in round brackets at the end of each entry indicate the page or pages of this volume on which the work in question is mentioned. In the case of the Freud entries, the letters attached to the dates of publication are in accordance with the corresponding entries in the complete bibliography of Freud's writings to be included in the last volume of the *Standard Edition*.

For non-technical authors, and for technical authors where no specific work is mentioned, see the General Index.]

ABEL., K. (1884) *Über den Gegensinn der Urworte,* Leipzig. (179–80, 229–30)

ABRAHAM, K. (1908) 'Die psychosexuellen Differenzen der Hysterie und der Dementia praecox', *Zbl. Nervenheilk. Psychiat.*, N.F. **19**, 521. (415)

[*Trans.:* 'The Psycho-Sexual Differences Between Hysteria and Dementia Praecox', *Selected Papers on Psycho-Analysis*, London, 1927, Chap. II.]

(1916) 'Untersuchungen über die früheste prägenitale Entwicklungsstufe der Libido', *Int. Z. (ärztl.) Psychoanal.*, **4**, 71. (327)

[*Trans.:* 'The First Pregenital Stage of the Libido', *Selected Papers on Psycho-Analysis*, London, 1927, Chap. XII.]

(1922) 'Die Spinne als Traumsymbol', *Int. Z. Psychoan.*, **8**, 470. (488)

[*Trans.:* 'The Spider as a Dream Symbol', *Selected Papers on Psycho-Analysis*, London, 1927, Chap. XIX.]

(1924) *Versuch einer Entwicklungsgeschichte der Libido,* Leipzig, Vienna, Zurich. (563, 564)

[*Trans.:* 'A Short Study of the Development of the Libido', *Selected Papers on Psycho-Analysis*, London, 1927, Chap. XXVI.]

ADLER, A. (1910) 'Der psychische Hermaphroditismus im Leben und in der Neurose', *Fortschr. Med.*, **28**, 486. (237)

(1912) *Über den nervösen Charakter,* Wiesbaden. (381)

[*Trans.: The Neurotic Constitution,* New York 1916; London, 1918.]

AICHHORN, A. (1925) *Verwahrloste Jugend,* Vienna. (610, 614)

[*Trans.: Wayward Youth,* New York, 1935; London, 1936; revised reprint, London, 1951.]

ALEXANDER, F. (1925) 'Über Traumpaare und Traumreihen', *Int. Z. Psychoan.*, **11**, 80. (491)

[*Trans.:* 'Dreams in Paris and Series', *Int. J. Psycho-Anal.*, **6**, 446.]

ANDREAS-SALOMÉ, L. (1916) ' "Anal" und "Sexual" ', *Imago*, **4**, 249. (315), (565)

ARISTOTLE, *De somniis* and *De divinatione per somnum.* (88)
    [*Trans.:* in *On the Soul,* Loeb Classical Library (trans. W. S. Hett),
    London and New York, 1935.]

ARTEMIDORUS OF DALDIS, *Oneirocritica.* (86, 236)
    [*Trans.* (Abridged): *The Interpretation of Dreams* (trans. R. Wood),
    London, 1644.]

BERNHEIM, H. (1886) *De la suggestion et de ses applications à la thérapeutique,* Paris. (448–9)
    (1892) *Hypnotisme, suggestion et psychothérapie: études nouvelles,* Paris.
    (449)

BETLHEIM, S. and HARTMANN, H. (1924) 'Über Fehlreaktionen des
Gedächtnisses bei Korsakoffschen Psychose', *Arch. Psychiat. Nervenkr.,*
72, 278. (486–7)

BINET, A. (1888) *Études de psychologie expérimentale: le fétichisme dans
l'amour,* Paris. (348)

BINZ, C. (1878) *Über den Traum,* Bonn. (86)

BLOCH, I. (1902–3) *Beiträge zur Ätiologie der Psychopathia sexualis* (2 vols.),
Dresden. (307)

BÖLSCHE, W. (1911–13) *Das Liebesleben in der Natur* (2 vols.), Jena. (354)

BREUER, J., and FREUD, S. (1893) *See* FREUD, S. (1893a)
    (1895) *See* FREUD, S. (1895d)

BRILL, A. A. (1912) *Psychoanalysis: Its Theories and Practical Application,*
Philadelphia and London. (2nd ed., 1914; 3rd ed., 1922.) (31, 52–3,
55)

BRUNSWICK, R. MACK (1928) 'Die Analyse eines Eifersuchtswahnes', *Int.
Z. Psychoan.,* **14,** 458. (594)
    [*English Text:* 'The Analysis of a Case of Paranoia', *J. nerv. ment.
Dis.,* **70** (1929), 177.]

BURLINGHAM, D. (1932) 'Kinderanalyse und Mutter', *Psychoan. Päd.,* **6,**
269. (520)
    [*English Text:* 'Child Analysis and the Mother', *Psychoanal. Quart.,* **4**
(1935), 69.]

DARWIN, C. (1872) *The Expression of the Emotions in Man and Animals,*
London. (2nd ed., 1899.) (396, 399)
    (1958) *The Autobiography of Charles Darwin,* London. (76)

DEUTSCH, H. (1926) 'Okkulte Vorgänge während der Psychoanalyse', *Imago,*
12, 418. (518)
    (1932) 'Über die weibliche Homosexualität', *Int. Z. Psychoan.,* **18,** 219.
    (595)
    [*Trans.:* 'Homosexuality in Women', *Int. J. Psycho-Anal,* **14** (1933),
    34.]

DEVEREUX, G. (1953) *Psychoanalysis and the Occult,* New York. (467)

DU PREL, C. (1885) *Die Philosophie der Mystik,* Leipzig. (133)

EISLER, M. J. (1919) 'Beiträge zur Traumdeutung', *Int. Z. (ärztl.) Psychoanal.,* **5,** 295.
    [*Trans.:* in *The Psychoanalytic Reader* (ed. R. Fliess), New York,
    1948, 378.]

EISLER, R. (1910) *Weltenmantel und Himmelszelt* (2 vols.), Munich. (488)

FECHNER, G. T. (1860) *Elemente der Psychophysik,* Leipzig. (2nd ed., 1889.)
(90)

FEDERN, P. (1914) 'Über zwei typische Traumsensationen', *Jb. psychoan.,*
6, 89. (155)

FERENCZI, S. (1913) 'Entwicklungsstufen des Wirklichkeitssinnes', *Int. Z. (ärztl.) Psychoanal.*, **1**, 124. (351)
  [*Trans.*: 'Stages in the Development of the Sense of Reality', *First Contributions to Psycho-Analysis*, London, 1952, Chap. VIII.]
  (1921) 'Die Symbolik der Brücke', *Int. Z. Psychoan*, **7**, 211. (488)
  [*Trans.*: 'The Symbolism of the Bridge', *Further Contributions to the Theory and Technique of Psycho-Analysis*, London, 1926, Chap. LXI.]
  (1922) 'Die Brückensymbolik und die Don Juan-Legende', *Int. Z. Psychoan.*, **8**, 77. (488)
  [*Trans.*: 'Bridge Symbolism and the Don Juan Legend', *Further Contributions to the Theory and Technique of Psycho-Analysis*, London, 1926, Chap. LXII.]
  (1925) 'Zur Psychoanalyse von Sexualgewohnheiten', *Int. Z. Psychoan.*, **11**, 6, (551)
  [*Trans.*: 'Psycho-Analysis of Sexual Habits', *Further Contributions to the Theory and Technique of Psycho-Analysis*, London, 1926, Chap. XXXII.]

FLIESS, W. (1906) *Der Ablauf des Lebens*, Vienna. (320)

FREUD, S. (1877a) 'Über den Ursprung der hinteren Nervenwurzeln im Rückenmarke von Ammocoetes (Petromyzon Planeri)', *S.B. Akad. Wiss. Wien* (Math.-Naturwiss. Kl.), III Abt., **75**, 15. (340)
  (1878a) 'Über Spinalganglien und Rückenmark des Petromyzon', *S.B. Akad. Wiss. Wien* (Math.-Naturwiss. Kl.), III Abt., **78**, 81. (340)
  (1885d) 'Zur Kenntnis der Olivenzwischenschicht', *Neurol. Zbl.*, **4**, Nr. 12, 268. (393)
  (1886b) With DARKSCHEWITSCH, L., 'Über die Beziehung des Strickkörpers zum Hinterstrang und Hinterstrangskern nebst Bemerkungen über zwei Felder der Oblongata', *Neurol. Zbl.*, **5**, Nr. 6, 121. (393)
  (1886c) 'Über den Ursprung des Nervus acusticus', *Mschr. Ohrenheilk.*, Neue Folge **20**, Nr. 8, 245, and 9, 277. (393)
  (1888–9) Translation with Introduction and Notes of H. Bernheim's *De la suggestion et de ses applications à la thérapeutique*, Paris, 1886, under the title *Die Suggestion und ihre Heilwirkung*, Vienna. (448–9)
  [*Trans.*: Introduction to Bernheim's *Die Suggestion und ihre Heilwirkung*, *C.P.*, **5**, 11; *Standard Ed.*, 71.]
  (1889a) Review of Forel's *Der Hypnotismus*, *Wien. med. Wschr.*, **39**, Nr. 28, 1097, and Nr. 47, 1892. (462)
  [*Trans.*: *Standard Ed.*, **1**, 89.]
  (1892a) Translation of H. Bernheim's *Hypnotisme, suggestion et psychothérapie: études nouvelles*, Paris, 1891, under the title *Neue Studien über Hypnotismus, Suggestion und Psychotherapie*, Vienna. (449)
  (1892–3) 'Ein Fall von hypnotischer Heilung nebst Bemerkungen über die Entstehung hysterischer Symptome durch den "Gegenwillen"', *G.S.*, **1**, 258; *G.W.*, **1**, 3. (72, 141, 499)
  [*Trans.*: 'A Case of Successful Treatment by Hypnotism', *C.P.*, **5**, 33; *Standard Ed.*, **1**, 115.]
  (1893a) With BREUER, J., 'Über den psychischen Mechanismus hysterischer Phänomene: Vorläufige Mitteilung', *G.S.*, **1**, 7; *G.W.*, **1**, 81. (257, 275)
  [*Trans.*: 'On the Psychical Mechanism of Hysterical Phenomena: Preliminary Communication', *C.P.*, **1**, 24; *Standard Ed.*, **2**, 3.]
  (1893f) 'Charcot', *G.S.*, **1**, 243; *G.W.*, **1**, 21. (145)
  [*Trans.*: 'Charcot', *C.P.*, **1**, 9; *Standard Ed.*, **3**, 9.]

FREUD, S. (1893*h*) 'Vortrag Über den psychischen Mechanismus hysterischer Phänomene' [shorthand report revised by lecturer], *Wien. med. Pr.*, **34,** Nr. 4, 121, and 5, 165. (555)
   [*Trans.*: Lecture 'On the Psychical Mechanism of Hysterical Phenomena', *Int. J. Psycho-Anal.*, **37,** 8; *Standard Ed.*, **3,** 27.]

(1894*a*) 'Die Abwehr-Neuropsychosen', *G.S.*, **1,** 290; *G.W.*, **1,** 59. (215, 336, 357, 480, 540, 557–8)
   [*Trans.*: 'The Neuro-Psychoses of Defence', *C.P.*, **1,** 59; *Standard Ed.*, **3,** 43.]

(1895*b* [1894]) 'Über die Berechtigung, von der Neurasthenie einen bestimmten Symptomenkomplex als "Angstneurose" abzutrennen', *G.S.*, **1,** 306; *G.W.*, **1,** 315. (386, 392, 398, 400)
   [*Trans.*: 'On the Grounds for Detaching a Particular Syndrome from Neurasthenia under the Description "Anxiety Neurosis"', *C.P.*, **1,** 76; *Standard Ed.*, **3,** 87.]

(1895*c* [1894]) 'Obsessions et phobies' [in French], *G.S.*, **1,** 334; *G.W.*, **1,** 345. (400)
   [*Trans.*: 'Obsessions and Phobias', *C.P.*, **1,** 128; *Standard Ed.*, **3,** 71.]

(1895*d*) With BREUER, J., *Studien über Hysterie*, Vienna. *G.S.*, **1,** 3; *G.W.*, **1,** 77 (omitting Breuer's contributions). (141, 257, 269, 274, 275, 279–80, 286, 292, 293–4, 296, 396, 431, 449, 504, 538, 584–5)
   [*Trans.*: *Studies on Hysteria*, London, 1956; *Standard Ed.*, **2.** Including Breuer's contributions.]

(1895*f*) 'Zur Kritik der "Angstneurose"', *G.S.*, **1,** 343; *G.W.*, **1,** 357. (245, 347, 386, 392)
   [*Trans.*: 'A Reply to Criticisms of my Paper on Anxiety Neurosis', *C.P.*, **1,** 107; *Standard Ed.*, **3,** 121.]

(1896*b*) 'Weitere Bemerkungen über die Abwehr-Neuropsychosen', *G.S.*, **1,** 363; *G.W.*, **1,** 379. (268, 554, 584)
   [*Trans.*: 'Further Remarks on the Neuro-Psychoses of Defence', *C.P.*, **1,** 155; *Standard Ed.*, **3,** 159.]

(1896*c*) 'Zur Ätiologie der Hysterie', *G.S.*, **1,** 404; *G.W.*, **1,** 425. (6, 584)
   [*Trans.*: 'The Aetiology of Hysteria', *C.P.*, **1,** 183; *Standard Ed.*, **3,** 189.]

(1897*b*) *Inhaltsangaben der wissenschaftlichen Arbeiten des Privatdozenten Dr. Sigm. Freud (1877–1897)*, Vienna. *G.W.*, **1,** 463. (141, 340 393)
   [*Trans.*: *Abstracts of the Scientific Writings of Dr. Sigm. Freud (1877–1897)*, *Standard Ed.*, **3,** 225.]

(1898*a*) 'Die Sexualität in der Ätiologie der Neurosen', *G.S.*, **1,** 439; *G.W.*, **1,** 491. (386, 391)
   [*Trans.*: 'Sexuality in the Aetiology of the Neuroses', *C.P.*, **1,** 220; *Standard Ed.*, **3,** 261.]

(1899*a*) 'Über Deckerinnerungen', *G.S.*, **1,** 465; *G.W.*, **1,** 531. (201)
   [*Trans.*: 'Screen Memories', *C.P.*, **5,** 47; *Standard Ed.*, **3,** 301.]

(1900*a*) *Die Traumdeutung*, Vienna. *G.S.*, **2–3;** *G.W.*, **2–3.** (75, 83–239 passim, 272, 287, 315, 329, 335, 342, 397, 428, 429, 467, 472, 474, 478, 480, 487, 490, 552, 553, 565, 603, 625)
   [*Trans.*: *The Interpretation of Dreams*, London and New York, 1955; *Standard Ed.*, **4–5.**]

(1901*a*) *Über den Traum*, Wiesbaden. *G.S.*, **3,** 189; *G.W.*, **2–3,** 643. (122)
   [*Trans.*: *On Dreams*, London and New York, 1951; *Standard Ed.*, **5,** 633.]

(1901*b*) *Zur Psychopathologie des Alltagslebens*, Berlin. 1904. *G.S.*, **4,** 3;

G.W., **4,** (4, 25–79 passim, 107, 111, 201, 202, 504)
[*Trans.: The Psychopathology of Everyday Life, Standard Ed.,* **6.**]
(1904*a*) 'Die Freud'sche psychoanalytische Methode', *G.S.,* **6,** 3; *G.W.,*
5, 3. (287)
[*Trans.:* 'Freud's Psycho-Analytic Procedure', *C.P.,* **1,** 264; *Standard
Ed.,* **7,** 249.]
(1905*a*) 'Über Psychotherapie', *G.S.,* **6,** 11; *G.W.,* **5,** 13. (6, 450, 451)
[*Trans.:* 'On Psychotherapy', *C.P.,* **1,** 249; *Standard Ed.,* **7,** 257.]
(1905*c*) *Der witz und seine Beziehung zum Unbewussten,* Vienna. *G.S.,*
9, 5; *G.W.,* **6.** (39, 118, 122, 172, 174–5, 197, 235, 236, 497, 504, 553,
562)
[*Trans.: Jokes and their Relation to the Unconscious,* London, 1960;
Standard Ed., **8.**]
(1905*d*) *Drei Abhandlungen zur Sexualtheorie,* Vienna. *G.S.,* **5,** 3; *G.W.,*
5, 29. (200, 303, 310, 323, 348, 373, 407, 415, 562, 565, 578, 579, 585)
[*Trans.: Three Essays on the Theory of Sexuality,* London, 1962;
Standard Ed., **7,** 125.]
(1905*e* [1901]) 'Bruchstück einer Hysterie-Analyse', *G.S.,* **8,** 3; *G. W.,* 5;
163. (156, 185, 222, 384–5, 431)
[*Trans.:* 'Fragment of an Analysis of a Case of Hysteria', *C.P.,* **3,** 13;
Standard Ed., **7,** 3.]
(1906*a*) 'Meine Ansichten über die Rolle der Sexualität in der Atiologie
der Neurosen', *G.S.,* **5,** 123; *G.W.,* **5,** 149. (246, 386, 585)
[*Trans.:* 'My Views on the Part played by Sexuality in the Aetiology
of the Neuroses', *C.P.,* **1,** 272; *Standard Ed.,* **7,** 271.]
(1907*b*) 'Zwangshandlungen und Religionsübung', *G.S.,* **10,** 210; *G.W.,* **7,**
129, (263, 309, 632)
[*Trans.:* 'Obsessive Actions and Religious Practices', *C.P.,* **2,** 25;
Standard Ed., **9,** 116.]
(1907*c*) 'Zur sexuellen Aufklärung der Kinder', *G.S.,* **5,** 134; *G.W.,* **7,**
19. (610)
[*Trans.:* 'The Sexual Enlightenment of Children', *C.P.,* **2,** 36; *Standard
Ed.,* **9,** 131.]
(1908*a*) 'Hysterische Phantasien und ihre Beziehung zur Bisexualität',
G.S., **5,** 246; *G.W.,* **7,** 191. (99, 371)
[*Trans.:* 'Hysterical Phantasies and their Relation to Bisexuality', *C.P.,*
2, 51; *Standard Ed.,* **9,** 157.]
(1908*b*) 'Charakter und Analerotik', *G.S.,* **5,** 261; *G.W.,* **7,** 203. (315,
555, 566)
[*Trans.:* 'Character and Anal Erotism', *C.P.,* **2,** 45; *Standard Ed.,* **9,**
169.]
(1908*c*) 'Über infantile Sexualtheorien', *G.S.,* **5,** 168; *G.W.,* **7,** 171. (317,
564)
[*Trans.:* 'On the Sexual Theories of Children', *C.P.,* **2,** 59; *Standard
Ed.,* **9,** 207.]
(1908*d*) 'Die "kulturelle" Sexualmoral und die moderne Nervosität',
G.S., **5,** 143; *G.W.,* **7,** 143. (310)
[*Trans.:* ' "Civilized" Sexual Morality and Modern Nervous Illness',
C.P., **2,** 76; *Standard Ed.,* **9,** 179.]
(1908*e* [1907]) 'Der Dichter und das Phantasieren', *G.S.* **10,** 229; *G.W.,*
7, 213. (99, 371, 377)
[*Trans.:* 'Creative Writers and Day-Dreaming', *C.P.,* **4,** 173; *Standard
Ed.,* **9,** 143.]

(1909a) 'Allgemeines über den hysterischen Anfall', *G.S.*, **5**, 255; *G.W.*, **7**, 235. (332, 384, 396)
[*Trans.*: 'Some General Remarks on Hysterical Attacks', *C.P.*, **2**, 100; *Standard Ed.*, **9**, 229.]

(1909b) 'Analyse der Phobie eines fünfjährigen Knaben', *G.S.*, **8**, 129; *G.W.*, **7**, 243. (176, 310, 317, 364, 400, 610)
[*Trans.*: 'Analysis of a Phobia in a Five-Year-Old Boy', *C.P.*, **3**, 149; *Standard Ed.*, **10**, 3.]

(1909d) 'Bemerkungen über einen Fall von Zwangsneurose', *G.S.*, **8**, 269; *G.W.*, **7**, 381. (85, 261, 266, 301, 337)
[*Trans.*: 'Notes upon a Case of Obsessional Neurosis', *C.P.*, **3**, 293; *Standard Ed.*, **10**, 155.]

(1910a [1909]) *Über Psychoanalyse*, Vienna. *G.S.*, **4**, 349; *G.W.*, **8**, 3, (6, 83, 294, 377)
[*Trans.*: 'Five Lectures on Psycho-Analysis', *Amer. F. Psychol.*, **21** (1910), 181; *Standard Ed.*, **11**, 3.]

(1910d) 'Die zukünftigen Chancen der psychoanalytischen Therapie', *G.S.*, **6**, 25; *G.W.*, **8**, 104. (164, 291)
[*Trans.*: 'The Future Prospects of Psycho-Analytic Therapy', *C.P.*, **2**, 285; *Standard Ed.*, **11**, 141.]

(1910e) ' "Über den Gegensinn der Urworte" ', *G.S.*, **10**, 221; *G.W.*, **8**, 214. (179)
[*Trans.*: ' "The Antithetical Meaning of Primal Words" ', *C.P.*, **4**, 184; *Standard Ed.*, **11**, 155.]

(1910f) Letter to Dr. Friedrich S. Krauss on *Anthropophyteia*, *G.S.*, **11**, 242; *G.W.*, **8**, 224. (162) [*Trans.*: *Standard Ed.*, **11**, 233.]

(1910h) 'Über einen besoderen Typus der Objektwahl beim Manne', *G.S.*, **5**, 186; *G.W.*, **8**, 66. (330)
[*Trans.*: 'A Special Type of Choice of Object made by Men', *C.P.*, **4**, 192; *Standard Ed.*, **11**, 165.]

(1910i) 'Die psychogene Sehstörung in psychoanalytischer Auffassung', *G.S.*, **5**, 310; *G.W.*, **8**, 94. (308)
[*Trans.*: 'The Psycho-Analytic View of Psychogenic Disturbance of Vision', *C.P.*, **2**, 105; *Standard Ed.*, **11**, 211.]

(1910k) 'Über "wilde" Psychoanalyse', *G.S.*, **6**, 37; *G.W.*, **8**, 118. (391)
[*Trans.*: ' "Wild" Psycho-Analysis', *C.P.*, **2**, 297; *Standard Ed.*, **11**, 221.]

(1911b) 'Formulierungen über die zwei Prinzipien des psychischen Geschehens', *G.S.*, **5**, 409; *G.W.*, **8**, 230. (190, 355, 357, 377, 553)
[*Trans.*: 'Formulations on the Two Principles of Mental Functioning', *C.P.*, **4**, 13; *Standard Ed.*, **12**, 215.]

(1911c) 'Psychoanalytische Bemerkungen über einen autobiographisch beschriebenen Fall von Paranoia (Dementia Paranoides)', *G.S.*, **8**, 355; *G.W.*, **8**, 240. (166, 422, 424, 563)
[*Trans.*: 'Psycho-Analytic Notes on an Autobiographical Account of a Case of Paranoia (Dementia Paranoides) ', *C.P.*, **3**, 387; *Standard Ed.*, **12**, 3.]

(1911e) 'Die Handhabung der Traumdeutung in der Psychoanalyse', *G.S.*, **6**, 45; *G.W.*, **8**, 350. (184, 478)
[*Trans.*: 'The Handling of Dream-Interpretation in Psycho-Analysis', *C.P.*, **2**, 305; *Standard Ed.*, **12**, 91.]

(1912b) 'Zur Dynamik der Übertragung', *G.S.*, **6**, 53; *G.W.*, **8**, 364. (149, 287, 292, 374, 431)

[*Trans.:* 'The Dynamics of Transference', *C.P.*, **2**, 312; *Standard Ed.*, **12**, 99.]

(1912*c*) 'Über neurotische Erkrankungstypen', *G.S.*, **5**, 400, *G.W.*, **8**, 322. (350)

[*Trans.:* 'Types of Onset of Neurosis', *C.P.*, **2**, 113; *Standard Ed.*, **12**, 229.]

(1912*f*) 'Zur Onanie-Diskussion', *G.S.*, **3**, 324; *G.W.*, **8**, 332. (317, 591, 619)

[*Trans.:* Contributions to a Discussion on Masturbation', *Standard Ed.*, **12**, 243.]

(1912–13) *Totem und Tabu*, Vienna. 1913. *G.S.*, **10**, 3; *G.W.*, **9**. (254, 267, 332, 335, 355, 629, 630, 641)

[*Trans.: Totem and Taboo*, London, 1950; New York, 1952; *Standard Ed.*, **13**, 1.]

(1913*a*) 'Ein Traum als Beweismittel', *G.S.*, **3**, 267; *G.W.*, **10**, 12. (182, 222, 227)

[*Trans.:* 'An Evidential Dream', *C.P.*, **2**, 133; *Standard Ed.*, **12**, 269.]

(1913*b*) Introduction to Pfister's *Die psychanalytische Methode*, *G.S.*, **11**, 224; *G.W.*, **10**, 448. (610)

[*Trans.: Standard Ed.*, **12**, 329.]

(1913*c*) 'Weitere Ratschläge zur Technik der Psychoanalyse: I. Zur Einleitung der Behandlung', *G.S.*, **6**, 84; *G.W.*, **8**, 454. (287)

[*Trans.:* 'On Beginning the Treatment (Further Recommendations on the Technique of Psycho-Analysis, I)', *C.P.*, **2**, 342; *Standard Ed.*, **12**, 123.]

(1913*h*) 'Erfahrungen und Beispiele aus der analytischen Praxis', *Int. Z. (ärztl.) Psychoanal.*, **1**, 377; partly reprinted *G.S.*, **11**, 301; *G.W.*, **10**, 40. (488)

[*Trans.:* 'Observations and Examples from Analytic Practice', *Standard Ed.*, **13**, 193 (in full). Also partly incorporated in *The Interpretation of Dreams, Standard Ed.*, **4**, 232, and **5**, 409f.]

(1913*i*) 'Die Disposition zur Zwangsneurose', *G.S.*, **5**, 277; *G.W.*, **8**, 442. (563)

[*Trans.:* 'The Disposition to Obsessional Neurosis', *C.P.*, **2**, 122; *Standard Ed.*, **12**, 313.]

(1913*j*) 'Das Interesse an der Psychoanalyse', *G.S.*, **4**, 313; *G.W.*, **8**, 390. (377)

[*Trans.:* 'The Claims of Psycho-Analysis to Scientific Interest', *Standard Ed.*, **13**, 165.]

(1914*c*) 'Zur Einführung des Narzissmus', *G.S.*, **6**, 155; *G.W.*, **10**, 138. 390, 414–15, 416, 426, 428, 429, 529, 596)

[*Trans.:* 'On Narcissism: an Introduction', *C.P.*, **4**, 30; *Standard Ed.*, **14**, 69.]

(1914*d*) 'Zur Geschichte der psychoanalytischen Bewegung', *G.S.*, **4**, 411; *G.W.*, **10**, 44. (83, 245, 286, 292, 346, 585, 601, 604–5)

[*Trans.:* 'On the History of the Psycho-Analytic Movement', *C.P.*, **1**, 287; *Standard Ed.*, **14**, 3.]

(1914*g*) 'Weitere Ratschläge zur Technik der Psychoanalyse: II. Erinnern, Wiederholen und Durcharbeiten', *G.S.*, **6**, 109; *G.W.*, **10**, 126. (444)

[*Trans.:* 'Remembering, Repeating and Working-Through (Further Recommendations on the Technique of Psycho-Analysis, II)', *C.P.*, **2**, 366; *Standard Ed.*, **12**, 147.]

(1915*a*) 'Weitere Ratschläge zur Technik der Psychoanalyse: III.

Bemerkungen über die Übertragungsliebe', *G.S.*, **6**, 120; *G.W.*, **10**, 306. (431)
[*Trans.*: 'Observations on Transference-Love (Further Recommendations on the Technique of Psycho-Analysis, III)', *C.P.*, **2**, 377; *Standard Ed.*, **12**, 159.]

(1915c) 'Triebe und Triebschicksale', *G.S.*, **5**, 443; *G.W.*, **10**, 210. (323, 350, 360, 375, 415, 428, 537, 561)
[*Trans.*: 'Instincts and their Vicissitudes', *C.P.*, **4**, 60; *Standard Ed.*, **14**, 111.]

(1915d) 'Die Verdrängung', *G.S.*, **5**, 466; *G.W.*, **10**, 248. (286, 404 (377)
[*Trans.*: 'Repression', *C.P.*, **4**, 84; *Standard Ed.*, **14**, 143.]

(1915e) 'Das Unbewusste', *G.S.*, **5**, 480; *G.W.*, **10**, 264. (22, 286, 297, 360, 374, 409, 410, 422, 528–9, 553)
[*Trans.*: 'The Unconscious', *C.P.*, **4**, 98; *Standard Ed.*, **14**, 161.]

(1915f) 'Mitteilung eines der psychoanalytischen Theorie widersprechenden Falles von Paranoia', *G.S.*, **5**, 288; *G.W.*, **10**, 234. (267, 348, 426)
[*Trans.*: 'A Case of Paranoia Running Counter to the Psycho-Analytic Theory of the Disease', *C.P.*, **2**, 150; *Standard Ed.*, **14**, 263.]

(1916c) 'Eine Beziehung zwischen einem Symbol und einem Symptom', *G.S.*, **5**, 310; *G.W.*, **10**, 394. (157, 268)
[*Trans.*: 'A Connection between a Symbol and a Symptom', *C.P.*, **2**, 162; *Standard Ed.*, **14**, 339.]

(1916–17) *Vorlesungen zur Einführung in die Psychoanalyse,* Vienna. *G.S.*, **7**; *G.W.*, **11**. (467–70, 472, 477, 479, 481, 488, 490, 491, 497, 527, 529, 535, 545, 549, 552, 555, 562, 563, 566, 568, 579, 582, 590, 597, 606, 609, 610, 613, 615)
[*Trans.*: *Introductory Lectures on Psycho-Analysis,* revised ed., London, 1929 (*A General Introduction to Psychoanalysis,* New York, 1935) ; *Standard Ed.*, **15–16**.]

(1917a) 'Eine Schwierigkeit der Psychoanalyse', *G.S.*, **10**, 347; *G.W.*, **12**, 3. (209, 285)
[*Trans*: 'A Difficulty in the Path of Psycho-Analysis', *C.P.*, **4**, 347; *Standard Ed.*, **17**, 137.]

(1917c) 'Über Triebumsetzungen insbesondere der Analerotik', *G.S.*, **5**, 268; *G.W.*, **10**, 402. (315, 565)
[*Trans.*: 'On Transformations of Instinct as Exemplified in Anal Erotism', *C.P.*, **2**, 164; *Standard Ed.*, **17**, 127.]

(1917d [1915]) 'Metapsychologische Ergänzung zur Traumlehre', *G.S.*, **5**, 520; *G.W.*, **10**, 412. (237, 372, 419, 497)
[*Trans.*: 'A Metapsychological Supplement to the Theory of Dreams', *C.P.*, **4**, 137; *Standard Ed.*, **14**, 219.]

(1917e [1915]) 'Trauer und Melancholie', *G.S.*, **5**, 535; *G.W.*, **10**, 428. (276, 427, 428)
[*Trans.*: 'Mourning and Melancholia', *C.P.*, **4**, 152; *Standard Ed.*, **14**, 239.]

(1918a) 'Das Tabu der Virginität', *G.S.*, **5**, 212; *G.W.*, **12**, 161. (267, 597)
[*Trans.*: 'The Taboo of Virginity', *C.P.*, **4**, 217; *Standard Ed.*, **11**, 193.]

(1918b [1914]) 'Aus der Geschichte einer infantilen Neurose', *G.S.*, **8**, 439; *G.W.*, **12**, 29. (7, 185, 363, 371, 452)
[*Trans.*: 'From the History of an Infantile Neurosis', *C.P.*, **3**, 473; *Standard Ed.*, **17**, 3.]

1919a [1918]) 'Wege der psychoanalytischen Therapie', *G.S.*, **6**, 136; *G.W.*, **12**, 183. (5, 290)

[*Trans.*: 'Lines of Advance in Psycho-Analytic Therapy', *C.P.*, **2**, 392; *Standard Ed.*, **17**, 159.]

(1919d) Einleitung zu *Zur Psychoanalyse der Kriegsneurosen*, Vienna. *G.S.*, **11**, 252; *G.W.*, **12**, 321. (274, 382)

[*Trans.*: Introduction to *Psycho-Analysis and the War Neuroses*, London and New York, 1921. *C.P.*, **5**, 83; *Standard Ed.*, **17**, 207.]

(1919h) 'Das "Unheimliche" ', *G.S.*, **10**, 369; *G.W.*, **12**, 229. (216)

[*Trans.*: 'The "Uncanny" ', *C.P.*, **4**, 368; *Standard Ed.*, **17**, 219.]

(1920c) 'Dr. Anton von Freund', *G.S.*, **11**, 280; *G.W.*, **13**, 435. (516)

[*Trans.*: 'Dr. Anton von Freund', *Standard Ed.*, **18**, 267.]

(1920g) *Jenseits des Lustprinzips*, Vienna. *G.S.*, **6**, 191; *G.W.*, **13**, 3. (7, 246, 274, 374, 395, 414, 415, 494, 538, 572)

[*Trans.*: *Beyond the Pleasure Principle*, London, 1961; *Standard Ed.*, **18**, 7.]

(1921c) *Massenpsychologie und Ich-Analyse*, Vienna. *G.S.*, **6**, 261; *G.W.*, **13**, 73. (7, 448, 504, 527, 531–2, 597, 598)

[*Trans.*: *Group Psychology and the Analysis of the Ego*, London and New York, 1959; *Standard Ed.*, **18**, 69.]

(1922a) 'Traum und Telepathie', *G.S.*, **3**, 278; *G.W.*, **13**, 165. (223, 237, 501)

[*Trans.*: 'Dreams and Telepathy', *C.P.*, **4**, 408; *Standard Ed.*, **18**, 197.]

(1922b) 'Über einige neurotische Mechanismen bei Eifersucht, Paranoia und Homosexualität', *G.S.*, **5**, 387; *G.W.*, **13**, 195. (457)

[*Trans.*: 'Some Neurotic Mechanisms in Jealousy, Paranoia and Homosexuality', *C.P.*, **2**, 232; *Standard Ed.*, **18**, 223.]

(1923b) *Das Ich und das Es*, Vienna. *G.S.*, **6**, 353; *G.W.*, **13**, 237. (7, 175, 227, 246, 337, 407, 409, 416, 428, 521, 527, 529, 536, 543, 544, 549, 553, 555, 567, 569, 573, 574)

[*Trans.*: *The Ego and the Id*, London and New York, 1962; *Standard Ed.*, **19**, 3.]

(1923c) 'Bemerkungen zur Theorie und Praxis der Traumdeutung', *G.S.*, **3**, 305; *G.W.*, **13**, 301. (117, 238, 475, 478)

[*Trans.*: 'Remarks on the Theory and Practice of Dream-Interpretation', *C.P.*, **5**, 136; *Standard Ed.*, **19**, 109.]

(1923e) 'Die infantile Genitalorganisation', *G.S.*, **5**, 232; *G.W.*, **13**, 293. 327, 563)

[*Trans.*: 'The Infantile Genital Organization', *C.P.*, **2**, 244; *Standard Ed.*, **19**, 141.]

(1924c) 'Das ökonomische Problem des Masochismus', *G.S.*, **5**, 374; *G.W.*, **13**, 371. (275, 528, 572, 574)

[*Trans.*: 'The Economic Problem of Masochism', *C.P.*, **2**, 255; *Standard Ed.*, **19**, 157.]

(1924d) 'Der Untergang des Ödipuskomplexes,' *G.S.*, **5**, 423; *G.W.*, **13**, 395. (317, 556)

[*Trans.*: 'The Dissolution of the Oedipus Complex', *C.P.*, **2**, 269; *Standard Ed.*, **19**, 173.]

(1925a) 'Notiz über den "Wunderblock" ', *G.S.*, **6**, 415; *G.W.*, **13**, 3. (540)

[*Trans.*: 'A Note upon the "Mystic Writing-Pad" ', *C.P.*, **5**, 175; *Standard Ed.*, **19**, 227.]

(1925d [1924]) *Selbstdarstellung*, Vienna, 1934. *G.S.*, **11**, 119; *G.W.*, **14**, 33. (90, 287, 450, 585)

[*Trans.: An Autobiographical Study*, London, 1935 (*Autobiography*, New York, 1935); *Standard Ed.* **20**, 3.]

(1925*f*) Preface to August Aichhorn's *Verwahrloste Jugend*, Vienna. *G.S.*, **11**, 267; *G.W.*, **14**, 565. (610, 614)

[*Trans.*: Preface to Aichhorn's *Wayward Youth*, *C.P.*, **5**, 98; *Standard Ed.*, **19**, 273.]

(1925*h*) 'Die Verneinung', *G.S.*, **11**, 3; *G.W.*, **14**, 11. (553)

[*Trans.*: 'Negation', *C.P.*, **5**, 181; *Standard Ed.*, **19**, 235.]

(1925*i*) 'Einige Nachträge zum Ganzen der Traumdeutung', *G.S.*, **3**, 172; *G.W.*, **1**, 561. (211, 232, 477, 504)

[*Trans.*: 'Some Additional Notes upon Dream-Interpretation as a Whole', *C.P.*, **5**, 150; *Standard Ed.*, **19**, 125.]

(1925*j*) 'Einige psychische Folgen des anatomischen Geschlechtsunter-schieds', *G.S.*, **11**, 8; *G.W.*, **14**, 19. (246, 317, 333, 529, 576)

[*Trans.*: 'Some Psychological Consequences of the Anatomical Distinction between the Sexes', *C.P.*, **5**, 186; *Standard Ed.*, **19**, 243.]

(1926*d*) *Hemmung, Symptom und Angst*, Vienna. *G.S.*, **11**, 23; *G.W.*, **14**, 113. (61, 526, 540, 549–52, 554–5, 558, 622)

[*Trans.*: *Inhibitions, Symptoms and Anxiety*, London, 1960 (*The Problem of Anxiety*, New York, 1936; *Standard Ed.*, **20**, 77.]

(1926*e*) *Die Frage der Laienanalyse*, Vienna. *G.S.*, **11**, 307; *G.W.*, **14**, 209. (6, 17, 296–7, 540)

[*Trans.*: *The Question of Lay Analysis*, London, 1947; *Standard Ed.*, **20**, 179.]

(1927*c*) *Die Zukunft einer Illusion*, Vienna. *G.S.*, **11**, 411; *G.W.*, **14**, 325. (6, 499, 610, 632, 635, 639, 643)

[*Trans.*: *The Future of an Illusion*, London, 1962; New York, 1928; *Standard Ed.*, **21**, 3.]

(1927*d*) 'Der Humor', *G.S.*, **11**, 402; *G.W.*, **14**, 383. (374)

[*Trans.*: 'Humour', *C.P.*, **5**, 215; *Standard Ed.*, **21**, 159.]

(1927*e*) 'Fetischismus', *G.S.*, **11**, 395; *G.W.*, **14**, 311. (349)

[*Trans.*: 'Fetishism', *C.P.*, **5**, 198; *Standard Ed.*, **21**, 149.]

(1930*a*) *Das Unbehagen in der Kultur*, Vienna, *G.S.*, **12**, 29; *G.W.*, **14**, 421. (23, 146, 372, 574, 575, 579, 597, 632, 643)

[*Trans.*: *Civilization and its Discontents*, London, 1930; New York, 1961; *Standard Ed.*, **21**, 59.]

(1930*b*) Preface to *Zehn Jahre Berliner Psychoanalytisches Institut*, Vienna. *G.S.*, **12**, 388; *G.W.*, **14**, 572. (616)

[*Trans.*: In 'Personal Memories', in *Max Eitingon In Memoriam*, Jerusalem, 1951, 47; *Standard Ed.*, **21**, 257.]

(1931*b*) 'Über die weibliche Sexualität', *G.S.*, **12**, 120; *G.W.*, **14**, 517. (333, 370, 576, 585)

[*Trans.*: 'Female Sexuality', *C.P.*, **5**, 252; *Standard Ed.*, **21**, 223.]

(1931*d*) 'Das Fakultätsgutachten im Prozess Halsmann', *G.S.*, **12**, 412; *G.W.*, **14**, 541. (338)

[*Trans.*: 'The Expert Opinion in the Halsmann Case', *Standard Ed.*, **21**, 251.]

(1931*e*) Letter to the Burgomaster of Příbor, *G.S.*, **12**, 414; *G.W.*, **14**, 561. (605)

[*Trans.*: *Standard Ed.*, **21**, 259.]

(1932*a*) 'Zur Gewinnung des Feuers', *G.S.*, **12**, 141; *G.W.*, **16**, 3. (566)

[*Trans.*: 'The Acquisition and Control of Fire', *C.P.*, **5**, 288; *Standard Ed.*, **22**, 185.]

(1933*a*) *Neue Folge der Vorlesungen zur Einführung in die Psychoanalyse*, Vienna. *G.S.*, **12**, 151; *G.W.*, **15**, 207. (5, 6, 157, 206, 227, 239, 246, 323, 333, 347, 365, 370, 388, 392, 395, 429, 434, 461)
[*Trans.: New Introductory Lectures on Psycho-Analysis*, London and New York, 1933; *Standard Ed.*, **22**.]

(1933*b* [1932]) *Warum Krieg?*, Paris. *G.S.*, **12**, 349; *G.W.*, **16**, 13. (643)
[*Trans.: Why War?*, Paris, 1933; *C.P.*, **5**, 273; *Standard Ed.*, **22**, 197.]

(1933*c*) 'Sándor Ferenczi', *G.S.*, **12**, 397; *G.W.*, **16**, 267. (617)
[*Trans.:* 'Sándor Ferenczi', *Int. J. Psychol-Anal.*, **14**, 297; *Standard Ed.*, **22**, 227.]

(1937*c*) 'Die endliche und die unendliche Analyse', *G.W.*, **16**, 59. (431, 445, 448, 554, 610, 620)
[*Trans.:* 'Analysis Terminable and Interminable', *C.P.*, **5**, 316; *Standard Ed.*, **23**, 211.]

(1937*d*) 'Konstrunktionen in der Analyse', *G.W.*, **16**, 43. (50)
[*Trans.:* 'Constructions in Analysis', *C.P.*, **5**, 358; *Standard Ed.*, **23**, 257.]

(1939*a* [1937–39]) *Der Mann Moses und die monotheistische Religion*, *G.W.*, **16**, 103. (161, 347, 536, 626, 632)
[*Trans.: Moses and Monotheism*, London and New York, 1939; *Standard Ed.*, **23**, 3.]

(1940*a* [1938]) *Abriss der Psychoanalyse*, *G.W.*, **17**, 67. (333, 338, 355, 374, 553, 576)
[*Trans.: An Outline of Psycho-Analysis*, London and New York, 1949; *Standard Ed.*, **23**, 141.]

(1940*b* [1938]) 'Some Elementary Lessons in Psycho-Analysis' [title in English: German text], *G.W.*, **17**, 141. (34, 277)
[*Trans.:* 'Some Elementary Lessons in Psycho-Analysis', *C.P.*, **5**, 376; *Standard Ed.*, **23**, 281.]

(1940*c* [1922]) 'Das Medusenhaupt', *G.W.*, **17**, 47.
[*Trans.:* 'Medusa's Head', *C.P.*, **5**, 105; *Standard Ed.*, **18**, 273.]

(1941*d* [1921]) 'Psychoanalyse und Telepathie', *G.W.*, **17**, 27. (495, 504–12, 518)
[*Trans.:* 'Psycho-Analysis and Telepathy', *Standard Ed.*, **18**, 177.]

(1950*a* [1887–1902]) *Aus den Anfängen der Psychoanalyse*, London. Includes 'Entwurf einer Psychologie' (1895). (201, 329–30, 357, 374, 384, 553, 585, 603)
[*Trans: The Origins of Psycho-Analysis*, London and New York, 1954. (Partly, including 'A Project for a Scientific Psychology', in *Standard Ed.*, **1**.)]

(1955*c* [1920]) Memorandum on the Electrical Treatment of War Neuroses', *Standard Ed.*, **17**, 211. (382)
[*German Text* (unpublished): 'Gutachten über die elektrische Behandlung der Kriegsneurotiker].

(1960*a*) *Briefe 1873–1939* (ed. E. L. Freud), Berlin. (4–5, 603)
[*Trans.: Letters 1873–1939* (ed. E. L. Freud) (trans. T. and J. Stern), New York, 1960; London, 1961.]

GRODDECK, G. (1923) *Das Buch vom Es*, Vienna. (536)

HALL, G.S. (1914) 'A Synthetic Genetic Study of Fear', *Amer. J. Psychol.*, **25**, 149. (398, 411)

HARTMANN, H., and BETLHEIM, S. *See* BETLHEIM, S., and HARTMANN, H.

HESNARD, A., and RÉGIS, E. (1914) *See* RÉGIS, E., and HESNARD, A. (1914)

HILDEBRANDT, F. W. (1875) *Der Traum und seine Verwerthung für's Leben*, Leipzig. (92-3)

HITSCHMANN, E. (1913) *Freuds Neurosenlehre*, Vienna (2nd ed.). (9)

HUG-HELLMUTH, H. VON (1915) 'Ein Traum der sich selbst deutet', *Int. Z. (ärztl.) Psychoanal.*, **3**, 33. (136-8)

JANET, PIERRE (1888) 'Les actes inconscients et la mémoire', *Rev. Philosoph.*, **13**, 238. (257)

    (1913) 'Psycho-Analysis. Rapport par M. le Dr. Pierre Janet', *Int. Congr. Med.*, **17**, Section XII (Psychiatry) (1), 13. (257)

JODL, F. (1896) *Lehrbuch der Psychologie*, Stuttgart. (87)

JONES, E. (1911) 'The Psychopathology of Everyday Life', *Amer. J. Psychol.*, **22**, 477. (31, 55, 56)

    (1912) *Der Alptraum in seiner Beziehung zu gewissen Formen des mittelalterlichen Aberglaubens* (tr. H. Sachs), Leipzig and Vienna. (514–16) [*English Text:* In *On the Nightmare*, London and New York, 1931.]

    (1916) Review of G. Stanley Hall's 'A Synthetic Genetic Study of Fear', *Int. Z. (ärztl.) Psychoanal.*, **4**, 55. (398)

    (1953) *Sigmund Freud: Life and Work*, Vol. 1, London and New York. (Page references are to the English edition.) (5, 274, 625)

    (1955) *Sigmund Freud: Life and Work*, Vol. 2, London and New York. (Page references are to the English edition.) (5, 349, 625)

    (1957) *Sigmund Freud: Life and Work*. Vol. 3, London and New York. (Page references are to the English edition.) (467, 495, 603)

JUNG, C. G. (1907) *Über die Psychologie der Dementia praecox*, Halle. (52, 269)

    [*Trans.: The Psychology of Dementia Praecox*, New York, 1909.]

KAPLAN, L. (1914) *Grundzüge der Psychoanalyse*, Vienna. (9)

LAMPL-DE GROOT, J. (1927) 'Zur Entwicklungsgeschichte des Ödipuskomplexes der Frau', *Int. Z Psychoan.*, **13**, 269. (594–5) [*Trans.:* 'The Evolution of the Oedipus Complex in Women', *Int. J. Psycho-Anal.*, **9**, (1928), 332.]

LEURET, F. (1834) *Fragmens psychologiques sur la folie*, Paris. (257)

LEVY, L. (1914) 'Die Sexualsymbolik der Bibel und des Talmuds', *Z. Sexualwiss.*, **1**, 274; 318. (162)

LICHTENBERG, G. C. VON (The Elder) (1853) *Witzige und satirische Einfälle*, Vol. 2 of New Enlarged Edition, Göttingen. (38-9)

LINDER, S. (1879) 'Das Saugen an den Fingern, Lippen, etc., bei den Kindern (Ludeln)', *Jb. Kinderheilk*, N.F., **14**, 68. (313–14)

MAEDER, A. (1906) 'Contributions à la psychopathologie de la vie quotidienne', *Archives de psychologie*, **6**, 148. (55)

    (1908) 'Nouvelles contributions à la psychopathologie de la vie quotidienne', *Archives de psychologie*, **7**, 283. (55)

    (1912) 'Über die Funktion des Traumes', *Jb. psychoan. psychopath. Forsch.*, **4**, 692. (236–7)

MAURY, L. F. A. (1878) *Le sommeil et les rêves*, Paris. (1st ed., 1861.) (86–7, 92, 94)

MAYER, C., and MERINGER, R. (1895) *See* MERINGER, R. (1895)

MEIJER, A. F. (1915) *De Behandeling van Zenuwzieken door Psycho-Analyse*, Amsterdam. (9)

MERINGER, R. (1895) with MAYER, C., *Versprechen und Verlesen, eine psychologisch-linguistische Studie*, Vienna. (32–4, 42, 43, 49)

NÄCKE, P. (1899) 'Kritisches zum Kapitel der normalen und pathologischen Sexualität', *Arch. Psychiat.*, **32**, 356. (416)

NORDENSKJÖLD, O., *et al.* (1904) *Antarctic. Zwei Jahre in Schnee und Eis am Südpol* (2 vols.), Berlin. (132–3)

BIBLIOGRAPHY 661

[*Trans.:* (abridged) : *Antarctica,* London, 1905.]

PLATO *Republic.* (146)

[*Trans.:* in *Dialogue,* Vol. 2 (tr. B. Jowett), Oxford, 1871.]

PFISTER, O. (1913) *Die psychanalytische Methode,* Leipzig and Berlin. (9, 610)

[*Trans.: The Psychoanalytic Method,* New York and London, 1917.]

RANK, O. (1909) *Der Mythus von der Geburt des Helden,* Leipzig and Vienna. (160–1)

[*Trans.: The Myth of the Birth of the Hero,* New York, 1914.]

(1910*a*) 'Ein Beispiel von poetischer Verwertung des Versprechens', *Zbl. Psychoan.,* **1,** 109. (37–8)

(1910*b*) 'Ein Traum der sich selbst deutet', *Jb. psychoan. psychopath, Forsch.,* **2,** 465. (185)

(1912*a*) 'Aktuelle Sexualregungen als Traumanlässe', *Zbl. Psychoan.,* **2,** 596. (134)

(1912*b*) *Das Inzest-Motiv in Dichtung und Sage,* Leipzig and Vienna. (208, 337)

(1924) *Das Trauma der Geburt,* Vienna. (551–2)

[*Trans.: The Trauma of Birth,* London, 1929.]

RÉGIS, E., and HESNARD, A. (1914) *La psychoanalyse des névroses et des psychoses,* Paris. (9)

REIK, T. (1915–16) 'Die Pubertätsriten der Wilden', *Imago,* **4,** 125; 189. (335)

(1920) 'Völkerpsychologische Parallelen zum Traumsymbol des Mantels', *Int. Z. Psychoan.,* **6,** 350.

(1942) *From Thirty Years with Freud,* London; New York, 1940. (5, 6)

SACHS, H. (1912) 'Traumdeutung und Menschenkenntnis', *Jb. psychoan. psychopath. Forsch.,* **3,** 568. (206)

(1945) *Freud, Master and Friend,* Cambridge (Mass.) and London. (Page reference is to the English edition.) (5)

SCHERNER, K. A. (1861) *Das Leben des Trammes,* Berlin. (95, 152, 153, 159)

SCHROTTER, K. (1912) 'Experimentelle Träume', *Zbl. Psychoan.,* **2,** 638. (486)

SCHUBERT, G. H. VON (1814) *Die Symbolik des Traumes,* Bamberg. (163)

SILBERER, H. (1909) 'Bericht über eine Methode, gewisse symbolische Halluzinations-Erscheinungen hervorzurufen und zu beobachten', *Jb. psychoan. psychopath. Forsch.,* **1,** 513. (487)

(1912) 'Symbolik des Erwachens und Schwellensymbolik überhaupt', *Jb. psychoan. psychopath. Forsch.,* **3,** 621. (487)

(1914) *Probleme der Mystik und ihrer Symbolik,* Vienna. (237, 304)

[*Trans.: Problems of Mysticism and its Symbolism,* New York, 1917.]

SPERBER, H. (1912) 'Über den Einfluss sexueller Momente auf Entstehung und Entwicklung der Sprache', *Imago* **1,** 405. 167)

STÄRCKE, J. (1916) 'Aus dem Alltagsleben', *Int. Z. (ärztl.) Psychoanal.,* **4,** 21; 98. (55)

STEKEL, W. (1911) *Die Sprache des Traumes,* Wiesbaden. (149, 237)

STRÜMPELL, L. (1877) *Die Natur und Entstehung der Träume,* Leipzig. (87, 90)

TOULOUSE, E. (1896) *Émile Zola: enquête médico-psychologique,* Paris. (260)

VIENNA PSYCHOANALYTIC SOCIETY, MINUTES OF, Vol. I, New York, 1962. (397–8)

VOLD, J. MOURLY (1910–12) *Über den Traum* (2 vols.) (*German trans.* by O. Klemm), Leipzig. (87, 92, 155, 238)

WUNDT, W. (1874) *Grundzüge der physiologischen Psychologie,* Leipzig. (87)

LIST OF ABBREVIATIONS

G.S.   = Freud, *Gesammelte Schriften* (12 vols.), Vienna, 1924–34
G.W.   = Freud, *Gesammelte Werke* (18 vols.), London, from 1940
C.P.   = Freud, *Collected Papers* (5 vols.), London, 1924–50
Standard Ed. = Freud, *Standard Edition* (24 vols.), London, from 1953
P.E.L.   = Freud, *The Psychopathology of Everyday Life, Standard Ed.,*
                Vol. VI
I. of D.   = Freud, *The Interpretation of Dreams, Standard Ed.,*Vols. IV
                and V

INDEX OF PARAPRAXES

The source of each parapraxis is given in brackets where it is other than Freud himself.

INDEX OF DREAMS

The names or descriptions in brackets are the dreamer's followed by the reporter's.

INDEX OF SYMBOLS

For things symbolized see the General Index

GENERAL INDEX

This index includes the names of non-technical authors. It also includes the names of technical authors where no reference is made in the text to specific works. For references to specific technical works, the Bibliography should be consulted.—The compilation of the index was undertaken by Mrs. R. S. Partridge and Miss Angela Richards.

Nancy, 103, 448

Narcissism, 7, 414 *n*. 2, 416–18, 529
  n. 1, 566–7, 596–7
  and egoism differentiated, 417–18
  and homosexuality, 426–7
  infantile, 204, 210, 424, 429, 446,
    455
  of sleep, 417, 420–1

Narcissistic
  identification, 427–8
  illness, 619
  libido, 414 *n*. 2, 416–22, 429–30, 447
  object-choice, 426

Narcissus, 566 *n*. 3

Nature, man's control over, 637, 641–
  642, 645

Nature-gods, 629

Necessity, 355, 357, 412, 430

Necrophilia, 305–6, 605

Negative does not exist in dreams,
  178

Negative therapeutic reaction, 573–4

Nestroy, J., 321 *n.,* 352

Neuroses (*see also* Actual neuroses
    Anxiety neurosis; Children,
    neuroses of; Hysteria; Obses-
    sional neurosis; Phobias; Trans-
    ference neuroses; Traumatic
    neuroses; War neuroses)
  aetiology of 521, 551, 590, 613
  and ego-psychology, 522
  and fixation of libido, 346, 348–9,
    352
  and frustration, 346, 348–9, 352
  and tendency to conflict, 352–4,
    378, 521
  compared to dreams, 479–80, 492
  curability of, 457, 617–20
  medical view of, 450
  Oedipus complex as nucleus of,
    329, 332, 335, 337, 341
  of society, 632 and *n*.
  onset of, 349, 359, 363, 380–4, 387
  physical treatment of, 616
  precipitating cause of, 382, 391,
    453
  predisposition to, 347, 364–6, 406
  prevention of, 364–5, 612–14
  religion and, 632 and *n*.
  sexual aetiology of, 22, 246 *n.,* 264,
    269, 298–301, 319, 328, 339, 348–
    352, 362–3, 380–403, 433

theory influences treatment of,
  607–8
theory of, 83, 168, 185, 222, 239,
  243, 291–2, 375, 379–81
traumatic aetiology of, 246 *n.,*
  273–6, 346–7
unconscious need for punishment
  in, 572–4

Neurotic symptoms (*see* Symptoms)

Neurotics
  characteristics of, 260, 291, 298,
    318, 378, 380–1
  compared to normal persons,
    297–8, 456–7
  infantile characteristics of, 552–3,
    612
  masturbation in, 591
  psycho-analysis of, 15, 167–8, 300,
    307, 326–7, 335, 453–4, 521, 572–
    574, 609, 611–12, 615–21
  psychological treatment of, 616–17
  tendency to transference in, 439–
    446

Neveu de Rameau, le (by *Diderot*),
  337–8

Newton, 637

Nietzsche, F., 536

Nihilism, intellectual, 639–40

Nimrod, 19

Nonsense, pleasure in, 497 and *n*. 2

Nordsee (by *Heine*), 577 and *n*.

Normal persons
  compared to neurotics, 297–8,
    456–7
  dreams of, 83–4, 98, 185, 297–8,
    456–7
  mental processes of, 368
  sexual development in, 309–10,
    317–19, 322–3, 339, 386, 391, 415

Numbers
  as symbols, 163–4, 220
  experiments with, 107
  in dreams, 182

Nutritive instinct, 313–14, 328–9

Oberländer, A., 385

Object-cathexes, libidinal, 561, 564–1
  identifications as precipitates of,
    528, 541
  infantile, 549–50, 581, 588
  source of, 541, 567 and *n*.

Object-choice
  anaclitic attachment, 426–7

Psychology
  experimental, 20
  female, 468, 527, 551, 576–99, 635
  group, 519, 531–2, 601–2, 604, 606,
    641–5
  'Individual', 529, 604–7
  sociology as applied, 643
Psychoneuroses (see Neuroses)
Psychoses (see also Dementia prae-
    cox; Manic depressive states;
    Melancholia; Paranoia; Para-
    phrenia), 257, 260, 415, 422 n.,
    423, 429–30, 457 n.
  compared to dreams, 479–80
  delusions in, 523
  psycho-analysis and, 618–19
  turning away from external re-
    ality in, 480, 523, 624
Psychotherapy, 471, 472, 616–17
Puberty, 190, 208, 311–12, 317, 319,
    327, 329, 336, 348, 353, 365, 369,
    403, 563
  -rites, 165, 335, 550–1
Pubic hair, 596
  symbols for, 156
Punishment, unconscious need for,
    572–4, 606
Punishment dreams, 219, 221, 491–2

Quality, 374–5, 457, 538–9
Quantity, 356, 358, 373–5, 418 n. 1,
    457, 538–9, 558, 618–19
Questenberg (in Schiller's Wallen-
    stein), 37

Radium, discovery of, 637
Railway phobia, 399–400, 407
Rank, O. (see also Bibliography), 5,
    168, 607 and n. 3
'Rat Man', case of, 266 n., 301 n. 2,
    337 n.
Rawlinson, H. C., 232
Reaction-formations of the ego, 375,
    381, 554–5, 566
Reality
  and anxiety, 393–4, 401, 404–9, 411,
    430, 468, 526, 542, 545–6, 548–51,
    557–9
  and the ego, 480, 539–43, 549, 557,
    574–5
  and phantasy, 367–8
  and science, 634–5, 638–40, 646
  frustration by, 314–15, 355, 359

-principle, 357, 366, 371–2, 412,
    416, 540
-testing, 372, 497 and n. 1, 539,
    553 n.
  turning away from, in psychoses,
    480, 523
  turning away from, in sleep, 480,
    483
Reason (see also Intellect)
  advance of, 635–6
  ego stands for, 540
  man's hostility to, 497–8
Recovery, instinct for, 570
Reflection, analyst curbs powers of,
    474 and n.
Regression
  and repression, 341–4
  in dreams, 180–1, 183, 185, 199,
    210–12, 223–4, 483–4
  of ego, 357
  of libido, 339–44, 359–66, 373–4,
    409–12, 527, 556, 563–4, 590,
    594–5
  two kinds of libidinal, 343
Reitler, R., 57 n.
Relatives of patient obstruct psycho-
    analysis, 458–62
Relativity, theory of, 608
Religion, 28, 167, 169, 332, 389, 468
  and Bolshevism, 644
  and occultism, 498
  and scientific Weltanschauung,
    498, 624–39
  science of, 609
Religious education, 610 n. 2
Repeat, compulsion to, 7, 270, 274,
    570–2, 572 n., 597, 607
Repressed, the, 521, 541, 542
  unaltered by time, 538
Repression, 603
  and anxiety, 401–4, 409–11, 425,
    547, 549–51, 553–6, 558
  and censorship, 217, 295–6, 344
  and civilization, 574
  and dreams, 217–18, 226, 297, 419,
    429, 456–7, 479–83, 493
  and regression, 341–4
  and self-preservative instinct, 561
  and symptom-formation, 294,
    297–301, 359–61, 365, 456–7
  as exclusion from consciousness,
    293–6, 331, 342, 403, 430